HEROPHILUS

THE ART OF MEDICINE IN

EARLY ALEXANDRIA

HEROPHILUS
The Art of Medicine in
Early Alexandria

Edition, translation and essays

HEINRICH VON STADEN

Professor of Classics and Comparative Literature

Yale University

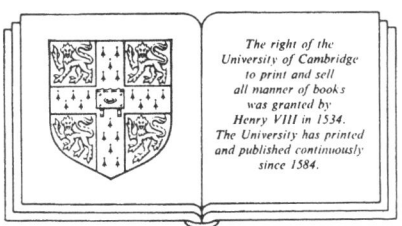

The right of the
University of Cambridge
to print and sell
all manner of books
was granted by
Henry VIII in 1534.
The University has printed
and published continuously
since 1584.

CAMBRIDGE UNIVERSITY PRESS

Cambridge

New York   New Rochelle

Melbourne   Sydney

CAMBRIDGE UNIVERSITY PRESS
Cambridge, New York, Melbourne, Madrid, Cape Town, Singapore, São Paulo

Cambridge University Press
The Edinburgh Building, Cambridge CB2 8RU, UK

Published in the United States of America by Cambridge University Press, New York

www.cambridge.org
Information on this title: www.cambridge.org/9780521236461

First published 1989
This digitally printed version 2007

A catalogue record for this publication is available from the British Library

Library of Congress Cataloguing in Publication data
Von Staden, Heinrich, 1939–
Herophilus: The art of medicine in early Alexandria.
Bibliography.
Includes indexes.
1. Herophilus, of Chalcedon, ca. 330 B.C.-ca. 260 B.C.
2. Medicine, Greek and Roman. 3. Medicine –
Egypt – Alexandria – History. I. Title.
R126.H373V66 1988 610'.932 87-6406

ISBN 978-0-521-23646-1 hardback
ISBN 978-0-521-04178-2 paperback

For Torben and Tamás

CONTENTS

PART 2 · THE HEROPHILEANS
(*c*. 250 B.C.–A.D. 50)

PREFACE

Discussions of ancient Greek views of human beings often tend to remain riveted to Athens – to the works of the philosophers, historians, playwrights, and visual artists who achieved prominence in Athens. The present work requires a shift of focus from the old citadel of learning to the new, from Athens to Alexandria, from the undisputed centre of philosophy to the burgeoning centre of science, from the Athenian 'philosophy of man' to the Alexandrian 'science of human beings'.

The first comprehensive presentation of the ancient evidence concerning the extraordinary accomplishments of one of the leading scientists of the ancient world hardly requires an apologia. Plunged into obscurity in part by the popularity of rival schools, in part by the durability and canonicity of Galen's subsequent system, the first and greatest Alexandrian representative of scientific medicine, Herophilus, had to wait long for his rehabilitation. Only in the Renaissance, when the tenacious authority of Galen became subject to sporadic challenges, were the achievements of Alexandrian physicians such as Herophilus accorded renewed recognition and respect. Thus the distinguished Renaissance physician Gabriello Falloppia exclaimed in his *Observationes Anatomicae* (Venice, 1561): 'Quando Galenus refutat Herophilum, censeo ipsum refutare Evangelium medicum', and 'Herophili . . . authoritas [*sic*] apud me circa res anatomicas est Evangelium.' Other Renaissance authors, though restricted (as are we) to a very fragmentary knowledge of Herophilus, called him 'the Vesalius of antiquity', and judgments like these were sounded increasingly as the Renaissance *agon* with Galen's *auctoritas* spasmodically but certainly swung in favour of the 'moderns' (but even while more than 600 editions of Galen's treatises printed between 1473 and 1599 continued making Galen a powerful force in the contest). As one classical patriarch – Galen – was vanquished, new ones had to satisfy the perennial need for the sanction of the past: Herophilus as the Gospel.

Although scholars of our century, too, have continued to recognize the scientific significance of several of the Alexandrian physicians who span the five murky centuries between Aristotle and Galen, a critical edition and evaluation of the ancient evidence about the methods, theories, and practices of Herophilus and his followers have remained a desideratum. Werner Jaeger's prediction that 'when a critical collection of the extant remains . . . of the doctrines of Praxagoras, Erasistratus, and Herophilus has become available, the history of Greek medicine *in the period of its greatest scientific progress* will have to be rewritten', has been echoed by a number of modern scholars. The Praxagorean gap – a Coan, not an Alexandrian gap – has been closed by F. Steckerl's edition; the present volume will, I hope, accomplish the same for Herophilus.

Since this book aims both at the non-specialist with an interest in the history of science and medicine and at the specialist, all the ancient evidence concerning Herophilus is presented in translation and in the original. Part 1 (Herophilus) aims at providing a complete set of texts and translations, along with interpretive essays and comments, but Part 2 (The Herophileans) has been restricted to two complementary purposes: first, to provide a brief account of major developments within the Herophilean 'school' after Herophilus, and secondly, to offer some sense of the distinctive characteristics of individual Herophileans. A complete enumeration of relevant ancient sources is provided in the chapters on each Herophilean in Part 2, but the texts and translations have been omitted. It is hoped that this restrictive approach to Part 2 will render the book more approachable, especially for the non-specialist. (In Part 2 the boundaries suggested by 'early Alexandria' are occasionally violated both geographically and chronologically, but the overwhelming majority of texts presented here were a product of early Alexandria.)

It remains controversial whether Erasistratus belongs mainly to the Alexandrian sphere, and the original intention of treating him and Herophilus in a single work has therefore been abandoned in favour of separate studies. Wherever Erasistratus might have practised, the similarities between his scientific interests and those of Herophilus are striking. Human dissection and vivisection are attributed to both Herophilus and Erasistratus; both are credited with the discovery of the nerves and with the distinction between motor and sensory nerves; they both displayed a keen interest in the structure and functions of the brain, the heart, and the vascular system. Moreover, both wrote on ophthalmology, respiration, reproductive physiology, therapeutics, and causal theory. Even the specifics on which they lavished attention are often remarkably similar – for example, the relation between fever and pulse frequency. While their pathophysiological systems display major differences, the concept of pneuma remains central to both, and their main therapeutic principle – treatment by 'contraries' – is the same. Reference will be made throughout this work to the relation between Herophilean and Erasistratean medicine, but a full discussion of the relation will have to await a critical edition of all the testimonia and fragments of Erasistratus.

The most notable exception to the general neglect of Alexandrian medicine has been K. Deichgräber's invaluable account of the Empiricist school of medicine (founded in Alexandria c. 250 B.C. by a renegade pupil of Herophilus). The only complete extant treatise of Hellenistic medicine, a first-century B.C. commentary by one Apollonius on the Hippocratic treatise *On Joints*, also belongs to the Empiricist school and has been edited admirably by J. Kollesch and F. Kudlien. Although frequent reference is made in this volume to the Alexandrian Empiricists, my primary purpose was to fill the most serious gap that remains in our knowledge of medicine in Alexandria, viz. Herophilus and his followers; for the Empiricists the reader will have to continue relying on Deichgräber.

It is my hope that the present work will not only provide access to a significant and neglected chapter in the history of medicine, but be of value for other reasons as well. For most scholars the main avenues of access to the 'views of human beings' in a given culture have tended to remain the literary, religious, and philosophical texts of the culture, its political and social history, its art, and its other artefacts. Yet from ancient Greece to the present, scientific theories and observations, too, have moulded our self-perception and self-depiction decisively. Scientific views, both about the nature of the external world and about the internal construction of humans, tend to become known outside the scientific community, even if in popularized or distorted versions, and sometimes they strongly influence attitudes and views displayed in non-scientific texts. From the anguished choral cry 'much cuts to the liver' in Aeschylus' *Agamemnon* to Shakespeare's 'a good sherris-sack . . . ascends me into the brain, dries me all the foolish and dull crudy vapours which environ it', and from Plato's account of the construction of the body (*Timaeus*) to Ezra Pound's 'the bone is in fact constructed | according to trigonometrical whichwhat . . .', a rich history of allusion, image, and fancy testifies to the impact of scientific and, in particular, of medical theories upon non-scientific texts. Alexandria is no exception, and a number of examples of the penetration of literary and philosophical texts by medical theories are pointed out in this volume; more examples will undoubtedly strike other readers of the texts presented here.

It is also my hope that this work will contribute to a more balanced and informed assessment of the accomplishments and complex character of what has come to be called the 'Hellenistic Age' – often with pejorative overtones – ever since the German schoolmaster and historian Johann Gustav Droysen coined the term 'Hellenistic' in the nineteenth century. Not that assessments of the Hellenistic Age have been uniformly negative: while Nietzsche characterized Hellenistic culture as feeding on degenerate 'air that was rank and overcharged with Aphrodisiac odours', Victor Ehrenberg found in it 'a climate of serenity'; and while Julius Beloch described it as an epoch in which the *demi-monde* saw its brightest times, Michael Rostovtzeff saw in the early Hellenistic period the birth of a sober *humanitas* and believed that 'the future proved that the pride of that age in its past and present was justified'. One thing these disparate, though by no means mutually exclusive, assessments tend to have in common is their failure to accommodate explicitly the contributions to medical science presented and analysed in this volume. (A laudable exception is P. M. Fraser's *Ptolemaic Alexandria*.) I hope it is not rash to suggest that any scholar who wishes to do justice to the complex dimensions and achievements of the period should also become cognizant of the remarkable scientific achievement which even now has become only partially unveiled through the fragmentary evidence presented in this volume.

H.v.S.

ACKNOWLEDGEMENTS

It is a pleasure to record, however inadequately, my warm gratitude to friends, colleagues, and institutions that offered scrutiny and encouragement.

Some of the ideas in this book profited from being presented to audiences at Boston University, Harvard University, Johns Hopkins University, McMaster University, University of California at Los Angeles, Wellesley College, Wesleyan University, Yale University, and to the Society for Ancient Medicine and the American Association of Ancient Historians. Professors Phillip De Lacy, David Furley, Geoffrey Lloyd, and Friedrich Solmsen read the manuscript in various stages of completion and revision. They generously offered numerous suggestions and rescued me from many a lapse. Professor De Lacy and Professor David Sider very kindly made some of their unpublished manuscript collations available to me. Dr Vivian Nutton graciously provided access to his forthcoming edition of Galen's *De sententiis*. The late Derek deSolla Price offered many useful suggestions, as did several colleagues in the Yale School of Medicine (especially Dr Elisha Atkins). Mr N. G. Wilson generously shared his redating of several MSS and gave the conspectus siglorum the benefit of his expert scrutiny. The sustained interest and warm support of Professors Evelyn Hutchinson, Donald Kagan, and Hugh Lloyd-Jones animated the project more than once. For assistance with various technical aspects of preparing the manuscript I am indebted to Martha Achilles, Thomas Crawford, Professor Michael Poliakoff, Brock Reeve, Dr Henry Schneiderman, and Professor David Tandy. Many others, too numerous to mention here, have my gratitude for their helpful suggestions. Pauline Hire of Cambridge University Press deserves special thanks for her enormous patience and constructive help. The flaws that remain are, of course, my responsibility. *Quae me fugerunt, alii facile reperient.*

I owe warmest thanks to my wife, Eve Ingalls, and to our sons, Torben and Tamás. Faith and forbearance are but two of the magnificent gifts they have given in most generous measure.

NOTE ON
TEXT, ARRANGEMENT AND TRANSLATION

I Criteria for inclusion

One of the more vexing problems facing an editor of fragmentary material is that of criteria for including and excluding texts. The guiding principle of this volume was to restrict the edition to texts in which Herophilus or his followers are explicitly mentioned by name. The severity of this principle will perhaps be no less controversial than was the lack of severity displayed in, for example, Hans von Arnim's selection of texts in *Stoicorum Veterum Fragmenta* or in Karl Reinhardt's liberal use of putative indirect testimonies to reconstruct Posidonius' philosophy. It could admittedly be argued that numerous passages in Soranus, Galen, Rufus, and other writers of the Imperial period stand in the shadow of early Alexandrian physicians, such as Herophilus, without any explicit acknowledgement by these later authors of the Herophilean provenance of their theories or observations. The decision to confine this edition to explicitly attested material at the expense of such indirect sources – to which reference is, however, made in the introductions to (and comments on) some chapters – was reached on several grounds. First, I believe that an edition limited in this way at present is the most crucial (and least misleading or confusing) contribution to the study of early Alexandrian medicine. What is lacking at present is, after all, a conservative presentation of the primary evidence on which any subsequent analysis of derivative, influenced, or dependent passages in authors of the Roman Imperial and Byzantine periods will have to be based. Second, the inclusion of large amounts of unattested but 'influenced' material might have brought with it the danger of reconstructing Herophilean theories mainly through the hypothetical victims or beneficiaries of influence, as has occurred, for example, with highly problematic results in scholarship on Posidonius and on Gnosticism. Several well-known discussions of the 'Posidonian' origins of treatises by Cicero and Philo

xvi

of Alexandria have illustrated how rapidly the supposed indirect sources tend to usurp the attested primary evidence. Third, as Felix Jacoby, among others, has suggested (*FGrH* I, p. viii), the selection of indirect testimonia tends to be as subjective and eclectic as an editor's notions of 'influence' and 'affinity' are. What to one critic seems a strong and central affinity, to another looks weak or peripheral; what to one seems a clear genealogical line, to another is an irregular pattern of thematic coincidences without any genetic implications. I do not mean to question the value of scholarship on indirect sources and on influence, but it seemed advisable first to offer a foundation on which such research must build, and to alert the reader to some potential indirect sources in the introductions and comments.

By restricting the texts to those which mention Herophilus and his followers by name, I do not wish to suggest, however, that authenticity is guaranteed by the presence of a name. Some ancient authors giving accounts of 'Herophilean' views may have been misinformed and some, as pointed out throughout this work, were certainly polemical, whereas others, including Galen, used Herophilus or one of his followers without naming them. But again, one could not analyse these problems adequately until all views and observations directly and explicitly ascribed to various Herophileans by ancient sources were first collected and subjected to a critical sifting. While attention is drawn to the questionable value of some such texts – and to the occasional need for emending others so as to deprive them of their value – all explicitly attested texts that have come to my attention are included on the grounds that the reader must be allowed to decide for her- or himself whether my conclusions about the value of a given text are merited. Texts included under the rubric *Dubia* (at the end of the collection of texts in some chapters) are the ones whose authenticity or relevance I doubt very strongly.

When Herophilus or one of his followers is referred to repeatedly in a continuous passage, or when the sense of reference (for example, of pronouns) in a text would be unclear or ambiguous in the absence of a larger context, I have thought it useful to print more than just the sentences explicitly mentioning a Herophilean and his views, so as to facilitate the reader's understanding of the passage. In all other cases I have tended to severity.

2 *Fragment and testimonium*

Where there is reason to believe that a literal quotation from an authentic work by Herophilus or a Herophilean is intended by an ancient source, this has been indicated by inverted commas. Such quotations are referred to throughout this volume as 'fragment' (Fr), although I must stress that it is not possible to determine in each case how closely or loosely even a putative 'fragment' is related to the original. All other texts will be referred to as 'testimonia' (T).

Every editor tends to be more exhilarated by the discovery of a 'fragment' than by a 'testimonium', and I am no exception, but one should guard against an undue exaggeration of the value of fragments. While it is true that paraphrases or polemical refutations of precursors' views (and many of the testimonia in this volume are culled from such polemical contexts) tend to transform the original texts to a greater degree, and in more ways (lexical, terminological, conceptual, perspectival, etc.) than does transmission by literal quotation, one should nevertheless remember that even if part of an Alexandrian text is preserved word for word in a fragment, the recovery of the true meaning of a fragment is often no easier than the recovery of a theory that is being paraphrased or refuted, inasmuch as the fragment is now dislodged from its original context. In short, an interpretation based on fragments, while different in kind – and while often based on a more transparent process of transmission – is frequently no less defective and partial than one based on testimonia. (The non-classicist should perhaps be warned that this view will not be shared by all classicists, but it is a conclusion which seems to be substantiated by the results presented in this volume.)

3 *Principles of arrangement*

In the ordering of fragmentary evidence a number of variations tend to be possible, and no two editors are likely to opt for identical sequences. A brief explanation of the principles which guided this edition might therefore be useful.

The Herophileans are introduced in chronological sequence, starting with Herophilus in the early third century B.C. and ending in the mid first century A.D. with Demosthenes Philalethes (probably no later than the Neronian period). In some cases chronological certainty is impossible, and the particular sequence of Herophileans I have settled on is, therefore, to be understood only as a provisional ordering device and not as a sequence on which one could insist dogmatically. The existing evidence is not always unambiguous, and further evidence might well necessitate a revision.

The bulk of the ancient evidence concerns the founding master of the school, Herophilus. Within the large corpus of texts about him I have first provided the testimonies about his life, about the books he wrote, about his theory of the parts of medicine, and about his views on method and causation. Then follow the central categories of his medical 'system': anatomy, for which he was perhaps most famous both in antiquity and in the Renaissance; physiology and pathology (here his area of special expertise, pulse theory, is most prominent); and therapeutics. These central chapters are finally followed by the controversial testimonia about his interest in, and perhaps exegesis of, some Hippocratic treatises. The sequence of the central chapters, from anatomy to therapeutics, seems compatible with Herophilus' own division of medicine (see Chapter IV), although it is not clear that he consistently separated these branches of medicine in his writings: anatomy and physiology would belong to the first branch ('healthy things'), pathology to the second ('things pertaining to disease'), and therapeutics to the third ('neutrals').

Perhaps the most controversial aspect of the arrangement of texts will be the decision not to present all the 'fragments' together in complete isolation from the 'testimonia', as, for example, in Hermann Diels' *Fragmente der Vorsokratiker*. This decision was reached only after much hesitation. The reasons for the arrangement include the following: first, it is not always clear that the evidential value of a fragment, at least in medical history, is greater than that of a testimonium, and often the meaning of the fragment remains impenetrable in isolation. Second, in many cases the reader would have to perform a constant shuttle between a given fragment and the many testimonia on the same subject in order to arrive at an understanding of the fragment. Third, the compromise solution adopted in this volume – clustering together, within each chapter, all fragments identified as belonging to a relevant book or books by Herophilus, and then grouping together all other evidence thematically related to these fragments – provides the reader with convenient, consecutive access to all evidence on a given subject, without violating the fundamental distinction between fragment and testimonium.

Finally, most chapters consist of two parts: A, *Introduction*; B, *Texts and Translation*. In some chapters a third part – C, *Comments*, consisting of minor points not covered in A – is included; however, when a necessary minimum of interprétive points has been made in the *Introduction* (A), C is omitted.

4 *Translation, cross-references*

All translations from Greek and Latin are my own and, to my knowledge, most are the first translations of these texts into English. In the few cases where earlier translations exist I have, however, not hesitated to learn from them. The translations of the medieval Arabic texts fall into two classes: where English translations of these texts exist, I availed myself of them, as acknowledged throughout; in other cases the translations are based on German and French translations whenever available. For help with some of the Arabic material I am grateful to Professors Manfred Ullmann, Franz Rosenthal, and Dimitri Gutas. Although I have probably not always succeeded, I have tried to be scrupulous within the bounds of intelligible English, and to take into account semantic, syntactic, and stylistic shifts in post-classical Greek and Latin. My interpretation of some phrases and constructions might seem implausible at first, at least to ears attuned mainly to fifth- or fourth-century B.C. Greek prose, but a check in LSJ, Lampe, Kühner–Gerth, Schwyzer, Blomquist, Rydberg, and others will often provide Hellenistic and later parallels that appear to confirm the interpretations I have offered.

One of the more serious problems for the translator is provided by the notoriously ambiguous phrases οἱ περὶ Ἡρόφιλον, οἱ ἀμφὶ τὸν Ἡρόφιλον, οἱ ἀπὸ τῆς Ἡροφίλου οἰκίας, οἱ ἀφ᾽ Ἡροφίλου, and so on. Whenever one of these phrases unequivocally refers to a view developed by Herophilus' followers but not by Herophilus himself, it is translated as 'the followers of Herophilus', 'the descendants of Herophilus', or a corresponding phrase; but when it refers to a view held by both Herophilus and later Herophileans, it is usually translated as 'Herophilus and his followers'. To ambiguous cases I have at times deliberately responded with ambivalent phrases such as 'those around Herophilus'. Perhaps further evidence, or further scrutiny of the evidence presented here, will result in a resolution of some of the ambiguities and an amendment of some of my translations.[1]

While the conventions governing the use of brackets and parentheses in classical texts are retained in the Greek and Latin passages, I have adhered to English usage in the translations: (   ) for a parenthetical remark which occurs in the *original* text; [   ] or [sc.   ] for the *translator's explanatory additions*, which are usually drawn from the immediate context in which a testimonium or fragment is imbedded.

In the occasional transliterations of Greek words, I have followed a traditional scholarly practice, i.e. rendering all Greek letters by their closest English equivalent, but using *y* for υ (unless υ is part of a diphthong). This use of *y* will not please those classicists who, with some justification, regard it as a Latinate intrusion, but it has the advantage of making readily recognizable to the Greekless reader modern terminological cognates which are known primarily through a Latinized medical nomenclature.

Finally, since a single passage in an ancient source is sometimes useful for the reconstruction of more than one of the dimensions of Alexandrian medicine treated in this volume, I have in a few cases found it necessary to reproduce a part or parts of a testimonium in more than one chapter. In all such cases a cross-reference to the most complete version of the text in this edition follows immediately upon the truncated version.

5 *Text*

The texts printed in this volume were culled from some hundred different works by more than fifty ancient authors, and only a deluded person could claim textual expertise covering so wide a range. Extensive use therefore has been made of the best editions currently available (see Sigla, editions and Bibliography). Texts from these editions are, however, not simply reproduced: the apparatus criticus is selective, eschewing mention of most minor orthographic slips and disagreements (except in the case of central concepts or proper names of Herophileans), but supplying the reader with enough important or characteristic variants to obviate recourse to the

[1] Cf. von Staden, 1982: 76–100, 199–206.

standard editions. In a number of cases I have returned to manuscript readings at the expense of an editor's conjecture, and in a few cases I have also ventured to offer my own conjectures, if those of previous editors have not seemed entirely satisfactory. While these decisions were all made in the interest of an intelligible text, and with a conservative respect for the manuscript evidence, they were not all made with the same degree of confidence; the reasons for this are often indicated either in the critical apparatus or in the comments.

In several cases it has, however, been possible to have recourse to unpublished manuscript evidence. The most important are Marcellinus' *De pulsibus*; Galen's *De semine, De tremore, palpitatione, convulsione et rigore, De pulsuum differentiis, De pulsuum dignotione, De venae sectione adversus Erasistratum*; and the pseudo-Galenic *Introductio sive medicus*. A few brief comments on the MSS traditions of these texts might therefore be useful.

For his edition of Marcellinus' *De pulsibus* Hermann Schöne used only three manuscripts: Vindobonensis med. gr. 16(*A*) of the fourteenth century and two incomplete and interdependent manuscripts of the fifteenth century, Vindobonensis med. gr. 15 (*V*) and Parisinus gr. 2332 (*P*). For these three texts Schöne relied exclusively on transcripts produced by acquaintances, and it is therefore perhaps not surprising that my report of *APV* sometimes differs from his. In addition to *APV*, I collated a fifteenth-century MS, Bononiensis gr. Bibliothecae Universitatis 3632 (*B*), which did not become known to Schöne until he had completed his edition, as well as three MSS not known at all to Schöne: Palatinus gr. 400 (*H*) of the fifteenth century, Mosquensis gr. 283 [283 Savva = 466 Vladimir = 270 Matthaei] of the sixteenth century (*M*), and Parisinus gr. 2260 (*F*), likewise a sixteenth-century manuscript. *BHMF* are all incomplete: *B* contains I. 1–III.83, V.114–48, IX.234–48, XI.254–60, XII.268–XIV.285, XV.288–90, XVI.295–9, XVII.302–4, XVIII.308–407, XXXI.417–23, XXXII.433–7, XXXIII.443–5 and 448–54, XXXIV.461–4, XXV.483–5. *H* contains XI.254–67 and XVIII.309–XXX.408. *M* supplies VIII.222–XXVI.510 (but omits lines 231–4 and some chapter headings), while *F* provides XI.254–XXXIV.473. *A* is the most complete and best source, and seems to depend on a different hyparchetype from the other MSS. *VP*, while belonging to a different line, share the same archetype or exemplar with *FH*, as does *M*. A third tradition seems to be represented by *B*, which contains numerous variants not resembling any of those in *A* or in *FHMVP*. My apparatus for texts drawn from Marcellinus is based on a collation of these seven manuscripts.

The apparatus to the texts from Galen's *De semine* I owe to the generosity of Professor De Lacy, who permitted me to examine his unpublished edition (in preparation for the *CMG*). The primary evidence, as Professor De Lacy reports, is provided by two independent sixteenth-century manuscripts, Parisinus gr. 2279 (*P*) and the same Moscow MS in which excerpts from Marcellinus occur, Mosquensis gr. 283 Savva [= 466 Vladimir] (*M*). Valuable subsidiary evidence is offered by the Latin translation of Niccolò da Reggio (extant in four manuscripts and in the Venetian *editio princeps* of 1490), but none of Niccolò's variants are of significance for the passages concerning Herophilus. More relevant for this edition is the evidence of the Aldine (*Ald*), which at times deviates from *PM*.

For the passages from Galen's *De venae sectione adversus Erasistratum* the text rests on two manuscripts I collated: Ambrosianus gr. 129 (B.108. sup.) of the fourteenth century (*A*) and Urbinas gr. 70 (*U*) of the fifteenth. *U* appears to depend indirectly on *A*. See Kotrč, 1973.

For texts culled from Galen's *De tremore, palpitatione, convulsione et rigore* I relied on Vaticanus gr. 1845 (*V*) of the twelfth century and Marcianus gr. 282 (*B*) of the fifteenth century. I am indebted to Professor David Sider for providing a complete list of the variants he recorded when collating these two manuscripts; they confirm my own collations without exception.

Two Galenic treatises, *De pulsuum differentiis* and *De pulsuum dignotione*, provide a wealth of information about Herophilus as well as his followers. For both works I relied primarily on collations of Vaticanus gr. 281 (*A*), s. XIV; Laurentianus plut. 74.18 (*L*), s. XII; Laur. plut. 74.28 (*B*) (early thirteenth century); the fifteenth-century Vulcanianus 43 in Leyden (*V*); and Harleianus 5625, of the fifteenth or sixteenth century, in the British Museum (*H*). Since a number of MSS still await collation, a comprehensive assessment of the MSS filiation is at present impossible, but the earliest MSS were examined, and among them *ABL* appear the more reliable and useful, *H* seems to depend on *A*, *V* on *L*. *BL* belong to the same tradition, while *A* is derived from a different hyparchetype. *ABHLV* deviate from Kühn's text to a limited degree, however.

Finally, the texts from the pseudo-Galenic *Eisagoge* (better known as *Introductio sive medicus*), a work which perhaps predates Galen and seems to be of Pneumatic provenance, are based on specimen collations of four manuscripts: Dresdensis Da I of the fifteenth century (*D*), the most important source; Lipsiensis 52 (*L*); Berolinensis Philippicus 1526 (*P*); and Monacensis 109 (*M*). *LPM* seem to belong to the sixteenth century. A more confident assessment of the MSS filiation will have to await the edition being prepared by F. Kudlien; in the meantime I have relied largely on the useful observations of Georg Helmreich, *Handschriftliche Studien zu Galen*, Part III (Programm Ansbach, 1914).

Details of other texts are given either in the index of sigla and editions below, or with the texts themselves. I have listed only those sigla relevant to my own apparatus. (Fuller discussions of the manuscript traditions can, of course, be found in the standard editions listed below or in the standard analyses of the MSS filiations.)

Conventional practice has been followed in the use of brackets and parentheses in the Greek and Latin texts, but papyrological conventions have been retained in the excerpts from papyri. My own explanatory additions, drawn from the larger contexts in which the testimonia and fragments occur, are introduced as follows: (sc. . . .). A different practice seemed advisable in the translation (see Section 4 above).

ABBREVIATIONS

Abh   *Abhandlungen* of the Learned Academies in Berlin, Göttingen, Leipzig, Mainz, Munich, Vienna (*philosophisch-historische* or *geistes- und sozialwissenschaftliche Klasse* unless otherwise specified)

AGM   *(Sudhoffs) Archiv für Geschichte der Medizin (und der Naturwissenschaften)*, (1907–) [Title varies; most recently, *Sudhoffs Archiv, Zeitschrift für Wissenschaftsgeschichte.*]

AM.   Apollonius Mys, the Herophilean (see Chapter xxiii)

An.   Andreas, the Herophilean (see Chapter xi)

Ant. Med.   *Antike Medizin (Wege der Forschung*, vol. 221), ed. Hellmut Flashar (Darmstadt, 1971)

AP.   Alexander Philalethes, the Herophilean (see Chapter xxii)

Ar.   Aristoxenus, the Herophilean (see Chapter xxv)

Ba.   Bacchius, the Herophilean (see Chapter xiv)

BHM   *Bulletin of the History of Medicine*

CIA   *Corpus Inscriptionum Atticarum* (Berlin, 1873–) [in the series *Inscriptiones Graecae*]

CIG   *Corpus Inscriptionum Graecarum* (Berlin, 1828–1877)

CIL   *Corpus Inscriptionum Latinarum*, ed. T. Mommsen et al. (Berlin, 1863–)

Cm.   Callimachus, the Herophilean (see Chapter xiii)

CMG   *Corpus Medicorum Graecorum* (Berlin/Leipzig, 1908–; Berlin, 1947–)

CML   *Corpus Medicorum Latinorum* (Berlin/Leipzig, 1915–)

Cn.   Callianax, the Herophilean (see Chapter xii)

Cr.   Chrysermus, the Herophilean (see Chapter xx)

Cy.   Cydias, the Herophilean (see Chapter xxvi)

DA.   Demetrius of Apamea, the Herophilean (see Chapter xvi)

DG   Hermann Diels (ed.), *Doxographi Graeci* (Berlin, 1879; repr. 1965)

Diocles fr., Wellmann M. Wellmann (ed., comm.), *Fragmentsammlung der griechischen Ärzte*, I. *Die Fragmente der sikelischen Ärzte Akron, Philistion und des Diokles von Karystos* (Berlin, 1901)

DK   Hermann Diels, Walther Kranz, *Die Fragmente der Vorsokratiker*, 6th (and later) ed., 3 vols. (Berlin/Zürich, 1951)

D.L.   Diogenes Laertius, *Vitae philosophorum* (see Sigla)

DP.   Demosthenes Philalethes, the Herophilean (see Chapter xxviii)

Ds.   Dioscurides Phacas, the Herophilean (see Chapter xix)

Dsc.   Dioscurides, Pedanius, *De materia medica* (see Sigla)

FGrHist   *Fragmente der griechischen Historiker*, ed. Felix Jacoby (Berlin/Leiden, 1923–) (F = Fragmente, Komm. = Kommentar)

Fr   Fragment

G.   Gaius, the Herophilean (see Chapter xxvii)

Galen, *Scr. Min.* *Galenus, Scripta Minora*, ed. J. Marquardt, I. Müller, G. Helmreich, 3 vols. (Leipzig, 1884–93; repr. Amsterdam, 1967)

GCS   *Die griechischen christlichen Schriftsteller der ersten Jahrhunderte* (Berlin, 1897–)

GMÄ   Hermann Grapow *et al.*, *Grundriss der Medizin der alten Ägypter* (Berlin, 1954–73)

HE.   Heraclides of Erythrae, the Herophilean (see Chapter xxiv)

Hg.   Hegetor, the Herophilean (see Chapter xvii)

Hp.   Hippocrates

IG   *Inscriptiones Graecae* (Berlin, 1873–)

K   C. G. Kühn, *Claudii Galeni opera omnia*, 22 vols. in 20 (Leipzig, 1821–33; repr. Hildesheim, 1965) = *Medicorum Graecorum opera*, vols. 1–20

Kl. P.   *Der kleine Pauly*, ed. Konrat Ziegler and Walther Sontheimer (Stuttgart, 1964–75)

Kühner–Gerth Raphael Kühner, *Ausführliche Grammatik der griechischen Sprache, Teil 2: Satzlehre*, 3rd edn, rev. B. Gerth, 2 vols. (Hannover/Leipzig, 1898–1904; repr. 1966)

Kw.   *Hippocratis opera*, ed. Hugo Kühlewein, 2 vols. (Leipzig, 1894–1902)

L   E. Littré (ed. and transl.), *Oeuvres complètes d'Hippocrate*, 10 vols. (Paris, 1839–61)

LAW	*Lexikon der Alten Welt*, ed. Carl Andresen, Hartmut Erbse, Olof Gigon *et al.* (Zurich/Stuttgart, 1965)
LSJ	H. G. Liddell, R. Scott, H. S. Jones, *A Greek–English Lexicon (with Supplement)* (Oxford, 1968)
Ma.	Mantias, the Herophilean (see Chapter xviii)
REG	*Revue des Études Grecques* (1888–)
RhM	*Rheinisches Museum* (Neue Folge, 1842–)
Sammelb.	*Sammelbuch griechischer Urkunden aus Ägypten*, ed. F. Preisigke, F. Bilabel, E. Kiessling, H.-A. Rupprecht (Strassburg / Berlin / Leipzig / Heidelberg / Wiesbaden, 1915–)
S.E., *M*	Sextus Empiricus, *Adversus Mathematicos* (see Sigla)
S.E., *P*	Sextus Empiricus, *Outlines of Pyrrhonism* (see Sigla)
Sitzb.	*Sitzungsberichte* of the Learned Academies in Berlin, Munich, Leipzig, and Vienna (*philosophisch-historische Klasse* unless otherwise specified)
SVF	Hans von Arnim, *Stoicorum Veterum Fragmenta*, 4 vols. (vol. 4 ed. M. Adler) (Leipzig, 1903–24; repr. Stuttgart, 1964)
T	Testimonium
Zn.	Zeno, the Herophilean (see Chapter xv)
Zx.	Zeuxis, the Herophilean (see Chapter xxi)

SIGLA, EDITIONS

Aëtius Amidenus, *Libri medicinales*, ed. A. Olivieri, *CMG* VIII.1-2 (Berlin, 1935-50)

A	Athous Laurae 718.Ω. 63, s.XV
A^t	Athous Laurae 719.Ω. 64, s.XIV
B	Parisinus gr. 2192, s.XV
C	Parisinus gr. 1883, s.XIV
C^p	Parisinus gr. 2228, s.XIV
D	Athous Vatopedi A.29, s.XIV
E	Parisinus gr. 2193 s.XV
G^a	Parisinus gr. 2194, s.XV
H^a	Parisinus gr. 2195, s.XIII
L^a	Laurentianus 75.20 et 5, s.XII
M^o	Marcianus gr. 291, s.XV
P	Vaticanus gr. 298, s.XIV
P^x	Palatinus gr. 199, s.XIII
Q	Marcianus gr. 596, s.XVI
S	Scorialensis ψ. IV. 14, s. XV (Books I-II. 96); s.XIII (II.81-VI)
T	Scorialensis T. II. 14, s.XVI
X	Parisinus gr. 2199, s.XVI
$Υ$	Parisinus gr. 2198, A.D. 1522
χ	$C^p P^x M^o X$
ψ	$A D P T B E Q$
ω	$S A^t G^a H^a Υ$

Aëtius Doxographus, *De placitis philosophorum*, ed. H. Diels, *Doxographi Graeci* (Berlin, 1879), pp. 267-444

M	Mosquensis gr. 352 (Savva) (= 339 Matthaei = 501 Vladimir), s.XII
E	Parisinus gr. 1672, s.XIV med.
B	Marcianus gr. 521, s. XIII/XIV

(Cf. etiam infra s.vv. 'Ps.-Plutarchus, *Placita Philosophorum*')

Agnellus Ravennas (?), *In Galeni De sectis commentaria*, ed. 'Seminar Classics 609', State University of New York at Buffalo (Arethusa Monographs 8, 1981)
A   Ambrosianus C 108 inf., s.IX
P   editio Galeni operum Papiensis (1515); vid. etiam infra s.vv. 'Iohannes Alexandrinus'

Anatolius, *De decade*, ed. J. L. Heiberg, in *Annales internationales d'histoire: Congrès de Paris, 1900, 5ᵉ section, Histoires des sciences* (Paris, 1901), 27–41

Anecdota Graeca, ed. I. Bekker, 3 vols. (Berlin, 1814–21)

Anecdota Graeca Oxoniensia, ed. J. A. Cramer, 4 vols. (Oxford, 1835–7)

Anecdota Graeca Parisiensia, ed. J. A. Cramer, 4 vols. (Oxford, 1839–41)

Anecdota Graeca et Graecolatina, ed. V. Rose, 2 vols. (Berlin, 1864–70)

Anonymus Bambergensis, ed. K. Sudhoff, *Archiv für Geschichte der Medizin* 8 (1915), 410–13
B   Bambergensis L.III.8 (med. 1), s.IX

Anonymus Bruxellensis, *Vita Hippocratis*, ed. H. Schöne, *Rheinisches Museum* N.F. 58 (1903), 56–66

Anonymus Laurentianus, ed. M. Wellmann, *Hermes* 35 (1900), 367–82

Anonymus Londinensis, *Menonia*, ed. H. Diels, *Supplementum Aristotelicum* III.1 (Berlin, 1893); W. H. S. Jones (Cambridge, 1947)
P   Papyri Londinensis CXXXVII scriptor (idemque corrector)

Apollonius Citiensis, *In Hippocratis De articulis*, ed. J. Kollesch, F. Kudlien, *CMG* XI.1.1. (Berlin, 1965)

Athenaeus, *Deipnosophistae*, ed. G. Kaibel (Leipzig, 1887–90); A. M. Desrousseaux, C. Astruc (Paris, 1956–)

Caelius Aurelianus, *Celeres sive acutae passiones, Tardae passiones*, ed. I. E. Drabkin (Chicago, 1950)
L   Zuiccaviensis lat., s.IX (the only manuscript; contains *Tardae passiones* 5.77–91 and 5.122–8)
S   J. Sichardus (ed.), *Tardae passiones* (Basel, 1529)
G   J. Guinterius Andernacus (ed.), *Celeres vel acutae passiones* (Paris, 1533)
R   G. Rovillius (ed. Lyon, 1567)
A   J. C. Amman (ed. Amsterdam, 1709)

Caesar, C. Julius, *Bellum Alexandrinum*, ed. J. Andrieu (Paris, 1954); R. Giomini (Rome, 1956)

Calcidius, *In Platonis Timaeum commentarius*, ed. J. H. Waszink, *Plato Latinus*
  IV, in *Corpus Platonicum Medii Aevi* (London/Leiden, 1962)
Br_1 Bruxellensis 9625-6, s.X
B_2 Vaticanus Barberinus lat. 22, s.XI
Vat_1 Vaticanus lat. 1544, s.XV
A   consensus Br_1 B_2 Vat_1

Val   Valentianus 293, s.IX
Am_2 Ambrosianus I.195.Inf., s.XI ex.
Λ consensus *Val*. Am_2

Lu   Lugdunensis 324, s.IX
P_5 Parisinus lat. 6282, s.XI
Σ consensus *Lu* P_5

P_8 Parisinus lat. 6570, s.XII
A_4 Londinensis (Mus. Britt.) Addit. 19968, s.XI
Ba   Bambergensis Bibl. publ. M.v.15 (class. 18), s.XI
Col   Coloniensis Eccles. Metropolit. 192 (Darmst. 2167), s.XI
Reg_8 Vaticanus Reginensis lat. 1861, s.XI
U_1 Vindobonensis lat. 443, s.XI
$\mathcal{N}$ Neopolitanus VIII. F.11, s.XII
Υ consensus P_8 A_4 *Ba Col* Reg_8 U_1 $\mathcal{N}$

Cam   Cantabrigiensis Coll. Sidney Sussex 31 (Δ.2.9), s.XIV

Reg_6 Vaticanus Reginensis lat. 1308, s.XI
L_3 Leidensis B.P.L. 64, s.XI
P_3 Parisinus lat. 6280, s.XI
Reg_5 Vaticanus Reginensis lat. 11114, s.XIV
Ξ consensus Reg_6 L_3 P_3 Reg_5
τ consensus Reg_6 P_3

F_3 Florentinus Bibl. Nat. Centr. San Marco I. IV.28, s.XI
La   Florentinus Gaddianus plut. 89.sup.51, s.XI
Π consensus F_3 *La*

Cassius Iatrosophista, *Problemata*, ed. J. Ideler,*Physici et Medici Graeci Minores*
  I (Berlin, 1841)

Celsus, A. Cornelius, *De artibus* 6–12 (= *De medicina* 1–6), ed. F. Marx, *CML* I
  (Leipzig/Berlin, 1915); prohoem. ed. P. Mudry (Rome, 1982)
F   Laurentianus 73.1, s.IX
V   Vaticanus lat. 5951, s.IX (contains lacunae)
J   Laurentianus 73.7, s.XV (copied by Nicolaus Niccoli from a lost
    codex)

Egnatius   ed. Aldina (Venice, 1528)
Caesarius   ed. (The Hague, 1528)

Censorinus, *De die natali*, ed. N. Sallmann (Leipzig, 1983)
  C   Coloniensis 166 (olim Darmstadiensis 2191), s.VIII
  P   Palatinus lat. 1588, s.IX
  V   Vaticanus lat. 4929, s.IX med.

Choeroboscus(?), Georgius, *De quantitate*, ed. J. A. Cramer, in *Anecdota Graeca e codd. manuscriptis Bibliothecarum Oxoniensium*, vol. II (Oxford, 1835)

Diogenes Laertius, *Vitae philosophorum*, ed. H. S. Long (Oxford, 1964)

Dionysius Aegeus, *Dictyaca*, in Photius, *Bibliotheca* III (cod. 211), ed. R. Henry, *Collection Byzantine* (Paris, 1962)
  A   Marcianus gr. 450, s.X
  M   Marcianus gr. 451, s.XII

Dioscurides, Pedanius, *De materia medica*, ed. M. Wellmann, 3 vols. (Berlin, 1906–14)

Erotianus, *Vocum Hippocraticarum Collectio cum Fragmentis*, ed. E. Nachmanson (Gothenburg, 1918)

Etymologicon Magnum, ed. T. Gaisford (Oxford, 1848)

Eusebius, *Praeparatio evangelica* (Die Griechischen Christlichen Schriftsteller der ersten Jahrhunderte: Eusebius 8.1–2), ed. K. Mras, 2nd ed. E. des Places (Berlin, 1982–3)

Eustathius Thessalonicensis, *Commentarii ad Homeri Odysseam*, ed. J. G. Stallbaum (Leipzig, 1825–6)

Fragmenta Poematum rem naturalem vel medicinam spectantium, ed. U. C. Bussemaker, in *Poetae Bucolici et Didactici, Bibliotheca Graecorum Scriptorum* (Paris, 1851)

Galenus: with the exception of the editions of Galenic works listed below, see C. G. Kühn, *Medicorum Graecorum Opera quae exstant: Claudius Galenus* 1–20 (Leipzig, 1821–33)

Galenus, *Adversus Iulianum*, ed. E. Wenkebach, *CMG* v.10.3 (Berlin, 1951)
  L   Laurentianus 74.3, s.XII

Galenus, *An in arteriis natura sanguis contineatur*, ed. F. Albrecht (Diss. Marburg, 1911); D. J. Furley, J. S. Wilkie (Princeton, 1984)
  L   Laurentianus 74.3, s.XII
  V   Marcianus gr. app. cl. v.4, s.XV

  Ald   ed. Aldina (Venice, 1525)

Galenus, *De causis procatarcticis*, ed. K. Bardong, *CMG Suppl.* 2 (Leipzig/ Berlin, 1937). Translated by Niccolò da Reggio (s.XIV)

P   Parisinus lat. 6865, s.XIV
D   Dresdensis Db.93, s.XV
v   ed. Venice, 1490 (vol. I, fols. 144ff.)

Galenus, *De emperica subfiguratione*, ed. M. Bonnet (Diss. Bonn, 1872); K.
   Deichgräber, *Die griechische Empirikerschule*, 2nd edn (Berlin/Zurich,
   1965), pp. 42–90. Translated (A.D. 1341) by Niccolò da Reggio.
pr   ed. Aldina [princeps] (Venice, 1502). (Monacensis lat. 465 was
         copied in the year 1503 from the Aldine edition.)

Galenus, *De experientia medica* (*'On Medical Experience'*), ed. R. Walzer
   (Oxford, 1944)

Ps.-Galenus, *De historia philosopha*, ed. H. Diels, *Doxographi Graeci* (Berlin,
   1879); J. Mau (in preparation)
A   Laurentianus 74.3, s.XII
B   Laurentianus 58.2, s.XV

Galenus, *De libris propriis*, ed. I. von Müller, *Scr. Min.* II (Leipzig, 1891)
Q   Ambrosianus gr. Q.3, sup., s.XVI in.
Ald   ed. Aldina (Venice, 1525)

Galenus, *De naturalibus facultatibus* III, ed. G. Helmreich, *Scr. Min.* III (Leipzig,
   1893)
L   Laurentianus 74.5, s.XII
M   Marcianus gr. 275, s.XV
O   Bodleianus Laud. gr. 58, s.XV
P   Parisinus gr. 2267, s.XV

Galenus, *De placitis Hippocratis et Platonis*, ed. Phillip De Lacy, 3 vols., *CMG*
   v.4.1.2 (Berlin, 1978–84)
H   Hamiltonensis 270, s.XII/XIII
C   Cantabrigiensis Caius coll. 47/24, s.XII
L   Laurentianus 74.22, s.XII

Caius   ed. (Basel, 1544)
recens. anon.   F. Hultsch, *Literarisches Centralblatt* (1875), cols. 49–51

Galenus, *De pulsuum differentiis* and *De pulsuum dignotione* (VIII, pp. 493–961K)
A   Vaticanus gr. 281, s.XIV
B   Laurentianus 74.28, s.XIII init.
H   Harleianus 5625, s.XV
L   Laurentianus 74.18, s.XII
V   Vulcanianus gr. 43, s.XV

Galenus, *De sanitate tuenda*, ed. K. Koch, *CMG* v.4.2 (Leipzig/Berlin, 1923)
M   Marcianus gr. 276, s.XII/XIII

V   Marcianus gr. 282, s.XV

R   Vaticanus Reginensis gr. 173, s.XV

Scal Scaliger (his *lectiones* entered in the margins of a copy of the Aldine edn)

Galenus, *De septimestri partu*, ed. R. Walzer, *Rivista di studi orientali* 15 (1935), 323–57

Galenus, *De semine*, ed. Ph. De Lacy, *CMG* (Berlin, forthcoming)

P   Parisinus gr. 2279, s.XVI

M   Mosquensis gr. 283 (Savva) (= 270 Matthaei = 466 Vladimir), s.XVI

Nicolaus Niccolò da Reggio (Latin translation, s.XIV)

Ald   ed. Aldina (Venice, 1525)

Galenus, *De tremore, palpitatione, convulsione et rigore* (VII, pp. 584–642K)

V   Vaticanus gr. 1845, s.XII

B   Marcianus gr. 282, s.XV

Galenus, *De usu partium*, ed. G. Helmreich (Leipzig, 1907–9)

A   Parisinus gr. 2253, s.XI/XII

B   Parisinus gr. 2154, s.XIII

C   Parisinus gr. 985, s.XV

D   Parisinus gr. 2148, s.XV

L   Laurentianus 74.4, s.XII

P   Palatinus gr. 251, s.XV

U   Vaticanus Urbinas gr. 69, s.X–XI

N   Niccolò da Reggio (Latin translation, s.XIV)

Ald   ed. Aldina (Venice, 1525)

Bas   ed. Basel (1538)

Ch   ed. R. Chartier [= Charterius] (Paris, 1679)

Galenus, *De usu pulsuum*, ed. D. J. Furley, J. S. Wilkie (Princeton, 1984)

S   Scorial. Φ III 11, s.XIV–XV

Ald   ed. Aldina (Venice, 1525)

Galenus, *De uteri dissectione*, ed. D. Nickel, *CMG* v.2.1 (Berlin, 1971)

V   Vaticanus gr. 1845, s.XII

C   Coislinianus gr. 228, s.XIV

P   Parisinus gr. 2165, s.XVI

P (Orib.) See below, s.v. Oribasius, *P*

F (Orib.) See below, s.v. Oribasius, *F*

Galenus, *De venae sectione adversus Erasistratum*, ed. C. G. Kühn, *Opera omnia*, vol. XI; R. F. Kotrč, *CMG* (in preparation)

A   Ambrosianus gr. 129 (B.108, sup.), s.XIV
U   Vaticanus Urbinas gr. 70, s.XV

Galenus, *Explanatio vocum Hippocratis*, ed. C. G. Kühn, *Opera omnia*, vol. xix
    (Leipzig, 1830); J. G. F. Franze (Leipzig, 1780)
A   Laurentianus 74.3, s.XII
L   Leidensis Vossianus Miscell. I pars 13, s.XV
M   Monacensis gr. 71, s.XVI
M°   Mosquensis gr. (apparently no longer extant, but used by Franze)
D   Dorvillianus x.1.1.3, s.XV ex.
R   Vaticanus gr. 277, s.XIV

Galenus, *In Hippocratis De natura hominis commentarii*, ed. J. Mewaldt, *CMG*
    v.9.1 (Leipzig/Berlin, 1914)
L   Laurentianus 59.14, s.XIV
V   Marcianus gr. 282, s.XV
R   Vaticanus Reginensis gr. 173, s.XV
R²   deperditus ab Opizone (Aldinae auctore) excussus

Galenus, *In Hippocratis Epidemiarum tertium librum commentarii 1–3*, ed. E.
    Wenkebach, *CMG* v.10.2.1 (Berlin/Leipzig, 1936)
L   Laurentianus 74.25, s.XII
M   Monacensis gr. 231, s.XV
P   Parisinus gr. 2165, s.XVI
Q   Parisinus gr. 2174, s.XVI
V   Marcianus gr. app. cl. v.5, s.XV
O   archetypus codd. *MQV*, fort. s.XIV

Galenus, *In Hippocratis Epidemiarum sextum librum commentarii 1–8*, ed. E.
    Wenkebach, F. Pfaff, *CMG* v.10.2.2 (Berlin, 1956)
U   Marcianus gr. 283, *c.* 1300–1320
H   Scorialensis arab. 805, s.XIII (Ḥunain's Arabic version, trans-
       lated by Pfaff)
Ald ed. Aldina (Venice, 1525)
Bas ed. Hieronymus Gemusaeus (Basel, 1538)
Cornarius Janus Cornarius (in his copy of the Aldine edn)

Galenus, *In Hippocratis Prognosticum commentarii*, ed. J. Heeg, *CMG* v.9.2
    (Leipzig/Berlin, 1915)
V   Vaticanus gr. 1858 et 1063, s.XIII
R   Vaticanus Reginensis gr. 175, s.XIV
P   Palatinus gr. 157, s.XIV
F   Parisinus gr. 2266, s.XII
F¹   Supplementa codicis *F*, s.XVI

Galenus, *In Hippocratis Prorrheticum commentarii*, ed. H. Diels, *CMG* v.9.2
  (Leipzig/Berlin, 1915)
  R   Vaticanus Reginensis gr. 175, s.XIV
  T   Trivultianus Mediolanensis gr. 685, s.XIII/XIV
  L   Laurentianus 75.5, s.XII

Ps.-Galenus, *Introductio sive medicus*, ed. C. G. Kühn, *Opera omnia*, vol. xiv, pp.
  674–797; F. Kudlien (in preparation)
  L   Lipsiensis gr. 52, s.XVI
  P   Berolinensis Philippicus 1526, s.XVI
  M   Monacensis gr. 109, s.XVI
  D   Dresdensis Da.I, s.XV

Galenus, *Thrasybulus (Utrum Medicinae sit an Gymnasticae Hygieine)*, ed. G.
  Helmreich, *Scr. Min.* iii (Leipzig, 1893)
  L   Laurentianus 74.3, s.XII
  P   Parisinus gr. 2164, s.XVI
  Ald   ed. Aldina (Venice, 1525)

Hyginus, *Fabulae*, ed. H. J. Rose, 2nd edn (Leyden, 1963)
  F   Micyllus (ed. Basel, 1535)

Iohannes Alexandrinus, *Commentaria in librum De sectis Galeni*, ed. C. D.
  Pritchet (Leiden, 1982)
  R   Parisinus lat. 6865, s.XIV
  B   Vaticanus lat. 2446, s.XIV
  V   Vaticanus lat. 2376, s.XIV
  U   Vaticanus Urbinas lat. 247, s.XIV
  E   Erfurtensis F 280, s.XIV
  C   Cesena Dextra Plut. 25, cod. 2, s.XIII
  Q   editio princeps, 1490
  S   editio Veneta, 1502
  P   editio Papiensis, 1515 (vid. supra s.vv. 'Agnellus Ravennas(?)')

Iohannes Alexandrinus, *Commentaria in sextum librum Hippocratis Epidemiarum*,
  ed. C. D. Pritchet (Leiden, 1975)
  P   Vaticanus lat. 1079, s.XV
  U   Vaticanus lat. 2417, s.XIV
  B   Vaticanus lat. 2446, s.XIV
  V   Vaticanus Reginensis 1305, s.XIII(?)
  E   Erfurtensis Amplonianus Q 201, s.XIV
  A   *Articella*, ed. Veneta 1483 (A^1) et 1523 (A^2)

Lydus, Ioannes Laurentiis, *Liber de mensibus*, ed. R. Wünsch (Leipzig, 1898)

Marcellinus, *De pulsibus*, ed. H. Schöne, *Festschrift zur 49. Versammlung deutscher Philologen und Schulmänner* (Basel, 1907), pp. 448–72; H. von Staden, *CMG* (in preparation)

    A   Vindobonensis med. gr. 16, s.XIV
    B   Bononiensis gr. Bibl. Universitatis 3632, s.XV
    V   Vindobonensis med. gr. 15, s.XV
    P   Parisinus gr. 2332, s.XV
    M   Mosquensis gr. 283 (Savva) (= 270 Matthaei = 466 Vladimir), s.XVI
    H   Palatinus gr. 400, s.XV
    F   Parisinus gr. 2260, s.XVI

Marcellus, *De medicamentis*, ed. M. Niedermann, 2nd edn E. Liechtenhan, tr. J. Kollesch, D. Nickel, *CML* v (Berlin, 1968)

Martianus Capella, *De nuptiis Philologiae et Mercurii*, ed. J. Willis (Leipzig, 1983)

    A   Harleianus 2685, s.IX
    B   Bambergensis Msc. class, 39, s.IX ex.
    D   Parisinus lat. 8670, s.IX
    P   Petropolitanus publ. bibl. class. lat. F. V.10 s.X.
    R   Reichenauensis 73, s.IX

Michael Italicus, *Epistulae*, ed. P. Gautier (Archives de l'Orient Chrétien 14, Paris, 1972)

Nonius Marcellus, *De conpendiosa doctrina*, ed. W. M. Lindsay, 3 vols. (Leipzig, 1903)

Oribasius, *Collectiones medicae*, ed. J. Raeder, *CMG* vi.1–3 (Leipzig/Berlin, 1926–31)

    P   Palatinus gr. 375, s.XII
    A   Parisinus gr. 2151, S.XVI
    C   Parisinus gr. 2262, s.XVI
    D   Parisinus gr. 2263, s.XVI
    E   Parisinus gr. 2321, s.XVI
    L   Londinensis Burneianus 94, s.XVI
    O   Vaticanus Ottobonianus gr. 235, s.XVI
    S   Scorialensis Φ. 1.2, s.XVI
    F   Parisinus gr. 2237, s.XIV (contains only Books 9.52–5; 10.19–36; 24.29–32)
    R   Vaticanus gr. 1885, s.XIV
    Morelius   ed. Paris, 1556 (contains Books 24.1–30; 25.2–58)

Palladius, *In Hippocratis Epidemiarum librum VI comment.* (cf. F. R. Dietz (ed.),
  Scholia in Hippocratem et Galenum (Königsberg, 1834; repr. Amsterdam,
  1966), vol. 2, pp. 1–204)
  A   Ambrosianus B. 113 sup., s.XIV
  L   Laurentianus 75.22, s.XV

Papyrus Coll. Goleniščev (Pack² 2347), ed. A. Bäckstrom, *Archiv für
  Papyrusforschung* 3 (1906), 158–62

Paulus Aegineta, *Pragmateia Iatrikē*, ed. J. L. Heiberg, *CMG* IX.1–2 (Leipzig/
  Berlin, 1921–4)
  A   Parisinus gr. 2205, s.XI
  B   Parisinus gr. 2206, s.XI
  D   Parisinus gr. 2208, s.XIV
  E   Parisini gr. 2216 et 2217, s.XI
  F   Parisinus gr. 2292, s.XIV
  G   Patmiacus 208, s.XI
  H   Laurentianus 74.29, s.XI
  K   Athous Vatopedi 535, s.X
  M   Athous Laurae 330, Γ. 90, s.XI

Philumenus, *De venenatis animalibus*, ed. M. Wellmann, *CMG* X.1.1 (Leipzig/
  Berlin, 1908)
  P   Vaticanus gr. 284, s.X
  Pr   Aelii Promoti *De venenatis animalibus* cod. Vaticanus gr. 299,
            s.XV

Physici et medici Graeci minores, ed. J.L. Ideler, 2 vols. (Berlin, 1841–2)

C. Plinius Secundus, *Naturalis historia*, ed. O. Jan–C. Mayhoff, 6 vols.
  (Leipzig, 1892–1909); A. Ernout, J. Beaujeu, R. Pepin, J. André
  et al. (Paris, 1947–85)
  M   Moneus rescriptus, s.V–VI
  D   Vaticanus lat. 3861, s.XI
  F   Leidensis Lipsii 7, s.X
  R   Riccardianus 488, s.X–XI
  E   Parisinus lat. 6795, s.IX–X
  e   Parisinus lat. 6796, s.XIII
  V   Leidensis Vossianus fol. 61, s.X
  p   Parisinus lat. 6796A, s.IX–X
  g   Parisinus lat. 6800, s.XII fin.
  d   Parisinus lat. 6797, s.XIII

X	Luxemburgensis 138 (pars altera), s.XII
a	Vindobonensis olim 234, nunc 10, s.XII–XIII
T	Toletanus 47–14, s.XIII
f	Chiffletianus (ex margine editionis Dalecampianae Lugdunensis, 1685)
r	codex a Dalecampio (ex *M* u.v.) excerptus
Pintianus	*Observationes in loca obscura Naturalis Historiae Plinii* (Salamanca, 1544), and *In C. Plinii Naturalem Historiam emendationes* (Lyon, 1593) ('Pintianus' is Fernando Núñez de Toledo y Guzmán)
Ha	ed. Hardouin (Paris, 1685)
Ma	Mayhoff (*vid. supra*)

Plutarchus, *De curiositate* (*Moralia*, vol. III), ed. M. Pohlenz (Leipzig, 1929)

A	Parisinus gr. 1671, s.XIII ex.
C	Parisinus gr. 1955, s.XI–XII
D	Parisinus gr. 1956, s.XI–XII
E	Parisinus gr. 1672, s.XIV med.
G	Vaticanus Barberinianus gr. 182, s.XI
J	Ambrosianus gr. 881, s.XIII
M	Mosquensis gr. 352 (Savva) (= 339 Matthaei = 501 Vladimir), s.XII
N	Mosquensis gr. 425 (Savva) (= 337 Matthaei = 502 Vladimir), s.XII
R	Mazarineus (Paris.) 4458, s.XIV
V	Marcianus gr. 427, s.XIV
X	Marcianus gr. 250, s.X/XI
Y	Marcianus gr. 249, s.XI–XII
Z	Marcianus gr. 511, s.XIV
a	Ambrosianus gr. 689, s.XV
b	Bruxellensis 18967, s.XV
h	Harleianus (Lond.) 5612, s.XV
w	Vindobonensis gr. 36, s.XV
α	Ambrosianus gr. 859, s.XIII ex.
β	Vaticanus gr. 1013, s.XIV
γ	Vaticanus gr. 139, s.XIII ex.
Θ	consensus *Zab*
Δ	consensus *D*Θ
Λ	recensio Byzantina, *c.* 1300 (Laurentianus 56.3)
Π	codices Planudei *AE*αβγ

Ps.-Plutarchus, *Placita philosophorum* (*Moralia*, vol. v.2.1, ed. J. Mau (Leipzig, 1971)

A
E
M
α   } *vid. supra* s.vv. 'Plutarchus, *De curiositate*'
β
γ
Π

B   Marcianus gr. 521, s.XIII/XIV

Plutarchus, *Quaestiones naturales*, ed. F. H. Sandbach, in *Plutarch's Moralia*, vol. xi (Cambridge, Mass./London, 1965)
U   Vaticanus Urbinas gr. 97, s.X
H   Palatinus Heidelbergensis 283, s.XI

Plutarchus, *Quaestiones symposiacae* (*Moralia*, vol. iv), ed. C. Hubert (Leipzig, 1938)
T   Vindobonensis phil. gr. 148, s.X–XI in. (the archetype of all the extant MSS)

Pollux, *Onomasticon*, ed. E. Bethe in *Lexicographi Graeci* ix.1–3 (Leipzig, 1909–37)
F   Falcoburgianus: Parisinus gr. 2646, s.XV
S   Schottianus: Salmanticensis (Hispan.) 1.2.3, s.XV
Π   consensus *FS*

A   Parisinus gr. 2670, s.XV
C   Palatinus gr. 375, s.XII

Polybius, *Historiae*, ed. T. Büttner-Wobst, 2nd edn (Leipzig, 1905–); Book 12, ed. P. Pédech (Paris, 1961)
M   Vaticanus gr. 73, s.X

Proclus, *In Platonis Rem publicam commentarius*, ed. W. Kroll (Leipzig, 1899–1901)
m^1 Librarius codicis Vaticani gr. 2197, s.IX
m^3 eius corrector, s.XI vel XII

Remigius Autissiodorensis, *Commentum in Martianum Capellam*, ed. C. E. Lutz, 2 vols. (Leiden, 1962–5)
L   Londinensis (Bibliothecae Regiae) xvA 33, s.X
P   Parisinus lat. 8786, s.X
Π   Parisinus lat. 14754, s.XII

G   Parisinus lat. (Bibliothecae S. Genev.) 1041–2, s.XIII
C   Caesenas (Bibliothecae Malatestianae) Plut. 16, cod. 1, s.XV

Rufus Ephesius (?), *De anatomia partium hominis*, ed. C. Daremberg, C. E.
      Ruelle (Paris, 1879)
A   Ambrosianus T.141, s.XVI

Rufus Ephesius, *De nominatione partium hominis*, ed. C. Daremberg, C. E.
      Ruelle (Paris, 1879)
L   Laurentianus 74.7, s.IX/X

Rufus Ephesius, *De satyriasmo et gonorrhoea*, ed. C. Daremberg, C. E. Ruelle
      (Paris, 1879)

Rufus Ephesius, *Quaestiones medicinales*, ed. H. Gärtner, *CMG Suppl.* IV
      (Berlin, 1962); ed. alt. (Leipzig, 1970)
M   Parisinus Suppl. gr. 637, s.XV
V   Vindobonensis med. gr. 8, s.XV

Rufus Ephesius (?), *Synopsis de pulsibus*, ed. C. Daremberg, C. E. Ruelle
      (Paris, 1879)
F   Laurentianus 75.7, s.XII
P   Parisinus gr. 2193, s.XIV
G   Latin translation, in R. Chartier's edition of Galen (Paris, 1679)

Scholia in Aristophanis Aves, ed. J. W. White (Boston/London, 1914)

Scholia in Hippocratem et Galenum (*Apollonii Citiensis, Stephani, Palladii . . .*), ed.
      F. R. Dietz, 2 vols. (Königsberg, 1834)

Scholia in Nicandri Alexipharmaca, ed. M. Geymonat (Milan, 1974)

Scholia in Nicandri Theriaka, ed. A. Crugnola (Milan, 1971)

Scribonius Largus, *Compositiones* (praefatio), ed. K. Deichgräber, *Abh.*
      Mainz, 1950, no. 9, pp. 855–79; S. Sconocchia (Leipzig, 1983)
P   Parisinus lat. 6880, s.IX
L   Laudunensis 420, s.IX–X
A   Arundelianus 166, s.X–XI
T   Toletanus Capit. 98. 12, s.XVI in.
M   Ps.-Marcellus Empiricus, ed. M. Niedermann, in *CML* V (Leipzig/
        Berlin, 1916; rev. E. Liechtenhan, 1968)
Ru   Joannes Ruellius, ed. princeps (Paris, 1528)

Sextus Empiricus, *Opera*, ed. H. Mutschmann, J. Mau (Leipzig, 1914–58)
N   Laurentianus 85.19, s.XIII
L   Laurentianus 85.11, s.XV

E   Parisinus gr. 1964, s.XV
Vr   Vratislavensis Rehdigeranus 45, s.XV ex.

A   Parisinus gr. 1963, s.XVI
B   Berolinensis Phillipicus 1518, s.XVI
V   Marcianus gr. 262 (olim 408), s.XV ex.
R   Regiomontanus 16^{b}12
ς   Consensus *ABVR*

C   Cicensis, s.XVI
Ac   Leningradensis Academicus xx.Aa/II, s.XV
G   consensus codicum omnium *Ac* excepto
T   Parisinus lat. 14700, s.XIV in. (Latin translation)

Gen   ed. Petrus et Jacobus Choueti (Geneva, 1621)
Fabr   ed. J. A. Fabricius (Leipzig, 1718)

Silvaticus, Matthaeus, *Liber Pandectarum Medicinae* (Venice, 1480)

Simon Ianuensis, *Synonyma medicinae sive Clavis sanationis* (Padua, 1474)

Soranus, *De signis fracturarum*, ed. J. Ilberg, *CMG* IV (Leipzig/Berlin, 1927), pp. 155–71
L   Laurentianus 74.7, s.IX–X

Soranus, *Gynaecia*, ed. J. Ilberg, *CMG* IV (Leipzig/Berlin, 1927), pp. 3–152
P   Parisinus gr. 2153, s.XV
p   papyrus Pistelli, ed. L. De Stephani (Florence, 1913)
P, F ap. Oribasium: vid. s.v. Oribasius, *supra*

Soranus, *Vita Hippocratis*, ed. J. Ilberg, *CMG* IV (Leipzig/Berlin, 1927), pp. 175–8

Stephanus Philosophus, *In Hippocratis Prognosticum commentaria* III, ed. J. M. Duffy, *CMG* XI. 1.2 (Berlin, 1983)
L   Laurentianus 59.14, s.XIV
M   Ambrosianus gr. 473 (L.30 sup.), s.XVI
P   Parisinus gr. 2296, s.XVI
V   Vaticanus gr. 2154, s.XVI
Υ   Yalensis Bibl. Medic. 50, s.XVI

Stobaeus, Joannes, *Eclogae* and *Florilegium*, ed. C. Wachsmuth, O. Hense (Berlin, 1884–1912)
S   Vindobonensis phil. gr. 67, s.X
M   Scorialensis gr. 90 (Σ.II.14), s.XII in.
A   Parisinus gr. 1984, s.XIV

corp. Par.   Corpus Parisinum gnomologicum codicis Parisini gr. 1168, s.XIII

Strabo, *Geographica*, ed. G. Kramer (Berlin, 1844–52); A. Meineke (Leipzig, 1877); F. Lasserre, R. Baladié, G. Aujac (Paris, 1966–). (The editions of F. Sbordone and Lasserre/Aujac have not reached Book 14, to which some of the testimonia belong.)

Suda ['Suidae' *Lexicon*], ed. A. Adler, *Lexicographi Graeci* I, vols. 1–5 (Leipzig, 1928–38)

Supplementum Hellenisticum, ed. H. Lloyd-Jones, P. Parsons (Berlin/New York, 1983)

Tertullianus, *De anima*, ed. J. H. Waszink (Amsterdam, 1947)
 A   Agobardinus (Parisinus lat. 1622), s.IX (main authority)
 B   ed. Martinus Mesnart (Paris, 1545), vulgo Gagneiana (e codice nunc deperdito)
 Gel ed. Sigismundus Gelenius (Basel, 1550) (*Gel* used *B* and the lost codex Masburensis)
 Rig ed. Nicolaus Rigaltius (Paris, 1634)
 Iun Franciscus Iunius (his notes in the second editio Pameliana, 1597)
 Lat Latini Latinii Bibliotheca Sacra et Profana, ed. Dominicus Macrus Melitensis (Rome, 1677)
 Scal Joseph Justus Scaliger (his annotations in a copy of the editio Iuniana, preserved in the library of the Koninklijke Akademie, Leiden)
 Urs Fulvius Ursinus' readings, in Johannes van Wouwer, *Ad Q. Septimii Florentis Tertulliani opera emendationes epidicticae* (Frankfurt, 1603), pp. 76–91

Theo Smyrnaeus, *Expositio rerum mathematicarum ad legendum Platonem utilium*, ed. E. Hiller (Leipzig, 1878); J. Dupuis (Paris, 1892)
 A   Marcianus gr. 307, s.XI vel XII

Theodoretus Cyrrhensis, *Graecarum affectionum curatio*, ed. P. Canivet (*Sources chrétiennes* 57, 2 vols. (Paris, 1958))
 K   Vaticanus gr. 2249, s.IX
 B   Bodleianus Auct. E.ii.14, s.XI
 L   Laurentianus X.18, s.XI
 M   Marcianus gr. 559, s.XII
 S   Scorialensis X.ii.15, s.XI
 C   Parisinus gr. Coislinianus 250, s.XI
 V   Vaticanus gr. 626, s.XIV init.

Theophilus Protospatharius, *De corporis humani fabrica*, ed. W. A. Greenhill (Oxford, 1842)
 E   Nanianus 246, s.X

C   Junius Paulus Crassus' Latin translation (Venice, 1536)
F   Fabricius, *Bibliotheca Graeca*, vol. 12 (1724)

Varro, M. Terentius, *Saturarum Menippearum Fragmenta*, ed. R. Astbury (Leipzig, 1985)

Vindicianus, *De semine* (Fragmentum Bruxellense), ed. M. Wellmann, *Fragmentsammlung der griechischen Ärzte*, I. *Die Fragmente der sikelischen Ärzte Akron, Philistion und des Diokles von Karystos* (Berlin, 1901), pp. 208 ff; W. Jaeger, *Diokles von Karystos* (Berlin, 1938, 1963) pp. 191–8
B   Bruxellensis lat. 1348–59, fol. 48r, s.XII

Neu Octavius Horatianus, *Res medicae*, ed. Heremannus comes a Neuenar (Strassburg, 1532)

Vindicianus, *Gynaecia*, ed. V. Rose, in *Theodori Prisciani Euporiston libri* III (Leipzig, 1894), pp. 425–66; K. Sudhoff, *AGM* 8 (1915), 410–13; J. Schipper, *Ein neuer Text der Gynaecia des Vindicianus* (Diss. med. Leipzig, 1921)
F   Laurentianus 73.1, s.XI
E   Parisinus lat. 11219, s.IX
D   Parisinus lat. 11218, x.VIII–IX
L   Lipsiensis lat. 1118, s.XIII
M   Monacensis lat. 4622, s.XII
G   Sangallensis 751, s.X
P   Parisinus lat. 4883, s.IX
C   Casinensis 97, s.X
B   Bambergensis L.III.9, s.XII–XIII in.

I · INTRODUCTION
Alexandrian and Egyptian medicine

'The situation of Alexandria is most curious.'

1 *Introduction*

Early in 331 B.C. a twenty-five year old Macedonian gave audacious political expression to a long-standing Greek fascination with Egypt. Having conquered Egypt, the young king, Alexander the Great, actively participated in laying out his new eponymous city, Alexandria, at the western extremity of the Nile Delta on the Mediterranean shore of Egypt.[1] Only a few decades later Alexandria was becoming the centre of the remarkable advances in scientific medicine recorded in the chapters that follow.

The rapid, exceptional development of medicine in a Greek city on Egyptian soil is particularly interesting in view of the almost legendary reputation which Egyptian medicine had acquired throughout the Mediterranean at least as early as the second millennium B.C. Hittite and Persian kings employed Egyptians as court physicians,[2] and Greek authors of the archaic and classical periods record the high esteem in which the medicine of the Pharaohs was held. It was from Egypt that Helen of Troy obtained the miraculous drug described in the *Odyssey*:[3]

---

[1] Cf. Arrian, *Anabasis of Alexander* 3.1.1–3.2.2. Of Alexander's personal role at the founding of Alexandria Arrian says *inter alia* (3.1.5): 'A longing for the task seized him, and he himself established the main marking points of the city . . .'

[2] Cf. Edel, 1976; Herodotus 3.1 and 3.129 (Egyptian physicians in Persia). Cf. also Yahuda, 1947.

[3] *Odyssey* 4.220–32. This passage became famous in later antiquity; cf., for example, ps.-Galen, *Introductio sive medicus* 1 (XIV, p. 675K); Pliny, *Natural History* 25.5.11–12. On the pseudo-Galenic text see Kollesch, 1973: 30–4; Hanson, 1985: 25–30.

I

And now she dropped into the wine they were drinking
a drug – an anodyne, bile-allaying, causing one to forget all ills.
Whoever swallows it when it's mixed in the wine bowl
would not drop tears down his cheeks for a day,
not even if his mother has died and his father too,
nor if they cut down with bronze his brother or his own son
right in front of him, and he saw it with his eyes.
Such cunningly good drugs the daughter of Zeus had;
drugs Polydamna, mistress of Thon, had provided her
in Egypt, where food-giving fields yield most
kinds of drugs: many good when mixed, many baneful.
And each physician there is knowledgeable beyond all
humans; for they are of the race of Paean [a healer-god] . . .

A few centuries later Herodotus describes Egypt as 'teeming with
physicians' and the Egyptians as 'the healthiest of all humans' next to
the Libyans.[4]

Egypt's medical fame endured until later antiquity. Thus, in the
first century B.C. a Greek historian, Diodorus of Sicily, includes in his
universal history a positive account of ancient Egyptian medicine,[5]
and in the first century A.D. Pliny the Elder, drawing ultimately on
Greek sources, entertains the possibility that the art of medicine was
invented by the Egyptians.[6] Only rarely was a disapproving voice
heard: in the second century A.D., for example, Galen, who like
Herodotus, Diodorus Siculus, and many other Greek intellectuals
spent some time in Egypt, criticizes the author of a Greek pharmacological treatise for 'diverting himself to some old wives' tales, to some
silly Egyptian spells with incantations, which the Egyptians [physi-
cians?] utter while picking their herbal drugs . . . I don't consider
such tales to be exactly useful, not even for small children, let alone for

[4] Herodotus 2.77.3; 2.84.
[5] Diodorus Siculus 1.82 (but see n. 12 below on Hecataeus).
[6] Pliny, *Natural History* 7.56.196 (but cf. 29.1 ff.); see also 29.30.93 and 26.3.4. At
the end of the second century A.D. Clement of Alexandria still refers to famous
Egyptian medical books used in Hermetic sacred processions, but the relation of
these books to the Pharaonic papyri and to the anatomical 'books of Athothis' in
Memphis, which Manetho (*Aegyptiaca, FGrHist* 609F2, 3a–b; pp. 18.2–7, 19.1–2)
mentions, is very uncertain, despite Clement's mention of ophthalmology and
gynaecology (disciplines strongly represented in Pharaonic papyri; see below);
see *Stromateis* 6.4.37.3 (*GCS*, Clemens II (1960), pp. 449–50 Stählin/Früchtel). Cf.
also Galen, *De compositione medicamentorum per genera* 5.2 (XIII, pp. 776-7K) – a
passage which does not necessarily have anything to do with what Clement or
Manetho describe.

those who strive to pursue the art of medicine.'[7] On the whole, however, Greeks of the archaic, classical, and Hellenistic periods display considerable appreciation of the achievements of native Egyptian medicine.

The enduring nature of this Greek esteem, combined with the relatively high standards displayed in parts of Egyptian medical papyri of Pharaonic times, has prompted modern claims that the debt of Greek medicine to Pharaonic Egypt was considerable.[8] Moreover, it has been suggested that the efflorescence of scientific medicine in Alexandria in the third century B.C. (documented below especially in Chapters VI–VII) is attributable in large measure to the Alexandrian physicians' direct exposure to native Egyptian medicine.[9] These views have, however, also met with radical scepticism.[10]

A clear resolution of this controversy is made difficult by several factors, three of which merit mention here.

First, a chronological gap: our main sources for indigenous Egyptian medicine are seven Pharaonic papyri, all of which are roughly 800 or 1,000 to 1,600 years older than the earliest Alexandrian medical fragments. Some Egyptian papyri, such as the Edwin Smith papyrus (written c. 1650 B.C.), transmit medical lore that is even more ancient, probably dating back to dynasties of the Old Kingdom – perhaps as early as 2600 B.C. And the very latest of the extant medical papyri of Pharaonic Egypt, Chester Beatty VI, was written during the New Kingdom, probably between 1300 B.C. and 1085 B.C.[11] This sizable chronological distance between Pharaonic

[7] Galen, *De simplicium medicamentorum temperamentis ac facultatibus* 6, prooem. (XI, pp. 792–3K).

[8] Cf., for example, Steuer & Saunders, 1959; Saunders, 1963; Lefebvre, 1956: 2; Breasted, 1930: vol. I, 16–17; Ghalioungui, 1973: 166ff.; G.E. Smith, 1914: 190; Iversen, 1953. See also n. 72 *infra*; Thivel, 1981: 472ff.

[9] Ghalioungui, 1968 (especially p. 104). So too Robert Littman, unpublished commentary (Seventh Annual Meeting, American Association of Ancient Historians, 8 May 1970, Stanford University), in response to a paper presented by the author. It is gratefully acknowledged that Professor Littman's comments contributed to a more precise definition of the views presented here. Leca, 1971: 443, advocates a more differentiating view (but without details or evidence): 'si la médecine préhippocratique peut avoir fait des emprunts à la médecine égyptienne, celle de l'époque hellénistique ne lui doit rien'.

[10] Cf., for example, Kudlien, 1967a: 13; Allbutt, 1921: 133, 329; Sigerist, 1951–61: vol. I, pp. 356–8; Fraser, 1972: vol. I, p. 345 (the debt of Alexandrian medicine to Egyptian medicine 'may be discounted as negligible').

[11] Gardiner, 1935: vol. I, pp. 53–4 (vol. II, Plates 30–2A). For a more complete account see Jonckheere, 1947.

texts and Alexandrian texts makes any attempt to demonstrate influence problematic, since the state of native Egyptian medicine in the third century B.C. remains shrouded in veils of silence.

Some scant help might be derived from Greek characterizations of Egyptian medicine. As will be shown below, the brief reports of Herodotus, Hecataeus,[12] and Diodorus Siculus, as well as the allusions in the Galenic passage cited above, contain nothing that is inconsistent with the content of the extant Pharaonic texts. The Greeks therefore might confirm, though only obliquely, a modern conjectural consensus that native Egyptian medical theory and practice did not change significantly between 1085 B.C. and 300 B.C. (or, for that matter, between the Middle Kingdom and 60–59 B.C., when Diodorus visited Egypt, or even the second century A.D., when Galen was in Alexandria). If this view is correct, it might not be senseless to explore the relation between Alexandrian and indigenous Egyptian medicine through recourse to Pharaonic papyri, despite the chronological gap and despite the lack of significant direct knowledge about Egyptian medicine either of the late period of Pharaonic rule (Dynasties XXI–XXXII, c. 1085–332 B.C.) or of the Ptolemaic period (c. 305–30 B.C.).

The amalgam of magic, law, and empiricism that characterizes the medicine of the Pharaohs might partially account for the extraordinary stability and inertia of Egyptian medicine implied by this view. It was noted above that, as late as the second century A.D., Egyptian pharmacology is still associated with magic spells and incantations, which indeed are richly represented in Pharaonic medical papyri (see below). When medical theories and practices are supported and sanctioned by ritual, by belief in magic, and by the priesthood, they can become relatively immune to the revisionary processes that tend to be associated with scientific growth. When, in addition, medical practices are frozen and protected through codification and punitive legal sanctions, as they were in Egypt (e.g. by means of the death penalty for physicians who violated codified therapeutic prescrip-

[12] Hecataeus (*FGrHist* 264, F 25), who visited Egypt in the third century B.C., deserves mention since Diodorus used him as a source (although Diodorus himself also visited Egypt in 60 or 59 B.C.). Some Coptic evidence also suggests that there was continuity in the Egyptian medical tradition (cf. Sigerist, 1951–61: vol. I, pp. 358–9). But Greek and Arabic infusions, as well as a reversion to a less advanced state of medical knowledge, characterize much of the Coptic material; see Till, 1951, and Chassinat, 1921.

tions, according to Diodorus[13]), the odds against significant change rise considerably.

A second factor which impedes a conclusive answer to the question what, if anything, Alexandrian medicine owes Pharaonic medicine is uncertainty about the precise meaning of numerous Egyptian and Greek words; names of diseases, anatomical and pathological nomenclature, measurements, and the names of drug ingredients are sources of scholarly headaches for which there are no easy cures. Thus one eminent Egyptologist translates a hieroglyphic cluster in the Ebers papyrus 'acacia thorn', while another renders it 'prepuce'.[14]

A third difficulty in tracing influence has its origin in the fact that a number of ideas, insights, and therapeutic or preventive practices are shared by several Mediterranean cultures, and sometimes also by other cultures. The occurrence of a similar general notion or of a readily available herbal drug in both Alexandrian and Egyptian texts therefore does not in and of itself constitute proof of Egyptian influence. Thus the Egyptian concept of pathogenic decay (*wḫdw*), which is central to their view of human pathology (see below), is not alien to Greek medicine. But 'decay' is a concept also used in the medicine of many other cultures – it even survives in the modern use of 'sepsis', an ancient Greek word for 'putrefaction', to refer to the presence of pathogenic organisms or their toxins in the blood or the tissues – and it might simply be a fairly obvious concept for explaining or describing diseased conditions. Similarly, Egyptian medicine makes extensive pharmacological use of myrrh, and so do Hippocratic, Alexandrian, and other Greek physicians. But myrrh is native to neither culture. In antiquity it was produced only on the South Arabian coast and the Horn of Africa, whence it was exported also to Persia, India and so on, for medical and other uses; 'Egyptian influence' here too would be only one of several possible explanations of a Greek practice.

Despite difficulties of this nature, and despite the caveat implicit in the preceding paragraphs, it seems reasonable to risk the generaliza-

---

[13] Diodorus Siculus 1.82.
[14] The notorious passage in question is Ebers papyrus 732. Ebbell's translation reads: 'Remedy for a prepuce [?] which is cut off [circumcised] and whence blood comes out', whereas von Deines–Grapow–Westendorf offer: 'Remedy for an acacia thorn, when it is cut out, inasmuch as blood comes out of it . . .' (*GMÄ* IV.1, p. 213). In his commentary Grapow interprets 'acacia thorn' as referring to an open wound made by an acacia thorn (*GMÄ* IV.2, p. 163). Cf. Ebbell, 1937: 103.

tions that follow concerning the relation of Alexandrian medicine to native Egyptian medicine.

2 *Magic, religion, and medicine*

The pervasive magico-religious dimension of Egyptian medicine is largely foreign both to Alexandrian and to pre-Alexandrian Greek medicine. In almost all the Egyptian medical papyri spells against a given disease alternate with drug prescriptions and with a brief description of the disease. Even the two papyri containing the best observations – Edwin Smith papyrus (*c.* 1650 B.C.) and Ebers papyrus (*c.* 1550 B.C.) – are not devoid of incantations and magical charms. A few examples should suffice.

When a bandage is loosened, the Egyptian physician or *swnw* characteristically chants:

Someone is being loosened, who is loosened by Isis; Horus is loosened by Isis from the evil done to him by his brother Seth, when he killed his father Osiris. Oh, Isis, great in sorcery, may you loosen me, may you save me from all evil, bad, red things . . . just as you were loosened, just as you were saved by your son Horus. For, I have entered into the fire, I have come forth from the water; no, I will not fall into this day's trap. I spoke when I still was a child, when I still was small. Oh, Re, speak of your body; Osiris, bemourn that which came forth from you . . . (Papyrus Ebers 2)[15]

While preparing a drug cure – turtle bile with honey – for an eye ailment (*sḥdw*), the Egyptian *swnw* chants:

There is loud noise in the southern sky ever since nightfall, and rough weather in the northern sky. A heap has fallen into the water. The crew of Re is knocking in its mooring pegs because the heads have fallen into the water. Who is it that will fetch it [a head], will find it? I am the one who will fetch it; I am the one who will find it. I fetched your heads, I tied [the heads] to your necks, I fastened your cut-off parts in their place. I have brought you to expel the effects of a god, of a dead man, of a dead woman . . . to be repeated at will. (Papyrus Ebers 360)[16]

A similar incantation, to stop bleeding, ends with the following

[15] *GMÄ* IV.1, pp. 308–9. (My translations of Pharaonic papyri are based on the German translation by Hildegard von Deines, Hermann Grapow, and Wolfhart Westendorf in *GMÄ* IV.1, unless otherwise specified.) Cf. also Grapow, *GMÄ* II, pp. 90–2, 114–33 (on pap. Ebers).
[16] *GMÄ* IV.1, p. 49.

instruction: 'This saying is recited over a red pearl of Carnelian, placed in the anus of the man or the woman. This is to dispel blood' (the 'London papyrus' (British Museum 10059), 37).[17]

Incantations with exorcizing power also were among the Egyptian physician's tools:

You should flow out, mucus, son of mucus, who breaks the bones, who destroys the brain, who chops around in the bone marrow, who causes the seven openings in the heads of the followers of Re to become ill, and they turn to Thoth in prayer. See, I have brought your cure against you, your preventive medicine against you: milk of a woman who has given birth to a boy, aromatic gum – this eliminates you, it removes you, and vice versa [i.e., it removes you, it eliminates you]. Come out on to the earth; putrefy, putrefy; four times. (Papyrus Ebers 763)[18]

In addition, amulets, charms made of linen knots or animal hair, and vulture plumes were recommended by Egyptian physicians for their power to heal or protect patients.

All of this might have had powerful psychosomatic benefits, but it is entirely alien to the medicine of Herophilus and his followers (as a glance at Chapters VIII or XI would confirm). In this central respect there can, therefore, be no question of 'Egyptian influence' on Alexandrian medicine.

This is not to deny that Greek culture also accommodated magico-religious forms of therapy. There is, for example, ample evidence, especially from the Hellenistic period, of Greek belief in the therapeutic efficacy of divine as well as human laying on of hands; of faith in the healing power of certain statues and amulets; and of a deep, abiding trust in incubation or curative sleep in the hundred or more temples of Asclepius that existed in ancient Greece.[19] Patients

[17] *Ibid.*, p. 158; cf. *GMÄ* IV.2, p. 134, ad loc., and II, pp. 94–5, 141 (on the London papyrus).
[18] *GMÄ* IV.1, p. 64. See also Grapow, *GMÄ* II, pp. 11–26, on Egyptian medical 'Zaubersprüche'.
[19] Cf. Thrämer, 1896: more than 180 sanctuaries of Asclepius are enumerated. But Thrämer, 1914: 550, says these are 'only a selection from among the 410' such sanctuaries of which he knew. With reference to the Hellenistic period E. J. & L. Edelstein, 1945: vol. II, p. 251, say 'hundreds of temples are still known'. For other magico-religious aspects of Greek therapeutics see Weinreich, 1909; E. J. & L. Edelstein, 1945: vol. I, chapter IV, and vol. II, chapters III, IV.1-2, and VI; Herzog, 1931; Meier, 1967; Behr, 1968, especially Chapters VII-VIII; Sudhoff, 1909: 213–33; Krug, 1985: 120–87.

who could not get help from mortal physicians could turn to the divine physician. At the temples of Asclepius they could listen to hymns and relax in the holy grounds until they lay down at night in the *a-baton* ('not to be walked upon') or sacred hall and waited for the god to grant them advice or cures in their dreams. The god would appear to them either in person or in the guise of one of the sacred animals kept at the temple – often a snake or a dog – which might lick the afflicted part of the suppliant's body.[20]

I know of no evidence that the Greek physicians of Cos, Cnidus, Magna Graecia, and Alexandria ever objected to the priestly assistance offered at the temples of Asclepius (although there is criticism of magic as early as the Hippocratic treatise on epilepsy known as *On the sacred disease*). Indeed, one of the later Hippocratic treatises, *Decorum*, concedes a place of honour to the gods.[21] (Whether Herophilus' celebrated statement that 'drugs are the hands of the gods'[22] represents a similar concession to divine healing power or, as seems more likely, is intended as a metaphorical evocation of the power and importance of drugs, is uncertain.)

Nevertheless, Alexandrian and Hippocratic medicine appear to eschew the spells, incantations, and charms which dominate many – and intrude upon all – Pharaonic medical papyri. In Greek society, priest and physician exercised their distinct functions in sharply different ways, even if they shared the same god; in Egypt many

---

[20] Cf. E. J. & L. Edelstein, 1945: vol. I, T392–T442 (pp. 197–254). T423.42 (Edelstein) (I, p. 237), e.g., describes the dream by which Nicasibule of Messena achieved the pregnancy she had been desiring: she dreamt that she had intercourse with the snake of Asclepius; and T423.26 provides an example of the healing power of the tongue of Asclepius' dog.

[21] Hp., *Decorum* 6 (*CMG* I.1, p. 27 Heiberg). Furthermore, in the Hippocratic *Oath* the physician swears by Asclepius among others (*ibid.*, p. 4). Hippocrates himself was, after all, thought of as a descendant of Asclepius (E. J. & L. Edelstein, 1945: vol. I, T213–16); but also see Hp., *On Sacred Disease* 1, concerning the limits of what is attributable to the gods (for an excellent analysis see G. E. R. Lloyd, 1979: 15–29). Later Galen still describes Asclepius as 'my ancestral god, whose servant I declared myself to be, ever since he saved me when I had a fatal condition of an abscess' (*De libris propriis* 2; *Scr. Min.* II, p. 99 Müller). Cf. also Galen, *De sanitate tuenda* 1.8.19–21 (*CMG* v.4.2, p. 20 Koch); *De morborum differentiis* 9 (VI, p. 869K): a certain Nicomachus of Smyrna had a body so badly swollen that he could not move himself until 'Asclepius cured this man'; *Protrepticus* 9 (*Scr. Min.* I, pp. 117–18 Marquardt). Cf. also Parker, 1983: 207–56.

[22] See below, Chapter VIII, T248a-c.

medical practitioners were also priests of the goddess Sekhmet,[23] and all of them engaged in practices which Greek physicians would have thought fit, at best, for priests and 'enchanters' alone.

3   *Anatomy and pathophysiology*

When one turns to the general theoretical foundations of Greek and Egyptian medicine, one encounters some of the bolder, more insistent modern claims of Egyptian influence.[24] Three distinctive features of Egyptian theory require brief discussion here: (i) the vascular system; (ii) the pathological principle of *wḥdw* ('decay' or pathogenic matter; *Schmerzstoff*, in Hermann Grapow's felicitous translation[25]); (iii) the pathophysiological significance assigned to the anal region.

First, a famous passage in the Ebers papyrus seems to reveal not only a knowledge of the pulse, but also an awareness of its connection with the heart, and the desire to measure the pulse:

There are vessels in him at every part of the body. As far as these [vessels] are concerned: if with reference to them any *swnw*-physician, any priest of Sekhmet, any magician gives both hands, his fingers on the head, on the back of the head, on the hands, on the place of the heart, on both arms, on both legs – then he is measuring for the heart. For its [the heart's] vessels [lead] to every part of his body. It is the case: it [the heart] speaks in front, in the vessels of every part of the body.[26]

A parallel passage in a somewhat earlier text, the Edwin Smith papyrus, confirms this account and offers some elaboration: 'He says "measuring" for applying his [hands] to the vessels of the head, of the back of the head, of both his legs. One "measures" the vessels of the heart to recognize the manifestations which take place in it. One says "one measures it" to recognize what takes place in it.'[27] Before introducing the parallel passage, the scribe of the Ebers papyrus also offers these comments: 'Concerning: you examine a man. That

---

[23]   Cf., in particular on the idea (now widely discredited) that the priests of Sekhmet were only surgical specialists, Lefebvre, 1956: chapter II (especially pp. 24–6); *id.*, 1952; Jonckheere, 1951a; *id.*, 1951b; *id.*, 1958, especially pp. 95ff.

[24]   E.g., Steuer & Saunders, 1959, especially on what they regard as affinities between Egyptian and Greek aetiological concepts of disease; on this see also Yoyotte, 1968.

[25]   See *GMÄ* IV.1, pp. 7–14; III, pp. 36, 55.

[26]   *GMÄ* IV.1, p. 1.

[27]   *Ibid.*, p. 172 (Edwin Smith papyrus, Case 1).

means: counting (*ip*) someone . . . like counting things with the *ip.t* measure. Counting something with one's fingers [occurs] in order to learn . . .[lacuna in text]. Measuring things with the *ip.t* measure is like counting a disease with it, just like measuring the disease of a man to recognize the course of his heart.'[28]

What renders these passages interesting is not only the relatively high level of insight and of quantifying aspiration they seem to represent, but the fact that sphygmology – the study of the pulse – is precisely the subject for which Herophilus in antiquity became at least as renowned as for his anatomical discoveries (see Chapter VII.A.4). The struggling but insistent Egyptian emphasis on counting or measuring is particularly interesting in view of Herophilus' use of a portable, adjustable water-clock – adjustable according to the age of the patient – to measure the pulse and, as suggested below (Chapter VII.A.4), to take the patient's temperature. Egypt was a land rich in time-measuring devices including, in particular, clepsydrae.[29] Although measurement, quantification, and the clepsydra were not unknown to pre-Alexandrian Greeks,[30] it is not inconceivable that the sophisticated Egyptian water-clock technology, the Egyptian interest in quantification (more on this *infra*), and the keen interest of Greek Alexandrians in technology and gadgetry[31] all combined to prompt or facilitate Herophilus' introduction of his measuring device.

As for pulse theory itself, the Egyptian view of the vascular system

[28] *Ibid.*

[29] Cf., for example, from the fourteenth century B.C. (the reign of Amenhotep III), the *merkhet* or alabaster water-clock designed to mark the hours of the night at any season: Neugebauer & Parker, 1969: 12–14 (Text) and Plate 2; see also pp. 42, 47, 60, 152. According to an autobiographical tomb inscription, Amenemhet, court astronomer to Amenhotep I, invented this device; see Borchardt, 1920: 6ff, 6ff.

[30] The most famous allusion to the clepsydra is probably Empedocles' simile (fr.100DK). See *infra*, Chapter VII, nn. 152–4, on Greek water-clocks. Among early Hellenistic scientists Archimedes and Ctesibius (*infra*, n. 31) gained fame for their clepsydrae. Hp., *On Diseases of Women* 1.6 (VIII, p. 30L) and *Epidemics* v.14, 18 (v, pp. 214–18L) provide examples of measurement. But also see *On Ancient Medicine* 9 (I, pp. 588–90L; *CMG* I.1, p. 41 Heiberg); *Regimen* 1.2.iii (VI, pp. 470–2L; *CMG* 1.2.4, p. 124.17ff. Joly/Byl). On the whole a 'reign of quality' (Joly, 1966: 102), not of quantity, governs the Hippocratic Corpus. (*On Nutrition* 35, on the difficulty of fitting quantity to faculty, is intriguing, but it probably post-dates Herophilus.)

[31] See *infra*, Chapter XI (Andreas). Cf. also Drachmann, 1963; *id.*, 1948; Brumbaugh, 1966; West, 1973.

does not inspire confidence that it had any significant influence upon
Herophilus or his followers. Although the Egyptians, like most
Greeks, recognize the heart as the main centre of the vessels (*mtw*),
they thought the vessels had a second key point of convergence in the
area of the anus. Thus, according to the Ebers papyrus (confirmed by
a similar passage in the Berlin medical papyrus (3038)), 'the vessels *all*
come to his heart, divide to his nose, and *all* unite at his anus . . .'[32]
Furthermore, the *mtw* carry not only blood but, depending on where
they are going, also air, water, tears, urine, semen, and faeces. Some
Greeks admittedly also allowed life-giving pneuma[33] and, in the case
of Aristotle,[34] seed into parts of the vascular system, but their
conception of the content of the vessels never was quite as licentious as
that of the Egyptians.

Even the six main vessels depicted by the Egyptians as leading to
the lower limbs are said to pass so close to the anus that they are
constantly threatened with becoming flooded with excrement. This
faecal material, often identified as a repository of the 'rot' or
Schmerzstoff (wḥdw) that constitutes the main pathogenic agent in
Pharaonic medicine,[35] could be absorbed into any vessels and thus
could travel anywhere in the body through the vascular system – even
to the heart. Wherever the *wḥdw* went, it could cause decay and hence
disease.

Rather than announcing a vascular tree, the two Pharaonic
statements introducing major descriptions of the vascular system
promise a god-given, miracle-working map of a human system full of
pathogenic rot:[36] 'Beginning of the Book of the roaming (*hbhb*) of the
rot (*wḥdw*) in every part of a man's body; the Book found among
writings under the feet of Anubis at Letopolis . . .' (Papyrus Ebers
856a);[37] and more elaborately:

Beginning of the collected manuscript of the wandering (*ht*) of the rot
(*wḥdw*), which was found among old writings in a case of books under the feet
of Anubis in Letopolis. Because of its excellence, it [this book] was brought to

---

[32] Ebers 856h and Berlin 163h; *vid. GMÄ* IV.1, p. 10.

[33] See *infra*, Chapter VII.A.4 (with notes); Verbeke, 1945, especially pp. 175–220;
Saake, 1974: especially cols. 391–5.

[34] See *infra*, Chapter VII.A.5; cf. Aristotle, *On Generation of Animals* 1.18–20.

[35] Cf. *GMÄ* IV.1, pp. 7–14; III, pp. 36–7, 55. (Grapow, *GMÄ* III, also offers rich
information on many other aspects of Egyptian pathology.)

[36] *Sic* Majno, 1975: 130.

[37] *GMÄ* IV.1, p. 7.

his majesty Sendi the Blessed, King of Upper and Lower Egypt; this book at that time loosened the two feet that were locked, [and it did so] through a scribe of divine words . . . What one did at that time [because of] this book was a procession at sunrise [and] a sacrifice of bread, beer, terebinth resin over flames, in the name of Isis the Great, Horus Khentekhtai, Khons Thoth, the god who is in the belly. (Papyrus Berlin (3038), 163h)[38]

Even a cursory glance at the evidence concerning Herophilus' theories about the vascular system (Chapters VI.6; VII.4 *infra*) – and at the pulse lore of his followers (Part 2 *infra, passim*; Chapter X.A) – would reveal how remote the Herophilean views are from the all-purpose Egyptian *mtw* with their anal and faecal focus. The Herophileans distinguished carefully between veins and arteries, and they did not confuse them with other tube-like structures in the body. Unlike the Egyptians, they did not use the same word (in Egyptian, *mt*) indiscriminately to designate blood vessels, nerves, the urinary tract, the reproductive tract, the rectum, tendons, and sinews. Nor did the Greek Alexandrians crowd the blood vessels with the constant putrefying threat of a faecal, disease-causing substance that could rise from the anal region to any part of the body.

The pathological preoccupation with the anus that seems to characterize Pharaonic medicine had consequences for regimen and therapy, and these, too, do not seem to have made a major impression on Alexandrian medicine. The Egyptians took loving but very anxious care of the anus, soothing it, washing it, fumigating it, refreshing it, manipulating it to keep it from slipping or twisting[39] – practices which, combined with the legendary Egyptian obsession with personal cleanliness,[40] are bound to elicit an ethno-psychoanalytic study of Pharaonic Egypt sooner or later. Herodotus reports that the Egyptians' preventive measures included purging themselves

---

[38] *Ibid.*

[39] Cf. *GMÄ* IV.1, pp. 124–32. These examples are drawn from a wide range of papyri: Ebers, Hearst, Berlin 3038, Chester Beatty VI, and Edwin Smith. The recto of the Chester Beatty papyrus no. VI is exclusively devoted to recipes for diseases of the anus. Cf. Jonckheere, 1947, especially pp. 16–72 (translation, commentary). See also Grapow, *GMÄ* III, pp. 62–3; II, p. 94.

[40] Cf. Herodotus 2.37: 'They [sc. the Egyptians] wear linen garments always freshly washed, and they take special care with this. They practice circumcision for the sake of cleanliness, preferring to be clean rather than very comely . . . They take baths twice every day in cold water, and twice every night . . .' Useful (and somewhat more realistic) summaries of ancient Egyptian hygiene and sanitation are provided by Leca, 1971: 379–402; Ghalioungui, 1973: 150–8.

with enemas and emetics three consecutive days every month;[41] Diodorus Siculus emends this to enemas, emetics, and fasting, 'sometimes every day and sometimes at intervals of three or four days'.[42] Although Hippocratic and Alexandrian physicians on occasion also made use of enemas, fumigations 'from below', and other forms of treating the anus, neither their pathophysiological theories nor their versatile practice reflects this Pharaonic emphasis.

The impression seems unavoidable that, even if Herophilus' pulse lore derived some stimulus from Egyptian water-clock technology and from the Egyptian emphasis on 'measuring', the Alexandrian development of vascular theory and, more specifically, of sphygmology received much greater impetus from the speculation and observation of Greeks such as Aristotle and Herophilus' teacher, Praxagoras of Cos,[43] who was the first to make a firm distinction between arteries and veins, than from Egyptian medicine.

Whether the Egyptian practice of mummification might have prompted human dissection in Alexandria will be considered below (see also Chapter VI.A.1: 'Dissection and Vivisection').

4 'Rational' wound care and pharmacology

Egyptian medicine did not consist only of magic, multi-purpose vessels, and pathogenic rot. The Egyptian physician also treated wounds in what historians of medicine have tended to label 'rational' ways. But the three most common 'non-magical' Egyptian techniques of wound care – putting a slab of fresh (*wadj*) or 'living' (*ankh*) meat (*ywf*) on a wound; applying a salve made either of honey and animal fat or of honey and aromatic resins; applying adhesive linen tape[44] – are not among the techniques that dominate Greek wound care. The Greeks instead washed the wound with wine or vinegar[45] – a basic

---

[41] Herodotus 2.77.

[42] Diodorus 1.82.

[43] For further details see below, Chapters II, VI.6, VII.4.

[44] Cf. especially the Edwin Smith papyrus (*GMÄ* IV.1, pp. 172–99). (Breasted, 1930; vol. 1, General Index, s.vv. 'Adhesive plaster, Grease, Honey, Linen, Lint, Meat', also provides simple access to the relevant passages.) See also Grapow, *GMÄ* II, pp. 44–80, and III, pp. 100–40 (especially 125–30); Buchheim, 1958; *ead.*, 1960. Honey has some value in wound care; see Majno, 1975: 115–20.

[45] Cf., e.g., Hp., *On Wounds* 17 (VI, p. 422L), on the use of hot vinegar; *id.*, *On the Use of Liquids* 5 (VI, pp. 128–30L), on wine; *ibid.*, 4 (VI, pp. 126–8L), on vinegar. The

antiseptic procedure apparently ignored in Egypt – or they sprinkled
'enhemes' (antiseptic styptic liquids or powders, often made of zinc
oxide with lead powder, of lead oxide, of copper oxide with copper
sulphate, or of alum) on the wound. Sometimes they bandaged
wounds with linen cloths soaked in wine, while at other times they
used a leaf-covered sponge or wool pad, soaked in oil and wine, often
in combination with various poultices.[46] Although we are less well
informed about early Alexandrian wound care than about Hippocratic techniques, the therapeutic practices and principles that emerge
below (Chapter VIII; Part 2, *passim*) do not suggest that the Pharaonic
meat-slab or honey-and-grease treatment had a significant impact on
Alexandrian medicine.

There are, however, some similarities between the therapeutics of
Greek and Egyptian physicians. Like his Greek counterpart, the
Egyptian practitioner made limited surgical incisions, used sutures,
achieved hemostasis by cautery, and made some attempt at antisepsis
by means of copper salts. And like the physicians of many other
countries, the Greeks and Egyptians both attached great medical
significance to their dietary prescriptions.[47] Furthermore, both the
Greek and the Egyptian physician explicitly and publicly acknowledged that certain wounds and diseases could be treated and others
not.[48] But it seems impossible to prove that such practices, pro-

external use of wine and vinegar never disappeared from Greek medicine: cf.,
e.g., Galen, *In Hp. De fracturis commentarius* 3.21 (XVIIIB, pp. 567–8K); and *infra*
Herophilus, T257 (Chapter VIII), An.31 (Chapter XI), Ma.10 (Chapter XVIII),
AM.11, 12, 14, 15, 16, 18, 19 (Chapter XXIII).

[46] Cf. Hp., *On Fractures* 24 (II, p. 81Kw); *On Joints* 63 (II, p. 216Kw); *On Wounds* 13,
14, 23 (VI, pp. 416–28L): *On Diseases* 2.33–7 (VII, pp. 50–2L). For a useful
summary see Majno, 1975: 185. On the putative parallels between Egyptian and
Greek treatments of head wounds (see Iversen, 1953) cf. Majno, 1975: 499, n.
283. See also Hdt.2.77.

[47] According to Diodorus Siculus (1.82.2) the ancient Egyptians viewed overeating
as the primary cause of disease. The Egyptian medical papyri are as replete as
Greek medicine with dietary allusions, although diet as *therapy* is not common.
This does not mean that there were no diseases of overeating in Egypt: cf. Darby,
Ghalioungui, Grivetti, 1977: vol. I, pp. 58–65. For the Greek tradition cf.
Edelstein, 1931a.

[48] In the Edwin Smith papyrus each case is given one of three labels, depending on
the chances of successful treatment: 'A disease which I shall treat. A disease with
which I shall struggle. A disease which one cannot treat'; see *GMÄ* IV.1, pp. 172ff.
For Greek examples see *infra* Herophilus, T51 (Chapter V); Hp., *Prognostic* 1 (I, p.
78Kw); *id., On Joints* 58 (II, p. 205Kw); *id., Art* 3 (*CMG* I.1, pp. 10–11 Heiberg).

cedures, and attitudes, whether in Cos, Cnidus or Alexandria, were the result of Egyptian influence.

A further striking feature of Egyptian wound care is the aggressive use of palpation, especially as described in the Edwin Smith papyrus (the main surgical text of Pharaonic Egypt).[49] The *swnu* uses his hand not only to search for fractures, to feel a lump, to measure a patient's temperature, and to feel the pulse. In a culture where soap was apparently unknown, the physician's bare hand frequently also is depicted as reaching deeply into a wound, which apparently had not been washed with an antiseptic, and poking around inside it. The Hippocratic physician, by contrast, often uses surgical probes to explore wounds which have been disinfected with wine or vinegar (both of these liquids have superb bactericidal qualities).[50] The Greeks' reliance on palpation is much more restrained and, when feasible, it is complemented with auscultation.[51] There is no evidence to suggest that the Alexandrians, with their keen awareness (and philological cultivation) of the Hippocratic tradition, abandoned these features of Hippocratic therapeutics. While the Egyptian practitioner's aggressive 'touch' in some cases might have been psychologically reassuring – the divine power of the healing hand? – it was not a particularly aseptic, let alone antiseptic, asset.

If any indigenous Egyptian ideas travelled to Greece or Alexandria, they did not travel alone; pharmacotherapeutic materials from Egypt also found a limited place in Greek culture fairly early, and indeed, the trade in materials might have facilitated the transport of ideas. Homer's Helen was not the only person in the Graeco-Roman sphere who drew on Egyptian pharmacology. From the classical period in Athens to the Roman Empire, Egyptian drugs continued to enjoy a remarkable reputation: Aristophanes refers to the fame of healing drugs from Egypt, and so does Aelius Aristides;[52] Josephus singles out poisonous drugs from Egypt; Pliny (*Natural History*) and Dioscurides (*Materia med.*) are familiar with efficacious Egyptian substances; and

[49] *GMÄ* IV.1, pp. 172–99; Breasted, 1930: vol. I, pp. 41, 56–7, 89, 92–3, 177, 417.

[50] See Majno, 1975: 186–8 (with notes): vinegar owes its bactericidal power to acetic acid, 'a powerful antiseptic', and wine contains malvoside or oenoside, a polyphenol ('a relative of phenol, the historic antiseptic').

[51] Cf. Hp., *On Diseases* 2.61 (VII, p. 94L).

[52] Aristophanes, *Peace* 1253; Aelius Aristides, *Oration* 36 (*Aegyptius*), §124 (II, p. 302 Keil).

Galen seems to praise Egyptian Thebes as the source of the best opium in the world.[53] But for present purposes, i.e. the question of Egyptian influence on Alexandrian medicine, it is more important to recognize that Egyptian drug ingredients entered Greek medicine well before the founding of Alexandria.

Ingredients labelled 'Egyptian' appear in a number of Hippocratic drug prescriptions. Egyptian *ntry* or *natron* (a sodium carbonate known to the Greeks as *nitron* or *litron*, and used by the Egyptians mainly for embalming) occurs in several drug prescriptions recommended in the Hippocratic treatises *Epidemics* II and *On Internal Affections*.[54] Alum (*stypteriē*) from Egypt likewise was a popular drug ingredient in the Greek world, recommended in no less than six Hippocratic treatises.[55] Dietary use of 'Egyptian beans' likewise is prescribed frequently.

The author or authors of Hippocratic gynaecological treatises seem to have been particularly keen on Egyptian ingredients – perhaps a reflection of the strong gynaecological tradition within Pharaonic medicine.[56] Thus, in addition to Egyptian alum, the author of *On Diseases of Women* I–II prescribes the use of the fruit of Egyptian thistle, white Egyptian oil, Egyptian salt, Egyptian saffron, and 'the purse tassels that are seen especially in Egyptian grain fields' for use in a variety of uterine purges, in pessaries to induce menstruation or childbirth, and so on.[57] Similarly, the author of *On the Nature of Women* recommends the use of Egyptian oil, Egyptian perfume, the

---

[53] Josephus, *Jewish Antiquities* 17.70 (= 17.iv.2); *id.*, *History of the Jewish War Against the Romans* 1.598–600 (= 1.xxx.7); Galen, *On Antidotes* 1.2 (XIV, p. 6K) – while *opos* here might mean 'silphium juice' or any 'acid juice' (*vid.* LSJ s.v.), the qualifier 'most potent' (ἰσχυρότατον) perhaps suggests *opion* or opium, which was already known in Pharaonic medicine.

[54] Cf. Hp., *Epidemics* II.6.9 and 29 (V, pp. 134, 138L); *On Internal Affections* 26, 31, 51 (VII, pp. 236, 248, 294L).

[55] *Vid.* Hp., *Epidemics* V.69 (V, p. 244L), *Epid.* VII.66 (V, p. 430L); *On Wounds* 14 and 17–18 (VI, pp. 416, 422L); *On Haemorrhoids* 7 (VI, p. 442); *On Fistulae* 7 (VI, p. 454L); *On Diseases of Women* I.75 (VIII, p. 166L). Objects from Egypt also are mentioned in 'Hp.', *On Hebdomads* 21 (VIII, p. 644L); *On Diseases* II.33 (VII, p. 50L); *On Fractures* 30 (II, p. 91Kw).

[56] Cf. *GMÄ* IV.1, pp. 267–95; Lefebvre, 1956: 89–109; *GMÄ* III, pp. 46–7, and II, p. 143.

[57] Cf. Hp., *On Diseases of Women* 1.37, 75, and 78; II.126, 181, and 203 (VIII, pp. 90, 166–8, 186–8, 270, 364, 390L). Cf. also Daumas, 1956: 174 (with n. 1) on a further gynaecological parallel.

fruit of Egyptian thistle, and Egyptian acorns in pessaries and douches.[58]

An influx of Egyptian ingredients into pre-Alexandrian Greek pharmacology is, therefore, solidly attested. It probably reflects an interest in exotica whose use would enhance the physician's prestige. But from the time of Herophilus and the early Empiricists to the time of Galen, Alexandrian pharmacology was significantly enriched – perhaps not always to good therapeutic effect – by a further assimilation of elements from native Egyptian drug lore, even though it retained its Greek roots. Some of the ramifications of this assimilation will be traced elsewhere; a few examples might suffice here.

Among the vegetable substances which do not appear in pre-Alexandrian Greek medicine but are used by the Herophileans are:[59]

Nile milfoil
castor-oil leaves (in poultices, for heat-stroke)
aloe (in emollients and lozenges)
'Cyrenaic juice' (for inflammation of the uvula)
plantain juice (in enemas; in potions to check expectoration of blood)
flower of wild pomegranate (in potions and emollients)
bdellium (an aromatic gum, used in emollients)
root of marsh mallow (in emollients)
salep (a starchy flour ground from the dried roots of orchids; used in plasters and poultices)
rhubarb (in a lozenge for stomach disorders)
comfrey root (in a potion to stop expectoration of blood)
ginger
ironwort
tragacanth (in lozenges for dropsy; for disorders of the stomach and the spleen)

It is independently attested that most of these 'new' substances were available in ancient Egypt,[60] even though some probably had to be

[58] Hp., *On the Nature of Women* 7, 32–4, 109 (VII, pp. 322, 360, 366, 372, 430L).

[59] Cf. *infra*, e.g. Herophilus, T258–9 (Chapter VIII); *An*.26, 28, 29, 30, 37, 38, 40 (Chapter XI): *Ba*.6 (Chapter XIV); *Ma*.9 (Chapter XVIII); *Cr*.6 (Chapter XX); *AM*. (Chaper XXIII), *passim*.

[60] Cf. *GMÄ* VI (even for the non-specialist the *Wörterverzeichnis*, pp. 625ff., is useful); II, pp. 44–80; cf. VII.1–2. Lucas & Harris, 1962, and Darby, Ghalioungui, Grivetti, 1977, provide further valuable information on substances available in ancient Egypt.

imported by the established spice and drug trade routes. But the
possibility that at least some of them also had become known to the
Greeks in the course of the eastern conquests of Alexander the Great
cannot be excluded.[61]

The vegetable kingdom dominates in Herophilean drug lore, as it
does in native Egyptian pharmacology – but so does it in Hippocratic
drug lore. Plants simply were easier to cultivate or obtain than most
mineral or animal substances. More than 300 different substances are
mentioned in the Hippocratic Corpus as having medicinal power,
and of these about 250 belong to the vegetable kingdom, whereas only
about forty each are drawn from the mineral and animal kingdoms.[62]
But in Alexandria, Egyptian animal substances also enter into Greek
pharmacology: hyena bile, crocodile dung, camel urine, the head of a
spotted lizard, and tortoise blood are among the drug ingredients
which now make their début in Greek medicine.[63] The mention of
urine and dung should not be misunderstood to mean that ingredients from the so-called *Dreckapotheke* – i.e. especially the urine and
excrement of various animals – were not represented in pre-Alexandrian Greek medicine. It is a fairly common practice in primitive
cultures to try to make medicinal use of such substances and, the
idealizing protestations of some modern scholars notwithstanding,[64]

[61] A number of pharmacological substances in the corpus of Herophilean texts are,
e.g., identified as 'Indian' (cf. Indian aloe, *An.*30; Indian spikenard, *An.*32). But
one should not jump to conclusions too rapidly; the Hippocratic Corpus likewise
recommends 'Indian' substances: *On Diseases of Women* 1.81; 11.158, 185, 205 (VIII,
pp. 202, 336, 366, 394L); all of these references might be a further reflection of an
obsession with prestige-enhancing, costly exotica. On the ancient drug trade cf.
A. Schmidt, 1927: 63–131.

[62] Cf. Dierbach, 1824; von Grot, 1887. Both are quite incomplete, but they remain
useful. Stannard, 1961, emphasizes the 'rational' aspects of the Hippocratic
application of many of these substances.

[63] Cf. *infra*: Herophilus, T260 (Chapter VIII); *AM.*11, *AM.*18, *AM.*25 (internal use
of donkey urine), all in Chapter XXIII.

[64] Cf. Dierbach, 1824: 80: 'Hoffentlich wird man es mir auch nicht verargen, wenn
ich von der Anwendung des Urins und des Kothes mancher Tiere, wovon in
einigen *untergeschobenen* Büchern die Rede ist, so wie von andern dergleichen
Mitteln ganz schweige.' Despite *AM.*11 (*infra*, Chapter XXIII) Galen himself still
resorted to dung and similar substances for wound dressings; cf. his chapter on
pigeon dung: *De compositione medicamentorum per genera* 3.6 (XIII, pp. 633–4K). Cf.
also Dsc. 2.80,100. In this respect – the usefulness of the *Dreckapotheke* –
Mesopotamian, Egyptian, Indian, Talmudic, Greek, and Roman physicians
were in general agreement. Some of the anthropological perspectives suggested
by Douglas, 1966, might aid our understanding of this aspect of ancient medicine;
particularly suggestive are her resurrection of the idea of dirt as matter out of
place and her emphasis on the unclean as potent for good.

Hippocratic physicians too made fairly liberal use of the excrement of pigeons, poultry, goats, cows, donkeys, and mules,[65] prescribing the external application of some and the internal consumption (in potions) of others. Of the latter – internal use – there are still examples in Herophilean medicine, but by the second century A.D. Galen expressed his aesthetic and scientific disgust even at the external application of urine by a Herophilean physician to combat dandruff.[66]

More significantly, Greek drug prescriptions of the pre-Alexandrian era are notoriously vague in their specification of the amount of each ingredient, whereas physicians of the Pharaonic times attempt to give the appearance of recording exact measures in their roughly 800 extant drug recipes.[67] Even the fragmentary remains of early Alexandrian pharmacology reveal a marked advance over Hippocratic medicine in this respect: for the most part, Herophileans and Empiricists from the third century B.C. on become meticulous in their specification of measures – ounce, drachm, obol, ladle, cup – in their prescriptions. Here again, the Egyptian emphasis on measuring and quantifying might have imparted some stimulus to Alexandrian medicine. The Egyptians of the Pharaonic papyri thought of drugs as an invention of the gods, and Herophilus said that 'drugs are the hands of the gods', but both recognized that, whatever the origin of the power of drugs, their preparation required some human science.

---

[65] E.g., Hp., *Fistulae* 6 (VI, p. 452L). The prescription of animal dung occurs with striking frequency in Hippocratic gynaecological treatises or contexts; cf., for example, the use of bird, goat, donkey, and mule excrement in *On the Nature of Women* 32, 82, 90 (VII, pp. 350, 406, 408L); *On Diseases of Women* II.177, 189, 192, 203 (VIII, pp. 360, 374, 390L); *On Barren Women* 245 (VIII, p. 458L); *On Superfetation* 32 (VIII, p. 500L); *On Places in Man* 47 (VI, p. 346L; a passage which deals with treatments for disorders of the uterus). In at least ten further prescriptions Hippocratic authors recommend fumigating the female genitalia with, *inter alia*, cow dung (*bolbiton*): *On the Nature of Women* 2, 34 (*bis*), 103 (VII, pp. 312–14, 372–4, 418L); *On Diseases of Women* I.86, 89 and II.195, 206 (thrice), 203 (VIII, pp. 210, 212, 378, 390, 398–400L). See also above, nn. 56–8, on gynaecological parallels.

[66] See Chapter XXIII, *AM*.11 (but cf. n. 64 *supra*). Dsc. 2.80–1 also reports many internal (as well as external) medicinal uses of dung and urine.

[67] Cf. *GMÄ* VI; IV.1, *passim*; II, pp. 44–81. See also *ibid.*, III, pp. 132ff. G. E. R. Lloyd convincingly suggests that much of this measuring activity amounts to pseudo-quantification, i.e. that it achieves nothing more than the spurious appearance of exactness (personal communication).

5 *Ophthalmology; 'birth prognoses'*

Ophthalmology represents another branch of Greek medicine in Alexandria that might have received some stimulus, however limited, from indigenous Egyptian medical lore. Herodotus already singles out Egyptian eye specialists for explicit mention,[68] and, of the seven medical papyri of Pharaonic provenance, three – Ebers, Carlsberg, and London – deal with eye diseases.[69] The Ebers papyrus alone offers 100 drug prescriptions to combat various forms and degrees of blindness, and until modern times Egypt has remained notorious for its enormous share of eye diseases.

If the treatise *On eyes* attributed to Herophilus is an authentic work of the great Alexandrian, as suggested below (Chapter III), it would be one of the earliest Greek treatises known to have been devoted exclusively to ophthalmology. (A subsequent example of the Herophilean interest in eyes is provided by Demosthenes Philalethes (Chapter XXVIII), who wrote the most influential ophthalmological work of antiquity.) It is perhaps significant that Herophilus' treatise prescribes ingredients that are distinctively Egyptian, also in their ophthalmological application, such as crocodile dung to treat day-blindness.[70] But other Herophilean ingredients, such as liver (a good source of vitamin A), had been in use both in Egypt and in pre-Alexandrian Greece to treat eye ailments.[71]

[68] Hdt. 2.84. Cf. also 3.1: the Persian king Cyrus requested the Pharaoh Amasis to send him the best eye-doctor in Egypt.

[69] Cf. *GMÄ* IV.1, pp. 41–61; IV.2, pp. 51–65; I, pp. 33–5; Lefebvre, 1956: 66–88; Waterman, 1958. But among the well-known later Egyptian terra cottas depicting diseases, eye disorders are curiously under-represented: cf. Panayotatou, 1929; Perdrizet, 1921: vol. I, pp. 161–9, and II, Plates CV–CXIX. For a brief discussion of rival interpretations of the meaning of these terra cottas see also Graindor, 1939: 37f. For evidence of the continuity between earlier (Pharaonic) and later (Coptic) Egyptian ophthalmology cf. Chassinat, 1921.

[70] Chapter VIII, T260; cf. papyrus Ebers 344, 378, 412 (*GMÄ* IV.1, pp. 43, 54). Instances of the application of excrement to the eyes in Hippocratic medicine are not known to me, whereas the excrement of pelicans (pap. Ebers 365), lizards (Ebers 370), deer (Ebers 339), and children (Ebers 349), as well as human urine (pap. Ramesseum III A.19–20) all belong to the ophthalmological materia medica of Pharaonic Egypt (*GMÄ* IV.1, pp. 41, 46, 53, 59). See also Pliny, *Nat. Hist.* 28.28.108; Dsc. 2.80.6. See also *Comments*, T260 *infra*.

[71] Cf. beef liver in papyrus Ebers 351, and pap. Londin. 35 (*GMÄ* IV.1, p. 49); goat liver in Herophilus, T260, for 'day'-blindness; Hp., *On Vision* 7 (IX, p. 158L); beef liver in a remedy for night-blindness. (Cf. also the Hippocratic use of sheep and goat liver in *On Diseases of Women* 1.34 (VIII, p. 80L).) Cf. *Comments* on T260 below.

The extent and exact nature of Egyptian influence on Herophilean ophthalmology therefore remains unclear. What is clear, however, is that Herophilus had a much more sophisticated, precise understanding of the anatomy of the eye than any Egyptian *swnw* or priest of Sekhmet. The Egyptians might have had a fairly good idea of the external anatomy of the eye, but Herophilus became the first to distinguish carefully between four coats of the eye and to introduce an influential nomenclature for them (Chapter vi, T84–9).

Both in Pharaonic Egypt and in classical Greece, as in many other cultures, there was a lively interest in so-called 'birth prognoses', i.e. in determining whether a woman or, less frequently, a man would be fertile or infertile, whether or not a woman was pregnant, whether a foetus would be a boy or a girl, and so on. In a study of fragments of an Egyptian papyrus of the nineteenth or twentieth dynasty (*c.* 1314–1085 B.C.), papyrus Carlsberg VIII, Erik Iversen established that there are some close parallels between Egyptian birth prognoses and prognoses in the Hippocratic Corpus.[72] I shall limit myself to one example, since the main concern here is Alexandrian, not Hippocratic, medicine.

A Pharaonic prognosis (papyrus Carlsberg VIII.4): 'Another, to distinguish a woman who will give birth from one who will not give birth: you shall let an onion bulb . . . remain the whole night (on her vulva?) until dawn. If the smell passes through her mouth, she will give birth; if . . . (lacuna), she will not give birth.'[73] 'Hippocrates', *On Barren Women* (= *On Diseases of Women* III) 214, describes a similar test to determine whether a woman will conceive: 'Another: clean off a clove of garlic all around, snip off its head, and apply it to the vagina; and on the following day see whether she smells (of garlic) through her mouth; and if she smells, she will conceive; if not, she won't.'[74]

These and similar prognoses[75] might be indicative of some influx of Egyptian ideas into Greek medicine before the founding of Alexandria (although one cannot exclude the possibility of two independent

[72] Iversen, 1939. Le Page Renouf, 1873, first drew attention to parallels between Egyptian and Greek birth prognoses on the basis of passages in pap. Berlin 3038 (Berl. 193, *GMÄ* IV.1, p. 274) and Hp., *On Barren Women* 214 (VIII, p. 414L).
[73] Iversen, 1939: 21–2.
[74] VIII, p. 416L.
[75] Cf., e.g., pap. Carlsberg VIII.5 (Iversen, 1939: 23) and Hp., *Aphorisms* 5.59 (IV, p. 174 Jones, Loeb; IV, p. 554L).

developments in Greece and Egypt). A number of these prognoses were absorbed into the Hippocratic aphoristic tradition, and this may account in part for their frequent recurrence in European folk medicine until modern times.[76] Aphorisms and gnomic sayings tend to have a long life span and to be relatively immune to social, political, and scientific change.

Although arguments from silence are notoriously dangerous, it is worth noting that there is no evidence that these popular, durable birth prognoses became part of the Herophilean tradition, despite the documented availability of copies of the Hippocratic *Aphorisms* – and perhaps of most of what then was the Hippocratic Corpus – in Alexandria in the third century B.C.[77] It is conceivable that Herophilus' careful study of reproductive anatomy and physiology and of obstetrics (Chapters VI.5, VII.5–6) convinced him of the absurdity and uselessness of these Egyptian intrusions into Greek medicine, and that he therefore abandoned what has been hailed as the most significant Egyptian element in Greek medicine. (Herophilus' interest in Hippocratic notions of prognosis and prediction is also attested,[78] but it was probably more of an exegetical or philological interest, and it does not seem to have focused on 'birth prognoses' as such.)

6 *Political, organizational, and social aspects*

While Greek physicians, including Herophilus, tended to be generalists, Egyptian physicians belonged to a sizable caste of medical specialists. Egyptian doctors of the eyes, the teeth, the belly, and 'hidden' (internal?) diseases are mentioned by ancient sources, along

---

[76] Among the Egyptian birth prognoses that recur more frequently in European folk medicine is the following: 'You shall put wheat and barley into purses of cloth; the woman shall pass her water on it every day, it being mixed with dates and sand. If both sprout, she will give birth; if the wheat sprouts, she will give birth to a boy . . . if the barley sprouts, she will give birth to a girl; if they do not sprout, she will not give birth at all' (Iversen, 1939: 14). Iversen provides several parallels from medical sources as late as the seventeenth century; cf. also ps.-Galen, *De remediis parabilibus* 2.26.5 (XIV, p. 476K). For further Egyptian birth prognoses see *GMÄ* IV.1, pp. 272–6.

[77] See *infra*, especially Chapters IX, XIV, XV.

[78] Chapter IX, T261–T266.

with the famous Shepherds of the Anus.[79] Even when native Egyptians became increasingly numerous and active in Alexandria in the later Ptolemaic period,[80] this distinctively Pharaonic specialization did not become extinct. A papyrus of the second century B.C., for example, refers to the Alexandrian practice of an indigenous Egyptian enema specialist[81] – a latter-day Shepherd of the Anus, who helped rid his Alexandrian clients of *wḥdw?*

Most of the physicians presented in the chapters that follow are representatives both of scientific and of clinical medicine, i.e. they did research, developed their own theories, modified those of their predecessors, and wrote medical books in addition to treating patients. But there also must have been a large number of general practitioners in Alexandria, and various specialists in the rest of Egypt, about whom only silence reigns today; they left no written record. Under the Pharaohs, all such Egyptian physicians were public officials, paid by the state, offering free treatment to their patients.[82] It seems likely that this practice was continued in the Ptolemaic period, since a medical tax (*iatrikon*) was collected by the Ptolemies too.[83] A similar tax had been imposed in at least some Greek communities outside Egypt,[84] but in this case the Ptolemies probably refined and perpetuated an existing Egyptian structure. Papyrological evidence of the Hellenistic period suggests that this system of public medicine was overseen at the provincial level by a

---

[79] Cf., e.g., Herodotus 2.84. But for examples of more versatile physicians see Junker, 1928: especially 68ff. Cf. also Lefebvre, 1956: 17–26, and Jonckheere, 1958: 125ff., 99–100; *id.*, 1951c. Whether the Shepherd of the Anus was a true physician-specialist or simply a person who administered enemas is a controversial issue; cf. Jonckheere, 1958: 99.

[80] Cf. Fraser, 1972: vol. I, pp. 70ff., 81–92, 115–18, 130–1, 256–66.

[81] Wilcken, 1927–37: vol. I, no. 148 (pp. 635–6). See infra, n. 91.

[82] Cf. Diodorus Siculus 1.82.3 (Hecataeus, *FGrHist* 264, F25); Jonckheere, 1958: 95–137. On administrative aspects see also Jonckheere, 1951c. See also n. 23 *supra.*

[83] Cf. Wilcken, 1899: vol. I, 170 (pp. 375–7); Préaux, 1939: 45, 132–3, 401, 421 (with n. 5); Nanetti, 1944; Kudlien, 1979: 19ff.

[84] See Pohl, 1905: 72ff. But the careful analysis by Cohn-Haft, 1956, seems to have established that Greek physicians normally received fees from patients. Cf. also Hp., *Precepts* 4–7 (*CMG* I.1, pp. 31–3 Heiberg), on how a 'good' physician should determine what to charge each patient; and see Deichgräber, 1965: 213–14 (fr. 293), 323, on earning money as the main motive of some physicians.

'royal physician', and that the entire system in turn was under the central control of an *archiatros* or a similar official.[85]

This basically Pharaonic organization of medicine prevailed outside Alexandria, but whether it was replicated in the capital itself is difficult to determine in the absence of adequate evidence. In a typical Greek *polis* the physicians, even if they belonged to a fraternal Asclepiad association, were free agents – free also to collect fees from patients and apprentices. In all probability this practice, like numerous other Greek customs, was transported to Alexandria. A papyrus of the second century B.C. records that one Sosicrates contractually apprenticed a certain Philon to the physician Theodotus for a period of six years, to learn the art of healing in exchange for a fee.[86]

As in Pharaonic Memphis and in the capitals of most ancient monarchies, the court physician played a considerable role in Alexandria. But most of the scientific or academic physicians of Alexandria – i.e. the Empiricists, perhaps Erasistratus, and the Herophileans – do not seem to have been closely affiliated with the Ptolemaic court, perhaps out of a desire to avoid the uncertainties endemic in political life, perhaps simply because their services were never solicited by the rulers. There were, however, some exceptions, also among the followers of Herophilus: Andreas (Chapter XI) seems to have been the court physician of Ptolemy IV Philopator, and Dioscurides Phacas (Chapter XIX) served the last Ptolemy, the famous Cleopatra, as an emissary. A distinguished Alexandrian Empiricist, Apollonius of Citium, also might have been fairly closely affiliated with the court of the flute-playing twelfth Ptolemy, Auletes,[87] but the

---

[85] Cf., from the late second century B.C., Wilcken, 1927–37: vol. II.1, no. 162, col. II, lines 25–6 (p. 62), on 'Tatas [an Egyptian?], the Royal (*basilikos*) Physician'. See also, from the first century B.C., *Sammelb.* 5216 (Athenagoras, the *archiatros*). Cf. Rostovtzeff, 1953: vol. II, pp. 1091–3; *infra*, Chapter XX (Chrysermus), especially notes 3–7; Kudlien, 1979: 73–81. On public physicians see Cohn-Haft, 1956; Kudlien, 1979: 18–40; Gil, 1973. As Vivian Nutton (1977) has pointed out, in the Imperial period *archiatros* can refer to royal as well as civic physician.

[86] See *infra*, Chapter II, n. 16 (and the texts mentioned *ibid.*, notes 14–15).

[87] Cf. Apollonius Citiensis, *In Hippocratis De Articulis Commentarius* I.1, II *init.*, III *init.* (*CMG* XI.1.1, pp. 10, 38, 64 Kollesch/Kudlien). I have found no good evidence to confirm P. M. Fraser's view that Apollonius' teacher, Zopyrus of Alexandria, was 'closely associated with Auletes' (1972): vol. I, p. 371); cf. Deichgräber, 1965, fr. 266–74 and pp. 261–3. Fraser (*loc. cit.*) makes the interesting observation that the Ptolemaic court physicians of the third century B.C. were all immigrants (Greeks

remaining physicians known to have been associated with the court do not seem to have been people of scientific distinction.

More problematic is the question of social and professional contact between Egyptian and Greek physicians in Alexandria as a possible avenue of influence. No Egyptians seem to have been active as scholars in the Museum and the Library or to have been numbered among the early Alexandrian intelligentsia. Manetho of Sebennytus, the earliest known native Egyptian to have written in Greek (c. 280 B.C.), has been aptly characterized as standing 'quite apart from the main stream of Alexandrian life . . . it is not likely that he lived much of his life in Alexandria'.[88] Although Manetho's *Aegyptiaca*, an account of Egyptian history, chronology, and religious customs, was addressed to Ptolemy II Philadelphus, it apparently made minimal impact on contemporary Alexandrian writers, who were singularly uninterested in Egyptian chronology and customs. Not until the Egyptian element predominated over the Greek in later Ptolemaic Alexandria did Greek writers in Egypt begin to show an inclination to read or emulate Manetho.[89] This points to a more general phenomenon.

In the first century of Alexandrian history the Greek community remained remarkably insulated from the Egyptian population. This is a social and cultural pattern that is consistent with the modern colonial experience: the colonizers import their own culture and, despite frequent contact with indigenous labourers, artisans, religious leaders, and other professionals, preserve the imported culture of their forebears virtually unchanged for generations. They likewise tend to preserve their ignorance of all but some exotic features of the indigenous culture, rarely even bothering to learn the local language. For all their assimilative pretensions, the Ptolemies themselves participated in this isolation: the last Ptolemy was the first one to learn to speak Egyptian.

Yet it seems likely that at least some Alexandrian Greeks engaged in a certain amount of intellectual tourism. At first the temples with

from Cos, Cnidus, and Carystus), whereas the court physicians of the second and first centuries B.C. were Greeks with Alexandrian citizenship. For further details cf. Gorteman, 1957 (for Alexandria); and Jonckheere, 1952 (Pharaonic Egypt).
[88] Fraser, 1972: vol. I, pp. 505, 510. On the relation of Greeks and Egyptians cf. also Barns, 1978; Hanson, 1985: 25–9; Lewis, 1986: esp. 3–15, 27–9, 92–4, 134–7, 153–6, 159 nn. 3–5; Kudlien, 1979: 65–72.
[89] Fraser, 1972: vol. I, pp. 510–11.

their syncretic potential and their social importance might have been more conducive to intercultural contact than the Museum, the Library, or the dissecting rooms of Herophilus. Furthermore, some Greek patients of the third century B.C. turned to shrines of Egyptian gods of healing – Osiris, Sarapis, Imhotep – much the way Greeks previously had turned to the temples of Asclepius.[90] Eventually Greeks apparently also sought the help of Egyptian physicians. In the second century B.C. the same Egyptian enema specialist mentioned earlier employed a well-paid Greek interpreter in his practice, presumably to facilitate communication with Greek-speaking patients.[91] But evidence of this kind is very rare, and the general cultural isolation of the Alexandrian community from indigenous Egyptians might have contributed to the limited nature of the impact Greek and Egyptian medicine had upon one another.

7 Patronage and the Museum

The Alexandrian Museum as a research institute, the massive Alexandrian Library, royal patronage of the sciences and letters, and spectacular advances in medical research: this presents the modern scholar with a tempting causal nexus. But there is in fact no evidence that Herophilus (or, for that matter, any of his followers) was a member of the Museum, or that he was a recipient of *financial* support from the royal court, or that he conducted his dissections and other research at the Museum or under its auspices. There is, however, one very significant suggestion of royal support (discussed more fully in Chapter VI.A.1): through Ptolemaic intervention human cadavers and possibly live prisoners might have been made available to Herophilus – and, if he practised in Alexandria, to Erasistratus – for dissection and vivisection in contravention of a pristine Greek taboo (see below).

[90] Cf. *Sammelb*. 7470 (from Upper Egypt, third–second century B.C., an inscription in praise of the god Amenothes for having healed the dedicator) and 1934 (inscription from the Serapeum in Memphis); D.L. 5.76 (= Demetrius of Phaleron, fr. 68 Wehrli). See also Dittenberger, 1903–5: vol. I, no. 98: Ptolemy V Epiphanes dedicated a temple on Philae, an island in the southern Nile, to Imhotep under the name of Asclepius. On the acceptance in Alexandria itself of Sarapis' healing power cf. Fraser, 1972: vol. I, pp. 257–8. See also Sudhoff, 1909: 213ff.

[91] Wilcken, 1927–37: vol. I, no. 148. For a useful analysis of the difficulties presented by this papyrus see Rémondon, 1964.

If any medical research ever was conducted at the Museum or sponsored by it, none of our ancient sources has bothered to record the fact. A Delian inscription of the second century B.C. admittedly identifies a certain Chrysermus as 'Exegete, Superintendent of Physicians, and Supervisor of the Museum'.[92] But there is no independent evidence to confirm that this Chrysermus was a research physician rather than a layman who had been appointed both central administrator of public medical services and Museum chairman by a Ptolemy. It would seem precipitate to conclude, on the basis of this inscription alone, that 'medical studies formed an important part of the work in the Mouseion'.[93]

Much modern scientific research relies on costly technology and hence requires substantial financial support. Perhaps for this reason it has become an almost obligatory cliché of history of science that there is a direct causal link between patronage and scientific progress. It is commonly assumed that any scientific endeavour that flourished in Alexandria must have done so because of Ptolemaic subsidies. While this might be correct, evidence of such patronage is virtually non-existent. And indeed, with the possible exception of some forms of technological research, Alexandrian science would not seem to have been vitally dependent on the material largess of royal benefactors.

Herophilus had apprentices, such as Philinus of Cos,[94] who probably paid him; and for treating patients Herophilus was presumably remunerated either by the state or by his patients themselves. For his research he did not need a modern laboratory with sophisticated, expensive equipment but, in addition to his physician's office (iatreion), only a room or rooms equipped for dissection and for relatively simple experiments. His office may have contained his famous pulse-measuring clepsydra, his 'embryo-slayer',[95] and the usual tools of the better Greek physicians: numerous containers full of pharmacological substances (including work-horse ingredients like wine, vinegar, and honey), a brazier to heat cauteries and drugs, perhaps surgical machinery for reducing

---

[92] Chapter xx, n. 4 (cf. *ibid.*, notes 5–7). Fraser, 1972: vol. I, pp. 371, 373, and Gorteman, 1957: 332, n. 2, raise important questions about the meaning of this inscription.

[93] Fraser, 1972: vol. I, p. 371.

[94] See below, Chapter II, T1 (= Deichgräber, 1965: 40, fr. 6).

[95] See below, Chapters VII.4 (T182); VIII (T247).

dislocations,[96] probes, pans, jars, blades, syringes, drills, linen bandages, needles, thread, linen cloths, wool, sponges, and so on. With the exception of space for dissection, and possibly for vivisectory experiments, Herophilus' professional needs therefore might not have exceeded those of other Greek physicians – and his clinical income probably did not suffer from his fame.

Institutionally, too, Herophilus might have been independent. Ancient sources seem to make pointed reference to the 'House (oikia) of Herophilus' when describing his immediate followers: they are 'Those from the House of Herophilus', whereas adherents of later centuries are referred to simply as 'Herophileans' or, in a more characteristic Greek expression, as 'those around Herophilus'.[97]

Moreover, a simplistic causal correlation between scientific progress and patronage appears to be challenged by the fact that the relatively high standard of scientific medicine set by Herophilus – and, wherever he practised, by Erasistratus – does not seem to have been maintained by the next generations of Alexandrian physicians (see Chapters VI.A.1 and X), even though Ptolemaic patronage neither disappeared nor radically diminished upon Herophilus' death. Even if some form of direct or indirect patronage were a necessary condition of medical progress, it certainly is not a sufficient cause.

The silence of our sources does not of course preclude the possibility that Herophilus received significant financial patronage from the first two Ptolemies or that he was a member of the Museum, yet two forms of what one might call 'indirect patronage' were possibly more significant for the remarkable development of medicine in early Alexandria.

First, the general intellectual climate encouraged by the early Ptolemies: the sense of scientific and literary frontiersmanship that attracted intellectuals from all over the Greek world to Alexandria in the early third century B.C. probably stimulated efforts to establish new frontiers in medicine too. The Macedonian rulers of Egypt inherited some of the appreciation of discovery and of learning with

---

[96] Cf. Chapter XI (Andreas) for an example of Herophilean interest in orthopaedic surgery.

[97] See below, Chapter XII (A, Introduction and Cn.1); Chapter XIII, Cm.7. The use of oikia is problematic and any institutional conclusions drawn from it must remain hypothetical. See also Chapter X.A and von Staden, 1982; Nutton, 1975.

which Aristotle had 'infused' Alexander the Great. By creating and nurturing the Library and the Museum, the early Ptolemies offered symbolically and historically significant versions of Alexander's archives and of Aristotle's Lyceum; and by opening Alexandria not only to scholars and poets, but also to scientists, they ensured the relative security of science within the political and social order for at least a century.

Secondly, the 'frontier' environment apparently made it easier to overcome some inveterate Greek taboos, particularly if their violation could be sanctioned, however tenuously, by appeals to time-honoured Egyptian tradition. The Hellenistic kings of Egypt, whose syncretistic opportunism led them to be crowned Pharaoh and Ptolemy at once, themselves set the best-known example of violating a deep-rooted Greek taboo with impunity: disregarding the Greek taboo against incest between uterine brothers and sisters, some Ptolemies followed Pharaonic custom and married their own sisters, beginning with the marriage of Ptolemy II Philadelphus ('Sister Lover') to his older sister Arsinoe II in about 276 B.C. (to which the Greek poet Sotades objected with his notoriously blunt verse: 'You're thrusting your prick [*kentron*] into an unholy hole'[98]). Herophilus' dissections and possibly vivisections, apparently made possible by the king's active intervention, violated the Greek taboo against opening a human body,[99] dead or alive, but this violation, too, might have been perceived, however mistakenly, by the Ptolemies and others as sanctioned by an Egyptian tradition: the practice of mummification. As I shall argue below (Chapter VI.A.1), mummification has very little to do with medicine, and Herophilus and Erasistratus probably did not gain any of their anatomical knowledge from Egyptian mummifiers. Authors ranging from Herodotus and Diodorus Siculus to modern historians of science have recognized that the level of anatomical knowledge required by Egyptian methods of embalming is closer to that of a skilled butcher than of a Hellenistic physician or biologist.[100] Furthermore, no native Egyptian physician ever seems

---

[98] Fr. 1 Powell (*Collectanea Alexandrina*, p. 238; from Athenaeus, *Deipnosophistae* 14.621A).

[99] There are, however, examples of Greeks who desecrated corpses, especially of enemies; cf. *infra*, Chapter VI.A.1.

[100] Both Herodotus and Diodorus treat medicine and mummification separately, as entirely different subjects: Herodotus 2.84 vs. 2.86; Diodorus 1.82 vs. 1.91. Cf.

to have misinterpreted the religious and legal sanction of mummification as licence to practise dissection, let alone vivisection. Yet the existence in Egypt of a priestly caste whose main task involved opening human corpses might have facilitated justifying a temporary[101] breach of the Greek taboo by Hellenistic king and Hellenistic physician, and this in turn made possible the emergence of human dissection as almost synonymous with early Alexandrian medicine.

On balance it seems reasonable to conclude that the open, restless intellectual climate of a 'frontier' capital, Alexandria, and the forms of indirect royal patronage discussed above, perhaps along with Ptolemaic control of Greek centres of medicine such as Cnidus and Cos (see Chapter II), contributed more to the extraordinary Alexandrian advances in scientific medicine than did native Egyptian medicine. For all the assimilative and syncretistic efforts of the Ptolemies, and for all the possible instances of influence discussed above, Egyptian medicine remained a deeply un-Greek amalgam of magic, religion, and science, largely isolated from early Alexandrian culture, and as perennially different from it as a summer breeze on a North Sea island from a sirocco. There is considerable accuracy in E. M. Forster's observation that Alexandria 'then, as now, . . . belonged not so much to Egypt as to the Mediterranean, and the Ptolemies realised this. Up in Egypt they played the Pharaoh, and built solemn *archaistic* temples like Edfu and Kom Ombo. Down in Alexandria they were *Hellenistic*.'[102]

Majno, 1975: 138–9, who uses the analogy of the butcher. For further details, also on secondary literature, see below Chapter VI.A.1 ('Dissection and vivisection') with notes 2–38; T63–T70. The pseudo-Galenic author of *Introductio sive medicus* had a more sanguine view: 'Among the first physicians (sc. in Egypt) many things belonging to surgery seem to have been discovered on the basis of ripping open (*anaschisis*) cadavers in the course of embalmings' (XIV, p. 675K). Cf. also Pliny, *Natural History* 19.26.86: 'in Aegypto regibus[!] corpora mortuorum *ad scrutandos morbos* insecantibus'.

[101] It will be argued below (Chapter VI.A.1) that dissection (and, if it ever took place in Greek antiquity, vivisection) of humans was a relatively short-lived phenomenon, even in Alexandria. That the taboo was still strong in Hellenistic times is suggested by several ancient sources. Cf., in the third century B.C., Teles, *On Exile* (p. 31.9–10 Hense, 2nd edn (1909)): 'We (Greeks) shrink from looking at and touching (corpses).' Perhaps in a similar vein Cicero, probably drawing on the Stoic philosopher Chrysippus (c. 281–208 B.C.), lists among the 'nationum varios errores' the Egyptian and Persian custom of embalming (*Tusculan Disputations* 1.45.108).

[102] Forster, 1961: 13–16. For a different view cf. Barns, 1978: 12–14. A growing consensus supports Forster's view; cf. Lewis, 1986: 4: 'Where people of two

In medicine, being 'Hellenistic' or 'Alexandrian', as opposed to 'archaistic' or 'Egyptian', clearly entailed being considerably more advanced in theory, and probably in practice as well. To the Greeks, this would not have been the first example of the superiority of Greek medicine. About two centuries before the founding of Alexandria, according to Herodotus,[103] a Greek physician from southern Italy, Democedes of Croton, was persuaded to treat the severely injured ankle of the Persian king Darius, after the king's Egyptian court physicians had succeeded only in making the injury worse. Democedes successfully applied remedies customary among the Greeks. King Darius had previously considered his Egyptian physicians the best physicians in the world, but because 'they were surpassed by a Greek, they [now] were about to be impaled' – only to be saved by Democedes' intervention with the king. In Ptolemaic Egypt, too, the superiority of Greek medicine did not signal the death of Egyptian medicine.

cultures, speaking different languages, live in close proximity, something of each is bound to rub off on the other. But what . . . becomes clearer with each new study, is that in Hellenistic Egypt such mutual influences were minimal.'
[103] Hdt. 3.129–38.

Part 1
HEROPHILUS

II

LIFE

A · INTRODUCTION

1 *General*

It is characteristic of the post-classical period in Greece that Herophilus, one of the greatest scientists of Greek antiquity, was not born in a traditional centre of culture such as Athens or Syracuse, or in a traditional centre of medical learning such as Cos, or even in the glittering new centre of poetry and science – Alexandria – but in a relatively obscure and deprived town on the Asiatic side of the Bosporus, opposite Byzantium: in Chalcedon (Testimonia 1–3), often ridiculed in pagan antiquity as *Oppidum Caecorum*.[1] From infancy near the Black Sea to celebrity status in Alexandria might seem an unlikely journey, but in the increasingly mobile societies of the Hellenistic world, the more renowned Greek cities, which had always tended to

---

[1] Herodotus 4.144: 'Megabazus left an immortal memory among the people of the Hellespont for something he said. For when he was in Byzantion and learned that the Calchedonians had founded their town seventeen years before the Byzantines founded theirs, he said that the Calchedonians . . . were blind; for had they not been blind, they would never have chosen the uglier site when the better one was available.' Pliny, *Natural History* 5.43.149, on 'Calchadon' (*sic*; see below and n. 4): 'and later it was called Blind Men's Town (*Oppidum Caecorum*) because they did not know how to choose a site, Byzantion–a site so much more felicitous in all respects – being only seven miles away'. Even in later antiquity, its insignificance apparently contributed to Chalcedon's choice as a relatively uncontroversial location for the fourth Ecumenic Council in A.D. 451 (*Acta Conciliorum Oecumen.* II.1–6: *Conc. Univ. Chalcedonense*, ed. E. Schwartz (Berlin, 1932–8)).

Ancient sources vacillate between 'Chalcedon' and 'Calchedon'. T1 and T3 both have 'Chalcedon' but 'Calchedon' is suggested by T2 (see textual apparatus) and is found in most inscriptions (*CIG* 3068B, *CIA* 1.229–30, 238–9, 244, 247, 259; *SEG* XI.414.23, XVII.540, 827). The literary tradition is initially ambivalent, but in time 'Chalcedon' becomes the dominant form. Cf. Ruge, 1919: col. 1555.

attract gifted outsiders,[2] became more crowded than ever with intellectual leaders who had no metropolitan roots and, in several prominent cases, could not even claim Greek as their native language. The dominant figures among the new intelligentsia now included numerous northerners and easterners such as Zeno of Citium, Chrysippus and Clearchus of Soli, Sphaerus of Borysthenes, Diogenes of Babylon, Antipater of Tarsus, Strato of Lampsacus, Autolycus and Arcesilaus of Pitane, Cleanthes of Assos, Aristarchus of Samothrace, and Apollonius of Perge. As some traditional walls of the polis collapsed, starting even before Alexander's conquests, and horizons expanded to include the cosmopolis and *kosmopolitēs* envisioned by some Hellenistic Greeks, an earlier patriotism, symbolized in its more rarified and perhaps idealized Athenian form by never leaving one's polis except in its service, became obsolescent. Herophilus' journey from obscurity on the Bithynian periphery to scientific fame in the greatest centre of learning in the Greek world, Alexandria, is accordingly emblematic of its time and indicative of the opportunities afforded by the breakdown of old orders and the establishment of new ones.

If Herophilus lived roughly from 330/320 to 260/250 B.C., as I shall argue *infra*, he might in his earlier years have experienced the political vicissitudes that rapidly swept his strategically perched birthplace from active support of the Persian cause through conquest by the expansionist Macedonians to an alliance with the new masters of Egypt.[3]

The relatively early contact between Chalcedon and Ptolemaic Egypt might not have been without significance for Herophilus' career. When the Bithynian ruler Ziboites (Zipoites, Zeipoetes)

---

[2] There had always been great travellers among the Greeks, for example Democritus, Herodotus, the Sophists (and lesser travellers like Aeschylus and Plato, who journeyed to Sicily), but the important point here is that the intellectual leadership in both Athens and Alexandria now consisted largely of 'foreigners' who had migrated to the metropolitan centres.

[3] To the bitter end of Alexander the Great's battles against the Persians, the Chalcedonians fought as mercenaries on the Persian side (Arrian, *Anabasis* 3.24.5). Eventually Chalcedon was captured by Alexander, and subsequently it became involved in the battles between the diadochi (Diodorus Siculus 18.72; Polyaenus 4.6.8; *Marmor Parium* for 317/16 B.C.). See also Diod. Sic. 19.60 (but cf. Plutarch, *Moralia* 302E–303A = *Quaest. Graec.* 49); Droysen, 1952–3: vol. II, 218–19; Rostovtzeff, 1953: vol. I, 35, 567ff., 585ff.

besieged Chalcedon in 315 B.C., Ptolemy I Soter not only forced him to lift the siege but also concluded a treaty with the Chalcedonians.[4] It was apparently at some point after this that Herophilus moved to Egypt and practised in Alexandria (cf. T4–T6). If Chalcedon's alliance with Ptolemy I produced significant contact between the Alexandrians and Chalcedonians, this early connection might well have affected or facilitated Herophilus' decision to emigrate to Alexandria. Whether Herophilus moved there in his youth or only after completing his medical apprenticeship in Cos (see below) and practising elsewhere, is, however, unknown.

Because it is documented that Herophilus practised in Alexandria, the kings who in T7 are 'credited' with releasing prison inmates to Herophilus and Erasistratus for vivisection (more on this controversial evidence in Chapter VI.A) have often been thought to be Ptolemy I Soter, the founder of the famous Library,[5] and his son Ptolemy II Philadelphus, whose promotion of scientific research is even more celebrated than that of his father. If, however, Julius Beloch's recently revived but controversial view that Erasistratus did not practise in Alexandria at all but in Antioch,[6] the capital of Seleucid Syria, is correct, 'kings' might well refer to Seleucid as well as Egyptian rulers. But this would not affect our general picture of Herophilus' life: given the independent evidence about Herophilus' activity in Alexandria (T4–T6), 'kings' in his case almost certainly refers to a Ptolemy or Ptolemies. A reference to Soter, who ruled 323–283/2 B.C., and to Philadelphus (he ruled 283/2–246 B.C.), or to both, would not be incompatible with the date suggested below for Herophilus or, for

---

[4] Between 306 and 281 B.C., however, Chalcedon seems to have become dependent on Lysimachus, as the legends ΒΑΣΙΛΕΩΣ ΛΥΣΙΜΑΧΟΥ and ΚΑΛΧΑ on Chalcedonian coins suggest (καλχαδών is a common Doric form of the name, occurring especially on coins – and to be expected in a town founded c. 685 B.C. as a Megarian colony). Cf. Waddington, Babelon, Reinach, 1904–25: 294 no. 21 (cf. also nos. 22–3), 288f. Subsequently the Chalcedonians established an alliance with Mithridates (Ktistēs) and others against Seleucus I and Antiochus I, and by the end of the third century B.C. they had become a member of the Aetolian Confederacy (Memnon of Heracleia (?), FGrHist 434F7 and 11; Polybius 15.23.8f.; Rostovtzeff, 1953: vol. I, 585 ff. and vol. III, 1356 n. 51). For the earlier history of Chalcedon cf. Merle, 1916: 1–49 and 73–6; Dionysius of Byzantium, Anaplus Bospori §48 (pp. 19f. Güngerich, 1927).

[5] Cf. Fraser, 1972: vol. I, pp. 321–2. (Cf. also ibid., pp. 314ff., on the Museum.)

[6] Beloch, 1904: vol. III.2, pp. 473–4; likewise 2nd edn (1927), 564–5. This view has been supported by Fraser, 1969, but countered by Lloyd, 1975b. Cf. also Fraser, 1972: vol. I, p. 347.

that matter, with what is known about their energetic encouragement of scientific research in Alexandria. (One must guard, however,
against the relatively common practice of using T7 itself, in particular
'regibus', as adequate evidence that Herophilus conducted his
research in Alexandria; this would, of course, entail circular reasoning.)

About Herophilus' birth in Chalcedon and his practice in
Alexandria one can be sure; but the Athenian setting of T8 should
give one pause: Hyginus, a mythographer of the second century A.D.,
reports that a young Athenian woman, apparently in reaction against
the exclusion of women from the medical profession, disguised herself
as a man and completed a medical apprenticeship with 'a certain
Herophilus'.

In the absence of any mention in ancient sources of other physicians
by the name of Herophilus,[7] one might reasonably conclude that the
mythographer is referring to the famous Alexandrian. In that case 'a
certain' ('cuidam') would admittedly be puzzling, since it deprives
Herophilus of his usual celebrity status. To Latin readers of
mythographic handbooks in the second century A.D. Herophilus
might, however, have been a mere *quidam*, despite his continuing fame
among medical writers of that period.

While Hyginus does not explicitly specify where Hagnodice's

[7] Valerius Maximus, *Facta et dicta memorabilia* 9.15.1, refers to an ophthalmologist
('ocularius medicus'; but some MSS have '(a)equarius medicus', a horse-doctor)
of the first century B.C. by the name of Herophilus, but he is not said to have been
an Athenian, and in any case he was a notorious impostor. A contemporary of
Caesar and Pompey, he falsely paraded as the grandson of C. Marius (elected
consul seven times) and of the celebrated orator L. Licinius Crassus; his ambitions
and flamboyant pretensions earned him not only the nickname 'pseudo-Marius'
but also death in prison. A fugitive slave, he was better known as 'Amatius' than as
'Herophilus'. Cf. Appian, *Civil Wars* 3.1.2–6; Cicero, *Letters to Atticus* 12.49.2 (*ad
loc.* see Shackleton Baily, 1965–70: vol. v, p. 339); Cicero, *Philippic* 1.2.5; Livy,
Periochae 116: C(h)a(r)mates *codd.*: C. Amatius *Sigonius* (vol. xxxiv.2, p. 41 Jal).
Valerius Maximus is alone in suggesting that this 'pseudo-Marius' – 'Herophilus' – 'Amatius' was a doctor of any kind. See also Münzer, 1930. This
'Herophilus' is erroneously split into two persons in *RE* 8.1 (1912), cols. 1104 (No.
1: Vonder Mühll's eye-doctor) and 1110 (No. 5: Gossen's horse-doctor).
'Herophilus, the son of Theodorus' also occurs in Egyptian sources, but he is
identified neither as a physician nor as an Athenian, and in any case only turns up
in a papyrus of the sixth century A.D. (Pap. Graec. Vindob. 25884, from Fayûm);
cf. *Sammelb.* 9608, verso. On Hierophilus see Appendix (II). The name 'Herophilus' is reasonably well attested; e.g. *CIG* 171, 2052, 3089, 3830, 6238, 7195; *SEG*
26.1241; Kaibel, *Epigr. ex lapid.* 587. See also Appendix (IV).

apprenticeship with Herophilus took place, he does insist on the Athenian context of the episode as a whole. Thus, in *Fabula* 274.13 (not included below in T8) Hyginus reports that Hagnodice, as a result of her popularity with female patients – who alone knew that she was a woman – had to appear before the Areopagus on charges of seducing and corrupting her female patients. When she raised her tunic and revealed to this Athenian court that she was a woman in male disguise, and when she also received aggressive support from other women, 'the *Athenians* amended the law so that free-born women (*ingenuae*) could learn the science of medicine'.

Without more evidence about his life, the possibility that Herophilus at some point did practise and teach in Athens, and that an incident during his sojourn there somehow became fictionalized into this anecdote, cannot be excluded with absolute certainty. While no longer enjoying unrivalled scientific or cultural primacy, Athens still had its allures and had not become a scientific wasteland. At least some of the biological research initiated by Aristotle was being carried on in Athens. Furthermore, Athens remained the undisputed centre of philosophical schools, most of which continued to be interested in physiology, psychology (Peripatos, Stoa, Epicurus), and, if the case of the Peripatetic Clearchus is representative, perhaps in anatomy as well.[8] It is a measure of the continuing attractiveness of Athens, for physicians too, that the distinguished Erasistratus, for example, seems to have studied there under Theophrastus and Strato. The Peripatos, moreover, provided strong links between the new citadel of learning and culture – Alexandria – and the old centre, Athens. (The influence of the Peripatos upon the organization of the Alexandrian Museum and Library, and on the other aspects of intellectual life in Alexandria,[9] seems to have been so considerable that 'Peripatetic' from the middle of the third century B.C. in certain contexts was used as an equivalent of 'Alexandrian'.[10])

While the idea of Herophilus in Athens is therefore not prima facie absurd, one should of course not give Hyginus' anecdote unqualified

---

[8] Clearchus wrote a treatise *On Bodies*: frs. 106–10 Wehrli. It apparently included a description of human bones and muscles and of their nomenclature.

[9] See Chapter IV. A and Fraser, 1972: vol. I, pp. 314–16, 320–1, 427, 445, 453–4, 478, 483–4, 718–19, 770, 783, etc. (with corresponding notes in vol. II).

[10] On the identification of 'Alexandrian' with 'Peripatetic' cf. Leo, 1901: 118–35; Brink, 1946: 11–12.

credence. Although it might well contain an historical residue –
women were in fact excluded from the medical profession in Athens
(see *infra, Comments* T8) – more than one factor militates against
uncritical credulity. First and most obvious, this text belongs to the
'fabula' genre and, since it is embedded in an enumeration of
mythical inventors and discoverers,. it probably underwent the
schematization and embellishment characteristic of ancient 'invention' literature. (Bonner's entirely different suggestion that it belongs
to the 'sexual exposure' literature is typologically appealing but fails
to account for its heurematistic context.[11]) Second, midwifery was
sufficiently well known in Athens by the mid fourth century for
Plato's Socrates to introduce his famous self-depiction as a midwife
who attends pregnant male psyches (*Theaetetus* 148e6–151e6), by
saying to the young mathematician Theaetetus: 'Haven't you heard,
ridiculous fellow, that I am the son of a very noble and burly midwife,
Phainarete?' (149a1–2). If midwifery was already a recognized part
of Athenian society by Plato's time (and undoubtedly much earlier),
it would of course be nonsense to depict Hagnodice as inventing it two
or three generations later at the time of Herophilus. Yet here, too, a
kernel of truth might lurk obliquely somewhere in the anecdote
inasmuch as Herophilus' treatise *Midwifery* (*infra*, T25–T26, and

---

[11] Bonner, 1920: esp. 257ff. He sees Hyginus' fable as a novella parallel to the
Christian legend of St Eugenia and to the story of Phryne's trial in Athenaeus
13.590E: a female defendant achieves acquittal by exposing her breasts or her
genitalia in court. This is a common enough gesture in ancient literature (e.g. also
Clytaemnestra when faced by the judgment of the avenging Orestes: Aeschylus,
Choephori 896–8, not noted by Bonner), and Bonner's comments are illuminating
from a *motivgeschichtliche* perspective. But this 'fable' clearly belongs to the
heurematistic genre, on the *topoi* and history of which cf. Kleingünther, 1933.
　　Because of the mention of Herophilus, Bonner's attempt to establish an
Egyptian origin for this anecdote is tempting. Bonner (a) refers to Graeco-
Egyptian female figurines in the act of pulling up their clothes to expose
themselves, and (b) he assumes that 'the story comes down to us in a work which is
undoubtedly a product of Alexandrian learning' (pp. 262–3). But his thesis
remains highly speculative and fails to take account of the heurematistic context.
See also Kremmer, 1890, and Cole, 1967: 5, 48–50, esp. 48 n. 2 and 50 n. 7, 66 n.
15. Cole and Kremmer (90–4) establish various parallels between Hyginus' *Fabula*
274 and Cassiodorus, Pliny, possibly also Diodorus and Vitruvius (Cole 66 n. 15),
etc.; but there is no mention of the Hagnodice story in other heurematistic writings
or, for that matter, in any other ancient sources. For the *topos* of a woman
disguising herself as a man in order to study with a famous person see, e.g.,
Diogenes Laertius 3.46 (= Dicaearchus fr. 44 Wehrli); Themistius, *Oration* 23
(*Sophistes*) 295c (p. 356 Dindorf; II, p. 90 Schenkl/Downey/Norman).

Chapter VII, T193–T202) is the earliest treatise known to have been devoted to this subject, and Herophilus wrote it at a time when uncomplicated deliveries were still primarily in the hands of midwives. Whatever a real Hagnodice might have accomplished – perhaps challenging the exclusion of women from the ranks of physicians – it was not exactly what Hyginus says. Disentangling fictional elaboration and factual grain in this testimonium, if indeed there was any fact, would require more evidence; meanwhile the possibilities raised above remain open.

It is doubtful that much else can be learnt from the extant evidence about Herophilus' background and residence, although some scholars are of a different view. Thus Marx (1838:2), perhaps inspired by Erasistratus' attested contact with some Peripatetics, maintains that Herophilus began his studies under Aristotle, but the ancient evidence that has come to light provides no basis for this view.

If Herophilus' apprenticeship with Praxagoras conformed to the little we know about medical education in the fourth and third centuries B.C.,[12] it probably included active clinical participation, attendance at Praxagoras' lectures, and the use of written medical treatises, at least some of which were composed by Praxagoras.[13] One may assume that the picture provided by Aeschines (in his speech *Against Timarchus*) of the aspiring young doctor Timarchus in the office or ἰατρεῖον of the physician Euthydicus is not representative, and that Timarchus represents an isolated instance of a medical student starting a career in male prostitution by exploiting the sexual potential of a physician's chambers.[14] There are other, perhaps less colourful, but more informative pieces of evidence about the ingredients of medical training in Greek antiquity, for example (a) references to medical apprentices both in the Hippocratic Corpus[15]

---

[12] Cf. the useful survey by Kudlien, 1970. Also Temkin, 1953; Cohn-Haft, 1956: 15–17; Drabkin, 1944; *id.*, 1957; Kollesch, 1979; Nutton, 1975; Krug, 1985: 190–3.

[13] The works of Praxagoras known by title include: *Physics, Anatomy, On Diseases, On Foreign Diseases, On Attendant Symptoms, Incidental Diseases, On Cures.* See Steckerl, 1958, for details.

[14] Aeschines, *Against Timarchus* 40–3 (for the subsequent string of intimacies see *ibid.* 44–76; cf. also 135ff.). Cf. J. R. Oliver, 1935 (p. 634 on Timarchus).

[15] For example *Decorum* 17, where the apprentices (τῶν μανθανόντων), especially those who have been initiated, are clearly distinguished from mere laymen (τοῖσιν ἰδιώτῃσι). Cf. also Democedes of Croton's dissembling – but to his audience perfectly credible – statement to the Persian king Darius that he did not have

and in a Ptolemaic papyrus containing the earliest legal contract for medical training (P. Heid, 226, dated 215–213 B.C.);[16] (b) mention of medical lectures (in the Hippocratic Corpus, in medical sources for the Hellenistic period, and in inscriptions);[17] and (c) numerous references to medical treatises by almost every significant leader of a medical school or faction. It might therefore be reasonable to conclude that Herophilus' training included these three ingredients.

It is unclear where Herophilus' training took place. His teacher, Praxagoras, was from the island of Cos, which had long been famous for its 'Hippocratic' medical school, and Herophilus probably went there for his medical education. Praxagoras' treatise *On Foreign Diseases* (*Peregrinae Passiones*; fr. 63 Steckerl) has been said, however, to prove that 'he left his native country . . . for a while' (Steckerl, p. 1). The itinerant teacher is familiar in Greece, and the medical profession with its *Wanderärzte* is no exception.

It is perhaps not without significance for this question that there was a lively contact between Cos and Alexandria: Ptolemy I Soter's son Philadelphus was born in Cos in 309 B.C., and Philadelphus' tutor was Philitas of Cos (perhaps more famous through Theocritus' seventh *Idyll* than for this significant educational role). P. M. Fraser, commenting on the new intelligentsia of Alexandria, says of Cos and Alexandria: 'So marked is the preponderance of persons from these cities [sc. Cos, Cyrene, Samos] that . . . the generalization may be hazarded that the intellectual achievement of Ptolemaic Alexandria was based on them' (1972: vol. I, p. 307). This statement does not give adequate credit to leading Alexandrian figures from other cities – Apollonius of Perge, Aristophanes of Byzantium, Alexander of Aetolia, Aristarchus of Samothrace, Herophilus of Chalcedon, and so

exact medical knowledge but had 'associated with a physician' (ὁμιλήσας ἰητρῷ) and thereby had gained some mediocre skill (τέχνην); Herodotus 3.130.

[16] Sattler, 1963: no. 2 (pp. 12–14); a financial contract for medical instruction. To my knowledge this is the earliest legal contract for educational purposes. The next extant one seems to be only from the year 18 B.C.; cf. Hermann, 1957–8.

[17] E.g. the Hippocratic *Precepts* 12. Galen mentions the lectures (ἀκροάσεις) of the Herophilean Bacchius (VIII, p. 732K). See also *Monumenti Antichi (Reale Accademia dei Lincei)* 23 (1914), 59ff., no. 48 for decrees in honour of a doctor, Asclepiades of Perge, who is praised for 'having set forth many useful things pertaining to health in his lectures in his school' (lines 7ff.; cf. lines 34–5); and *Supplementum Epigraphicum Graecum* 19.467 (second century B.C., Histria), in honour of a physician, 'Diocles of Cyzicus, son of Artemidorus', whose ἀκροάσεις (lectures) are mentioned in line 8.

on – but it does emphasize an important point. Since the contact between Cos and Alexandria became firmly established much earlier than, for example, that between Alexandria and Samos, it is not inconceivable that Herophilus' medical education could have taken place under Praxagoras in Alexandria. In the absence of any firm evidence about a visit to Alexandria by Praxagoras, however, it seems more likely that Cos was the location of Herophilus' training, and that the impact upon Herophilus of the early contact between Chalcedon and Alexandria was reinforced during Herophilus' sojourn in Cos by the lively contact between Cos and Alexandria.

One final biographical point requires brief comment. It has been argued, with reference to T10, that Herophilus' 'humble origins appear to be indicated by Galen's description of him . . . as "he who was reared beside the looms", i.e. in a weaving establishment. This is perhaps more likely in Alexandria than in Chalcedon' (Fraser, 1972: vol. II, p. 503 n. 55). The judgment about Alexandria vs. Chalcedon is purely conjectural. But of more serious consequence is the fact that the person to whom Galen in T10 refers as 'nurtured at the looms' is in fact not Herophilus but a 'Methodist' physician of the Neronian period, Thessalus.[18]

The sociologically provocative suggestion that Herophilus was of 'humble origins' therefore seems to be without textual foundation.

2 Date

Trying to determine with accuracy when Herophilus lived is a frustrating undertaking; there are many tantalizingly suggestive and apparently informative pieces of evidence which, upon closer examination, turn out to be inconclusive. I shall consider them one by one.

(i) A significant clue seems to be provided by T9 and T11, which inform us that Herophilus was a pupil of Praxagoras of Cos. Further confirmation of this relationship is offered by T10 (at least if one reads, as one probably should, the 'his' (*autou*) accompanying

---

[18] Galen, *Methodus medendi* 1.2 (x, p. 10K): . . . ὦ τολμηρότατε Θεσσαλέ, . . . κρῖναι γοῦν ἀδύνατον ἦν σοι, τραφέντι μὲν ἐν γυναικωνίτιδι παρὰ πατρὶ μοχθηρῶς ἔρια ξαίνοντι . . . ; *id.*, *De crisibus* 2.3 (ix, p. 657K): . . . ἐν τῇ γυναικωνίτιδι τρεφόμενος ὁ ληρώδης Θεσσαλὸς ὑπὸ πατρὶ μοχθηρῶς ἔρια ξαίνοντι κακῶς ἐτόλμα λέγειν . . . See also n. 41 below.

'teacher' (*didaskalon*) as referring to Herophilus, not to Phylotimus).[19]

The date of Praxagoras is, however, still disputed. E. D. Baumann places Praxagoras' prime as early as 340–320 B.C.; Fridolf Kudlien puts it at 325 B.C.; Fritz Steckerl, Kurt Bardong and P. M. Fraser at 300 B.C.; Werner Jaeger at 300 B.C. or 'shortly after 300 B.C.'.[20] The later date – 300 B.C. or after – has become more widely accepted, but it is dependent on acceptance of Jaeger's contention that Diocles of Carystus (who was somewhat older than Praxagoras and is said to have influenced him) became a significant figure only at the very end of the fourth century B.C.[21] or, in Jaeger's own revised version,[22] in the first decades of the third century B.C., under Peripatetic influence.

It is significant for our purposes that Jaeger's revised date for Diocles (340–260 B.C.) depends in part on his conviction that Diocles lived long enough to engage in polemics against Herophilus. Herophilus' prime Jaeger ascribes to the 270s or 260s, but without discussing his only evidence (T14; see below) in more than passing fashion. If Diocles' date depends upon that of Herophilus, and Praxagoras' in turn depends on Diocles' – as in Jaeger's theory – then we clearly could not use the references to Praxagoras as Herophilus' teacher in T9–T11 to date Herophilus; this would simply complete the vicious circle Herophilus–Diocles–Praxagoras–Herophilus.

But can Herophilus in fact be used to reconstruct the date of Diocles, as Jaeger maintained? The answer must be largely negative. In his earlier work, *Diokles von Karystos*, Jaeger actually conceded that the only direct evidence for a reply by Diocles to Herophilus – Vindician's account (fourth century A.D.) of their views on the generation of sperm (see below, Chapter VII, T191) – is typical of the synchronistic schematization of compilatory literature in later antiquity and that it is therefore without value for reconstructing the dates of Herophilus or Diocles. I could not agree more.

Why then did Jaeger do a somersault in his slightly later articles on this issue (nn. 20, 22), and claim that the passage in Vindician proves

[19] Although both interpretations are possible, it is almost certainly correct to read this as 'Herophilus' teacher Praxagoras' in view of Phylotimus' designation as 'fellow student' (συμφοιτητής).

[20] Bauman, 1937; Kudlien, 1972b, and *id.*, *LAW* 2427; Steckerl, 1958: 2–3; Bardong, 1954; Jaeger, 1938b (esp. Anhang I). Cf. Sherwin-White, 1978: 102.

[21] Jaeger, 1938a: Diocles is a pupil of 'the older Aristotle' and died between 300 and 288/7 B.C.

[22] Jaeger, 1938b and 1940: Diocles lived from *c.* 340 to 260 B.C.

that Diocles tried to refute Herophilus? Apparently mainly because the territory Galatia is mentioned – though only once, and in an entirely different context – by Diocles (fr. 125 Wellmann = Athenaeus 2.59a). Since the first incursions of the Celtic Galatians into Asia Minor took place in 278 B.C., Jaeger argues, the name 'Galatia' could not have been used before 270 or 260 B.C. (a questionable conclusion at best); hence Diocles lived at least until 260 B.C. and could have 'replied' to Herophilus, as Vindician claims. Yet Kaibel, in his edition of Athenaeus, had already observed that καὶ Γαλατίᾳ ('and in Galatia') seems to be a corrupt reading ('videtur corruptum'), and Felix Jacoby on grounds of both content and style called it 'obviously a later insertion' into the text;[23] Ludwig Edelstein, too, advanced significant objections to using 'Galatia' for chronological reconstructions.[24] Equally inconclusive for Jaeger's chronological hypothesis are, as Kudlien points out,[25] the reference to 'a certain Diocles' in the will of the Peripatetic Strato of Lampsacus (†269 B.C.) and other indirect evidence about Diocles' date cited by Jaeger. In fact, the claim that Diocles lived long enough to polemicize against Herophilus seems to be refuted by most of the evidence, which places Diocles firmly between Hippocrates and Praxagoras within the sequence of great physicians (more on this below).

Furthermore, Jaeger operates with a concept of 'influence' – Aristotle and the Peripatos 'influenced' Diocles, hence Diocles could not have lived before the very end of the fourth century – which is so flexible and broad that it fails to establish beyond doubt that it was in fact Aristotle who influenced Diocles, and not the other way around. Theoretical affinities alone provide no proof of chronological priority. And even if Aristotle is 'the influencer' and Diocles 'the influenced', this does not necessarily entail that the 'influencer' *must* be a generation older, or even a day older, than his victim. Such are the fallacies of an *Entwicklungsgeschichte* that draws its central concepts and metaphors from biological models. Jaeger played the dating game – as well as the 'influence' and 'development' game – with a

[23] In a letter to Jaeger, mentioned in Jaeger, 1960: vol. II, 203 n. 1. On the Galatian incursions, see Rostovtzeff, 1953: vol. I, 578–84; Droysen, 1952–3: vol. III, 57, 166ff., 174f., 181, 204ff.; vol. II, 257ff.
[24] In his review of Jaeger's book on Diocles: Edelstein, 1940 = Edelstein, 1967: 145–52.
[25] Kudlien, 1963b. Cf. also Torraca, 1965.

confidence in general not warranted by his evidence;[26] more scepticism and less assertive certitude is needed in dealing with these questions.

If Werner Jaeger's chronological suppositions concerning Diocles cannot be established by the evidence he adduces,[27] then the chronology he offers for Praxagoras, Herophilus, and other physicians, being entirely dependent upon his thesis about Diocles, also becomes suspect. In the absence of firm evidence that Diocles' sun set near the middle of the third century, it seems reasonable to restore him to his traditional doxographic position as a figure belonging to the fourth century B.C., perhaps a contemporary of Aristotle (384–322 B.C.), although absolute certainty is at present impossible. This would make room for Diocles' younger contemporary, Praxagoras, in the last half of the fourth century, rather than rendering Praxagoras – as Jaeger would have us do – an exact contemporary of Diocles, in flagrant contradiction of most of the ancient evidence.

If this hypothesis has any merit, Herophilus 'the student of Praxagoras' might well have been born between 330 and 320 B.C. and have completed his medical training under Praxagoras around the turn of the century. This would be compatible with further considerations raised below.

(ii) Indirect corroboration that Herophilus belongs to the generation after Praxagoras is provided by T12 and T13, which seem to assign the physician Chrysippus to the same generation as Herophilus' teacher Praxagoras, and Erasistratus to the next (while also making Herophilus a contemporary of Erasistratus). If this Chrysippus is identical with Erasistratus' teacher by that name,[28] and if Erasistratus was indeed a contemporary of Herophilus (as T12 and, more explicitly, T14 confirm), one might have hoped to learn something from the dates of Chrysippus and Erasistratus. The chronology and

---

[26] In fairness to Jaeger it must be pointed out that he was aware of some of the problems I mentioned and at times conceded that he was on uncertain ground. Yet this did not prevent him from drawing precise chronological conclusions which, in subsequent scholarship, were widely accepted without regard for Jaeger's own caveats.

[27] The reader should be warned that not all current scholars share my scepticism. Cf., e.g., Longrigg, 1975b: 228: 'Jaeger has convincingly demonstrated' the chronological thesis advanced in his *Diokles* (Jaeger, 1938a).

[28] Diogenes Laertius 7.186; Galen XI.221 and 230K; *id.*, *CMG* v.10.2.2, p. 44.14–16 Wenkebach.

identity of the several physicians called Chrysippus remains chaotic, however,[29] and the name is therefore not of much help.

(iii) For Erasistratus, on the other hand, we do have firmer though by no means uncontroversial evidence. Passages in Plutarch, Valerius Maximus, and Appian suggest that Erasistratus was active in Antioch as a physician at the court of Seleucus I Nicator about 293 B.C.,[30] and this date is not incommensurate with the rest of what we know about his life. It is, however, incompatible with Max Wellmann's influential thesis that Erasistratus was as much as thirty years younger than Herophilus. Wellmann's view is based in part on the fact that Eusebius and Jerome assign Erasistratus' floruit to the third and fourth years of the 130th Olympiad, i.e. 258–257 B.C., under Ptolemy Philadelphus.[31] Eusebius' chronicle is, however, notoriously unreliable, as its editor Helm emphasizes (GCS 47, pp. lxiiff.). Wellmann's other arguments in favour of placing Erasistratus' birth between 310 and 300 B.C. have been shown in a detailed analysis by P. M. Fraser (1969; cf. n. 30) to be inconclusive as well, and this leaves us with 293 B.C. as our most firm evidence. A date of c. 330 to 255/250 B.C. for Erasistratus' life therefore does not seem implausible. If this is correct, Galen's designation of Erasistratus as a contemporary of Herophilus (T14) would square with the date I have proposed for Herophilus (330/320)–260/250 B.C.).

It would also be consonant with the doxographical tradition which makes Herophilus and Erasistratus members of the same generation. One must nevertheless guard against an uncritical acceptance of a chronological schematization that seems to have entered the doxographic tradition fairly early, perhaps under Empiric influence. The doxographers consistently used the following chronological sequence in their systematization of medical history:

1. Hippocrates
2. Diocles

[29] Cf. Wellmann, 1899 and id., 1900a; Fraser, 1969, and 1972: vol. I p. 347, vol. II, p. 502 n. 45.
[30] Fraser, 1969; cf. also Lloyd, 1975b; infra p. 142 n. 7.
[31] Eusebius, vol. 7 (Chronicon), ed. R. Helm, GCS 47 (1956), 131. 18–19 (Ol.130.4): 'Erasistratus medicus agnoscitur'; and vol. 5, ed. Karst, GCS 20 (1911), 200: 'Erasistratos war als berühmter Arzt gekannt' (under Ol.130.3). Wellmann, 1900a: 380 (further references to other articles by Wellmann in Fraser, 1969).

3. Praxagoras and Chrysippus
4. Herophilus and Erasistratus

(although Erasistratus is sometimes also listed as postdating Herophilus). With slight variations this sequence occurs, for example, in Celsus (T12), Pliny (T13), the pseudo-Galenic *Introductio sive medicus* (T1), the Anonymus Laurentianus (cod. Laur. Lat. 73, 1, eleventh century; T3), and the Anonymus Bambergensis (cod. Bamb. L. III. 8 med. 1, ninth century; T16a).

While not entirely invalid, such neat generational 'histories' fail to accommodate age differences between contemporaries or relative closeness in the ages of members of two different 'generations'. To put it differently, a doxographic sequence of ἀκμαί does not guarantee that there is a neat interval of twenty-five or thirty years between each ἀκμή and the next. Even if Erasistratus were twenty or thirty years younger than Herophilus, as Wellmann (in my view erroneously) suggests, he could have surfaced as a 'contemporary' of Herophilus in a doxographical list.

The stronger and harder evidence is, then, that which testifies to Erasistratus' activity as a court physician in 293 B.C., and this provides at least some corroboration for the date proposed here for Herophilus (although its significance could be compromised by considerations such as those just raised).

In addition to Erasistratus, three persons are mentioned as 'contemporaries' of Herophilus: Phylotimus[32] (T14, T10), Eudemus (T14), and Diodorus Cronus, the master of the 'dialectic' school (T15).

(iv) Eudemus, whom Galen more than once mentions with Herophilus, usually in anatomical contexts, provides no firm chronological pegs on which one could hang conjectures about the date of Herophilus.[33] (See below (*Comments*, T14) for a more detailed discussion of Eudemus.)

(v) Two inscriptions from Cos, dated 300–260 B.C., mention a

---

[32] More often written 'Philotimus' – which is also a more common name – but Diller, 1941: col. 1030, cites better MSS support for 'Phyl-'. Cf. Steckerl, 1958: 108–23.

[33] Cf. also Wellmann in Susemihl, 1891–2: vol. I, p. 811, and Wellmann, 1907b.

Phylotimus. If Rudolf Herzog's conclusion[34] that this Phylotimus is identical with the physician is correct, it would corroborate my suggestion that Herophilus' main activity occurred in the first half of the third century. While plausible, Herzog's theory is, however, not demonstrable, and again we are left with a tantalizing but inconclusive piece of evidence.

(vi) Diodorus Cronus' floruit is probably c. 315–285 B.C. His famous 'debate' with the Megarian Stilpon in the presence of Ptolemy I Soter probably occurred in Alexandria in the early third century B.C. (although this, too, is a disputed view).[35] If Diodorus was a contemporary of Herophilus *and* already famous before the turn of the century – this is also implied by the fact that the Stoic Zeno of Citium (*c.* 350/335–263 B.C.) was one of his students (Suda s.v. Zeno; D.L. 7.25) – Diodorus would seem to have been older than Herophilus. While Sextus (T15) seems to imply that both Herophilus and Diodorus were already famous when Diodorus sought Herophilus' medical help and instead received some dialectical flak, there is no reason why the older dialectician could not have consulted the younger 'dialectician' (T10) a few years after the turn of the century, when Herophilus, too, had established his reputation. (Efforts to use Bentley's reconstitution of Callimachus' epigram on Diodorus (fr. 393 Pfeiffer) to reconstruct the date of the encounter between Diodorus and *Herophilus* seem doomed to inconclusiveness.)

The evidence about this encounter might contain fabricated elements and does not provide decisive chronological help, but it warns against dating Herophilus too late in the third century.

Every piece of evidence about the date of Herophilus accordingly

[34] Herzog, 1928: 37–8. Deichgräber, 1933: 144f., has shown that not all of Herzog's conclusions are tenable. Paton & Hicks, 1891, do, however, include the text of an inscription referring to 'Phylotimus, son of Biton' (no. 387, line 24), and suggest *c.* 240 B.C. as its date (Appendix C, p. 336). Cf. Sherwin-White, 1978: 105 n. 116, 195, 280; Fraser, 1972: vol. I, p. 345; vol. II, p. 501 n. 34; Steckerl, 1958: 108–23; Diller, 1941.

[35] D.L. 2.111–12 = Döring, 1972: fr. 99 (fr. 100 = Pliny, *Nat. Hist.* 7.53.180, probably has more anecdotal than historical value). Cf. Döring, 1972: 124–8, on Diodorus' life. According to D.L. 2.115 (fr. 150 Döring) Stilpon refused to accept Ptolemy's invitation to Egypt, and this makes it possible that the debate occurred when Ptolemy himself conquered Megara (307 B.C.). But see Sedley, 1977: esp. 78–83 (Diodorus *fl.* 315–284 B.C.).

turns out to be open to more than one interpretation or to lead down a dead-end alley (or, at best, to provide only approximate dates). The frustrating search for firm, independent anchors has uncovered mostly slippery, elusive strands, several of them so interlinked that they fail to provide genuinely independent criteria. Nevertheless we do have (a) the fact that Praxagoras was Herophilus' teacher, (b) the doxographic tradition which locates Herophilus in the 'generation' after Praxagoras, (c) his fame as an *Alexandrian* physician, and (d) the mention of Erasistratus, Phylotimus, and Diodorus Cronus as his contemporaries; all of this suggests that 330/320-260/50 B.C. would not be an implausible conjecture. But this conclusion is as tentative as the evidence on which it rests is tenuous.

B · TEXTS

1 Ps.-Galenus, *Introductio sive medicus* 4 (xiv, p. 683K)

προέστησαν δὲ τῆς μὲν λογικῆς αἱρέσεως Ἱπποκράτης Κῷος, ὃς καὶ αἱρεσιάρχης ἐγένετο καὶ πρῶτος συνέστησε τὴν λογικὴν αἵρεσιν, μετὰ δὲ τοῦτον Διοκλῆς ὁ Καρύστιος, Πραξαγόρας Κῷος, Ἡρόφιλος Χαλκηδόνιος, Ἐρασίστρατος Κεῖος, Μνησί-
5 θεος Ἀθηναῖος, Ἀσκληπιάδης Βιθυνός Κιανός, ὃς καὶ Προυσιεὺς ἐκαλεῖτο . . . τῆς δὲ ἐμπειρικῆς προέστηκε Φιλῖνος Κῷος, ὁ πρῶτος αὐτὴν ἀποτεμόμενος ἀπὸ τῆς λογικῆς αἱρέσεως, τὰς ἀφορμὰς λαβὼν παρὰ Ἡροφίλου, οὗ καὶ ἀκουστὴς ἐγένετο.

4 Χῖος: *corr. Wellmann*   5 Κιανός: *del. Wellmann sed cf. Rawson, 1982:359*   Προυσίας: *corr. Wellmann*   6 προέστηκε *Schöne*: προέστησαν *LPM*: προέστησε *cett.*   7 ἀποτεμόμενος *Deichgräber*: ἀποτεμνόμενος *P vett.*

1 At the head of the rationalist school [sc. of medicine] stood Hippocrates of Cos, who was also the principal leader of the school and first established this rationalist school, and, after him, Diocles of Carystus, Praxagoras of Cos, Herophilus of Chalcedon, Erasistratus of Ceos, Mnesitheus of Athens, and Asclepiades the Cian of Bithynia, also called Asclepiades of Prusias. . . At the head of the Empiricist school, on the other hand, stood Philinus of Cos, who was the first to have severed it from the rationalist school, after getting the impulse for doing so from Herophilus, whose pupil he was.

2 Galenus, *De usu partium* 1.8 (I, p. 15 Helmreich)

... οὕτω δ' οὐκ ὀλίγοις ἄλλοις ἰατροῖς τε καὶ φιλοσόφοις, ἧττον μὲν ἴσως 'Αριστοτέλους, καλῶς δ' οὖν καὶ αὐτοῖς, ὥσπερ ἀμέλει καὶ 'Ηροφίλῳ τῷ Καλχηδονίῳ (sc. εἴρηται περὶ χρείας μορίων). (*Vid. Herophili T136 infra.*)

2 ἀριστοτέλους *U*: ἢ ἀριστοτέλει *CD*   3 Καλχηδονίῳ *scripsi*: καρχηδονίῳ *codd.*: Χαλκηδονίῳ *Marx, Helmreich (sed cf. infra comm., adn. 1, et eandem mutationem apud Diog. Laert. 2.106 et Hdt. 4.144.2)*

2 Thus several other physicians and philosophers also [sc. expressed themselves about the usefulness of the parts of the body], perhaps less fully than Aristotle, but competently too, among them of course Herophilus of Chalcedon ... (*See Chapter* VII, *T136 infra.*)

3 Anonymus Laurentianus: *Codex Laurentianus Latinus* 73, 1 (s.XI), fol. 143r, col. 2 (*Hermes* 35 (1900), 370 (Wellmann))

(fol. 142v.: nomina auctorum medicinae Aegyptiorum vel Graecorum et Latinorum ...)
... Praxagoras Nicharchi filius,
Herophilus Chalcedonius,
5 Erasistratus Cleombroti filius Ceius ...

4 Herofilius calcedonius *cod.*: *corr. Wellmann*

3 (Names of Egyptian, Greek, and Latin authors of medicine ...)
... Praxagoras the son of Nicharchus,
Herophilus of Chalcedon,
Erasistratus of Ceos, son of Cleombrotus ...

4 Galenus, *De anatomicis administrationibus* 9.5 (II, p. 731 K)

... καὶ μάλιστά γε κατὰ τὴν 'Αλεξάνδρειαν οὕτω γλύφουσι τοὺς καλάμους οἷς γράφομεν, ἔνθα διατρίβοντα τὸν 'Ηρόφιλον ... (*Vid. Herophili T79 infra.*)

4 Particularly in Alexandria they carve the pens with which we write this way, and since Herophilus lived there ... (*See Chapter* VI, *T79 infra.*)

5a Vindicianus, *Gynaecia*, praef. (vel 2), cod. *L* (K. Sudhoff, *AGM* 8 (1915), pp. 417–18)

(See Chapter VI, *T64a infra.)*

5b Vindicianus, *Gynaecia*, praef. (vel 2), cod. *M* (J. Schipper, *Ein neuer Text der Gynaecia des Vindician* (Diss. med. Leipzig, 1921), p. 13)

maioribus enim auctoribus hoc est prioribus in Alexandria agentibus medicinam id est Rufo et Philippo, Lupo et Erasistrato, Pelope, et Erophilo, Hypocrate et Apollonio et ceteris anathomicis licuit mortuos exenterare . . .

1–4 maiores enim nostri hos est priores vel antiquis in Alexandria gentibus medicinae lupione vel opphi et erofilo herasque servatus asclepiades et yppocras et apollonio et ceteris anatomicis. id est securioribus quibus licuit mortuus aperire . . . *G. (Cf. etiam alios codd. dett. apud V. Rose, Theodori Prisciani Euporiston et Vindiciani Afri reliquiae, Lips. 1894, pp. 428–9 et p. 427 sub cod. D, col. III.)*   2 Arasistrato *M: corr. e LF*   3 Ereophilo *M: corr. e LG*

5b For our ancestral, i.e., the earlier, experts who practised medicine in Alexandria, namely Rufus, Philip, Lycus, Erasistratus, Pelops, Herophilus, Hippocrates, Apollonius, and other anatomists were allowed to disembowel the dead.

6 Galenus, *De anatomicis administrationibus* 14.5 (II, p. 133 Simon; p. 201 Duckworth)

(See Chapter VI, *T90 infra.)*

7 A. Cornelius Celsus, *Medicina* 1 (*Artes* 6), prohoem. 23 (*CML* 1, p. 21 Marx)

. . . Herophilum et Erasistratum, qui nocentes homines a regibus ex carcere acceptos vivos inciderint . . . *(Vid. T63 infra.)*

1 a regibus ex *FV*: quia regibus *J*

7 . . . Herophilus and Erasistratus, who laid open living criminals

whom they had received out of prison from the kings . . . *(See Chapter* VI, *T63 infra.)*

8 Hyginus, *Fabula* 274 (quis quid invenerit) 10–11, p. 167 Rose

> 10. antiqui obstetrices non habuerunt, unde mulieres verecundia ductae interierant. nam Athenienses caverant ne quis servus aut femina artem medicinam disceret. Hagnodice quaedam puella virgo concupivit medicinam discere, quae cum concupis-
> 5 set, demptis capillis habitu virili se Herophilo cuidam tradidit in disciplinam. 11. quae cum artem didicisset, et feminam laborantem audisset ab inferiore parte, veniebat ad eam, quae cum credere se noluisset, aestimans virum esse, illa tunica sublata ostendit se feminam esse, et ita eas curabat.

3 Hagnodice *Rose*: Agn- *F*   5 Hierophilo *F*: *corr. M. Schmidt*

8 10. The ancients had no midwives, and therefore women died [sc. in childbirth], led on by their sense of shame. For the Athenians had taken heed that no slave or woman should learn the science of medicine. A certain girl, Hagnodice, as a young women desired to learn the science of medicine. Because of this desire, she cut her hair, put on male clothing, and entrusted herself to a certain Herophilus for her training. 11. After learning this science, when she heard that a woman was having labour-pains, she used to go to her. And when the woman refused to entrust herself [to Hagnodice], thinking that she was a man, Hagnodice lifted her undergarment and revealed that she was a woman. In this way she used to cure women.

9 Galenus, *De tremore, palpitatione, convulsione et rigore* 1 (VII, pp. 584–5K)

> διὰ τοῦτο ἔδοξέ μοι κοινῇ περὶ πάντων αὐτῶν (sc. σφυγμοῦ καὶ παλμοῦ καὶ σπασμοῦ καὶ τρόμου) ἐν τῷδε τῷ γράμματι διελθεῖν, οὐχ ἵνα ἐλέγξαιμι Πραξαγόραν ἐν οἷς σφάλλεται, τοῦτο μὲν γὰρ αὐτάρκως Ἡρόφιλος ἔπραξε, μαθητὴς αὐτοῦ γενόμενος, ἀλλ’
> 5 ἵν’ οἷς ὀρθῶς ἐκεῖνος ἔγραψε τὰ λείποντα προσθῶ.

9 For this reason I decided to deal with all these things [sc. pulse, palpitation, convulsion, and trembling] together in this treatise, not in order to refute Praxagoras where he took false steps – for this has been done adequately by Herophilus, who was his pupil – but in order to add what is missing to what he wrote correctly.

10 Galenus, *Methodus medendi* 1.3 (x, pp. 27–8K)

ἢ εἴπερ ἑτέραν τινὰ βελτίω (sc. μέθοδον) τῆς παρ' ἐκείνων (sc. Πλάτωνος, Ἀριστοτέλους, Χρυσίππου, κτλ.) γεγραμμένης ἐξεῦρες (sc. ὦ Θέσσαλε, ἐχρῆν) αὐτὸ τοῦτο πρότερον ἀγωνίσασ-θαι, καὶ δεῖξαι καὶ διδάξαι τοὺς Ἕλληνας ὡς ὁ παρὰ τοῖς ἱστοῖς
5 τραφεὶς ὑπερεβάλετο μὲν Ἀριστοτέλη καὶ Πλάτωνα μεθόδοις λογικαῖς, κατεπάτησε δὲ Θεόφραστόν τε καὶ τοὺς Στωϊκοὺς ἐν διαλεκτικῇ, φανερῶς δ' ἐξήλεγξε τοὺς ἑταίρους αὐτῶν ἅπαν-τας, οὐδὲ τίνα ποτ' ἐστὶ τὰ πρῶτα νοσήματα γιγνώσκοντας, τὸν Ἡρόφιλον ἐκεῖνον τὸν διαλεκτικόν, καὶ τὸν συμφοιτητὴν
10 αὐτοῦ Φυλότιμον καὶ τὸν διδάσκαλον αὐτοῦ Πραξαγόραν τὸν ἀπὸ Ἀσκληπιοῦ, καὶ σὺν τούτοις τε καὶ πρὸ τούτων Ἐρασίσ-τρατον, Διοκλέα, Μνησίθεον, Διευχῆ, Φιλιστίωνα, Πλειστόνικον, αὐτὸν Ἱπποκράτην.

10 Or if indeed, [Thessalus], you discovered some better [method] than the one described by them [sc. by Plato, Aristotle, Chrysippus, etc.], you should have argued for it first and shown and taught the Greeks that the person nurtured at the looms [sc. Thessalus] surpassed Aristotle and Plato in rational methods, that he trampled down Theophrastus and the Stoics in dialectic, and that he convicted all their colleagues (i.e., the dialectician Herophilus, his fellow student Phylotimus, and his teacher Praxagoras, a descendant of Asclepius; also – contemporary with them as well as prior to them – Erasistratus, Diocles, Mnesitheus, Dieuches, Philistion, Plistonicus, and Hippocrates himself) of not even recognizing which the primary diseases are.

11 Galenus (ex Aristoxeno?), *De pulsuum differentiis* 4.3 (viii, p. 723K)

οὐ σμικρὰ δ' ἀντιλογία ... γέγονεν Ἡροφίλῳ πρὸς τὸν διδάσκαλον Πραξαγόραν ... (*Vid. Herophili T150 infra.*)

11 No paltry dispute arose between Herophilus and his teacher
Praxagoras ... *(See Chapter* VII, *T150 infra.)*

12 A. Cornelius Celsus, *Medicina* 1 (*Artes* 6), prohoem. 8 (*CML*
1, p. 18 Marx)

> huius (sc. Democriti) autem, ut quidam crediderunt, discipulus
> Hippocrates Cous, primus ex omnibus memoria dignus, a studio
> sapientiae disciplinam hanc (sc. medicinam) separavit ... post
> quem Diocles Carystius, deinde Praxagoras et Chrysippus, tum
> 5 Herophilus et Erasistratus sic artem hanc exercuerunt, ut etiam
> in diversas curandi vias processerint. *(Vid. Herophili T49 infra.)*

> 1 discipulos *V*   2 Chous *FJ*   *ex omnibus FV*: quidem *J*   2 dignis
> *Caesarius*   4 quam *V*   *tum FV*: et *J*   5 sic *om. J*   *ut FV*: atque
> *J*   6 processerunt *J*

12 But it was, as some believed, a pupil of Democritus, Hippocrates
of Cos, a man first and foremost worthy of being remembered, who
separated this branch of learning [sc. medicine] from the study of
philosophy ... After him Diocles of Carystus, next Praxagoras and
Chrysippus, and then Herophilus and Erasistratus, practised this
science in such a way that they made progress also towards various
methods of treatment. *(See Chapter* IV, *T49 infra.)*

13 C. Plinius Secundus, *Historia naturalis* 26.6.10–11

> Hippocratis certe, qui primus medendi praecepta clarissime
> condidit, referta herbarum mentione invenimus volumina, nec
> minus Diocli Carysti, qui secundus aetate famaque extitit, item
> Praxagorae et Chrysippi ac deinde Erasistrati Cei, Herophilo
> 5 quidem, quamquam subtilioris sectae conditori, ante omnis
> celebratam rationem eam paulatim, usu efficacissimo rerum
> omnium magistro, peculiariter utique medicinae, ad verba
> garrulitatemque descendentem.

> 4 Cei *Pintianus e Strabone*: co *codd.*: Coi *Sillig*   6 ab usu *? Ma*
> 8 defendentem *VRE*: -te *Ha*

13 Certainly we find the works of Hippocrates, who was the first to establish with great brilliance the rules for medical treatment, crammed with mention of herbs, and no less so the works of Diocles of Carystus, who was second in time and reputation. Likewise the works of Praxagoras and Chrysippus, and next those of Erasistratus of Ceos; indeed [we find] this method [sc. the herbal] used above all others by Herophilus, even though he was the founder of a more exact school of medicine. But gradually [we find it] descending to mere words and chattering, although experience is the most effectual teacher in all things and especially in medicine.

14 Galenus, *In Hippocratis Aphorismos commentarius* 6.1 (XVIII A, p. 7K)

τοῦτο γὰρ οὐδεὶς προσέθηκεν οὔτε τῶν κατὰ τὸν αὐτὸν αὐτῷ (sc. τῷ Ἐρασιστράτῳ) γεγονότων χρόνον ἐπιφανεστάτων, οἷον Φυλότιμος, Ἡρόφιλος, Εὔδημος, οὔτε τῶν μετ᾿ αὐτὸν γενομένων τις ἄχρι τῶν νεωτέρων τούτων τῶν περὶ τὸν Ἀρχιγένην.
5 (*Vid. T220 infra.*)

2 χρόνων *Kühn, edd.: corr.*

14 This, you see, no one added: neither any of the most illustrious [doctors] who lived at the same time as he [sc. Erasistratus], for example Phylotimus, Herophilus, and Eudemus, nor any of those who lived after him, until these more recent followers of Archigenes. (*See Chapter* VII, *T220 infra.*)

15 Sextus Empiricus, *Hypotyposes Pyrrhoneae* 2.245

φέρεται δὲ καὶ Ἡροφίλου τοῦ ἰατροῦ χαρίεν < τι > ἀπομνημόνευμα· συνεχρόνισε γὰρ οὗτος Διοδώρῳ, ὃς ἐναπειροκαλῶν τῇ διαλεκτικῇ λόγους διεξῄει σοφιστικοὺς κατά τε ἄλλων πολλῶν καὶ τῆς κινήσεως. ὡς οὖν ἐκβαλών ποτε ὦμον ὁ Διόδωρος ἧκε
5 θεραπευθησόμενος ὡς τὸν Ἡρόφιλον, ἐχαριεντίσατο ἐκεῖνος πρὸς αὐτὸν λέγων "ἤτοι ἐν ᾧ ἦν τόπῳ ὁ ὦμος ὢν ἐκπέπτωκεν ἢ ἐν ᾧ οὐκ ἦν· οὔτε δὲ ἐν ᾧ ἦν οὔτε ἐν ᾧ οὐκ ἦν· οὐκ ἄρα ἐκπέπτωκεν", ὡς τὸν σοφιστὴν λιπαρεῖν ἐᾶν μὲν τοὺς τοιούτους λόγους, τὴν δὲ ἐξ ἰατρικῆς ἁρμόζουσαν αὐτῷ προσάγειν
10 θεραπείαν.

1 τι *add. T* (gratum quid)   2 ἐναπειροκαλῶν *Bekker*: ἐν ἀπειροκάλω *G*: in dyalectica inexpertus *T* (*sed cf.* ἀπειρολογία *S.E. P 2.151*)   3 κατὰ *G*: de *T*   5 *ad* ἐχαριεντίσατο *L in marg.* habet εὐτραπελίσατο, ἔσκοψεν 6 λέγων *Ac T* (dicens): λέγω *G*   ὢν om. *T*

15 A lovely reminiscence concerning the physician Herophilus is also transmitted. He was a contemporary of Diodorus, who, invoking dialectic endlessly, used to expound sophistical arguments against motion as well as many other things. So, when Diodorus dislocated his shoulder once and came to Herophilus for medical treatment, Herophilus with charming wit said to him: 'Your shoulder was dislocated either being in the place where it was or being where it was not; but [it was dislocated] neither where it was nor where it was not; therefore it has not been dislocated.' As a result the sophist implored him to drop such arguments and to apply instead a suitable treatment based on medicine.

16a Anonymus Bambergensis: *Cod. Bambergens.* L.iii.8 (med. 1) [s.IX], fol. 6r (K. Sudhoff, *AGM* 8 (1915), 411)

posteriores autem eius (sc. Hippocratis) qui successerunt hic sunt: Thessalus, Dracon, Hippocrates iunior, Polybus, quorum libri non apparuerunt. subsequente autem tempore facti sunt rationabiles potentes medici Diocles, Praxagoras, Herophilus, 5 Erasistratus, Asclepiades, Athenaeus, Agathinus, Ariston, Archigenes, Herodotus, Philumenus, Antyllus.

2 Draccus *B*   Epocratis *B*   Polybus *scripsi (cf. comm.)*: Poliemmius *B* 4 Dioclex *B*   Praxacoras *B*   Herophilos *B*   5 Agatheneus *B* 6 Philominus Antillus *B*

16a The ones after Hippocrates who succeeded him are these: Thessalus, Draco, Hippocrates the Younger, Polybus, whose books have not made their appearance. But in the ensuing period these 'rationalist' physicians became powerful: Diocles, Praxagoras, Herophilus, Erasistratus, Asclepiades, Athenaeus, Agathinus, Ariston, Archigenes, Herodotus, Philumenus, Antyllus.

16b Iohannes Alexandrinus, *Commentaria in librum De sectis Galeni*, prooem. 2ra (pp. 15–16 Pritchet)

Sed nunc videamus qui medicinam constituerunt et eos auctores secundum sectas suas nominemus. empericam namque sectam Serapion et Apollonius senior et Apollonius iunior et Eraclides Nicomachus Glaucias Menedotus Sextus Afer; logicam sectam
5 Ypocras Praxagoras Diocles Erasistratus Crisippus Erofilus Leufastus Asclipiades Galenus. illi empiricam, isti logicam constituerunt. methodicam sectam Themison Thesalus . . .

1 eos] eius *R fort. recte*   3 Eraclitus *codd.*, *Pritchet*: Eraclides (*sc.*
Heraclides Tarentinus) *scripsi*

16b But now let us look who established medicine and let us name those authors according to their schools. Serapion, Apollonius the elder, Apollonius the younger, Heraclides [sc. of Terantum], Nicomachus, Glaucias, Menedotus, and Sextus Afer established the Empiricist school. The Rationalist school [was established by] Hippocrates, Praxagoras, Diocles, Erasistratus, Chrysippus, Herophilus, Leufastus, Asclepiades, and Galen. The former established the Empiricist school, the latter the Rationalist school. The Methodist school by Themison, Thessalus . . .

C · COMMENTS

T1 The idea of a 'rationalist school' of medicine is a doxographic convenience which has limited historical justification. Hippocrates no more established such a school than Herophilus joined it or formally 'stood at the head' of it. Like other authors of later antiquity, Galen in his *De sectis ad eos qui introducuntur* 1 (*Scr. Min.* III, p. 2 Helmreich)[36] and elsewhere employs 'rationalist' and 'dogmatic' interchangeably. Sometimes these authors could be misunderstood to imply that the 'dogmatics' or 'rationalists' represent a relatively cohesive school or sect in the same sense as the Empiricist and the Methodists.[37] 'Rationalist' or 'dogmatic' is in fact a classificatory factotum

[36] καλεῖν δ' εἰσὶν εἰθισμένοι . . . τὴν . . . λογικὴν δογματικήν . . . Cf. also Galen, *De libris propriis* 1 (*Scr. Min.* II, p. 94.5–6 Müller); S.E., *M* 8.156; Celsus, 1 praef. 13.
[37] The label 'rationalist' or 'dogmatic' survived well beyond Graeco-Roman antiquity. Cf. T16a (ninth century): 'rationabiles medici'; Schubring, 1962: 297. Charles Patin in the seventeenth century advocated 'dogmatic' medicine as the 'optima secta'; cf. Creutz, 1935. Modern scholars have not always used these labels with adequate differentiation; cf., e.g., Deichgräber, 1937: Pelops was 'Dogmatiker'; Meyer-Steineg & Sudhoff, 1921: 71ff.; Jaeger, 1938b: *passim*. But Diepgen, 1949: 91, and Kudlien, 1965, provide counterexamples. Cf. also Temkin, 1973: 15 n. 20; von Staden, 1982; Lloyd, 1983: 165–6, 183–8, 191–2, 198–9; Scarborough, 1969: 12; Thivel, 1981: 44n. 100.

applied to many post-Hippocratic physicians who have in common only that they did not confine themselves to observation and passive experience, but also tried to develop the theoretical and more speculative branches of medicine such as physiology and pathology. A consequence of this broad, indiscriminate application of 'rational' is that physicians with strongly divergent theories are depicted as comfortable bedfellows.[38] In this testimonium and in T16a (rationabiles medici), for example, Herophilus, who made a version of humoral pathology the basis of his system, and Erasistratus, who strongly opposed the theory of the humours and instead introduced something closer to a corpuscular pathology, are presented as members of the same sect or school.

The main value of this testimonium therefore lies not in its claims about the 'school' history but in its inclusion of Herophilus' city-ethnic and in its general chronological implications.

αἱρεσιάρχης: a term popular especially in medical doxography. Cf. *IG* 14.1759. See also Galen, *De sanitate tuenda* 5.11.44–5 (*CMG* v.4.2, p. 164 Koch) on physicians' 'damnable ambition' (ἐπίτριπτος ἐπιθυμία) to have the reputation of being an αἱρεσιάρχης. The term is, however, also used in philosophical history, for example by S.E., *P* 3.245 (of Zeno as first leader of the Stoic school).

Diocles: fr. 3 Wellmann. **Praxagoras:** fr. 1 Steckerl. **Mnesitheus:** fr. 2 Bertier. **Asclepiades:** see below on T16a. **Philinus:** fr. 6 Deichgräber.

ἀποτεμόμενος: very rare in this usage, which is not listed in LSJ, but cf. Philo, *De cherubim* 4 (Analdez/Pouilloux/Mondésert III, p. 20): τὴν μετέωρον . . . φιλοσοφίαν . . . ἣν φυσιολογίας τὸ κράτιστον εἶδος ἀποτέτμηται μαθηματική; and Athenagoras, *Pro Christianis* pp. 6–7 (ed. Schwartz, *Texte und Untersuchungen zur Geschichte der altchristlichen Literatur* 4.2 (Leipzig, 1891)): οἶδα γὰρ ὅτι ὅσον συνέσει καὶ ἰσχύϊ τῆς βασιλείας πάντων ὑπερέχετε, τοσοῦτον καὶ τῷ πᾶσαν παιδείαν ἀκριβοῦν πάντων κρατεῖτε, οὕτω καθ' ἕκαστον παιδείας μέρος κατορθοῦντες ὡς οὐδὲ οἱ ἐν αὐτῆς μόριον ἀποτεμόμενοι. Cf. also *separavit* in T12.

T2 Καλχηδονίῳ scripsi: καρχηδονίῳ codd.: Χαλκηδονίῳ Marx et Helmreich. While Χαλκ- eventually became the dominant form in literary texts, Καλχ- is common too, especially in the epigraphical evidence (see n. 1). Since the corruption καρχ-, requiring only the confusion of -ρ- and -λ-, is more likely to have supplanted an original Καλχ- than Χαλκ-, I have restored Καλχηδονίῳ. Cf. Arrian, *Anab* 3.24.5 (cod. A); *SEG* 33.1211.

---

[38] Galen (e.g. *De libris propriis* 1, *Scr. Min.* II, pp. 93–4 Müller) is, however, aware of the need to distinguish between different branches of 'dogmatism': the dogmatics belong together only *kata genos*, and there are *diaphorai tines* within this and the other 'sects'.

T3 comes from the famous Laurentian MS of Celsus, in which this enumeration of physicians follows immediately upon the text of Celsus. The origin of the list is unclear, but none of the authors mentioned postdates the sixth century A.D.: Muscio or Mustio, a contemporary of Caelius Aurelainus and Cassius Felix, is the latest (cf. Rose, 1882: p. iv). Wellmann, 1900a, has shown that the author of this list is knowledgeable about medical history and that the information he provides – in this case confirmation of Herophilus' city-ethnic – is, in general, reliable (pp. 367–82).

T4 διατρίβοντα: in Hellenistic Greek διατρίβω can mean 'reside' (and not just 'spend time'); cf. P. Hal. 1.182; P. Strassb. 22.6.

T5a–b The problems encountered in any attempt to estimate the evidential value for Herophilus' life of streamlined historiography such as this later (fourth century A.D.) report quickly become apparent when one scrutinizes Vindician's claim that the physicians here classified with Herophilus were all 'Alexandrian anatomists'. Although a majority – but not all – of the famous 'Alexandrian anatomists' among whom Vindician numbers Herophilus in T5 are independently attested to have been distinguished anatomists,[39] it cannot be shown that all of them actually practised in Alexandria. Only Rufus, Herophilus, and Apollonius – whether Apollonius Mys or the Empiricist or the Erasistratean from Memphis – are independently known to have had Egyptian connections,[40] and this compromises the value of T5. T4 and T6, however, confirm independently that Herophilus was active in Alexandria. Perhaps T5 reflects one significant impact of Herophilus' spectacular anatomical discoveries upon medical doxography: the general identification of anatomical excellence with Alexandria.

---

[39] For details on Rufus, see Ilberg, 1930. Lycus is probably the Macedonian to whose 'book on anatomy' Galen refers critically in *On Anatomical Procedures* 14.1 (p. 148 Duckworth); cf. also *id.*, *De musculorum dissectione*, XVIIIB, pp. 926–7, 935, 940, 943, 956K, etc. Pelops was Galen's mentor in Smyrna, and his books on anatomy receive high praise from Galen; cf., e.g., *On Anatomical Procedures* 14.1 (p. 184 Duckworth); see also *ibid.*, 1.1 (II, p. 217K), *De musc. dissect.* XVIIIB, pp. 926–7, 935K, and *infra* Chapter VI, T115. 'Apollonius' probably refers to the Erasistratean from Memphis, whose work on anatomical nomenclature is mentioned in the pseudo-Galenic *Introductio sive medicus* 10 (XIV, p. 700K). I do not know of an anatomist among the several physicians called Philip.

[40] Though he was not an 'Alexandrian anatomist', Rufus visited Egypt (but Tzetzes' claim that he was Cleopatra's physician and beautician is chronologically impossible; *Historiarum variarum chiliades* 6.300), and Apollonius of Memphis may well have practised in Alexandria. But Lycus is invariably associated with Rome, and Pelops with Smyrna. The Empiricist Philip of Smyrna may have practised in Alexandria, but he was almost certainly not an anatomist (Deichgräber, 1965: fr. 23a and pp. 21, 266, 408). Less is known about another 'Philip', a Pneumatic physician; cf. Diller, 1938, and Kudlien, 1968d: 1099.

T7 On the background and method of Celsus' introduction see Temkin, 1935a; Mudry, 1982.

T8 servus aut femina: on the validity of Hyginus' claim that women and slaves were barred from the medical profession in Athens see Kudlien, 1970: 8, and 1968c. Plato, *Laws* 720A–E, 857C–D where free-born physicians are depicted as treating free-born patients, and slaves as treating slaves, present notorious problems; the possibility that these passages do not have their roots in historical fact but in Platonic philosophy remains strong . Cf. Laín-Entralgo, 1962: 194f., but see also Sinclair, 1951; Forbes, 1955: 343f.; Robert Joly's criticisms of Kudlien, 1969: 1–14; Gil, 1973. Further Comments on T8 *supra*, II.A.1; see also, n. 11. (On female doctors cf. *IG* II/III².6873 (= W. Pleket, *Epigraphica* II (1969).1); also Pleket II.12, 20, 26–7; Krug, 1985: 195–7; Kudlien, 1979: 88–9.)

T9 Praxagoras: fr. 27 Steckerl.

T10 Some better method: Galen's point is that the 'founder' of the Methodist school, Thessalus,[41] in contrast to Herophilus and others whom Thessalus tries to refute, in fact has no defensible method. If Galen's characterization is correct, Thessalus had to offer something perceived as revolutionary in order to attain popular success, but his claim to novelty (and to a better method) is in fact 'established' only by charlatanism and by invective against famous predecessors. Cf. Galen, *Methodus medendi* 1.3 (x, pp. 18–19K). But see Frede, 1982; Harig, 1976; Lloyd, 1983: 182–200.

In addition to Galen's chronological information about Herophilus, T10 therefore provides confirmation of the esteem in which Herophilus was held in the Imperial period: his authority was great enough for him to be attacked by a 'revolutionary'.

colleagues (hetairous) does not have chronological significance; it does not imply that Herophilus and all the other 'comrades', 'associates' or 'colleagues' were contemporaries of the Stoics, etc., but simply that they all belonged to a 'club' to which Thessalus, in Galen's view at least, could never gain admission, *viz.* the 'club' of those whose intellectual achievements are superior.

the dialectician: Whether fact or fiction, episodes such as Herophilus' quick-witted use of 'dialectic' (T15) to prove to the Megarian philosopher Diodorus Cronus that his dislocated shoulder could not have been dislocated (since motion is, after all, impossible according to one of Diodorus' own arguments), might have given rise to this reputation. Herophilus' division of medicine (see Chapter IV.A.1 *infra*), his subdivision of 'neutrals', and his

---

[41] On Thessalus see Meyer-Steineg, 1910; Diller, 1936b. See also below, Chapter XXIII, n. 22, on the Methodist school.

elaborate and often subtle sphygmological distinctions may have buttressed this reputation. Pliny's descriptions of Herophilus as a 'subtilioris sectae conditor' (T13) and as 'nimiam propter subtilitatem desertus' (T186) probably belong in the same context as 'dialectician'. (It is, however, also possible that Galen is simply referring to an epithet used pejoratively by Thessalus in his polemics against Herophilus.) Cf. Kudlien, 1974a: 192.

Phylotimus: see n. 34 and Steckerl, 1958: 108–23. **Praxagoras:** fr. 45 Steckerl. **Mnesitheus:** fr. 4 Bertier. **Dieuches:** fr. 2 Bertier. **Philistion:** cf. Wellmann, 1901: 109–16, 68–71. **Plistonicus:** cf. Steckerl, 1958: 124–6.

T11 Praxagoras: fr. 27 Steckerl.

T12 Diocles: fr. 4 Wellmann. **Praxagoras:** fr. 3 Steckerl. **Chrysippus:** on the confusion concerning the various Chrysippi cf. Fraser, 1969; *id.*, 1972: vol. I, p. 347; Wellmann, 1899; *supra* pp. 46–7 and n. 6.

T13 Diocles: fr. 5 Wellmann. **Praxagoras:** fr. 4 Steckerl.

ante omnis celebratam: Pliny's claim that Herophilus used herbs more than any other therapeutic treatment cannot be verified, but that Herophilus used pharmacology is confirmed by T248ff. (Chapter VIII).

T14 Phylotimus: not included in Steckerl's edition. See II.A.2 (above, pp. 48–9) and n. 34.

Eudemus: More than one Eudemus was known in medical circles in Galen's time. (1) Galen's older contemporary Eudemus, a Peripatetic philosopher (not to be confused with Eudemus of Rhodes or with Aristotle's friend Eudemus of Cyprus), whom Galen, on his first visit to Rome in A.D. 161/2, cured of quartan fever with spectacular success (Galen, *De praenotione ad Epigenem* 2–5 (*CMG* v.8.1, 74–94)),[42] can be eliminated, since Galen is referring to a contemporary of Erasistratus (cf. also *PIR*² III, p. 90 no. 109). (2) Eudemus, a Methodist expert on hydrophobia and pharmacology, who became better known as the lover of Livia – and as one of the murderers of her husband Drusus in A.D. 23 (Pliny, *Natural History* 29.8.20; Tacitus, *Annals* 4.3,11; cf. *PIR*² III, p. 90 no. 108) – likewise can be eliminated for chronological reasons. (3) The 'drug seller' of Aristophanes' *Plutus* (884) and Theophrastus' *History of Plants* (9.17.2) is also an unlikely candidate since (a) Galen refers only to 'most illustrious' physicians, not drug vendors, and (b) this Eudemus predates Herophilus and Erasistratus by perhaps as much as three quarters of a century. (4) The Eudemus of whom Galen reports in his last major work, *Methodus medendi* (6.6 (x, p. 454K)), that he was 'an old man' who had successfully applied the famous 'Isis Plaster' (or 'Epigonus' plaster', Galen XIII, pp. 774–8K, excerpted from Heras) to cuts resulting from trepanation, can also be disqualified on chronological grounds.

[42] Cf. Ilberg, 1905 (esp. pp. 286f.); Spoerri, 1966.

(5) This leaves us with a distinguished anatomist, whom Galen and other ancient authors usually mention *with Herophilus*, usually as Herophilus' fellow initiator of advanced anatomical investigations (e.g. Herophilus' and Eudemus' anatomy of the nerves , their study of the pancreas, their use of dissection, their anatomy of the uterus, their embryology).[43] The dates of this anatomist are, however, never independently mentioned – Galen only says that Eudemus, too, is an early post-Hippocratic physician – and the mention of Eudemus as Herophilus' contemporary in T14 therefore does not contribute to a reconstruction of the date of Herophilus.

T15 On the date of Diodorus see p. 49 above (and n. 35). His attempts to disprove motion, which Herophilus parodied according to this testimonium, are discussed by Sextus, *P* 3.71-5, and *M* 1.309-12; 10.48, 85–101, 112–17, 142-3, 347 (see Döring, 1972: fr. 121-9 and pp. 129-31).

ἐκβαλών: Other terms are more commonly used in medical literature for dislocating or displacing joints or bones, for example – all, however, in the passive sense 'to *be* dislocated' – ἐκπίπτειν (Hp., *On Joints* 57), ἐκβαίνειν (*ibid.*, 54), κινεῖσθαι (with or without ἐκ τῆς χώρης; Hp., *On Fractures* 9, 10), ἐξαρθρεῖν (*On Joints* 8, 29, 53, 63, 67). ἐκβάλλειν is sometimes used as the active counterpart of these passively used terms, a usage perhaps partly inspired by the common use of ἐμβολή and ἐμβάλλειν for the reduction of dislocated joints. Good examples are Hp., *On Fractures* 31: ἐκβάλλων τὸ ὀστέον; and *On Joints* 67: ἐκβάλλειν τὸ ἄρθρον. This active function of ἐκβάλλειν is not acquired by default, however, since ἐξαρθρεῖν can also be used transitively: 'Some tell the story that the Amazons dislocate (ἐξαρθρέουσιν) the joints of their male infants right away in early infancy . . . ' (Hp., *On Joints* 53). (Many other uses were found for ἐκβάλλειν in medical literature, for example 'to expel' the afterbirth, Hp., *Diseases of Women* 1.78: προσθετὸν ἐκβάλλον χόριον ἀπολελειμμένον,[44] or 'to abort', *ibid.*, 1.60, *Epidemics* 4.25.)

T16a The Bambergensis appears to distinguish chronologically between three groups of physicians: to the first and earliest only Hippocrates belongs: to the second, Hippocrates' relatives, including his sons, a grandson, and – if my emendation of *Poliemmius* to *Polybus* (see below) is correct – a son-in-law; to the third, some post-Hippocratic 'rationalist' physicians ranging in date from the fourth century B.C. (Diocles and Praxagoras) to the second century A.D. (see below). The broad span of time covered by the third group reduces the value of T16a for determining Herophilus' date; but since the sequence

---

[43] See below, Chapter VI, T67-9, 80, 84, 95; cf. also the continuation of T113 in Soranus, *Gynaecia* 1.57 (*CMG* IV, p. 42 Ilberg). There is no clear evidence for Fraser's suggestion (1972: II, pp. 1112–13) that Eudemus was a pupil of Herophilus.

[44] On *chorion* cf. Kudlien, 1964d.

within this group is strictly chronological, it does provide some general confirmation by placing Herophilus between his teacher Praxagoras and his contemporary Erasistratus.

Thessalus probably refers to the 'son of Hippocrates' mentioned by several sources, sometimes also as the author of certain Hippocratic treatises. Cf. Soranus, *Vita Hippocratis* 15 (*CMG* IV, p. 178 Ilberg); Codex Laurentianus 73.1, fol. 143r, line 13 (cf. Wellmann, 1900a: 370); Galen, *In Hippocratis De natura hominis comment.* 2.1 (*CMG* v.9.1, p. 58 Mewaldt); Suda, s.v. 'Hippokrates'; Tzetzes, *Historiarum variarum chiliades* VII. 968 ff. (Ps.-Galen, *In Hippocratis De humoribus comm.* 1.1 (XVI, pp. 3 and 5K) has little evidential value; see n. 49.) Cf. also Schöne, 1903: 57.

Draco, like Thessalus, is known as 'son of Hippocrates'; cf. Schöne, 1903: 57; Suda, *loc. cit.* (but s.v. 'Drakon' a different Draco is also said to be the son of Thessalus); Soranus, *loc cit.*; Galen, *CMG* v.9.1, p. 58 (Mewaldt): δύο γὰρ υἱεῖς οὗτοι γεγόνασιν τοῦ μεγάλου Ἱπποκράτους, Θεσσαλὸς καὶ Δράκων . . . Like his brother Thessalus, Draco is sometimes cited in ancient sources as the author of the Hippocratic *Prorrhetic* 1: cf. Galen, *In Hippocratis Prorrheticum* 2.17 (*CMG* v.9.2, p. 68 Diels).

Hippocrates iunior: according to Galen, *In Hippocratis De natura hominis* 2.1 (*CMG* v.9.1, p. 58 Mewaldt), both Thessalus and Draco had sons called Hippocrates; ancient sources attribute Hippocratic treatises to them, too. Galen, for example, reports (*loc. cit.*): ταῦτα μὲν ὁ Διοσκορίδης ἔγραψεν εἰκάζων εἶναι τὴν προκειμένην ῥῆσιν Ἱπποκράτους τοῦ Θεσσαλοῦ υἱέος.

Polybus. The MS reads *Poliemmius*, a name which to my knowledge does not recur in any other ancient or medieval text dealing with Greek medicine. I have presented the case for emending *Poliemmius* to *Polybus* elsewhere.[45] As the son-in-law of Hippocrates, Polybus belongs both chronologically and contextually in the ranks of Thessalus, Draco (the sons of Hippocrates), and Hippocrates the Younger (a grandson of Hippocrates). **Quorum libri non apparuerunt** alludes to the attribution of several treatises in the Hippocratic Corpus to these Hippocratic kinsmen – attributions which already in antiquity were controversial, and remain so today, despite Hermann Grensemann's impressive efforts to establish that Polybus was the author of some Hippocratic treatises.[46]

After physicians of the fourth and third centuries B.C., the author turns to a group of eight later physicians:

---

[45] See von Staden, 1976b.
[46] Grensemann regards Polybus as the author of *On the Nature of Man* and *On Birth in the Eighth Month.* Cf. Grensemann, 1968a; *id.,* 1974. There is, however, by no means universal agreement on these attributions; cf. Jouanna, 1969a; *id.,* 1969b; Joly, 1970; Kudlien, 1969c: 150; Deichgräber, 1971: 180; Phillips, 1970: 23–4; von Staden, 1976b; Jouanna, 1975: 55–9.

Asclepiades: Probably Asclepiades of Prusias, a famous Bithynian physician of the early first century B.C.[47] On Prusias vs. Prusa cf. Rawson, 1982: 359–60.

Athenaeus: of Attaleia (in Pamphylia), founder of the Pneumatic school of medicine in the mid or later first century B.C. Cf. Kudlien, 1962 (but see *infra* Chapter IV n. 68); *id.*, 1968d; Wellmann, 1895a: 5–11, 131–7, and *passim*.

Agathinus of Sparta was a Pneumatic physician who studied with Athenaeus and in turn became the teacher of the most famous of all Pneumatics, **Archigenes** of Apamea, and of **Herodotus**: Galen, *De pulsuum differentiis* 4.11 (VIII, pp. 750–1K); ps.-Galen, *Definitiones medicae* 14 (XIX, p. 353K). (Herodotus in turn seems to have been a teacher of Sextus Empiricus.[48]) See also Chapter VII, T160, *infra*.

Ariston. The putative author of the Hippocratic *Regimen in Health* (Galen, *In Hippocratis De victu acutorum* 1.17 (*CMG* v.9.1, p. 135 Helmreich); *id.*, *In Hipp. Aphorismos* 6.1 (XVIIIA, p. 9K)) cannot be meant, since *subsequente tempore* introduces the third group, thought of as postdating not only Hippocrates but also all figures recognized in ancient criticism as 'Hippocratic authors' (Thessalus, Draco, Polybus). This leaves the possibility that Ariston is the later physician whom Celsus (*De medicina* 5.18.33) and Galen (*De compositione medicamentorum secundum locos* 9.4 (XIII, p. 281K)) mention as an author or adherent of fairly 'advanced' drug recipes for podagra and colic (the *terminus ante quem* is provided by Celsus).

Philumenus. Since he mentions Archigenes, Soranus, Marcellus, and the Pneumatic Herodotus, but not Galen, Philumenus' floruit probably belongs to the mid-second century A.D. His only surviving work, *On Poisonous Animals* (*CMG* x.1.1, ed. M. Wellmann), exhibits a strong compilatory tendency and little originality. This further confirms that the choice of later authors in this group is fairly arbitrary, and that we cannot make much of the fact that Herophilus is placed in the company of this group of physicians.

Antyllus. The Pneumatics dominate the third group, and Antyllus is yet another. He too seems to belong to the second century A.D., postdating Archigenes, to whom he refers (cf. Oribasius, *Collectiones medicae* 9.23.18–19 (*CMG* VI.1.2, p. 26 Raeder)), but possibly – though by no means certainly – somewhat earlier than Galen, to whom Oribasius' extensive excerpts from Antyllus' works on dietetics, surgery, general therapeutics, and climatology never refer.[49]

---

[47] Wellmann, 1908; von Vilas, 1903; Lonie, 1965a; Rawson, 1982; Gottschalk, 1980: 48–56. See also ch. XXII, n. 5 (*infra*); ed. by J. T. Vallance (forthcoming).
[48] Cf. Kudlien, 1963a.
[49] The failure of one medical author to mention another rarely constitutes a reliable chronological indicator, although medical historians still make frequent use of

A survey of the authors with whom Herophilus is listed here as a 'rationalist' (*rationabilis medicus*) therefore reveals once again (see above, T1, on τῆς λογικῆς αἱρέσεως) the potentially misleading nature of the label 'rationalist'. The list is dominated by Pneumatics – Athenaeus, Agathinus, Archigenes, Herodotus, Antyllus – and that probably points to a Pneumatic source for this doxographical summary; but the remaining physicians have nothing of significance in common either with each other or with the Pneumatics, except (a) that they postdate the early Hippocratic family, and (b) that they are not Empiricists.

argumenta ex silentio. Furthermore, those who use Antyllus' silence about Galen to date Antyllus usually fail to add that Galen, in turn, never refers to Antyllus either. The resourceful Renaissance forger or forgers who wrote 'Galen's' commentary on the 'Hippocratic' *On Humours* (xvi, pp. 1–488K) made extensive use of Antyllus, as Valentin Rose and others have noticed. Cf., for example, ps.-Galen xvi, pp. 147–8K with Oribasius, *Collectiones medicae* 8.12–15, and ps.-Galen xvi, pp. 400–1K with Oribasius 9.7–9 and 9.11. (About xvi, pp. 394–416K Rose wrote with justifiable indignation: 'die ganze Abhandlung gibt . . . ein hübsches Beispiel ab für die Buchmacherei des Galenus' (Rose, 1864–70: vol. 1, p. 23), but he failed to recognize that it is a Renaissance forgery.)

III
WRITINGS

A · INTRODUCTION

1 *Context and transmission*

By the early Hellenistic period the written word had not only become more firmly entrenched than ever before in a culture which, as late as the mid fourth century B.C., had still been manifesting complex tensions between its deep oral roots and the usurping potential of literacy. Written texts had by now also become a widely used educational tool which was systematically employed in medical, philosophical,[1] and rhetorical training. In training his apprentices, the good physician, or at any rate the physician who left a discernible mark on history, did not rely on books written by famous predecessors but also wrote his own handbooks for use by his students and followers. It is in this pedagogic context, too, and not only in the more obvious context of making public one's scientific views, that Herophilus' writings belong. In subsequent centuries, when a branch of the school of Herophilus also flourished outside Egypt, the works of the founding master seem to have continued to play a central pedagogic role, and this undoubtedly aided their survival for some centuries.

Herophilus wrote at least eight books, and for several centuries after his death some of these apparently won the usual battles for transmission, surviving well beyond – and perhaps in part because of – the expulsion of large numbers of the Alexandrian intelligentsia

---

[1] There were, however, some famous exceptions, such as two leaders of the Platonic Academy during its sceptical phase (i.e. the 'New Academy'), Arcesilaus of Pitane (*c.* 316–241 B.C.) and Carneades of Cyrene (*c.* 214–129 B.C.). Cf. D.L. 4.32 (on Arcesilaus): 'Because he suspended judgment on all matters, some say he never wrote a book'; 4.65 (on Carneades): apart from some letters 'he himself left nothing' in writing.

by Ptolemy VIII Euergetes II in 145/4 B.C. A striking depiction of the effects of this diaspora upon the rest of Greece is given in the polyhistoric *Deipnosophistae* of Athenaeus (*c.* A.D. 200). What makes it particularly interesting is that Athenaeus drew on a first-hand account by an apparent victim of the expulsion order, the historian Menecles of Barca.[2]

A rejuvenation of all *paideia* was again brought about in the reign of the seventh[3] Ptolemy who ruled Egypt, the one appropriately named Malefactor (Kakergetes)[4] by the Alexandrians. For he slaughtered many of the Alexandrians and exiled not a few who had grown up with his brother [sc. Ptolemy Philometor], thereby causing the islands and cities to be jammed with philologists, philosophers, mathematicians, musicians, painters, physical educators, *as well as physicians* and many other professionals (τεχνῖται). On account of their poverty they taught what they knew and instructed many distinguished men. (*Deipnosophistae* 4.83.184b–c)

The exiled intelligentsia probably took important books with them – and Herophilus' works ranked among the more esteemed in Alexandria – so that this dispersion, and the founding of a Herophilean school in the first century B.C. near the great East–West trade route in Asia Minor, may have aided the transmission of at least some of Herophilus' treatises until well after the burning of the Alexandrian Library in 48 B.C. Authors of the second century A.D. still seem to have had access to some of Herophilus' treatises, as is shown below.

The fact that a Byzantine court physician and medical encyclopaedist of the early sixth century A.D., Aëtius of Amida in Mesopotamia, in his *Libri medicinales* 7.48 (*CMG* VIII.2, p. 303 Olivieri) quotes a

---

[2] For Menecles of Barca (second century B.C.), see *FGrHist* 270. ἔτι δὲ ˝Ανδρωνα (as a source for Athenaeus' account) was probably added by Athenaeus, unless Andron excerpted or summarized Menecles' account (cf. Jacoby, *Komm.* ad *loc. cit.*, p. 223; *FGrHist* 246 (Andron von Alexandreia), and 370; also Fraser, 1972: vol. II, pp. 745–6, nn. 198–201).

[3] By modern count Euergetes II is Ptolemy VIII, not VII. Athenaeus is, however, probably not counting Ptolemy VII Neos Philopator (the second son of Ptolemy VI Philometor) who as a teenager was king for less than a year (145–144 B.C.) under the regency of his mother Cleopatra II, but was murdered on Euergetes II's orders, perhaps on the day of his mother's forced marriage to Euergetes II. Cf. Otto, 1934:12, 128, 129, 131; Otto & Bengtson, 1938: 23ff., 29, 107, 110ff.; Fraser, 1972: vol. I, pp. 119–23, 86–8, 332–3, 360, 423, 462, 467–70, 485, 517–18, 538–9, 550, 552, 806, 808, 810 and corresponding notes in vol. II; Samuel, 1962: 144–7; Skeat, 1954: 14. (On Euergetes II see also *FGrHist* 234.)

[4] Obviously a play on 'Euergetes' ('Benefactor').

passage from Herophilus' treatise *On Eyes* (*Fr*260, pp. 423–4) without mentioning any intermediate source – although he often mentions his proximate sources – might suggest, at least prima facie, that one or more of Herophilus' works survived into the early Byzantine period. It could be argued that the possibility that Aëtius did not draw the quotation from a post-Herophilean source but from Herophilus himself is strengthened by the fact that the quotation from Herophilus is not recorded by Galen or by any other post-Herophilean source used by Aëtius. Arguments *ex silentio* are, however, notoriously insidious. In this case the silence of other ancient authors is perhaps all the more inconclusive, because several Galenic, pseudo-Galenic, and other ophthalmological works, from which Aëtius might have excerpted the Herophilean quotation, are not extant.[5] One such work is a famous treatise by an Herophilean of the first century A.D., Demosthenes Philalethes. His *Ophthalmicus*, which perhaps drew in part on Herophilus' *On Eyes*, became a major source of later ophthalmological discussions, and almost no one made more extensive use of it than Aëtius, although the Byzantine physician did not always acknowledge Demosthenes as his source (see Chapter XXVIII below). Demosthenes' work was not only widely used in the Imperial period – for example, by Galen and Rufus of Ephesus[6] – but in fact seems to have survived in some form or other until the fourteenth century.[7] In the tenth century Pope Sylvester II repeatedly refers to a book 'qui inscribitur Ophthalmicus', written by 'Demosthenes philosophus' (i.e. a copy of a Latin translation of Demosthenes' book) of which a manuscript was kept in Bobbio; in the thirteenth century Simon of Genoa used the Latin translation of Demosthenes' work in his *Synonyma medicinae sive Clavis sanationis*, and in the fourteenth Matthaeus Sylvaticus drew on it in his *Liber pandectarum medicinae*. It is therefore possible that Aëtius did not know Herophilus' work directly

---

[5] Cf. Meyerhof, 1928; Hirschberg, 1919b: 610–12, 620–3 (pseudo-Galenic). If the rather speculative observations of Wellmann, 1895a: 115–30, are correct, a lost Pneumatic source also might have been used by Aëtius. See also ch. II, n. 7; p. 72.

[6] Cf., e.g., Rufus in Oribasius, *Synopsis ad Eustathium* 8.49 (*CMG* VI.3, p. 266, lines 15–20 Raeder), with Demosthenes Philalethes in Aëtius, *Libri medicinales* 7.52 (*CMG* VIII.2, p. 308, lines 3–8, 13–14 Olivieri = *DP*. 20). The pseudo-Galenic *Introductio sive medicus* and *Definitiones*, Oribasius, Aëtius, Paul of Aegina, Theophanes Nonnus, and others used it as a primary source for ophthalmological questions and definitions. Details in Chapter XXVIII below on Demosthenes.

[7] For documentation of what follows see Chapter XXVIII *infra* (Demosthenes Philalethes).

but only through Herophilus' follower Demosthenes or through
another author who had quoted either Herophilus or Demosthenes.
Yet Aëtius' failure to make explicit mention of such an intervening
source remains striking and one cannot exclude with certainty the
possibility that some of Herophilus' works survived beyond the
Antonine period.

When one turns to the Antonine period, one can tread on firmer
ground. That Herophilus' books were not known by title alone in the
later second century A.D. seems clear both from extensive direct
quotations, which are uncharacteristic of earlier medical doxography, and from certain turns of phrase used especially by Galen. Thus,
in T38, Galen says Herophilus 'wrote lucidly' about certain phenomena relating to the pulse, '*at least for those who don't have just a cursory
encounter with his books*'. In T39 he likewise talks disparagingly of 'those
who are ignorant of Herophilus' writings', and elsewhere he suggests
that these *writings* make clear the comprehensive nature of Herophilus' interest in the human body (T37). Again, according to T41,
'Galen' found certain definitions 'scattered' throughout the *books* of
Herophilus. In the first century A.D. Pliny, too, seems to imply that he
had Herophilus' works available as a source for parts of Book XI of his
Natural History – although Pliny's enumeration of sources is highly
problematic (see *Comments* on T40) – and Soranus, a distinguished
physician under Trajan, quotes and paraphrases Herophilus liberally.

Although at least some texts by Herophilus therefore seem to have
been accessible to authors of the first and second centuries A.D., most
of the major sources were greatly indebted for details of Herophilus'
theories and observations to doxographical and other works by later
Herophileans such as Aristoxenus (especially on pulse theory),
Alexander Philalethes (on reproductive theory), and Demosthenes
Philalethes (ophthalmology). There was a strong doxographical
interest within the Herophilean 'school' of medicine almost from the
outset, and the founding master retained a place of honour in this
tradition (see Chapter X.A). Galen and other authors seem to have
made extensive use of these doxographic works for their presentations
of Herophilus' views. Hermann Schöne's study (1893) of Galen's *De
pulsuum differentiis* 4.2–10 (VIII, pp. 699–750K) suggests, for example,
that Galen might have depended to some extent on Book XIII of
Aristoxenus' *On the School of Herophilus* for his analysis of the pulse
theories of his Herophilean predecessors (see Chapter XXV.A; *Ar.* 1–2).

A further significant transmission of Herophilus' views occurred in the context of the Empiricists' polemics against the Herophileans. Ever since a renegade pupil of Herophilus, Philinus of Cos, founded the Empiricist school of medicine in the mid third century B.C., the Herophileans and Empiricists engaged in a protracted feud in which Herophilus' views, too, were often at issue. Philinus' work in six books against the Hippocratic lexicon of the Herophilean Bacchius (*Ba.* 13), the treatise in three books against Bacchius by the Empiricist Heraclides of Tarentum (*fl. c.* 75 BC.), the latter's work against Herophilus' treatise *On Pulses* (see T24), and the polemical books by two early Empiricists against the interpretation which the Herophilean Zeno had offered of enigmatic letter-symbols in the Hippocratic treatise *Epidemics* III (*Zn.*5–6) – all of these are examples of Empiricist vehicles of transmission which imparted colourations of the feud to some of the testimonia recorded in this volume.

Yet another prism through which some Herophilean theories may have passed is the Pneumatic school of medicine (founded in the mid first century B.C.), which seems to have had a lively doxographic interest. Among our sources for Herophilus and his school, a pseudo-Galenic treatise, *Introductio sive medicus* [*Eisagoge*], has often been thought to bear the mark of the Pneumatic school, but this view has not been established conclusively. More significant is the fact that Galen more than once explicitly identifies a Pneumatic physician of the first century A.D., Archigenes, as a source on whom he drew for Herophilean views, especially concerning pulse-lore (e.g. Chapter VII, T163). A further source, the pseudo-Galenic treatise, *Definitiones medicae*, has also been said to be of Pneumatic provenance, but an analysis by Jutta Kollesch has cast serious doubt on this hypothesis.[8]

The Peripatetic contribution to the preservation of Herophilus' works and views seems to have been less significant. Aëtius' famous doxographic work, the *Placita philosophorum* (*c.* A.D. 100), which depends in part – but only in part – on Peripatetic doxography, does provide some valuable morsels (especially T143a), but unfortunately it often presents Herophilus' views in a telegraphic and schematized form (e.g. Chapter VII, T137a and T202a). A famous papyrus of Peripatetic provenance, the *Anonymus Londinensis* (British Museum), likewise offers invaluable glimpses especially into some physiological theories of Herophilus (e.g. Chapter VII, T146) and of his followers

[8] See Kollesch, 1973: especially 66ff.

(e.g. Chapter xxii, *AP*.5–8). Parts of this work are perhaps dependent
on the main Peripatetic work on medical doxography, Menon's
Iatrika, and hence might go back to the third century B.C., but other
parts depend on much later sources, as the mention of Alexander
Philalethes (late first century B.C. or early first century A.D.; cf.
Chapter xxii) demonstrates. The evidence it offers is invaluable but
unfortunately very limited, and, in the case of Herophilus, the main
burden of transmission clearly was carried by other currents of
medical doxography.
A schematization of the main lines of transmission might accordingly
look as sketched in Figure 1, although it must be stressed that this
diagram inevitably runs the usual risks of oversimplification and
selectivity that a graphic representation entails.

2 *Genuine and spurious works*

Eleven works are explicitly ascribed to Herophilus by ancient sources.
Of these, six mentioned by title seem to be of indisputable authenticity:

1. *Anatomy*, T17–T19 (cf. Chapter vi, especially Fr60–Fr62)
2. *On Pulses*, T21–T24 (cf. Chapter vii, T144–T188, especially T148, T150, Fr162)
3. *Midwifery*, T25–T26 (Chapter vii, T193–T202; cf. also Chapter vi, T105–T114, and Chapter viii, T247)
4. *Therapeutics*, T27–T28 (cf. Chapter viii, T231–T259, especially T231 and T252)
5. *Dietetics*, T29 (Chaper viii, T230; cf. also T227–T229)
6. *Against Common Opinions*, T30 (Chapter vii, T203–T204)

A seventh treatise, *On Eyes* (T20),[9] might be considered suspect,
since an apparently different (but otherwise unknown) 'Herophilus
ocularius medicus' is mentioned once by a Roman historian.[10] But at
least seven considerations seem to speak in favour of the famous
Alexandrian's authorship. First, Celsus,[11] Rufus,[12] and Galen[13] all
mention 'Herophilus' as a physician who won renown for his
anatomy of the eye, but none of them distinguishes him from the

[9] See also Chapter viii, Fr260; Chapter vi, T84–T89; Chapter vii, T140a–c.
[10] Valerius Maximus; for details see Chapter ii, n. 7, *infra* n. 16, Appendix iv.
[11] Chapter vi, T88.   [12] T87, T89.   [13] T84–T85; cf. T140a.

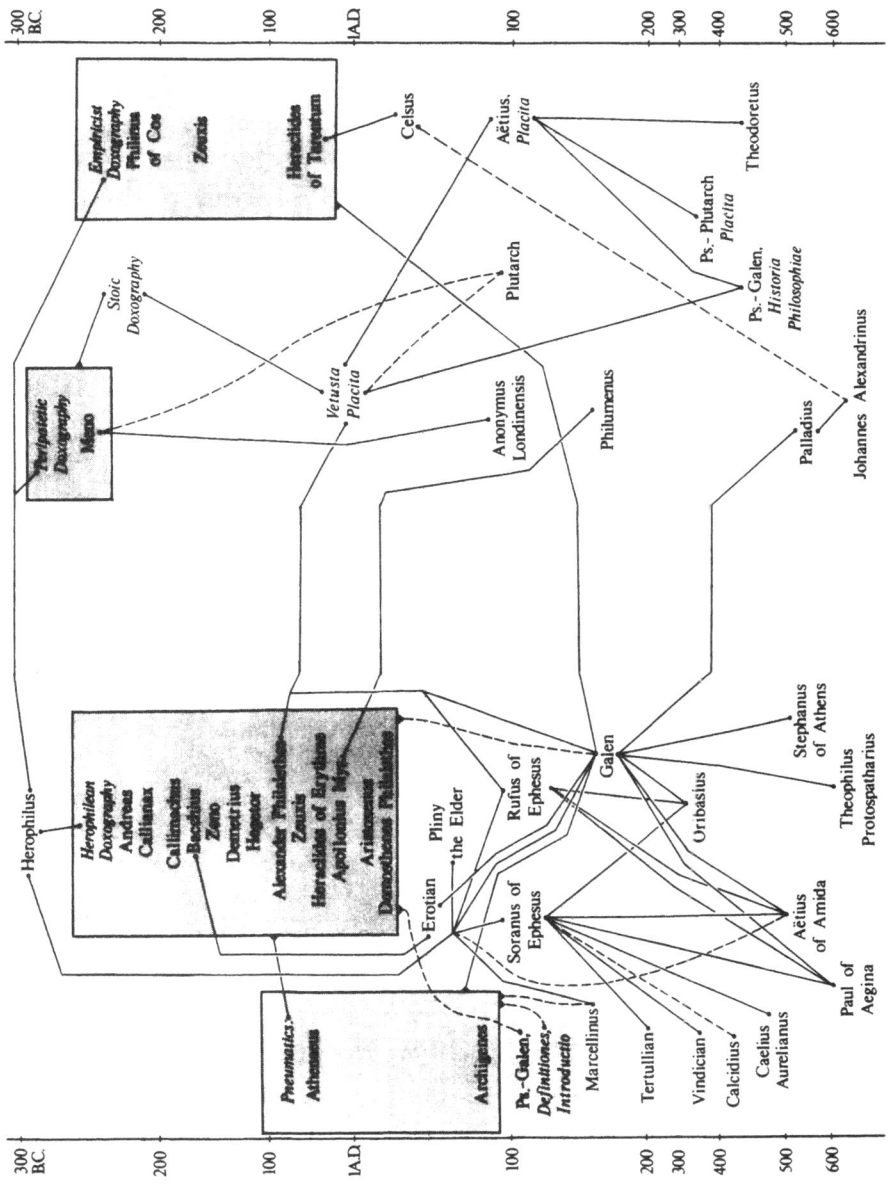

famous Alexandrian anatomist, whom they mention frequently in other contexts. Second, Herophilus' speculation about the optic nerve[14] is perfectly compatible not only with a larger ophthalmological interest but also with the Alexandrian's well-attested exploration of the brain and of the nervous system.[15] Third, the manuscript evidence for 'Herophilus ocularius medicus' is not unambiguous: a manuscript variant reads 'Herophilus the horse-doctor' instead of 'Herophilus the eye-doctor'.[16] Fourth, the drug prescription preserved in the fragment from *On Eyes*[17] is consistent with Herophilus' statements on pharmacology;[18] fifth, this fragment contains ingredients, such as crocodile dung,[19] which suggest an Egyptian context; sixth, there is an allusion to Herophilus' anatomy of the eye as early as the *Hymn to Artemis* by Callimachus (see *Comments*, T87–T89, ch. VI); and, finally, this 'Herophilus ocularius medicus' was a notorious impostor (see ch. II, n. 7).

An eighth work is described by a physician of the fifth century A.D., Caelius Aurelianus (T31, T261), as 'the book Herophilus wrote against Hippocrates' *Prognostic*'. Since Caelius Aurelianus is dependent on a normally reliable Greek source, Soranus of Ephesus (whom he often, but not always, simply translates into Latin), there is no compelling prima facie reason to distrust this testimony. It might be the same work by Herophilus to which Galen refers when he mentions 'what was said against Hippocrates' *Prognostic* by Herophilus' (T32), and 'the things written so poorly by Herophilus against Hippocrates' prognoses (*prognōseis*)' (T33). It is unlikely that the latter refers to the Hippocratic *Coan Predictions* in the absence of the word 'Coan', especially since this work also was known simply as αἱ Κῳακαί.

Edelstein expressed doubt about the existence of such an anti-Hippocratic work by Herophilus, arguing that the vacillation in the two Galenic passages between 'against Hippocrates' *Prognostic*' and 'against Hippocrates' prognoses' does not point to the title of a book,

---

[14] T84–T86, T140a.   [15] T75–T83.
[16] *Vid.* Chapter II, n. 7: ocularius medicus *Par., A* (in marg.): (a)equarius medicus *LA*.
[17] Chapter VIII, Fr260.
[18] *Ibid.*, T248a–T259. Several of the ingredients in Fr260 recur in other Herophilean testimonia, e.g. gum in T258; Cyprian copper in *AM*.18 (Chapter XXIII) and in *DP*.25a, 43 (Ch. XXVIII); honey in *AM*.16–22, 25, 26, 28, 38, 40, 42, 44 (Ch. XXIII) and in *DP*.5, 22, 30 (Ch. XXVIII).
[19] On the use of the *Dreckapotheke* in Greece and Egypt, see Chapter 1.4.

but only to Herophilus' critical comments on what were regarded in Alexandria as Hippocratic prognoses.[20] While I agree that one cannot be absolutely certain that Herophilus wrote a treatise called *Against Hippocrates' Prognostic*, Edelstein apparently overlooked the unequivocal, though not entirely conclusive, testimony of Caelius Aurelianus (or Soranus?) that Herophilus not only wrote against Hippocrates' *Prognostic*, but wrote a *book* against it: 'libro quem ad Hippocratis Prognosticum scripsit' (T31, T261). Although the Latin word *libro* might be more explicit than the Greek original – which might, for example, have been τὰ ὑφ' Ἡροφίλου πρὸς τὸ Ἱπποκράτους Προγνωστικὸν γεγραμμένα – it could equally well be an accurate translation (e.g. of *pragmateia*). Furthermore, like Galen (T32), Caelius Aurelianus specifically reports that Herophilus wrote against Hippocrates' *Prognostic*, and not merely against Hippocratic *prognoses*.

Edelstein's further point that Herophilus could not have written on what we know as the Hippocratic *Prognostic*, since the view Herophilus criticizes in T261 does not occur at all in the text of the *Prognostic* as it has been transmitted to us, deserves serious consideration (see Chapter IX, *Comments*, T261). Other hypotheses are, however, no less plausible than Edelstein's. Herophilus could, for example, have possessed a different recension of the Hippocratic treatise (as Regenbogen suggests), or a lacuna could have occurred at a subsequent stage in the transmission of the text of the *Prognostic*, as Wellmann maintains.[21] (It would, however, have been a considerably larger lacuna than Wellmann assumes.) It does not seem impossible that Herophilus wrote a book against a text that was known in the Hellenistic period as Hippocrates' *Prognostic*, and that this is the eighth treatise reliably attributed to Herophilus.

There are references to three further works by Herophilus. First, if Kühn's text is left intact, Galen numbers Herophilus among those who wrote commentaries on the Hippocratic *Aphorisms* (T34; see

---

[20] Edelstein, 1935a: col. 1309.

[21] On the hypothesis of two different recensions, see Regenbogen, 1931: 132 n. 1. But cf. also Diller, 1933b: 77; Alexanderson, 1963: 17. On the hypothesis that there was a lacuna, see Wellmann, 1929. Regenbogen, 1931, and Edelstein, 1935a: col. 1309, advance persuasive arguments against Wellmann's attempt to fill the lacuna. The lacuna must have been substantial enough to allow omission of more than just the sentence Wellmann wants to reinsert; as it stands, his reconstruction remains incompatible with the content of the rest of the treatise. On the solution of W. D. Smith, 1979: 191–3, see below, Chapter IX, *Comments* on T261–T266.

Ba.9). Here we are on somewhat less certain ground. As noted in the critical apparatus to T34, Cobet and Klein (apparently independently of one another) emended Kühn's text to eliminate Herophilus from such authorship, by rolling Herophilus and his adherent Bacchius of Tanagra into one person: 'the Herophilean Bacchius'[22] instead of 'Herophilus, Bacchius'. This emendation has been supported by several scholars.[23] I too am inclined to accept it, mainly for stylistic reasons, rather than on the grounds advanced by Cobet, Wellmann, and Edelstein, viz. that Herophilus could not have engaged in Hippocratic exegesis before the time of Bacchius or Xenocritus.[24]

A different case is presented by T35, T36a, and T36b, all of which report that some, but not all, ancient critics attribute the Hippocratic treatise *On Nutriment* (*Peri trophēs*) to Herophilus. Ancient *Echtheitskritik*, which often concerned itself with the 'Hippocratic Question',[25]

[22] Cobet, 1860: 21–2; none of the subsequent discussions of this passage give Cobet the recognition he deserves as primus coniector. Klein, 1865: xxii, n. 25.

[23] E.g. Wellmann, 1929: 17–18; W. D. Smith, 1979: 130; Fraser, 1972: vol. II, p. 541 n. 250; Diller, 1950: 231. But Dobson, 1925: 19, and Susemihl, 1891–2: vol. I, p. 797, apparently retain the transmitted text since they maintain, without qualification, that Herophilus actually wrote a commentary on the *Aphorisms*. See also von Staden, 1976a.

[24] The appearance of the definite article before Bacchius, and before Bacchius alone, in K's enumeration of proper names in T34 (= *Ba*.9, Chapter XIV) is jarring, although it could be an example of the anaphoric-emphatic use of the article; cf. Kühner–Gerth II.I, pp. 598–602.

[25] The canonization of fifty-eight treatises (in the Middle Ages, however, sometimes sixty-two) as the Hippocratic Corpus occurred relatively late. The edition of the Hadrianic period by Artemidorus Capiton and a somewhat enigmatic Dioscurides (not Pedanius) is the only comprehensive one mentioned unambiguously by ancient sources (cf. *CMG* v.9.1, pp. 13–16; v, 10.2.2, p. 4), but there is no broad agreement among modern scholars on how important it was for the formation of our Corpus. Earlier editions of a number of treatises are also referred to in ancient sources; see the section on Herophilus' Hippocratic exegesis (Chapter IX below) and Chapters XIV and XV below. If Galen's lost treatise *On Genuine Hippocratic Treatises* was authentic, it might also have played a role in the stabilization of the Corpus; see Mewaldt, 1909; Diller, 1933a; *id.*, 1933b: 70–8. Cf. on the Hadrianic edition Ilberg, 1890; Edelstein, 1935a: cols. 1310–17 (important col. 1314, bottom, on the possible role of Bacchius); *id.*, 1939; Pfaff, 1932. Also, a useful summary of the transmission by Hartmut Erbse in Erbse, 1961: 240–2. On criteria for distinguishing genuine from spurious (as well as earlier from later) works in the Hippocratic Corpus cf. Schöne, 1910; Regenbogen, 1921; Joly, 1961; Grensemann 1975: 217; Diller, 1959b. Lloyd, 1975c, offers a penetrating analysis of both the external and the internal evidence for authenticity and reaches largely negative conclusions. Cf. also W. D. Smith, 1979, especially Chapters 2 and 3.

correctly concluded, apparently in the early Imperial period and certainly no later than Galen, that this treatise could not have been written by Hippocrates himself. (There were, however, exceptions among the ancient critics: Erotian and Gellius seem to have thought of it as authentic; see critical apparatus to T36a.) This opened the gates to speculation about its authorship. There cannot be much doubt that *On Nutriment* is one of the later treatises in the Hippocratic Corpus, and several additional factors might have given rise to the identification of Herophilus as its author. First, in view of the absence of serious research on the pulse before Herophilus (see below, Chapter VII.A, *Introduction*, pp. 267–71), and in view of Herophilus' enormous sphygmological renown (Chapter VII, T144–T188), the mention of pulsation in Chapter 48 of *On Nutriment*, though only of a general nature, might have suggested to some critics that Herophilus was the author. A second factor which might have been interpreted as indicative of Herophilean authorship is that the author of *On Nutriment*, like Herophilus, has a certain amount in common with the Stoics (but see Chapter IV.A, *Introduction*, pp. 92–8). Third, Herophilus' reputation in antiquity for *subtilitas* and for being a 'dialectician' might have seemed compatible with the manneristic style of this treatise.[26] Fourth, Sextus Empiricus confirms that Herophilus was in fact interested in dietetics and even wrote a treatise on it (T29; cf. Chapter VIII, T230).

While these factors might have been thought by some critics of later antiquity to render Herophilus a suitable candidate for the authorship of *On Nutriment*, there can be little doubt that the work in fact postdates Herophilus, probably belonging to the second or first century B.C. Its Heraclitean tone and mannerisms are those of a self-consciously archaizing author, its aphoristic brachylogy is an unsuccessful attempt at 'Hippocratic' authenticity, and its Stoic or Pneumatic elements provide a reasonably firm *terminus post quem*. (Although pneuma played an important role in medicine much earlier, as Werner Jaeger showed, the first Pneumatist, Athenaeus of Attaleia, lived in the first century B.C.) The careful analyses by Diller[27] and Deichgräber,[28] in particular, have provided a number of

---

[26] Cf. commentary on T10, pp. 61–2 *supra*.
[27] Diller, 1936a which has become the foundation of all subsequent discussions.
[28] Deichgräber, 1973. Deichgräber's comments on style and general intellectual background seem to provide conclusive support for this date. Cf. also Kudlien, 1968d: col. 1101. See also Robert Joly, Budé edn (*Hp.*, VI.2), pp. 131–7.

other reasons for accepting this late date, and Herophilus can therefore be eliminated safely from candidacy for the authorship of *On Nutriment*.

Finally, the medieval *Epistula Herophili ad regem Antiochum*, briefly discussed in the Appendix to this edition, is not a genuine letter but a clear case of a 'pseudepigraphon', similar in character to the pseudepigraphic *Epistula Paraxagorae* [*sic*] in the same Brussels MS (3701–3715).[29] It is a brief, introductory medical handbook, clothed in a flimsy epistolographic disguise, of a kind that is well known in medieval medicine.

B · TEXTS

17 Galenus, *De anatomicis administrationibus* 6.8 (II, p. 571K)

τοῦτ' οὖν ὀρθῶς εἶπεν ὁ Ἡρόφιλος, ἔτι τε καὶ πρὸς τούτοις . . . ἀληθῶς ἔγραψεν ἐν αὐτῷ τούτῳ τῷ βιβλίῳ τῷ δευτέρῳ τῶν ἀνατομικῶν . . . (*Vid. Herophili Fr60 infra.*)

17 Herophilus therefore said this correctly and, in addition, . . . wrote truthfully in this, the second book of his *Anatomica* . . . (*See Chapter* VI, *Fr60 infra.*)

18 Galenus, *De semine* 2.1 (IV, p. 596K)

Ἡρόφιλος δὲ οὐκ οἶδ' ὅπως ἐκτὸς ἐκχεῖσθαί φησι τὸ τῶν θηλειῶν σπέρμα, καίτοι γε περὶ τῶν ὄρχεων ἀκριβῶς ἔγραψε τῶν κατ' αὐτὰς (sc. γυναῖκας) ἐν τῷ τρίτῳ τῆς ἀνατομῆς . . . (*Vid. Herophili Fr61 infra.*)

2 περὶ *Ald*: πως *P*   τῶν κατ' αὐτὰς *P*: τῆς κατ' αὐτοὺς *Ald*

18 Herophilus says the seed of females is somehow discharged to the outside, even though he wrote with accuracy about the 'testicles' [ovaries] in females in the third book of his *Anatomy* . . . (*See Chapter* VI, *Fr61 infra.*)

[29] Published by Schubring, 1962.

19 Galenus, *In Hippocratis Epidemiarum 2.4.1. Commentarius 4* (ad v.120 sq. L) (*CMG* v.10.1, p. 318 Pfaff) (From Ḥunain's Arabic translation)

... Herophilus ... said in Book IV of his treatise *On Anatomy* ... *(See Chapter VI, Fr62 infra.)*

20 Aetius Amidenus, *Libri medicinales* 7.48 (*CMG* VIII.2, p. 303, 4–5 Olivieri)

Ἡρόφιλος δὲ τὸ ἀνάπαλιν ἐν τῷ περὶ ὀφθαλμῶν φησι ... *(Vid. Herophili Fr260 infra.)*

20 Herophilus says the reverse in his work *On Eyes* ... *(See Chapter VIII, Fr260 infra.)*

21 Galenus, *De pulsuum differentiis* 4.2 (VIII, p. 716K)

ἐναντίως δ' αὐτῷ (sc. Αἰγιμίῳ) τὸν Ἡρόφιλον εὕροις ἂν εὐθὺς ἐν ἀρχῇ τῆς περὶ σφυγμῶν πραγματείας διορίζοντα σφυγμὸν παλμοῦ. *(Vid. Herophili T148 infra.)*

21 You would find that Herophilus, in contrast to him [sc. Aegimius], right at the beginning of his treatise *On Pulses* distinguishes pulsation from palpitation. *(See Chapter VII, T148 infra.)*

22 Galenus (ex Aristoxeno?), *De pulsuum differentiis* 4.3 (VIII, p. 724K)

... Ἡρόφιλος εὐθέως ἐν ἀρχῇ τῆς περὶ σφυγμῶν πραγματείας ἀνατρέπειν πειρᾶται τὴν τοῦ διδασκάλου (sc. Πραξαγόρου) δόξαν .... ὥστε εἰ μνημονεύω νῦν αὐτῆς Ἡροφίλου ῥήσεως, ἣν ἐν ἀρχῇ τοῦ πρώτου περὶ σφυγμῶν ἔγραψεν, ἢ τῶν εἰρημένων
5 τοῖς ἀπ' αὐτοῦ, μέγεθος ἑνὸς βιβλίου γενήσεται περὶ μόνων τούτων ἐπιμελῶς διερχομένου ... *(Vid. Herophili T150 infra.)*

22 ... Right at the beginning of his treatise *On Pulses* Herophilus tries to overturn his teacher's [sc. Praxagoras'] belief ... So if I now

were to recall the statement Herophilus recorded at the beginning of the first book of his *On Pulses*, or of the things said by his followers, it would be the size of a whole book even if it explained only these things carefully . . . *(See Chapter* VII, *T150 infra.)*

23 Galenus, *De pulsuum dignotione* 4.3 (VIII, p. 956K)

πρῶτον δ' ἀπ' αὐτῆς ἄρξομαι τῆς λέξεως, ἧς ἐκεῖνοι προβάλλουσιν, ἐν τῷ πρώτῳ [περὶ] τῶν Ἡροφίλου περὶ σφυγμῶν γεγραμμένης, ἣν καὶ μόνην ἀνεγνωκέναι μοι δοκοῦσιν. *(Vid. Herophili T162 infra.)*

2 περὶ *delevi (cf. Gal. ibid.* VIII, *p. 959K)*

23 First I shall start from the passage they put forward: the one recorded in the first book of Herophilus' *On Pulses*, which is also the only passage they seem to me to have read . . . *(See Chapter* VII, *T162 infra.)*

24 Galenus (ex Aristoxeno?), *De pulsuum differentiis* 4.4 (VIII, p. 726K)

καὶ λέγει (sc. ὁ Ἡροφίλειος Ἀλέξανδρος ὁ Φιλαλήθης ἐπικληθείς) γέ τινας λογισμοὺς ἐπ' αὐτοῖς, ὡς οἴεται, πιθανοὺς ἐν τῷ ε' τῶν ἀρεσκόντων, ὥσπερ καὶ ὁ Ταραντῖνος Ἡρακλείδης ἐν οἷς ἀντιλέγει πρὸς τὸ περὶ σφυγμῶν Ἡροφίλου. *(Vid. AP.3 infra.)*

24 And he [sc. the Herophilean Alexander, called 'Philalethes' or 'Truth-lover'] mentions some additional arguments – persuasive ones, as he thinks – in Book V of his *Opinions*, just like Heraclides of Tarentum in his arguments against Herophilus' *On Pulses*. *(See Chapter* XXII, *AP.3 infra.)*

25 Soranus, *Gynaecia* 3, prooem. 3.4 *(CMG* IV, p. 95 Ilberg)

καὶ Ἡρόφιλος ἐν τῷ Μαιωτικῷ φησι τὴν ὑστέραν ἐκ τῶν αὐτῶν τοῖς ἄλλοις μέρεσι πεπλέχθαι . . . *(Vid. T193 infra.)*

25 Herophilus too says in his book *Midwifery* that the womb is woven together from the same things as the other parts . . . *(See Chapter* VII, *T193 infra.)*

26 Soranus, *Gynaecia* 4.1 [53]. 4 (*CMG* IV, p. 130 Ilberg)

Ἡρόφιλος δὲ ἐν τῷ Μαιωτικῷ λέγει . . . *(Vid. Herophili Fr196 infra.)*

1 ἐν *Ermerins*: ἐπὶ P

26 But Herophilus says in his book *Midwifery* . . . *(See Chapter* VII, *Fr196 infra.)*

27 Caelius Aurelianus, *Tardae passiones* 2.13.186

. . . Herophilus primo libro Curationum . . . *(Vid. T231 infra.)*

27 . . . Herophilus, in Book One of his *Therapeutics* . . . *(See Chapter* VIII, *T231 infra.)*

28 Galenus, *De simplicium medicamentorum temperamentis ac facultatibus* 6, prooem. (XI, p. 795K)

See Chapter VIII, *T252 infra.*

29 Sextus Empiricus, *Adversus Mathematicos* 11 (= *Adv. Ethicos*).50

Ἡρόφιλος δὲ ἐν τῷ διαιτητικῷ . . .*(Vid. T230 infra)*

29 Herophilus [says] in his *Regimen* . . . *(See Chapter* VIII, *T230 infra.)*

30 Soranus, *Gynaecia* 1.27.2–3 (*CMG* IV, p. 17 Ilberg)

καὶ Ἡρόφιλος ἐν τῷ πρὸς τὰς κοινὰς δόξας ἐμνημόνευσεν . . . *(Vid. Herophili T203 infra.)*

30 ... Herophilus also mentioned in his book *Against Common Opinions* ... *(See Chapter* VII, *T203 infra.)*

31 Caelius Aurelianus, *Tardae passiones* 4.8.113

Herophilus vero libro quem ad Hippocratis Prognosticum scripsit ... *(Vid. T261 infra.)*

31 In the book Herophilus wrote against Hippocrates' *Prognostic* ... *(See Chapter* IX, *T261 infra.)*

32 Galenus, *In Hippocratis Prognosticum commentarius* 1.4 *(CMG* v. 9.2, p. 205 Heeg)

κάλλιον οὖν μοι δοκεῖ διὰ τῶνδε τῶν ὑπομνημάτων αὐτὰ τὰ χρήσιμα μόνα διεξελθεῖν, ἐξετάσαι δὲ αὖθις ἐπὶ σχολῆς πλείονος ἐν ἑτέρᾳ πραγματείᾳ καὶ διασκέψασθαι περὶ τῶν ὑπὸ Ἡροφίλου πρὸς τὸ Προγνωστικὸν Ἱπποκράτους ἀντειρημένων. *(Vid. Herophili T264 infra.)*

2 διελθεῖν *ab Aldo edd.*   3 ὑπὸ *om.* RP   4 ἀντειρημένον *F*[1]

32 I therefore thought it better to expound only the useful details through these commentaries [at present], but at a time of greater leisure to examine and scrutinize again in another treatise the things said by Herophilus in opposition to Hippocrates' *Prognostic. (See Chapter* IX, *T264 infra.)*

33 Galenus, *In Hippocratis Prognosticum comment.* 1.4 *(CMG* v.9.2, p. 207 Heeg)

ὅπερ οὖν εἶπον ἔμπροσθεν, ὡς οὐ χρὴ μνημονεύειν ἐν τοῖσδε τοῖς ὑπομνήμασι τῶν μοχθηρῶς εἰρημένων ἁπάντων, ἀλλ' ὅσα πιθανοῦ τινος ἔχεται (διὸ καὶ τὰ κακῶς ὑπὸ Ἡροφίλου γεγραμμένα πρὸς τὰς Ἱπποκράτους προγνώσεις ἀνεβαλλόμην
5 ἐπισκέψασθαι), τοῦτο καὶ νῦν καὶ καθ' ὅλον τὸν ἐφεξῆς λόγον αὐτός τε ποιήσω ... *(Vid. T262–266 infra.)*

1 ὡς *om. F*[1]   2 μοχθηρῶν *F*[1]   4 ἀνεκαλλόμην *P*   5 ἐπισκέψεσθαι *Aldus*

33 Both now and in the whole subsequent book I myself shall therefore do exactly what I said previously, namely that not all the badly written comments [sc. of previous commentators?] should be mentioned in these commentaries, but only those to which there is something plausible – for which reason I have also postponed examining the things written so poorly by Herophilus against Hippocrates' prognoses . . . *(See Chapter* IX, *T262–265 infra.)*

34 Galenus, *In Hippocratis Aphorismos commentarius* 7.70 (XVIIIA, pp. 186–7K)

διὰ τοῦτο ἀναγκάζονται προσγράφειν τοῖς ἐξ ἀρχῆς εὑρεθεῖσιν ἢ ἀφαιρεῖν ἢ μεταγράφειν, ὥσπερ ἀμέλει καὶ κατὰ τόνδε τὸν ἀφορισμόν (sc. Ἱπποκράτους 3.ξθ'), οὗ τὴν λέξιν οἱ πρῶτοι τῶν ἐξηγησαμένων τοὺς ἀφορισμούς, ὧν ἐστιν ὁ Ἡροφίλειος Βακχεῖος, Ἡρακλείδης τε καὶ Ζεῦξις οἱ ἐμπειρικοί, τοιαύτην τινὰ γράφουσιν· ὁκόσοις ἂν κάτω ὠμὰ ὑποχωρέῃ, χολῆς μελαίνης ἐστίν . . . '

4 ὁ Ἡροφίλειος Βακχεῖος *coni. Cobet, Klein:* Ἡρόφιλος, ὁ Βακχεῖος *Kühn* 6 διαχωρέῃ (*aut* ὑποχωρέῃ) ἀπὸ *codd. Hippocratis.*

34 For this reason [sc. because what a transmitted text says is not true] one is compelled to write things in addition to what was discovered at the beginning, or to subtract from it, or to rewrite it; just as, to be sure, in the case of this aphorism [sc. Hippocratic *Aphorism* 7.69], the first of those who interpreted the *Aphorisms,* among them the Herophilean* Bacchius, and the Empiricists Heraclides and Zeuxis, give the following reading: 'In all patients whose alvine discharges are crude, this is caused by black bile . . . '

35 Galenus, *De septimestri partu* 2 (45 sqq.). (From the Arabic translation; cf. Richard Walzer, *Rivista di studi orientali* 15 (1935), p. 345.)

Some people are of the opinion that the book *On Nutriment* [sc. in

* C. G. Cobet and J. Klein, probably correctly, emend the text to read 'Bacchius the Herophilean' instead of Kühn's reading '*Herophilus,* Bacchius'; cf. *supra,* pp. 75–6, and *infra,* Chapter IX.A; cf. T270, pp. 438–9.

the Hippocratic Corpus] is not by Thessalus but rather that the author is someone from Herophilus' circle, whereas others are of the opinion that the author is unknown.

36a *Scholium M* in Hippocratis *De alimento* (init.), Codex Marcianus graecus 269 (s.XI), fol. 77v (apud I. L. Heiberg, *Hippocratis opera* I.1, *CMG* I.1 (1927), p. 79)

τοῦτο (sc. τὸ περὶ τροφῆς βιβλίον) ἀνδρὸς οὐ τοῦ τυχόντος καὶ τάχα ἴσως τοῦ Θεσσαλοῦ, δοκεῖ δέ τισιν ὑπὸ Ἡροφίλου συγκεῖσθαι, φησὶν ὁ Γαληνός.

2 Ἡροφίλου *M*: Ἡροδίκου *Deichgräber (Abh. Berlin 1933.3, p. 63 adn. 1, sed cf. comm. supra III.A.2). Aulus Gellius (Noct. Att. 3.16) autem et Erotianus (Vocum Hippocraticarum coll. p. 9.16 Nachmanson) hunc librum ab Hippocrate scriptum esse censuerunt.*

36a Galen says this work [sc. the Hippocratic *On Nutriment*] is not by any chance person, and perhaps by Thessalus, but some think it was composed by Herophilus.*

36b *Scholia E et F* in Hippocratis *De alimento* (init.), Codex Parisinus graecus 2255, fol. 170v, et cod. Par. gr. 2144, fol. 74 (apud E. Littré, *Hippocratis opera* IX, p. 98 adn. 1)

τοῦτο σύγγραμμά (sc. περὶ τροφῆς) φησιν ὁ Γαληνὸς μὴ εἶναι Ἱπποκράτους, πλὴν ἀλλ' οὐδὲ παλαιοῦ τοῦ τυχόντος σοφοῦ, καὶ ἴσως εἴη τοῦ Θεσσάλου. δοκεῖ δὲ ὑπὸ Ἡροφίλου συγκεῖσθαι.

36b Galen says this treatise [sc. the Hippocratic *On Nutriment*] is not by Hippocrates – but also not just by any chance learned figure of ancient times – and perhaps it could be by Thessalus. But it seems to be composed by Herophilus.

37 Galenus, *Thrasybulus (Utrum medic. an gymn. hygieine)* 47 (*Scr. min.* III, p. 99 Helmreich)

. . . Ἱπποκράτης καὶ Διοκλῆς καὶ Πραξαγόρας καὶ Φιλότιμος

* Deichgräber emends the MS reading 'Herophilus' to 'Herodicus'; cf. above, pp. 76–8.

καὶ Ἡρόφιλος ὅλης τῆς περὶ τὸ σῶμα τέχνης ἐπιστήμονες ἦσαν, ὡς δηλοῖ τὰ γράμματα αὐτῶν ... (Vid. Herophili T227 infra.)

1 φιλότιμος codd. edd.: corr. Wellmann   3 γράμματα P Ald: συγγράμματα L

37 ... Hippocrates, Diocles, Praxagoras, Phylotimus, and Herophilus were knowledgeable about the whole science concerning the body, as their *writings* make clear... (See Chapter VIII, T227 infra.)

38 Galenus, *De pulsuum dignotione* 2.3 (VIII, p. 869K)

ἀλλὰ μικρὸν μὲν τὸν τοῦ παιδὸς εἰρήκασι σφυγμόν, ὡσαύτως δὲ καὶ τὸν τοῦ γέροντος μικρόν, ὁπότερος δ' αὐτῶν μικρότερος, οὐκέτι γράφουσιν, καίτοι σαφῶς Ἡροφίλου τοῖς γε μὴ παρέργως ἐντυγχάνουσιν αὐτοῦ τοῖς βιβλίοις ὑπὲρ ἀμφοτέρων
5 γεγραφότος. (Vid. Herophili T184 infra.)

3 γε ABL: τε vulg.

38 They have said the pulse of a child is small, and likewise that the pulse of an old man is small; but they do not record at all which of the two is smaller, although Herophilus wrote clearly about both, at least for those who don't have just a casual encounter with his *books*. (See Chapter VII, T184 infra.)

39 Galenus, *De pulsuum dignotione* 4.3 (VIII, p. 954K)

ταῦτ' οὖν αὐτοὶ μὲν λεγέτωσαν, Ἡροφίλου δὲ μὴ καταψευδέσθωσαν, μηδὲ δυσωπείτωσαν ὀνόματι σεμνῷ τοὺς ἀμαθεῖς τῶν Ἡροφίλου γραμμάτων, μηδ' ἐκ τούτου τὴν πίστιν τῷ λόγῳ πορίζεσθωσαν. (Vid. Herophili T162 infra.)

39 Let them then say this themselves, but do not let them falsify Herophilus, let them not put to shame with a revered name those who are ignorant of Herophilus' *writings*, and let them not procure belief in their argument on this basis. (See Chapter VII, T162 infra.)

40 C. Plinius Secundus, *Naturalis historia* I (Argumentum ad Librum XI)

ex auctoribus externis: . . . Apollodoro qui de bestiis venenatis. Hippocrate. Herophilo. Erasistrato. Asclepiade. Themisone.

40 [Excerpts] from foreign *authors*: . . . from Apollodorus who wrote about poisonous animals, from Hippocrates, Herophilus, Erasistratus, Asclepiades, Themison . . .

41 Ps.-Galenus, *Definitiones medicae*, prooem. (XIX, pp. 347-8K)

μετὰ δὲ τοὺς τούτου (sc. Ἱπποκράτους) χρόνους οἱ γενόμενοί τινες συνέγραψαν ὅρους, καὶ οὗτοι δὲ οὐ πάντας. δοκοῦσι δὲ ἐπιμελεῖς γεγονέναι ἐν τῇ τοιαύτῃ θεωρίᾳ οἵ τε ἀπὸ τῆς Ἡροφίλου αἱρέσεως καὶ Ἀπολλώνιος ὁ Μεμφίτης, ἔτι δὲ καὶ
5 Ἀθηναῖος ὁ Ἀτταλεύς, ἀλλὰ καὶ οὗτοι οὔτε τῇ τάξει τῇ δεούσῃ ἐχρήσαντο οὔτε συνήγαγον τὴν πραγματείαν, ἀλλὰ διεσπαρμένως ἐν τοῖς βιβλίοις συνέγραψαν. ἔτι δὲ καὶ ἐνδεῶς ἀνεγράφησαν. οὔτε γὰρ πάντες ὡρίσαντο τὰ κατὰ τὴν ἰατρικήν.

41 Certain authors who lived after the times of Hippocrates composed definitions, but not all definitions. The members of the school of Herophilus seem to have been fastidious in speculation of this kind, as was Apollonius of Memphis, and also Athenaeus of Attaleia. They too, however, neither employed the required order nor collected [their definitions into] a treatise, but rather composed them in a scattered fashion in their *books*. Furthermore, they [sc. the definitions] were described inadequately, for they [sc. the authors] did not all define them in accordance with medical science.

C · COMMENTS

T24 Schöne, 1893, has argued that this Galenic testimonium is directly dependent on Book XIII of Aristoxenus' treatise *On the School of Herophilus* (for details see Chapter XXV.A below).

Heraclides of Tarentum: a distinguished member of the Empiricist school in the first half of the first century B.C. The 'arguments against

Herophilus' *On Pulses'*, which Deichgräber (1965: 259 and fr. 171–2) interprets as a book with the title *Against Herophilus' On Pulses*, might have its origins in an attempt to justify his conversion from Herophileanism (cf. Chapter xviii, *Ma.* 2, *infra*) to Empiricism. This testimonium is not uncharacteristic of the mediated nature of much of the evidence about Hellenistic medicine:

3rd cent. B.C.: Herophilus, *On Pulses*
↓
early 1st cent. B.C.: Heraclides, *Against Herophilus' On Pulses*
↓
c. birth of Christ (?): Aristoxenus, *On the School of Herophilus*
↓
later 2nd cent. A.D.: Galen, *On Pulse Differences*

T27 See Chapter viii, *Comment* on T231.

T28 See Chapter viii, *Comment* on T252.

T30 See Chapter viii, *Comment* on T203.

T34 Zeuxis, Heraclides: Deichgräber, 1965: fr. 365. See also Chapters ix, xiv, and xv *infra* for examples and discussions of Hippocratic philology in the Herophilean school.

ἀναγκάζονται: 'one is compelled'; on the popularity of this use of the third person plural in Hellenistic prose see Rydbeck, 1967: 27–45.

ἀμέλει: 'to be sure'; on the growing number of uses of ἀμέλει in Hellenistic prose see Blomquist, 1969: 103–7.

T35, T36a–b Thessalus: not the Neronian Methodist from Tralleis but the 'son of Hippocrates', on whom see p. 64, *Comment* on T16.

T36b πλὴν ἀλλ': on the adversative–eliminative and other uses of πλήν in Hellenistic prose cf. Blomquist, 1969: 75–100.

T37 Diocles, fr. 144 Wellmann; Praxagoras fr. 43 Steckerl.

T40 Much of Book xi of Pliny's *Natural History* is devoted to human and animal physiology, but the only mention of Herophilus occurs in Pliny's discussion of arteries and veins (xi.89.219; see T186; cf. T185). Whether Pliny actually had access to any of Herophilus' works is difficult to determine. The *Indices auctorum* provided for each book in Book i of the *Natural History* are not enumerations of written sources directly consulted by Pliny – although these sources are also included – but rather inaccurate lists of the authors mentioned or quoted in Books ii–xxxvii, and of authors quoted by his sources. In his *praefatio* (17) Pliny claims that he drew his material 'Ex exquisitis auctoribus centum', but in the *Indices* he lists no less

than 473 authors. F. Münzer, H. Stadler, and others have shown that the
Indices are not much more than lists of all authors of whom Pliny knew that
they had written on the topics treated in a given book of the *Natural History*.
Not even Brunn's Law (*Plinium eodem ordine, quo in componendis libris usus est,
auctores etiam in indices rettulisse*) is observed religiously, and the sequence in
which the 'sources' for Book XI are enumerated is therefore not conclusive
proof that a work by Herophilus – his *On Pulses* would be the most likely
candidate – was used after a work by Hippocrates and before one by
Erasistratus. (For 'Brunn's Law' see Brunn, 1856). Cf. Stadler, 1891: 31ff.;
Münzer, 1897: 128–33; Kroll, 1951: cols. 424–8.

IV · THE PARTS OF
THE ART OF MEDICINE

A · INTRODUCTION

1 *Historical background*

Herophilus' tripartite division of 'the art of medicine' into knowledge of things concerning health, knowledge of things concerning disease, and knowledge of neutral things is an intriguing manifestation of a taxonomic passion shared by many Greeks.

The interest in the relation of the whole to its parts – the 'whole' often being an art, a science, or any class, genus or species of animate or inanimate things – increased especially from the fourth century B.C. onwards. Not only in medicine and biology, but also in rhetoric, philosophy, and educational theory an ordering urge can be seen at work, using many different structures: *diairesis* (as in Plato's *Statesman* and *Sophist*, and in a fragment of the physician Mnesitheus of Athens[1]); *ephexēs*-relations (as in Aristotle's account of the relation of the parts of the psyche to each other[2]); genus and species classifications (as in Aristotle's *Categories, Topics, Metaphysics*, and in the 'Hippocratic' *On Nutriment*[3]); a wide variety of classifications by

[1] Mnesitheus, fr. 10–11 Bertier.
[2] Arist., *De anima* 2.3.414b20–415a13 (ἐφεξῆς, 414b29). Cf. *id.*, *Metaphysics* 4.2.1004a2–9, 11.12.1068b31–1069a13, 13.9.1085a3–9 for similar 'successive' relations.
[3] *Topics* 1.5.102a31–2; 2.4.111a25–32; 4.1.120b11–4.5.128b10. *Metaphysics* 7.12.1037b27–1038a35; 7.14.1039a24–b19; 10.7.1057b4–7; 11.1.1059b25–1060a2, etc. *Categories* 3.1b10–24; 5.2a35–3b9; 13.14b33–15a7. In his zoological works Aristotle uses γένος for a number of different modern concepts (class, order, family, genus, species) – and at times he also uses εἶδος and γένος interchangeably – but the principles of classification on each occasion are essentially similar. Cf. *Historia animalium* 1.6.490b7–23 (and 2.15.505b26); *De partibus animalium* 1.1.639a15–19; 1.2.642b5–4.644b21; 4.5.679b16ff. But see n. 4 and cf. A. C.

89

differentiae (as in Aristotle's zoological works[4]); comprehensive correlational and analogic models (e.g. elements: qualities: humours: seasons), and so on.[5] Herophilus' division is therefore but one of the many taxonomic endeavours that had become characteristic of his age.

The only sources which explicitly attribute a tripartite division to Herophilus – Galen and pseudo-Galen[6] – refer to it in passing comments scattered through five different treatises (T42–T46), and details of the division remain correspondingly murky. This much is, however, reasonably clear:

(i) 'Knowledge of things related to health' is knowledge of everything concerning the construction and proper, harmonious functioning of a healthy body and its parts (T42), i.e. anatomy and physiology. It would therefore seem to include one of Herophilus' areas of special expertise, sphygmology, at least as it pertains to normal pulse functions. His treatise *Anatomy* and at least part of his *On Pulses* apparently belong to this branch. If Herophilus took a non-pathological view of normal childbirth, as the fragments from his *Midwifery* suggest, parts of this treatise too would seem to fall under the 'healthy' branch of medicine, namely those dealing specifically with the anatomy and physiology of the female body, and hence with its natural functions in health. (The passages from *Midwifery* which deal with difficult childbirth are more problematic from this classificatory perspective, especially since Herophilus did not always distinguish clearly between form and function.)

Not so clear is whether regimen for the healthy also belongs to this category. Dietetics had an important hygienic or preventive function in antiquity (and not only a therapeutic function), as, for example,

---

Lloyd, 1962; Balme, 1962. In the Hippocratic Corpus 'genus and species' also recur frequently. Cf., e.g., *On Nutriment* 1, 17 (μία–πολλαί), 28 (ὅλον–μέρος), 51, and Deichgräber, 1973: 15, 33, 51–2, 67. See also Diller, 1973: 28, on 'das Streben nach Einteilung'. (But cf. pp. 76–7 *supra*.)

[4] Ever since J. B. Meyer's famous *Aristoteles' Thierkunde* (Berlin, 1855) modern scholarship has been at pains to emphasize that Aristotle's zoological treatises are not essays in taxonomy, and this is undoubtedly correct (cf., e.g., Peck, 1965–: vol. I, v-xiii). One should not, however, stress this point at the expense of the strong classificatory thrust in many parts of these Aristotelian works. See Balme, 1962, and 1961; G. E. R. Lloyd, 1961.

[5] Cf. Schöner, 1964, for numerous examples.

[6] T42–T45. (T46–T47 are dependent on the earlier sources.)

the Hippocratic *Regimen in Health* confirms.[7] In the first century A.D.[8] this hygienic-preventive function was again reaffirmed: '*Most* people define medicine this way: it is an art which is capable of providing a *diet* for the *healthy* and cures for the ill' (ps.-Galen, *Definitiones medicae* 9, vol. XIX, p. 351K). Like Herophilus' 'neutrals', dietetics was, however, also widely used for two other purposes: (a) for therapeutic goals (as in the Hippocratic *Regimen in Acute Diseases*), and (b) for preventing the deterioration of morbid conditions (cf. the Hippocratic *Regimen*, with its emphasis on anticipatory or prophylactic treatment: προδιάγνωσις, προμηθεῖσθαι, etc.[9]). These multiple functions of dietetics are alluded to in the relativistic theory of δύναμις ('power', 'capacity') applied to food in the Hippocratic treatise *On Nutriment*: all foods and drinks are good or bad only πρός τι, i.e. in relation to something – a view also found in the Hippocratic *Aphorism* 7.66: the same food can be 'strength to the healthy but disease to the ill'.

If Herophilus' characterization of 'neutrals' as *all* the aids applied *in diseases* is to be taken at face value, regimen, including both diet and exercise, would therefore seem to have an ambivalent status, with its therapeutic foot in the 'neutral' camp and its purely 'hygienic' foot in the 'healthy' camp of things related to the harmonious functioning of a healthy body. A similar ambivalence is suggested by the Empiricists' subdivision of hygiene (which they separated completely from therapeutics) into that which preserves perfect health and that which helps convalescents to reattain full health.

(ii) 'Knowledge of things related to disease' is knowledge of whatever disrupts or destroys the healthy harmony of the body and causes dysfunctions (T42), i.e. pathology. Some of Herophilus' treatises – for example, *On Pulses*, *Midwifery*, and *On Eyes* – probably straddled the first two branches of medicine, since they dealt not only with pathological but also with physiological and anatomical details.

---

[7] Cf. Edelstein, 1931a = 1967: 307: 'Medicine in Hellenistic times, like earlier medicine, is concerned with the dietetics of the healthy. Indeed, at this time the doctrine of health is considered to be not only as important as therapeutics; it seems to be even more important than healing the sick'.

[8] The pseudo-Galenic *Definitions* were probably written in the first century B.C. Cf. the analysis by Kollesch, 1973.

[9] On this treatise cf. Diller, 1959a. The so-called 'Cnidian' treatises also emphasize the relation of aetiology, diagnosis, and therapy, but the prophylactic orientation which dominates especially the third book of *Regimen* is missing in them.

(iii) 'Knowledge of the neutrals' is identified as knowledge of the aids applied in disease and the material substances of which they are composed. Since the emphasis here is on '*all* the remedial measures applied in diseases' (T42), it would seem reasonable to conclude that this branch of medicine includes not only pharmacology, a part of which (materia medica) is explicitly identified, but also surgery, and, to the extent that it is used for therapeutic purposes, dietetics. Herophilus' treatise *Therapeutics* clearly belongs to this branch, and his *Regimen* possibly too. A therapeutic fragment from his work *On Eyes* (Fr 260 below) also survives, but, as suggested above, this work probably contained anatomical, physiological, and pathological sections as well.

While this leaves us with some unanswered questions – for example, where in this scheme prognostic, Hippocratic exegesis, and doxography might belong – it does provide an apparently authentic framework for ordering most of the testimonia, even though several of Herophilus' treatises straddled more than one of his main branches of medicine.

An assessment of the historical position of Herophilus' classificatory scheme might be facilitated by a brief consideration of divisions developed by other physicians and by philosophers. While a number of trichotomous divisions became entrenched in the late fourth century and the early Hellenistic period,[10] those most directly

[10] Cf., for example, *Metaphysics* 6.2.1026b27–37 (with Jaeger's conjecture in b30; *vid.* OCT edn, and Jaeger, 1960: vol. i, pp. 223–4), 1027a8–16; 11.8.1064b32–6; 6.1.1025b18–28; 11.7.1064a10–b2; *id., Topics* 6.6.145a15–16; 8.1.157a10–11, etc. See also Chapter vii, T223a–b, *infra,* and p. 305; Deichgräber, 1965: 309–10; Kollesch, 1968, who, however, does not discuss Herophilus with reference to the tripartite division of the interpretation of signs into those concerning the past, present, and future. Deichgräber (1965: 289) claims that the Empiricists invented this trichotomy, and that 'Herophileans' subsequently took it over from the Empiricists. The reverse might be closer to the truth; see Chapter vii (T223b). Cf. a similar temporal trichotomy (which might have inspired Herophilus to resort to his notion of τρίχρονος σημείωσις) in the Hippocratic *Epidemics* 1.11 (i, pp. 189–90Kw): λέγειν τὰ προγενόμενα, γινώσκειν τὰ παρεόντα, προλέγειν τὰ ἐσόμενα ... (in the context of σημαίνειν), and *Prognostic* 1 (i, p. 78Kw): προγινώσκων γὰρ καὶ προλέγων παρὰ τοῖσι νοσέουσι τά τε παρεόντα καὶ τὰ προγεγονότα καὶ τὰ μέλλοντα ἔσεσθαι ... One of the more influential trichotomous divisions – of philosophy into three parts – was introduced by Herophilus' fellow Chalcedonian, Xenocrates, fr. 1 Heinze = 82 Isnardi Parente (S.E., *M* 7.16). It was accepted by most Stoics; cf. S.E., *ibid.* (where it is also attributed to the Peripatos) = *SVF* ii, 38; cf. *SVF* i, 45–6 and ii, 35–44. For Epicurus' similar tripartite division see *Vita* 30 (D.L.10.30; p. 21 Arrigh.).

relevant to Herophilus' scheme seem to be two famous Stoic divisions.

First, the Stoics divided dialectic into 'knowledge of things that are true, false, and neither of these'.[11] 'Art of medicine' parallels 'art of dialectic'; 'health-related' and 'disease-related' parallel 'true' and 'false'; 'knowledge' and 'neither' ('neutral') are the same in both definitions.

Also closely analogous to Herophilus' division is a second Stoic division, of 'the things that are' into those that are good, those that are bad, and those that are 'neither': τῶν δ' ὄντων τὰ μὲν ἀγαθά, τὰ δὲ κακά, τὰ δ' οὐδέτερα ... (D.L. 7.101 = SVF III, 117). (In some accounts of Stoicism 'indifferent things', ἀδιάφορα, is substituted for 'neither' or 'neutral', οὐδέτερα, but in other respects the divisions remain similar.) While the parallels are again striking, and 'good' and 'evil' seem to be an ethical version of Herophilus' 'healthy' and 'diseased', an important Stoic distinction between physical and moral states complicates the analogy.[12] According to the Stoics, health and disease are not 'good' or 'bad' but belong among the 'neutral' or 'indifferent' things.[13] The good things comprise only virtues like justice, courage, and prudence, while the bad things refer to their harmful opposites: injustice, cowardice, folly, and so on. The neutrals or indifferents, by contrast, neither benefit nor harm a person morally[14] and hence do not contribute either to one's happiness, eudaimonia, or to its opposite, kakodaimonia.

In the Stoic view health and disease are therefore 'neutrals' or

---

[11] D.L.7.62 (from Diocles of Magnesia?) = SVF II, 122 and Posidonius fr. 188 Edelstein–Kidd = 454 Theiler; S.E., M 11.187 = SVF II, 123. See also S.E., P 2.94 and 2.247, and D.L. 7.42 (= SVF II, 48).

[12] Cf. the Stoic tripartite subdivision of the 'good' things, which tries to establish that all 'bodily goods', such as health, in fact are not 'goods': 'The Stoics ... declared that there are three classes of goods ...: some concern the psyche [e.g. virtues, right actions], some are external [e.g. friends, good children, parents], some neither psychical nor external [e.g. the virtuous person's relation to himself]; and they eliminate the class of goods concerning the body as not being goods ...'(S.E., M 11.46 = SVF III, 96).

[13] Already Zeno called health an 'indifferent' (ἀδιάφορον): SVF I, 190 (cf. also III. 70). So too Ariston of Chius (ibid., I, 359, p. 81, line 33); Diogenes of Babylon (ibid., III, Diog. 39); Apollodorus of Seleucia, Chrysippus, and Hecaton (cf. ibid., III, Apollod. 14; III, 117–23, 138–9, the latter however with critical apparatus). For further details on the role of the 'indifferents' in Stoic ethics cf. Kidd, 1971; and Reesor, 1951. On the problems inherent in this Stoic classification of health and disease, and on differences between individual Stoics, see Kudlien, 1974b.

[14] SVF III, 117ff.

'indifferents', just like wealth or poverty, a good or a poor reputation, high or low birth, and handsomeness or ugliness, whereas Herophilus follows an earlier tradition which regards health as a good.[15] Like the lyric poets Simonides (*PMG* 604), Licymnius (*PMG* 769), Ariphron (*PMG* 813), and others,[16] he seems to have awarded health the highest rank among the goods: even wisdom, science, wealth, and rationality, Herophilus says in what has almost become an obligatory cliché of popular value systems, are useless possessions in the absence of health (cf. Chapter VIII T230 *infra*).

Despite these differences, the analogies and correspondences between the Stoic and Herophilean divisions remain striking, even to the point that both include ternary subdivisions of their 'neutrals'. Herophilus' subdivision of the neutrals is not without its difficulties – and there might have been more than one such subdivision (see *Comments, infra,* on T45) – but it is at least attested (T44) that he divided the neutrals into (a) those which participate equally in both extremes,[17] (b) those which participate in neither of the extremes, and (c) those which participate now in this, now in that extreme. The Stoics likewise introduced tripartite subdivisions of their neutrals: first, into (a) those neutrals capable of arousing impulse (ὁρμή), (b) those capable of arousing repulse (ἀφορμή), and (c) those arousing neither impulse nor repulse (for instance, whether one has an odd or even number of hairs; Stobaeus, *Eclogae* 2.7.7c = II, p. 82 = *SVF* III, 121). Secondly, the Stoics subdivided neutrals into (a) those which contribute neither to happiness nor to unhappiness (this is the primary sense of 'indifferent' according to Sextus Empiricus, *M* 11.61[18]); (b) those with reference to which impulse and repulse occur equally; and (c) those which cause neither impulse nor repulse.[19] A

---

[15] Cf. below, Chapter VIII, T230. Interesting on the history of the question whether or not health is a 'good' (ἀγαθόν) is the survey in S.E., *M* 11.47–67. Particularly striking is the mediating solution of the Academic philosopher Crantor (*c.* 335–275 B.C.), who awards second place among the goods to health, after virtue (of which courage is the only example given), but before the third-ranking pleasure and last-place wealth (*ibid.*, 57–9).

[16] Cf. also *Carmen popularium* (*PMG* 882); the anonymous paean preserved in an inscription from Erythraea (*PMG* 934); Pindar, *Paean* 6.180–1 (but see also *Pythian* 3.73); Aristophanes, *Birds* 603, 877–8.

[17] In Galen's *Ars medica* I (I, pp. 308–9K) this first part of the subdivision is treated somewhat differently; for details see IV.A.2 and *Comment,* T44. Cf. Ottoson, 1984: 68–9, 166–7.

[18] κατὰ δὲ ... τελευταῖον τρόπον φασὶν ἀδιάφορον .... (S.E., *M* 11.61 = *SVF* III, 122).   [19] *SVF* III, 122.

third Stoic subdivision of neutrals or indifferents is into (a) neutrals that are advanced above the zero point of indifference (προηγμένα); (b) those below the zero point (ἀποπροηγμένα); and (c) those that are 'neither' above nor below zero indifference.[20] In this relativistic subdivision, health is sometimes ranked among the indifferent things above point zero.

In other areas, too, the Stoics found many uses for antithetical divisions that include 'neutrals', 'indifferents', or 'intermediates' (expressed through οὐδέτερος, ἀδιάφορος, μεταξύ or οὔτε . . . οὔτε), and in view of the prolific use of these divisions in Stoicism it is not surprising that scholars have tended to give the Stoics exclusive credit for first putting the concepts 'neutral' and 'indifferent' to significant use.[21]

Not only the unusual prominence of 'neutrals' in both the Herophilean and the Stoic divisions, but especially the fact that Herophilus was a contemporary of the earliest Stoics gives rise to the question: which of the two originated this use of neutrals? Who influenced whom? The genealogy traditionally offered – that Herophilus' division is a child of the Stoic division – is the answer to a question which has prejudicial suppositions built into it, inasmuch as it assumes that only a relation of dependence or derivation could exist between Stoic and Herophilean texts. The following observations are aimed at showing that other possibilities remain open, and that they make a precipitate embrace of the traditional answer inadvisable.

While the Stoics might have 'influenced' Herophilus' decision to use 'neutrals', as is usually assumed,[22] the reverse is certainly possible too, especially given the well-documented Greek tendency to use medical models in ethics.[23] It is perhaps significant that Stoicism was not represented strongly in Alexandria. Furthermore, while the intellectual contact between Athens and Alexandria was by no means confined to the Peripatos, the roles of other localities such as Cos, Samos, and Cyrene in Alexandrian cultural life were considerably greater than that of Athens (cf. Chapter II.A). For all its magnetic

[20] *Ibid.* (*fin.*). More common among the Stoics is a dichotomous division of τὰ ἀδιάφορα or τὰ μεταξὺ τῶν ἀγαθῶν καὶ τῶν κακῶν into προηγμένα and ἀποπροηγμένα. Cf. *SVF* III, 127–39; and Zeno, *SVF* I, 192–4.

[21] For a further example see the table of a Stoic division of *phantasia* ('impression, presentation') in von Staden, 1978: 107 (repeated use of 'neither . . . nor').

[22] E.g. Deichgräber, 1929; cf. *id.*, 1965: 290.

[23] Cf., for example, Jaeger, 1957; Longrigg, 1963.

impact upon the rest of Greece, Alexandria attracted surprisingly few Greeks of Athenian origin as residents in the third century B.C.;[24] and Stoics of this period, though they frequently left Athens to advise other kings, were notoriously reluctant to go to the Alexandrian court. Cleanthes and Chrysippus, for example, both refused invitations from Ptolemies to visit Alexandria.[25]

On the other side of the scale one could put the possibility that Herophilus visited Athens[26] and came into direct contact with Stoicism, and the more relevant consideration that authors of theories are of course not themselves the only vehicles of influence; whether the 'flow' was from Herophilus or to him, texts and oral or written accounts by third parties could also have served as vehicles of influence. The invitations to Cleanthes and Chrysippus might indicate that the Ptolemies recognized the Stoics' stature. But none of this is conclusive. Most other considerations, such as chronology, are equally inconclusive. Thus 'moral indifferent' is a concept already attested for the earliest Stoic, Zeno,[27] and, if the dates suggested in Chapter II for Herophilus are even only approximately correct, Zeno and Herophilus were contemporaries.[28] None of these factors

[24] Unless Euclid was an Athenian, Demetrius of Phaleron seems to have been the only Athenian prominent in the intellectual life of Alexandria. 'Athenian' is also rare among the city-ethnics found in early Alexandria. A few examples are *Sammelb.* 398 (third century B.C.), 453, 1271 (third or second century B.C.), 10680 (300–275 B.C.) = *Supplementum Epigraphicum Graecum* 24.1166. Cf. also Callimachus' description, in his *Aetia* (fr. 178), of a banquet given by a certain Pollis, an Athenian resident of Alexandria, on the occasion of the Attic festival of Aiora (to commemorate the death of Erigone). In subsequent periods, however, mention of Athenians is less rare.

[25] D.L. 7.185. The Stoic Sphaerus of Borysthenes, a pupil of Zeno (*SVF* I, 622) and Cleanthes (D.L. 7.37), who was famous as a tutor and adviser of the Spartan king Cleomenes (cf. Plutarch, *Cleomenes* 2, 11, etc.), seems to have undertaken a journey to Egypt on invitation of a Ptolemy (D.L. 7.185; Athenaeus 8.354E), but by that time Herophilus' system might already have been worked out. On the date of Sphaerus' Egyptian journey cf. Hobein, 1929: cols. 1685–90.

[26] See T8 and the relevant comments in Chapter II.

[27] *SVF* I, 190–5.

[28] Zeno's dates are approximately 334/3-262/1 B.C. The date of his death is more certain than that of his birth; cf. *Pap. Herc.* 339, col. IV.9–14, and Mayer, 1912; also, off by two years, Eusebius' *Chronicle* of Jerome (*GCS* 47 (1956), p. 131, Ol.129.1). If Persaeus' report (D.L. 7.28) that Zeno died at age 72 is correct, the date suggested above stands. There are, however, also problematic reports that Zeno lived to 98 or 101 years old. Cf. the detailed discussion by von Fritz, 1972: 83–5.

therefore conclusively establishes the traditional view that the Stoics must have provided the model for Herophilus' trichotomy.

A third possibility is that of relatively independent developments in Athens and Alexandria. This hypothesis seems worth considering particularly in view of the fact that significant and explicit use of 'neutrals' and 'indifferents' was made well before the Stoics and Herophilus. Aristotle, for example, says in his discussion of pleasure in *Nicomachean Ethics* 10.5: 'Since activities differ with respect to goodness and depravity, some being worthy to be chosen, others to be avoided, and others *neither* (οὐδετέρων), so too are the pleasures . . . ' (1175b24–6). A foreshadowing of this distinction already occurs in Protagoras' relativistic discussion of the advantageous, the disadvantageous, and the 'neutral', also in an ethical context: 'I know of many things that are disadvantageous to man . . ., of some that are advantageous, and of some that are neither (οὐδέτερα) for man – but advantageous to horses . . . ' (Plato, *Protagoras* 334a3–6).[29] Furthermore, in his logic too Aristotle found use for 'indifferents' (whereas the Stoic 'indifferents' lack ethical differentia, Aristotle's indifferents are individual objects in logic, and the designation 'indifferent' refers to their lack of logical differentia).[30]

Earlier models therefore exist for the use of neutrals in conjunction with antithetical divisions, and it might only have remained for Herophilus and the Stoics to put 'neutrals' to new and more elaborate uses. The Peripatetic presence in Alexandria was, as mentioned earlier, strong.[31] Aristotle's successor Theophrastus was invited to teach in Alexandria (D.L. 5.37), and Theophrastus' pupil and successor Strato was one of Ptolemy II Philadelphus' tutors (D.L. 5.58). The role of the Peripatetic Demetrius of Phaleron in Alexandrian intellectual life was also powerful. Aristotle's school was accordingly the only philosophical school that played a significant role both in Athens and in Alexandria, and its possible role as a dual

---

[29] Cf. the echoes in Hp., *On Nutriment* 11 (and a similar use of two antithetical concepts plus a neutral, *ibid.*, 19). Striking though the similarity with Protagoras is, this use of 'neither . . . nor' probably occurred under Stoic influence; cf. Chapter III.A (with nn. 27–8) *supra*. Cf. also Plato's use of *oudetera* in *Euthydemus* 281D2–E5 (and see 292B4–C1).

[30] Cf. *Topics* 1.7.103a10–12, 4.1.121b15–23; *Metaphysics* 5.6.1016a17–19. But none of these uses of ἀδιάφορος occurs in the antithetical, trichotomous contexts characteristic of Stoicism.

[31] Cf. II. A; Brink, 1946; and further literature cited in Chapter II, nn. 9–10.

provider of models – for Stoics in Athens, for Herophilus in Alexandria – merits consideration. At the very least it is clear that it is erroneous to conclude that whoever used trichotomies consisting of two antithetical concepts plus 'neutrals' must have done so under Stoic influence.

Herophilus was not the first to apply taxonomy to medicine and its branches. A few examples of pre-Herophilean efforts might provide further historical context for evaluating his system. First, the antithetical definition of medicine in Plato's *Charmides* (171a8–9) as 'knowledge of the healthy and of the diseased' is strikingly close to Herophilus' division, although it still left to the Alexandrian the significant addition 'and of neutral things'. Another antithetical definition occurs in the Hippocratic – or, as some critics argue, 'Sophistic' – essay *On Breaths* 1: 'The art of medicine is the subtraction of excesses and the addition of things that are lacking'. A restoration of the balance between excess and deficiency will result in health: this view occurs frequently in Greek medicine and is also expressed as *isonomia* or *isomoiria*,[32] an equal balance between the various elements, humours, properties of the body, or as a climatic equilibrium, or again as the right harmony or blend (εὐκρασία) of opposites enclosed in the body. Its enormous significance as a model for Greek legal, political and ethical philosophy has been pointed out, especially by Werner Jaeger,[33] and its resemblance to Aristotle's theory of virtue as an intermediate state (μεσότης) between excess (ὑπεροχή) and deficiency (ἔλλειψις) has been noted.[34]

A third antithetical definition is reflected in the attempt by Mnesitheus of Athens (probably later fourth century B.C.[35]) to

[32] Cf. Hp., *Airs, Waters, Places* 12 (*CMG* 1.1.2, p. 54.16 Diller), on the superiority of Asia over Europe: τὸ δὲ αἴτιον τουτέων ἡ κρᾶσις τῶν ὡρέων, ὅτι τοῦ ἡλίου ἐν μέσῳ τῶν ἀνατολῶν κεῖται πρὸς τὴν ἠῶ τοῦ τε ψυχροῦ πορρωτέρω, τὴν δὲ αὔξησιν καὶ ἡμερότητα παρέχει πλεῖστον ἁπάντων, ὁκόταν μηδὲν ᾖ ἐπικρατοῦν βιαίως, ἀλλὰ παντὸς ἰσομοιρίη δυναστεύῃ. See also MacKinney, 1964. For a characteristic later example see Galen, *De temperamentis* 1.4 (I, p. 534K): ἡ τῆς τῶν τεττάρων κράσεων ἰσομοιρία τῆς τε εὐκρασίας αὐτοῦ καὶ τῆς ὑγιείας αἰτία.
[33] Jaeger, 1947 (esp. 358ff.); *id.*, 1945: vol. III, pp. 6, 20, 293 n. 11; *id.*, 1957; Longrigg, 1963.
[34] Cf. Jaeger, 1960: vol. II, pp. 502ff.
[35] As in the cases of Diocles and Praxagoras, Jaeger tries to push Mnesitheus' date down well into the third century B.C., since he believes Mnesitheus was dependent upon the Peripatos. But again all depends on (a) the questionable validity of his arguments about the date of Diocles (on which see Chapter II) and (b) Jaeger's liberal use of the idea of 'Peripatetic influence'. Cf. Jaeger, 1938b: Anhang

systematize medicine (μεθόδῳ τὴν ἰατρικὴν συστήσασθαι, fr. 11 Bertier = 4 Hohenstein; μεθόδῳ τὴν ἰατρικὴν τέχνην ἀσκεῖν, fr. 10 Bertier = 3 Hohenstein). Starting from the first and highest genera, Mnesitheus divides medicine by genus, species, and differentiae, but his primary division of the physician's function is into (a) preserving the health of the healthy by means of similars and (b) curing the diseases of the diseased by means of opposites. Again, an antithetical structure. A different kind of pre-Hellenistic definition is Aristotle's teleological view of the science of medical treatment as a road from potential health to the actual telos of health, or as an example of the entelechy of the moved.[36]

Two divisions have been attributed to one of Herophilus' more influential predecessors, Diocles of Carystus.

(a) In T49, following immediately upon T12, Celsus says (*Medicina, prohoem.* 9; *CML* 1, p. 18 Marx):

Isdemque temporibus in tres partes medicina diducta est, ut una esset quae victu, altera quae medicamentis, tertia quae manu mederetur. Primam διαιτητικήν, secundam φαρμακευτικήν, tertiam χειρουργίαν Graeci nominarunt.

During the same times the art of medicine was divided into three parts, so that there was one that cures through diet, another through medicaments, a third by the hand. The first is called dietetics, the second drug therapy, the third surgery.

Wellmann includes this passage under Diocles fr. 4, but since Celsus uses the phrase *isdem temporibus*, this division seems to be assigned generally to the 'times' of Diocles, Praxagoras, Chrysippus, and Herophilus, all of whom have just been mentioned (cf. T12), and not to any one of them in particular. It seems to be one that was generally regarded as acceptable at the end of the fourth century B.C. Cf. T56.

(b) A fourfold division of medicine which occurs in the Brussels fragment attributed to Vindician (codex Bruxellensis 1348–59, fol.

---

11 = 1960: vol. II, pp. 235–41. A more balanced assessment, which restores Mnesitheus to the fourth century B.C., is offered by Bertier, 1972: 1–10; so too, before Jaeger's influential work, Hohenstein, 1935, and Deichgräber, 1932.

36 *Nicomachean Ethics* 1.1.1094a6-22 (esp. a6–9). But *De partibus animalium* 1.1.639b16–21 adds a significant qualification (cf. also 640a3–8 and 25–35); *Metaphysics* 11.9.1065b17–32, 12.4.1070b30–5 (cf. 12.3.1070a29–30); see also 5.12.1019a15ff.; *Physics* 2.1.193b12-17; 3.1.201a16-23, 3.3.202b23-9.

48rff.), is likewise attributed to Diocles by both Wellmann (Diocles fr. 4) and Deichgräber:[37]

Divisam esse dicimus medicinam in partes quatuor: regularem, quam diaetam vocamus; manuum officium, quod chirurgiam vocamus; medicamen, quod farmaciam vocamus; praenoscentiam, quam prognosin dicimus.[38]

We say the art of medicine is divided into four parts: regulative, which we call diet; the task of the hands, which we call surgery; medication, which we call pharmacology; precognition, which we name prognosis.

While the suggestion of Valentin Rose,[39] Hermann Diels,[40] and Max Wellmann[41] that most of the doxographical material in the second part of Vindician's fragment (to which this fourfold division belongs) ultimately depends on Diocles has much in its favour, this is still no proof that Diocles, and not some doxographer, is the author of this particular division – which in any case is not compatible with the division reported by Celsus. It might well, however, go back to the fourth or third century B.C., like much of the Brussels fragment.

When measured by previous definitions, Herophilus' definition of medicine is therefore striking for two major innovations in particular: the introduction of a third element into what had been primarily antithetical divisions, and the subsumption of *all* therapeutic measures and tools under neutrals, so that what seem to have been three main branches in some previous traditions – surgery, drug therapy, and dietetic therapy for example – are now lumped together as only one main branch of medicine. This contraction of three earlier branches into one probably reflects Herophilus' need to make room in his system for the theoretical areas of his major accomplishments:

---

[37] Deichgräber, 1929: 1766: 'die Einteilung der Medizin *bei Diokles* von Karystos (im Vindicianus Kap. 40)' (italics added).
[38] Vindician, *Fragmentum Bruxellense* 40 (Wellmann, 1901: 233).
[39] Rose, 1863: 379f.
[40] *DG*, pp. 185–6: 'ibi [sc. in the *Physica* of 'Theodorus Priscianus', i.e. of Vindician] porro Dioclis maxime doctrina explicatur, num ex eodum Alexandro [sc. Philalethe], incompertum nobis.' The possible intermediary between Diocles and Vindician to which Diels refers in this case is Alexander Philalethes' *De semine* (on which see below, Chapter xxii). (Wellmann (1901) argues persuasively that 'Theodorus Priscianus' here is identical with Vindician; see Jaeger, 1938a: 187–211.) Cf. also *DG*, p. 435 appar. ad 9: 'Theodor. Priscian. *ex Diocle* ut videtur' (italics added); Deichgräber, 1961: esp. cols. 34–6.
[41] Wellmann, 1901: 4ff.

physiology and anatomy, neither of which is explicitly accommodated in the earlier tripartite division.

Although Herophilus' division had its impact (see *infra*), it did not become the accepted Hellenistic model but soon encountered firm opposition from the Empiricist school of medicine. The Empiricists' relatively passive empiricism[42] left no room for systematic anatomy, let alone for physiology and pathology, both of which inquire into those 'hidden causes' that were anathema to the Empiricists.[43] While Galen seems to suggest in his *Subfiguratio emperica*[44] that some Empiricists took over the Herophilean division – even though it is not particularly compatible with Empiricist doctrine – the Empiricists more commonly divided medicine into 'semiotic' (σημειωτικόν), 'therapeutic', and 'hygienic' branches.[45] The 'semiotic' part in turn is subdivided into diagnosis and prognosis; the therapeutic into surgery, pharmacology and, according to some testimonia, dietetics; and the 'hygienic' branch sometimes into that which preserves perfect health and that which helps restore convalescents to full health.[46] These divisions are all subsumed under one branch of a 'higher' Empiricist division of medicine into the 'constituent' and 'final' parts of medicine.[47] The division into 'constituent' and 'final' parts might have been inspired by a popular distinction between two classes of goods that was employed by their Stoic contemporaries, viz. between the instrumental or 'causative' (ποιητικά) and the 'final' (τελικά) parts of happiness (friends, for example, are a 'causative' or instrumental good, whereas justice and courage are 'final' or actual goods), though a parallel distinction between instrumental and final goods had already been used by Plato and Aristotle.[48] In the Empiricist division the 'constituent' parts (συστατικά) are the methods recognized as having scientific validity, e.g. personal

---

[42] See von Staden, 1975, especially Part III, pp. 186–93; Deichgräber, 1965: 269–308.

[43] Cf. Galen, *De sectis ad eos qui introducuntur* 5 (*Scr. Min.* III, ed. G. Helmreich), p. 10.14ff.; Deichgräber, 1965: fr. 17–38 and pp. 269–88.

[44] Deichgräber, 1965: 52.24ff.; p. 42.7ff. Bonnet.

[45] Galen, *Subfiguratio emperica* 5 (Deichgräber, 1965: 51ff.); cf. also Deichgräber, 1965: 288ff., and fr. 39–40.

[46] Deichgräber, 1965: 288ff. Cf. Kollesch, 1968.

[47] Deichgräber, 1965: fr. 39–65 and pp. 288–91; cf. Galen, *Subfiguratio emperica* 4 and 5.

[48] *SVF* III, 106–8. For Plato see, for example, *Republic* II. 357a–358a; for Aristotle, *Nicomachean Ethics* I.7.1097a25–34.

observation, use of transmitted information, etc., whereas the 'final' parts are the semiotic, therapeutic, and hygienic branches of medicine. This influential Empiricist system accordingly leaves no room for two of Herophilus' main branches of medicine – 'health-related things' (anatomy and physiology) and 'disease-related things' (pathology) – and it was apparently developed in deliberate opposition to what was regarded as Herophilus' unempirical rationalism.

The question of *divisio artis medicae* remained alive in subsequent literature. It was discussed, for example, by Polybius in his comparison of medicine and history (in the mutilated section on the historian Timaeus),[49] by the Pneumatic physician Athenaeus of Attaleia (probably first century B.C.),[50] by the Empiricist Theodas of Laodiceia (very early second century A.D..),[51] on whom much of the doxography about medical divisions seems to depend, by Celsus, by later Alexandrian commentators on Galen, and by others.[52] With the exception of passages mentioned below, these later developments are, however, not immediately relevant to an understanding of Herophilus' division.

An exception is the Antonine period, when Herophilus' division seems to have been held in such regard that it was accepted by some as virtually canonical. Thus Sextus Empiricus, without explicit reference to Herophilus, provides one definition, and one only, of

[49] Polybius 12.25d2ff. See Chapter v *infra*, T56.

[50] Wellmann, 1895a: 67, 131. See below for details of Athenaeus' fivefold division.

[51] Cf. Galen, *Subfiguratio emperica* 5 (p. 53.11–17 Deichgräber; p. 42.18–21 Bonnet), and Capelle, 1934.

[52] E.g., Galen, *Thrasybulus* (*Scripta Minora* III, 33ff. Helmreich); *De partibus artis medicativae*, ed. H. Schöne (Schöne, 1911), and M. C. Lyons, *CMG Suppl. Orient.* II; *Ars medica* (see below); and the treatises from which T42–T46 are drawn. Also ps.-Soranus, *Quaestiones medicinales* 23 (trichotomous division into physiology, pathology, and therapeutics), in V. Rose, 1870: vol. II, p. 251; S.E., *M* 1.95: some say the parts of medicine are dietetics, surgery, and pharmacology (i.e. a division identical with that attributed to the end of the fourth century B.C. by Celsus, and expropriated for Diocles by Wellmann); cf. Celsus, procoem. 9. Temkin, 1935b: 420 also discusses divisions of medicine in Codex Vindobonensis gr. med. 35 (fol. 329) into (a) theoretical and practical branches (i.e. corresponding to Erasistratus' division, which Temkin overlooked), and (b) physiology, aetiology, semiotics (semiotics is subdivided into diagnostic, prognostic, and 'anamnestic', probably under the influence of the Herophilean-Empiricist τρίχρονος σημείωσις), hygiene, and therapeutics. The latter division is close to that attributed to the Pneumatics (see below, and n. 68), but semiotics, in its Empiricist-Herophilean version, takes the place of the Pneumatics' emphasis on materia medica as a distinct branch.

medicine: 'The art of medicine is said to be knowledge of things concerning health, of things concerning disease, and of neutrals, οὐθετέρων' (M 11.186; M 1.95 and 2.8 are not presented as definitions). More significantly, in the opening pages of his *Ars medica* Galen employs an elaboration of the Herophilean division as if it were his own, or as though it had become so widely accepted that it required neither identification of Herophilus as its author nor any historical introduction or defence. T47 confirms that Galen accepted Herophilus' division, and Galen's presentation of his own division of medicine in *Ars medica* 1 therefore deserves closer scrutiny.

2   *Galen, Ars medica 1*

The elaborate amplification of Herophilus' basic tripartite division in *Ars medica* 1 (1, pp. 307–9K) has been attributed to Herophilus by several scholars – including Hermann Schöne, Karl Deichgräber, and Manfred Fuhrmann[53] – but following the principle of severity developed above (pp. xvi–xvii), it has not been included among the testimonia in this edition, because Galen fails to mention Herophilus by name. To allow readers to judge for themselves how much of this passage might be attributable to Herophilus, the text is translated in full:

Medical science is knowledge of health-related, disease-related, and neutral things (but it would make no difference if someone said 'concerning sickness' instead of 'disease-related').[54] The word 'knowledge' must therefore be understood as a common denominator and not in the particular senses. 'Healthy', 'diseased', and 'neutral' each is predicated in three ways: as body, as cause, and as symptom. For that which is capable of receiving health is the body, while that which produces and preserves health is its cause, and that which is indicative of it, its symptom; all these things the Greeks call 'health-related'. In the same manner the bodies capable of receiving diseases and the causes producing and preserving diseases and the indicative symptoms [of disease] are all 'disease-related'. And indeed by the same definition 'neutrals' too are bodies, causes and signs [symptoms].

Now in the first place, by definition medical knowledge is of the causes of

---

[53] Schöne, 1893: 24–7; Deichgräber, 1965: 290, and *id.*, 1929: 1766; Fuhrmann, 1960: 178 ('Man hat . . . *glaubhaft* vermutet, dass das auf dieser Trichotomie aufbauende verzweigte System . . . bereits von Herophilos . . . geschaffen sei'). Talamonti, 1968, illustrates the later influence of the *divisio Herophilea*.

[54] The parenthetical statement might be a post-Galenic gloss.

things related to health, and by reason of them also of the others. Secondly, it is of the [causes of] disease, third of the [causes of] neutrals. Furthermore, after this [it is knowledge] of bodies; here too first of the healthy, subsequently of the diseased, then of the neutrals. And in the case of symptoms the same way.

In practice, however, the diagnosis of bodies is prior, on the basis of signs, of course, and after this [comes] the discovery of their causes.

But since the causative, the indicative, and the receptive are each predicated two ways – 'absolutely' and 'at the present moment' – one must know that the art of medicine is knowledge of both. 'Absolutely' is in itself also predicated two ways: 'completely' and 'for the most part'. The art of medicine is also knowledge of both of these.

The neutral cause, neutral symptom, and neutral body are predicated absolutely and at the present moment each in three ways: *qua* not participating in either of the opposites, *qua* participating in both opposites, *qua* participating now in this one and then in that. The second of these again is said in two ways: *qua* now participating in each of the two extremes equally, but then participating more in one of the two.

Through the whole definition there is a certain ambiguity in the words, which one must resolve. For the statement that the art of medicine is knowledge of health-related, disease-related, and neutral things, can mean [that it is] of all, taken as particulars, but it can also mean [that it is] of their qualities, and it can mean [that it is] of some. But the first is indefinable and impossible, the last is deficient and does not belong to this science. The question of qualities[55] both belongs to the science and is adequate to all the particulars of the science, and we say it is encompassed in our definition of medicine.

We shall therefore start with bodies first, [asking] what kinds of bodies happen to be healthy, ill, and neutral. After that let us go through our argument about signs as well as causes in detail.

The core of this elaborate division, on which Galen proceeds to build in susequent chapters of his *Ars medica*,[56] is undoubtedly Herophilean, but the distinctions between body, sign, and cause, between receptive, indicative, and causative elements, and between 'absolutely' and 'at the present moment', are not explicitly attributed

---

[55] ὁμοίων *vulg.: correxi e* qualium (*versio latina Charterii*), i.e. ὁποίων

[56] But Galen not only provides a more articulated version of the *divisio Herophilea*; he also classifies this division as only one of three ways of systematizing the art of medicine: it is (a) ἡ ἐξ ὅρου διαλύσεως διδασκαλία, in additiion to which there are also (b) ἡ ἐκ τῆς τοῦ τέλους ἐννοίας κατ' ἀνάλυσιν γινομένη and (c) ἡ ἐκ συνθέσεως τῶν κατὰ τὴν ἀνάλυσιν εὑρεθέντων (*Ars medica*, I, pp. 305–7K).

to Herophilus in any testimonium or fragment (see *Comments*, T45 *infra*). While the silence of ancient sources cannot be regarded as conclusive, it seems likely that these distinctions were introduced in a later elaboration of Herophilus' basic trichotomy. This impression is reinforced by the fact that Galen – who elsewhere, in three different treatises, never fails to identify Herophilus explicitly as the author of the basic tripartite division (T44–T46) – here refrains from mentioning Herophilus even once, and this in a lengthy passage of fundamental importance to the structure of his entire *Ars medica*.

If the amplification does indeed postdate Herophilus, as I believe, there are several candidates for its authorship.

First, it could have been developed in part or whole by a later Herophilean (or Herophileans) whose work Galen knew. As pointed out above, Galen probably relied on Aristoxenus' treatise *On the School of Herophilus*, Book XIII, for the fourth book of his own *De pulsuum differentiis*.[57] In his account of the Herophilean school Aristoxenus[58] included a collection of definitions developed by various members of Herophilus' school. It is possible that Galen in his *Ars medica*, too, plundered Aristoxenus for this elaborate definition and division of medicine.

There had been a strong doxographic interest within the Herophilean school before Aristoxenus as well. His teacher Alexander Philalethes wrote a treatise *On the Opinions of Physicians*,[59] Herophilus himself wrote *On Common Opinions*, and the Herophileans Bacchius, Heraclides of Erythrae, and Apollonius Mys[60] likewise wrote treatises on Herophilus' school that were known to Galen either directly or indirectly. Galen might well have found elements of his elaboration in these or other Herophilean sources. The fact that Galen, shortly before he launches into the elaborate division quoted above, refers to two kinds of attempts to systematize medicine (including the definitory kind used in *Ars medica*) developed by 'Herophileans'[61] – and not by 'Herophilus' – lends further plausibi-

---

[57] Especially VIII, pp. 699–715, 720–49K. Cf. Schöne, 1893.
[58] Aristoxenus: see below, Chapter XXV.
[59] See Chapter XXII.A and B (*AP*.3). Cf. also Diels, *DG*, pp. 185–6.
[60] See Chapters XII (*Cn.*1); XIV (*Ba.* 78); XXIII (*AM*.4,5,17); XXIV (*HE*.3); XXV (*Ar.* 3).
[61] *Ars medica*, prooemium (I, pp. 305–6K): 'Some of the Herophileans, like Heraclides of Erythrae, tried to produce this kind of instruction' (sc. based on analysis or resolution or explication of definition); and 'the Herophileans themselves, some of the Erasistrateans, and Athenaeus of Attaleia also attempted

lity to the hypothesis that a later Herophilean source lurks in the background of *Ars medica* 1.

Secondly, an Empiricist influence is possible. Empiricists such as Philinus of Cos and Heraclides of Tarentum[62] had been pupils of members of Herophilus' school and, as was indicated above, some Empiricists actually took over the Herophilean division. Furthermore, the *alii* ('others') of whom Galen says in T45 that they introduced sign, cause, and body into the subdivision of neutrals, might well be Empiricists (but see *Comments*, T45). Yet the fundamental incompatibility established above between the Empiricist and Herophilean divisions, the prominence of aetiology (which the Empiricists wanted to exclude from medical science) in Galen's version of the division, and Galen's frequently polemical posture toward the Empiricists[63] render the possibility of an Empiricist influence considerably weaker than my first hypothesis.

A third hypothesis worth mentioning, and one indirectly advocated by Max Wellmann,[64] is that the Pneumatic school of medicine is a source of *Ars medica* 1. This possibility is suggested by the fact that Galen lumps together 'Herophileans' and the founder of the Pneumatic school, Athenaeus of Attaleia, at the beginning of his *Ars medica*, with specific reference to their attempts to systematize medicine on a 'synthetic' basis (see nn. 56, 61). Three further factors weigh in favour of a Pneumatic source: (a) many Pneumatics were, as has often been pointed out,[65] eclectics, who might have tried to

(a systematization of medicine) by means of synthesis' (sc. a synthesis of all the parts discovered through analysis; see n. 56). Cf. below Chapter xxiv, *HE*.11.

[62] Cf. Chapter xviii, *Ma.* 2: the Empiricist Heraclides of Tarentum was a pupil of the Herophilean Mantias; Chapter ii, T1: Philinus of Cos, founder of the Empiricist school, was a pupil of Herophilus. See also Chapter xxiv, *HE*.8, where the Empiricist Zeuxis and the Herophilean Heraclides of Erythrae are lumped together.

[63] E.g. Deichgräber, 1965: fr. 32 (esp. 32F), 37, 38, 76 (especially p. 138.7ff.), 310. Galen's assessment of the pharmacological achievements of the Empiricists was, however, more positive. Deichgräber, 1965: 3–5. But cf. also Frede, 1981.

[64] Wellmann, 1895a: 67, regards the Pneumatic physician Athenaeus as the source of T43: 'die herophileische Definition von *iatrikē*(def. 9, 351) . . . geht . . . auf Athenaios zurück'.

[65] Wellman, 1895a: *passim*; Diller, 1936a: 195, especially the final paragraph (= *Kl. Schr.* 30); Kudlien, 1968d: 1098–100. But not all Pneumatics were equally eclectic. Thus Agathinus and Archigenes seem to have had very strong eclectic tendencies, whereas Aretaeus was more of a 'Hippocratic'.

assimilate Herophilean views to their own; (b) the pseudo-Galenic *Definitiones medicae* (probably first century B.C.),[66] from which the Herophilean definition in T43 is drawn, has been said to depend at least in part upon Athenaeus (but see Chapter III.A, especially p. 71), and the pseudo-Galenic *Introductio sive medicus*, which provides T42, seems to be of Pneumatic provenance; (c) more significantly, in connection with an excerpt from Galen's *De sectis*, the Codex Palatinus graecus 297, fol. 53, attributes Herophilus' basic trichotomy to Athenaeus: 'What is the art of medicine? This is the definition Athenaeus of Attaleia gave: "The art of medicine is knowledge of things concerning health, of things concerning disease, and of neutral things."'[67]

While Athenaeus at one time, in the course of raking in his eclectic harvest, might have adopted an Herophilean division, possibly under Stoic influence,[68] it seems more likely that the elaboration did not originate with the Pneumatics but was merely transmitted by them. Several considerations militate against assuming a Pneumatic origin for the division presented in *Ars medica*: (a) the 'Pneumatic' author of the pseudo-Galenic *Introductio* explicitly identifies Herophilus, not a Pneumatic, as the originator of the basic division. (b) Galen himself also never attributes the Herophilean division to any Pneumatic–neither in his numerous discussions of Pneumatic doctrines nor in his discussions of Herophilus' division. (c) The value of the Palatine evidence for determining the source of *Ars medica* 1 declines in the absence of any evidence of the Galenic elaboration in it. (d) Sources normally attribute a division of medicine into five, not three,

[66] This date is suggested by Kollesch, 1966; see especially pp. 204ff., where resemblances between the pseudo-Galenic *Definitiones* and Celsus are described. Cf. also Kollesch, 1973: 60ff.

[67] See Wellmann, 1895a: 67 n.2.

[68] There is considerable kinship between the Pneumatic physicians and the Stoics, and some scholars give credence to Galen's statement (*De causis contentivis* 2, p. 8 Kalbfleisch (*CMG Suppl. Orient.* II, p. 134)) that the Posidonius with whom Athenaeus studied was actually the famous Stoic (e.g. Kudlien, 1962; *id.*, 1968d:1097). The argument that Posidonius the Stoic should not be confused with the 'Posidonius medicus' quoted by Aëtius of Amida has, however, also been made, notably by Flashar, 1966: 121–4, and Diller, 1967: 656 (= *id.*, 1973: 261).

Although the Stoic and Herophilean assessments of the status of health and disease are strongly divergent, as pointed out above, it is possible that the Stoics were taken with the affinity between their own use of 'neutrals' and Herophilus', and that they therefore passed on Herophilus' division to their Pneumatic pupils. Such a mediated transmission might be behind the Palatine evidence.

branches to Athenaeus, viz. into physiology, pathology (or aetiology), regimen (or hygiene), materia medica, and therapeutics;[69] the classificatory orientation of this Pneumatic division is clearly very different from that of the Herophilean trichotomy. Together, these considerations place a serious hurdle in the way of postulating a Pneumatic origin for the division in *Ars medica* 1, although a Pneumatic account of the Herophilean division might have been known to Galen.

A final possibility, which seems to vie with the first for the highest degree of probability, is that Galen himself is solely responsible for all elements of this elaboration. However, the considerations raised in the discussion of the first hypothesis, in particular Galen's mention – twice – of 'the Herophileans' and of their systematizations of medicine in the introductory passage leading up to *Ars medica* 1, seem to give an edge to the hypothesis that Galen built upon a later Herophilean elaboration. This view might receive support from T45: *corpora, causae, signa*.[70]

B · TEXTS

42 Ps.-Galenus, *Introductio sive medicus* 6 (xiv, p. 688K)

Ἡροφίλῳ δὲ (sc. δοκεῖ) ὅτι ἰατρική ἐστιν ἐπιστήμη ὑγιεινῶν καὶ
νοσωδῶν καὶ οὐδετέρων. τριῶν γὰρ τούτων γνῶσιν ἔχει,
ὑγιεινῶν μὲν ὅσα τῶν κατασκευαζόντων τὰ ἐν ἀνθρώπῳ οὕτως
ἔχειν, ἐξ ὧν εὖ ἡρμοσμένων πρὸς ἄλληλα τὸ ὑγιαίνειν συνίστα-
5 ται, νοσωδῶν δὲ τῶν τὴν ὑγιεινὴν ἁρμονίαν διαλυόντων,
οὐδετέρων δέ ἐστιν ἅπαντα τὰ προσφερόμενα ἐν ταῖς νόσοις
βοηθήματα καὶ ἡ ὕλη αὐτῶν.

---

[69] Ps.-Galen, *Introductio sive medicus* 7 (xiv, p. 689K). Cf. ps.-Galen, *Definitiones medicae* 11 (xix, p. 351K). See also Wellmann, 1895a: 131f.; Englert, 1929: 21ff., 24ff. (and the review by Deichgräber, 1929).

[70] Cf. also Galen, *De sanitate tuenda* 4.1.2 (*CMG* v. 4.2, p. 103 Koch) – where Herophilus again is not named – on the classification of the *symptoms* of diseases and their possible membership in the neutral camp: αὐτίκα γέ τοι περὶ τῶν νοσωδῶν συμπτωμάτων ὑπὲρ ὧν ἐν τῷδε τῷ λόγῳ πρόκειται διελθεῖν, οὐ μικρὰ ζήτησίς ἐστι, πότερον ἐκ τῆς ὑγιεινῆς ὑπάρχει πραγματείας ἢ ἐκ τῆς θεραπευτικῆς ἢ τούτων μὲν οὐδετέρας, ἄλλης δέ τινος ἀμφοῖν τρίτης, ἣν δὴ καὶ μέσην ὑγείας τε καὶ νόσου τίθενταί τινες οὐδετέραν ὀνομάζοντες. See also the *Comments* on T45 and T46.

42 Herophilus [sc. thinks] that medical science is the knowledge of things relating to health, of things relating to disease, and of things that are 'neither of these two' ['neutral']. For medical science possesses knowledge of these three: 'relating to health' are all things that equip the parts in man to be such that, if they are harmoniously fitted to each other, the state of being healthy is constituted as a result; 'disease related' are the things that dissolve this healthy, harmonious arrangement [sc. of the body], while all the remedies applied in diseases and the substances of which they are made [sc. materia medica] are 'neutral'.

43 Ps.-Galenus, *Definitiones medicae* 9 (XIX, p. 351 K)

ἄλλως (sc. ὁρίζεται ἡ ἰατρική) κατὰ Ἡρόφιλον· "ἰατρική ἐστι τέχνη ὑγιεινῶν καὶ νοσερῶν καὶ οὐδετέρων". ἢ οὕτως· "ἰατρικὴ τέχνη ἐστὶ περιποιητικὴ ὑγιείας."

43 According to Herophilus [sc. medicine is defined] differently: 'Medical science is the science of things relating to health, things relating to disease and "neutral" things.' Or this way: 'Medicine is a science capable of producing health.'

44 Galenus, *De simplicium medicamentorum temperamentis et facultatibus* 1.23 (XI, pp. 421–2K)

τριχῶς δὲ τῶν οὐδετέρων λεγομένων, ὥσπερ καὶ Ἡρόφιλος διῃρεῖτο, τῶν μὲν τῷ μετέχειν ἴσον ἀμφοτέρων τῶν ἄκρων, τῶν δὲ τῷ μηδετέρου, τῶν δὲ νῦν μὲν τοῦδε νῦν δὲ τοῦδε, πάντως που καὶ ταῦτα (sc. τὸ ὄξος καὶ τὸ ῥόδινον) ἢ κατά τι τῶν
5 σημαινομένων ἤ τινα τῆς τῶν οὐδετέρων ἐστὶ φύσεως.

44 And since 'neutral' is predicated in three ways, as indeed Herophilus also used to divide it – some things being neutral through equal participation in both of their extremes, some through participation in neither extreme, and some through participation now in this then in that – these things [sc. the 'simple' remedies vinegar and rose-oil] are at any rate certainly of the nature of the 'neutrals' either in one or in some of these senses.

45 Galenus, *De emperica subfiguratione* 5 (p. 42 Bonnet; pp. 52–3 Deichgräber)

sunt autem alii qui totius quidem medicative dicunt illas (sc. signativam, curativam et sanativam) esse particulas, fieri autem ex incisione neutrorum que esse volunt tria (hec autem sunt corpora et cause et signa) preter sanativa et egrotativa. et
5 Herophylus ita ponebat, totam medicativam dicens scientiam esse sanorum et neutrorum et egrorum. sunt autem utique et in signis et in causis neutra.

45 There are others who say that these [sc. semiotics or diagnosis–prognosis, therapeutics, and hygiene] are the subdivisions of medical science as a whole, but that these come about through a division of its 'neutral parts' which they want to be threefold – bodies, causes, and signs [symptoms] – and separate from the 'healthy' and the 'diseased'. Herophilus too used to make this kind of assumption, saying that the whole of medical science consists of 'health related', 'neutral', and 'disease related' things. But the 'neutrals' are also [to be found] both among signs [symptoms] and among causes.

46a Iohannes Alexandrinus, *Commentaria in librum De sectis Galeni* (ad 1 p. 64K), 2va (p. 24 Pritchet)

46b Agnellus Ravennas(?), *In Galeni De sectis comm.* 10 (p. 44, S.U.N.Y., Arethusa Monogr. 8)

Hec Erofili diffinitio, que dicit: 'Medicina est disciplina sanorum et egrotantium atque neutrorum'. hic duo commemoravit (sc. Galenus), sanitatem et egritudinem; neutrum dimisit, sed tamen ipsum inferius commemoravit . . .

1 hec sed *P*: *om. R*: ista *A (Agnelli)*   que *om. P*: ubi *A(Agn.)*
3 neutralitatem *SP*   4 tamen *om. A(Agn.)*   ipsum *BAQ(Agn.)*:
ipsam *SP*: ipse *UR*: ipsa *rell. Pritchet*   memoravit *B*

46a–b This is Herophilus' definition – where he says: 'Medicine is the science of the healthy, the ill, and the neutral.' Here he [sc. Galen] mentions [only] two, health and illness; he omits the neutral. But subsequently he mentions it . . .

47 Iohannes Alexandrinus, *Commentaria in Librum De Sectis Galeni*, proemium, 2ra (p. 15 Pritchet)

(*2ra.25*) Erofilus autem sic diffinivit medicinam: 'medicina est disciplina sanorum languentium et neutrorum.' Cui videtur Galenus consentire. Et hec diffinitio sibi dicitur placere. . .

47 Herophilus, however, defined medicine this way: 'Medicine is the science of the healthy, the weak, and the neutral.' With this Galen seems to agree. And this definition is said to have been his [Galen's] view . . .

48 Galenus, *De sanitate tuenda* 6.2.20–1 (*CMG* v.4.2, p. 171 Koch)

ἔστι δὲ καὶ τρίτη τις διάθεσις σώματος, ἣν οἱ περὶ τὸν Ἡρόφιλον οὐδετέραν ὀνομάζουσι, τοῖς τε ἐκ πυρετῶν χαλεπῶν διασωθεῖσιν ὑπάρχουσα κατ᾽ αὐτὸν τὸν τῆς ἀναλήψεως χρόνον καὶ τῇ τοῦ γήρως ἡλικίᾳ· τὸ μὲν ἔξω νόσου τοῖς γέρουσιν εἶναι πάντως
5 ὑπάρξει, τὸ δὲ τὰς ἐνεργείας ἰσχυρὰς ἔχειν ὁμοίως τοῖς ἀκμάζουσιν οὐχ ὑπάρχει.

1 ἔστι: εἰ *R*: ἢ *V*   *post* τις *add.* ἐστι *VR*   2 τοῖς τε] τὴν τοῖς *VR*
4 καὶ *post* ἡλικίᾳ *add.* Mewaldt

48 There is a third state of the body, to which Herophilus and his followers give the name 'neutral'; it exists in those who have been saved from severe fevers, at the very time of their recovery, and also at the time of old age. While the state of being completely free from disease will exist in the elderly, the ability to engage in strenuous activities, in the same kind of way as people at their prime, does not exist.

49 A. Cornelius Celsus, *Medicina* (*Artes* 6), prohoem. 8–9 (*CML* i, p. 18 Marx)

post quem (sc. Hippocratem Coum) Diocles Carystius, deinde Praxagoras et Chrysippus, tum Herophilus et Erasistratus sic artem hanc (sc. medicinam) exercuerunt, ut etiam in diversas curandi vias processerint. Isdemque temporibus in tres partes
5 medicina diducta est, ut una esset quae victu, altera quae

medicamentis, tertia quae manu mederetur. primam ΔΙΑΙΤΗ-
ΤΙΚΗΝ secundam ΦΑΡΜΑΚΕΥΤΙΚΗΝ tertiam ΧΕΙΡΟΥΡΓΙΑΝ
Graeci nominarunt.

1–4 *cf. T12 supra*   5 diducta] divisa *J*   6 ΔΙΑΤΙΗΤΙΚΗΝ *F*:
ΘΗΛΥΤΗΤΙΚΗΝ *J*   7 ΧΕΙΡΟΥΡΥΡΓΙΑΝ *F*   8 nominaverunt *J*

49 After him [sc. Hippocrates of Cos], Diocles of Carystus, next
Praxagoras and Chrysippus, and then Herophilus and Erasistratus,
practised this art [of medicine] in such a way that they made progress
also towards various methods of treatment. During those same times
the art of medicine was divided into three parts, so that one was that
which heals through diet, another through medicaments, the third by
hand. The Greeks gave the name 'art of dietetics' to the first, 'art of
pharmacology' to the second, and 'art of surgery' to the third.

C · COMMENTS

T42 βοηθήματα: while often restricted to drugs (e.g. Dioscurides 4.83),
βοήθημα is also used for other kinds of remedies and, as the translation
indicates, for remedial measures in general. Cf., for example, its use for
general dietary measures in the Hippocratic *On Ancient Medicine* 13 (*CMG*
1.1, p. 44 Heiberg). See also Diodorus Siculus 1.25.2–3 (on Isis as healer and
provider of *boēthēmata*); S.E., *P* 3.280; Hp., *Diseases of Women* 2.167 (VIII, p.
346L).

T43 The second definition is probably not by Herophilus. Ps.-Galen is
offering a series of definitions of medicine, most of them introduced
anonymously by ἄλλως. The one introduced here by ἢ οὕτως possibly
belongs among these anonymous definitions. The novel adjective περιποιη-
τικός ('able to produce') was popular with medical authors; cf., e.g.,
Mnesitheus fr. 38.36 Bertier; Dioscurides 2.104.

T44 This text provides further evidence of Herophilus' application of
'neutrals' to materia medica, since Galen cites vinegar and rose-oil as
examples of the useful flexibility and range permitted by Herophilus'
threefold subdivision of the neutrals. On rose-oil and vinegar, see Chapter
VIII (*Comments*, T257, T259).

On the relation of the tripartite subdivision of neutrals here to Galen's *Ars
medica* 1 and to Stoic subdivisions of neutrals see above, IV. A, pp. 94–8, 103–
8. While Herophilus mentions only neutrals which participate *equally* in both

extremes, Galen introduces 'neutrals participating in both extremes' and then further subdivides them into (a) those which participate *equally* (ἐξ ἴσου) in both and (b) those which, while participating in both extremes, have *greater* part in one than in the other (πλέον θατέρου). This discrepancy reinforces the view advanced above that Galen's version in *Ars medica* 1 originated only after Herophilus' death.

Deichgräber's claim (1965: 290) that Herophilus subdivided neutrals into four groups (and not three) is presumably based on combining the (unattributed) dichotomy of 'neutrals partaking of both extremes' in *Ars medica* 1 with the (attested) trichotomous subdivision of neutrals. T44 suggests explicitly (τριχῶς) that Deichgräber's quaternary combination is erroneous or at least inapplicable to Herophilus himself.

T45 Herophylus ita ponebat: It is unclear exactly to what *ita* refers, since it can, of course, either refer to a preceding thought or introduce a thought which follows. If it refers to all of what precedes, it could be claimed – as it is by Deichgräber (1965: 381, Wortindex s.v. σημεῖα) – that Herophilus already introduced the distinction between body, cause, and sign which I characterized above (IV.A.2) as part of a *later* Herophilean elaboration. It seems more likely, however, that Galen at first refers in very general terms to a similarity between *alii* and Herophilus ('ita ponebat'), and then zeros in on the points of resemblance more precisely in the epexegetical *dicens*-phrase (totam medicativam . . . egrorum').

alii: since (a) the division by *corpora*, *causa*, and *signa* corresponds exactly to one of the trichotomies in Galen's *Ars medica* 1, and (b) Galen here attributes it to *alii*, not to himself, this text lends further support to the contention developed above that not all parts of the elaborate division in *Ars medica* 1 were written by Galen. The identity of *alii* is somewhat obscure. Deichgräber, who wants to attribute 'sunt alii . . . egrotativa' to Herophilus, apparently thinks *alii* deprives this attribution of its certainty, and hence athetizes it in his Greek translation (ἄλλοι, 1965: 52.24). Since *alii* cannot be said with certainty to mean 'other Empiricists', especially inasmuch as the Empiricists were allergic to speculation about *causae* of any kind, the possibility that the distinction between body, cause, and sign originated with later Herophileans, as I suggested above, remains open.

T46, T47 Both of these testimonia apparently originated with iatrosophists of the sixth or seventh century A.D. and were produced in the context of the late Alexandrian commentaries on Galen's *De sectis* ('Agnellus'). The relation between Johannes Alexandrinus and the Ambrosian codex, as well as the relation between these two testimonia and the other texts of similar provenance, is discussed in a useful analysis by Temkin (1935b). See also below, ch. VI, *Comments* on T63b–c; ch. XXIV, *HE.* 12, 14; ch. XXII, *AP.* 17–18.

T48 Here 'neutral' is not applied to the third main subdivision of medicine, comprising all remedial measures (surgery, drugs, regimen), but to a condition of the body. Neutrals *qua* remedies (such as materia medica) are clearly different in kind from neutrals *qua* physical conditions of the body, and the use of 'neutral' here therefore seems to derive from a different Herophilean trichotomy, which, however, also used 'healthy', 'ill', and 'neutral'.

The dilemma of a physician who tries to classify these οὐδέτεραι διαθέσεις is described vividly by Galen in his *De sanitate tuenda* 4.1.3 (*CMG* v.4.2, p. 103 Koch, just after the important passage quoted in n.70): ἐγὼ δ' ἐπιστάμενος μὲν ὡς εἴτ' ἐν τοῖς ὑγιεινοῖς τις εἴτ' ἐν τοῖς θεραπευτικοῖς αὐτῶν (sc. τῶν νοσωδῶν συμπτωμάτων) μνημονεύσειεν, ὁμοίως ὑπὸ τῶν σοφιστῶν ἐπηρεασθήσεται, γινώσκων δ' οὐδὲν ἧττον ὡς εἰ καὶ τρίτης τις αὐτοῖς ἀναθείη γενέσθαι πραγματείας ὑπὲρ τῶν οὐδετέρων διαθέσεων ἐπιγράψας, ἔτι καὶ μᾶλλον ἐπιγελάσονταί τε καὶ τωθάσονται καὶ ἐρήσονται, περὶ τῶν ἀρρενικῶν καὶ θηλυκῶν ἐν ποίᾳ πραγματείᾳ διδάσκομεν, εἱλόμην ἐν τῷ νῦν ἐνεστῶτι λόγῳ διελθεῖν ὑπὲρ αὐτῶν.

διάθεσις for a bodily state, condition, or disposition subject to fairly quick and abrupt change had become a terminus technicus of medicine and biology by the time of Herophilus. Cf. Hp., *On Ancient Medicine* 7 (*CMG* I, p. 40 Heiberg): ἡ διάθεσις ἐν οἵῃ ἂν ἑκάστοτε ἕκαστος τύχῃ διακείμενος; Aristotle, *De generatione animalium* 5.1.778b32-5. In philosophy, διάθεσις also played an increasingly important role in ethics and psychology, where the distinction between it and ἕξις (a somewhat more stable condition) was worked out mainly by Aristotle and the Stoics. Cf., for example, Aristotle, *Categories* 8.8b25–9a13, and *De anima* 2.5.417b9–18 (esp. 15–16); *SVF* III, 104–5: again a characteristic Stoic tripartite division including neutrals: διαθέσεις, ἕξεις, οὔτε διαθέσεις οὔτε ἕξεις.

ἀνάληψις: for the meaning 'recovery from illness, convalescence', cf. Plato, *Timaeus* 83E7; the Hippocratic treatises *Aphorisms* 4.27 and *On Nutriment* 50; Soranus, *Gynaecia* 3.38.2–3 (*CMG* IV, p. 117 Ilberg); Galen, *De sanitate tuenda* 5.9.15 (p. 154 Koch), etc. Similarly, ἀναληπτικὴ ἐπιμέλεια, 'restorative care', Soranus, *loc. cit.*; ἀναληπτικὸς κύκλος, 'cycle of convalescent treatment', *ibid.*, 4.39.3 (p. 151 Ilberg); τὸ μέρος τῆς τέχνης ἀναληπτικόν, Galen *op. cit.*, 5.4.2 (p. 142 Koch); *id.*, *Subfiguratio emperica* 5 (p. 52.22 Deichgräber, p. 42.6 Bonnet) where *resumptivam* (sc. *partem artis medicativae*) is correctly understood by Deichgräber as τὸ ἀναληπτικόν.

V · THEORY OF
METHOD AND CAUSE

A · INTRODUCTION

In *The Structure of Scientific Revolutions* Thomas Kuhn argues persuasively that the methodological theories and standards of an epoch affect its scientific practice and therefore cannot be dismissed a priori as irrelevant to scientific history. The history of Greek medicine seems to bear out this contention: it displays a frequent isomorphism between theory of method and method in practice, although here too there are instances of discrepancy between medical scientists' theoretical formulations of their method and the methods they use in practice. In an earlier contribution[1] attention was drawn to the theory and practice both of Erasistratus and of the Empiricists as important instances of such isomorphism. In the case of Herophilus similar patterns of correspondence are discernible, but here they are part of a more paradoxical and ambiguous picture.

Herophilus' statements about method display three distinct and, at least prima facie, not entirely consistent emphases. First, some of the texts in this chapter seem to confirm the ancient doxographical tradition which ranks Herophilus among the so-called 'rationalist' physicians (*logikoi*) – i.e. physicians who attached great value to causal explanation and to the deductive or inductive construction of medical theories – rather than among the so-called medical 'empiricists' (*empeirikoi*) who emphasized above all a relatively passive form of observational experience (*empeiria*) at the expense both of theories about invisible factors and of causal explanation. Thus Herophilus seems to have stated, in characteristic 'rationalist' fashion, that certain invisible faculties or causes can be grasped only by means of inference from appearances to the invisible. Galen attributes to

---

[1] Von Staden, 1975.

Herophilus the view (T57) that invisible faculties which control or
manage us are discovered, not simply through direct observation of
the parts of the body in dissection, but also through inference from (or
'on the basis of') other things which appear to us (*phainomena*). Purely
descriptive anatomy is very useful, but in itself it does not contribute
to the development of those general notions (*prolēpseis*) that are
necessary to theory formation (and, on this view, perhaps also to
reliable clinical judgments). Herophilus himself without question
adhered to some such 'general notions' about things which are not
seen. Thus he proposed a form of humoral pathology – perhaps a
version of 'Hippocratic' humoral pathology[2] – and Galen stresses
(T58–T59) that he is at times found to engage directly in aetiological
speculation. Indeed, Chapter VII (*infra*) provides rich documentation
of Herophilus' use of causal explanation both for physiological and for
pathological purposes. Furthermore, Polybius' ascription of the
origin of 'theoretical medicine' to the Alexandrian Herophileans
seems to be an unequivocal recognition of Herophilus' insistence on
the value of theory (T56), especially of anatomical and physiological
theory. In T55, too, Galen suggests that Herophilus, unlike the
Alexandrian Empiricists, did not rely only on empirical data derived
directly from sensory experience (or, for that matter, on transmitted
empirical data), but also insisted on the sustained use of abstract
reasoning (*logismos*). All of this would suggest that the doxographic
tradition (Chapter II, T1) which portrays Herophilus as a prime
mover of 'rationalist' or 'dogmatic' medicine is correct in some
respects.

A different perspective on Herophilus' methodological posture is,
however, suggested by other texts. Thus, according to a medieval
Arabic translation of one of Galen's treatises on empiricism, Herophilus granted experience (in the lost Greek presumably *empeiria* – the
cornerstone of the medical Empiricists' theory of method), and not
causal explanation or functional theory, an all-important role (T52).
In ancient medical literature, this kind of statement tends to be made
only about Empiricists, not about the so-called 'rationalists' who
engage in theoretical medicine. Elsewhere, too, Galen seems to imply
that there are significant affinities between Herophilus and the
Empiricists, saying that Herophilus emphasized observation and
experience (*empeiria*) at the expense of a 'rational' method. Support

---

[2] See below, Chapter VII.A.8.

for this characterization of Herophilus also seems to come from a text which describes him in terms normally reserved for adherents of the Empiricist movement: Herophilus went by what one can see and made 'the examination of *appearances*' (τὴν τῶν φαινομένων ἐξέτασιν), not opinions, the basis of his statements (T54).

A third group of texts in this chapter reveal a more sceptical emphasis, and some of these led Kudlien to proclaim, perhaps somewhat precipitately, that Herophilus 'can lay claim to a place of honour in the history of medical scepticism'.[3] Thus one learns from Galen that 'Herophilus expressed doubt about every cause [i.e. causal explanation] with many strong arguments' and that he said: 'Whether or not a cause exists is by nature undiscoverable . . .' (T59a *infra*). A sceptical echo, but a less assertive one, is also perhaps audible in one of Herophilus' more intriguing fragments preserved in a papyrus of the British Museum: 'Let the appearances [*phainomena*] be described first *even if they are not first*' (Fr50a). In his *Methodus medendi* Galen ascribes what might be a mutilated version of this same imperative to Herophilus: 'Let these things be first *even if they are not first*' (Fr50b).

In polemics directed against later Herophileans' views of 'cohesive cause', Galen in his *De plenitudine* seems to allude to some of these apprent inconsistencies, saying that the Herophileans' 'leader on the one hand was in doubt about many things for which proofs are at hand, and on the other hand made pronouncements in other matters in which proofs were impossible and the hypothesis false' (cf. Chapter x, T280, *infra*).

One could either resort to a genetic explanation of these three groups of texts, according to which Herophilus started out as a 'rationalist' and then developed into an 'empiricist', finally maturing into a sceptic (or however one wishes to juggle the sequence), or the apparently divergent emphases in these texts could be examined for internal consistency and compatibility. Since there is no basis in the ancient evidence for a developmental explanation – which therefore would have to rely upon a priori assumptions about what would be a plausible methodological evolution – the second alternative seems called for.

A useful starting-point might be the apparently Aristotelian overtones of Herophilus' phrase 'the appearances (*phainomena*) first'

[3] Kudlien, 1964c: 13.

(Fr50a). In his biological treatises Aristotle frequently sounds the refrain 'first the *phainomena*, then the causes or principles'. Thus, in a famous discussion of the method appropriate to biology at the beginning of his *On the Parts of Animals*, Aristotle asks whether the natural scientist should first consider the *phainomena*, and only subsequently treat causes and reasons. His answer is an unqualified 'yes'.[4] Later in the same work he emphasizes again: 'First the phenomena must be grasped . . . then their causes discussed' (πρῶτον τὰ φαινόμενα ληπτέον . . . , εἶτα τὰς αἰτίας λεκτέον).[5] In *On Heavens* 3.7 a similar point is developed. Ingemar Düring, in an analysis of Aristotle's method in biology,[6] traces Aristotle's use of these and similar formulations in the biological treatises, showing that Aristotle is quick to castigate those who do not begin with observable *phainomena* when they are dealing with the terrestrial world. It might be objected that Aristotle himself, in blatant contrast to the isomorphism mentioned earlier, often based his reasoning on a priori principles rather than on observation (and to a great extent relied on reported and transmitted observations rather than on autopsy), but this does not, in itself, disqualify him as a prime inspiration of Herophilus' 'the appearances first'. It is the formulation of the methodological principle, not Aristotle's violations of his own principle, that would have influenced Herophilus. Furthermore, though perhaps less prone to a priori reasoning than Aristotle, Herophilus himself, for all his insistence on the priority of phenomena, was also not immune to apriorism, as parts of his physiological and pathological theory (Chapter VII), including his dream theory (T226), reveal. Historically, an Aristotelian influence on Herophilus is also quite plausible: as was pointed out in Chapter II, the Peripatetic presence was the only significant philosophical element in Alexandria, and Aristotle's views, especially on biology, might well have become known there in scientific medical circles by the early third century B.C.

A more serious objection to viewing Herophilus' formulation of method as inspired by Aristotle might be that Aristotle and Herophilus perhaps do not mean the same thing by *phainomena*. G. E. L. Owen has pointed out[7] that Aristotle often used the term to refer not to observable phenomena but to generally accepted opinions

---

[4] *De partibus animalium* 1.1.639b3 ff.   [5] *Ibid.*, 640a14–15.
[6] Düring, 1961.   [7] Owen, 1961.

on a given issue (τὰ ἔνδοξα) or to what is commonly said about a subject (τὰ λεγόμενα), i.e. the way things 'appear' to people in the non-sensory, metaphorical sense of 'appearing' to the mind. Owen's examples are, however, drawn mostly from the *Nicomachean Ethics* and the *Physics*; in his biological treatises Aristotle often makes clear, when using *phainomena*, that he is talking about observable phenomena (for example, by adding to *phainomena* the phrase 'to our senses', κατὰ τὴν αἴσθησιν), and not about general opinions (*endoxa* or *doxai*). It is striking that Galen (T54), in talking about Herophilus, preserves this distinction between observable *phainomena*, which Herophilus examined, and opinions (*doxai*) in which he did not put his trust. Although one cannot be sure that Galen's usage goes back to Herophilus, it does confirm that Herophilus' first concern was with the observable. Not only does Herophilus seem to have used *phainomena* in the perceptual sense reserved for it in Aristotle's biological treatises; he also made it the basis of scientific investigation and associated it with an activist standard of observation, much like Aristotle – and in clear contrast to the more passive brand of empiricism which emerged in the Alexandrian school of medical Empiricists in the generation after Herophilus.[8]

The first part of Herophilus' dictum, 'first the phenomena', therefore seems to coincide with the first half of Aristotle's methodological refrain, but the physician and the philosopher part ways when it comes to the second component: Aristotle had said 'then the causes', whereas Herophilus changes this to a more guarded 'even if they are not first'. While Herophilus' phrase concedes the possibility that there might be more to reality than can be observed – for example, 'hidden causes' or invisible faculties, a possibility more explicitly affirmed in his physiology and pathology (see Chapter VII) – he does not seem to have felt bound to swear unqualified allegiance to the second or causal step of Aristotle's biological method: Herophilus does not deny the importance of causal explanation for theory formation, but he is not as sanguine as Aristotle about attaining knowledge of causes. Support for this interpretation of Herophilus' formulation comes from one of his above-mentioned fragments (Fr59a) preserved in Galen's *De procatarcticis causis*: 'Whether or not cause exists, is by nature undiscoverable, but it is on the basis of a *supposition* that I *think*

---

[8] Cf. Deichgräber, 1965: 291–308; von Staden, 1975: Part III, on the Empiricists' theory of method.

that cooling, heating, and being replenished occur' (sc. as causes of certain physical states?). Elsewhere in the same work Galen reports: 'Some people say that nothing exists as a cause of anything, others . . . dispute whether or not there is a cause, and still others, like Herophilus, accept it on a suppositional basis (*ex hypothesi*)' (T58). Herophilus' acceptance of 'hypothetical' or 'suppositional' causes is not part of a traditional hypothetico-deductive system or of hypothesis-formation only for the sake of a subsequent sublation of the hypothetical nature of the premise by means of experimental or empirical verification or falsification. Rather, this seems to be a radical hypotheticalism which denies that any causal explanation could ever be verified in such a way that it would no longer be purely hypothetical, even if cause is logically prior to phenomenon.

Yet even here, where Herophilus seems to be departing from Aristotle's view of knowledge of causes in biology, it is conceivable that an Aristotelian use of 'hypothetical', in part inspired or buttressed Herophilus' insistence on the suppositional nature of causal explanation in medicine. Aristotle distinguishes, for example in *On the Parts of Animals*[9] and in his *Physics*,[10] between 'absolute necessity' (ἀνάγκη ἁπλῶς) and 'hypothetical necessity' (ἀνάγκη ἐξ ὑποθέσεως). Whereas 'absolute necessity' governs the supramundane sphere of eternal things, 'hypothetical necessity' governs all things subject to generation, such as the human body. And it is, of course, precisely the kinds of causal 'necessities' governing the human body which Herophilus tries to accommodate within his hypotheticalism. A Herophilean allusion to the Stoic theory of 'hypothetical' or elementary syllogisms also is a possibility, but in this context it seems less likely.

Herophilus' acceptance of cause only *ex hypothesi* is, furthermore, consonant with the keen pragmatic caution which is sounded *inter alia* in Fr51: a perfect physician would be one 'who is capable of knowing the possible from the impossible'. This kind of caution, often coupled with an articulated reluctance to indulge in dogmatic, unqualified generalization, is not uncommon even within 'dogmatic' or 'rationa-

---

[9] *De partibus animalium* 1.1.639b21–640a6 (where health is specifically introduced as an example of what falls under hypothetical necessity). Cf. 642a33–4; *De Somno* 2.455b26–8; *Metaphysics* E.2.1026b27ff.
[10] *Physics* 2.9.

list' medicine from the fourth century B.C. onwards. Thus Diocles of Carystus, in his famous fragment on method,[11] reflects the pragmatic caution one might expect from a *technitēs* (such as a physician) rather than from a *physikos* (such as a biologist): through a subtle analysis of why things with similar qualities do not necessarily have similar effects, Diocles warns against precipitate generalizations and encourages a flexible adaptation of theory to experience.

Whatever the provenance of Herophilus' insistence on phenomenal priority, it seems clear that he eagerly walks along the phenomenal road with Aristotle, but has radical reservations about then proceeding to generalizable causes on more than a hypothetical basis.

To return to the three different methodological emphases – 'rationalist', empiricist, and sceptical – presented at the outset: how does the apparently Aristotelian background of part of Herophilus' formulation affect one's assessment of the internal consistency of these three characterizations of his method? First, it has become clear that Herophilus is not the Pyrrhonian sceptic that some scholars have made him out to be.[12] Although he gives causal explanation a status of provisionality which is radically different from the epistemic status granted knowledge of causes by Aristotle, Herophilus frequently resorts to causal explanation and engages in nomothetical statements without much apparent hesitation. The pejorative sense which one major Hippocratic authority on method, the author of *On Ancient Medicine*, had attached to 'hypothetical' reasoning in his attacks on theoretical medicine and, in particular, on causal explanation,[13] is not accepted by Herophilus. Instead, Herophilus finds in the provisionality which a 'suppositional' (*ex hypothesi*) causal explanation can accommodate a key to reconciling his extensive empirical or observational activity with a guarded form of theory formation.

Secondly, not only is the view that Herophilus was a Pyrrhonian sceptic incorrect, but so is the characterization of Herophilus in terms normally associated with the Empiricists – at least if 'Empiricist' is used in the sense attributed to it throughout Hellenistic and later antiquity: a physician whose methodological credo allows the use only of (i) relatively passive experience or *empeiria* (often defined as aggregates of similar observations), with 'involuntary chance experience' ranked even higher than 'voluntary' or directed experience; (ii)

[11] Jaeger, 1938a: 25–30.   [12] E.g. Kudlien, 1964c.
[13] E.g. *On Ancient Medicine* 20, 1, 13, 15.

transmitted empirical data (*historia*); (iii) a relatively restricted use of analogy or 'transition from similars' (*metabasis*),[14] permitted only as a last resort. Equally important, in Hellenistic and later medicine, an 'Empiricist' is invariably understood to be a physician opposed to theory, to causal speculation – and even to the use of dissection and experimentation in medicine, inasmuch as these constitute active interventions against nature and hence represent a radical departure from the passive norms of 'experience' advocated by the Empiricists. To the Empiricist, anatomy (which had to rely on dissection) and physiology (which had to rely on causal explanation) were accordingly taboo, whereas observation of the effects of various drugs was acceptable. Herophilus, for all his emphasis on sustained observation, and for all the other empirical dimensions of his method (inference only from the observable, sensory verification, and so on), clearly does not fit this Empiricist mould. To put it in perhaps more familiar Aristotelian terms:[15] the Empiricist deals mostly in *empeiria* or acquaintance with particulars (although some Alexandrian Empiricists might insist on the qualification 'along with some generalizing statistical differentiation'), whereas Herophilus deals also in *technē* and hence in generalization or acquaintance with universals.

Not only are Herophilus' statements of method therefore incompatible with the Empiricists'; the repeated methodological attacks by the Empiricists on Herophilus and his followers from the third to the first century B.C. bear unequivocal witness to a sharp division between the methods of these two schools.

Viewed in isolation, Galen's claim that Herophilus made experience all-important (T52) at the expense of 'rational method' (T53) is therefore misleading. It might well be a reflection of Herophilus' insistence on 'first the phenomena', but in itself it certainly does not provide a characterization that is complex, full, and subtle enough to accommodate both the 'empirical' and the 'rationalist' dimensions of his method, let alone his embrace of causal explanation *ex hypothesi*.

A glance at Herophilus' contemporary Erasistratus might further define the Aristotelian shadow in which the emphasis on phenomenal priority in early Hellenistic discussions of scientific method seems to

[14] This empirical 'tripod' is analysed in Deichgräber, 1965: 288–301 (cf. *ibid.* 121–30); von Staden, 1975: 188ff.; cf. Frede, 1981: 73ff.; *id* ., 1982: 1–7. 13, 17.
[15] Cf., for example, Aristotle, *Metaphysics* A.1.980b28–982a3 on differences between *empeiria*, directed at particulars (*hekasta*), and *technē*, which is γνῶσις τῶν καθόλου.

stand. In a brief discussion of scientific method in a treatise from the second or third century A.D., *On Venomous Animals*, transmitted under the name of Pedanius Dioscurides,[16] Erasistratus is warmly commended for having rejected the anti-aetiological views of the Alexandrian Empiricists. Erasistratus, it is said, granted that one must start with the observation (παρατήρησις) of phenomena, but he also maintained that one must proceed beyond observation to a comprehension of 'hidden' causes 'visible' only to reason. Causal explanation is not only possible but also highly desirable, since the causes of individual afflictions are comprehensible as a class or generically (κατὰ γένος), and a knowledge of such generic causes can have an important bearing on clinical decisions. Aristotle's correlation of cause, the generic or universal, and the knowable,[17] seems to lurk behind Erasistratus' argument; here the Peripatetic background is perhaps even more apparent than in the case of Herophilus.

That the 'shadow' is indeed Aristotelian perhaps becomes still clearer when one considers other theories of scientific method that might have been within the purview of the earliest Hellenistic physicians. (i) Diocles' well-known fragment on method, mentioned earlier, displays a cautious approach to generalization, not unlike Herophilus', but there the affinity ceases. (ii) The Empiricists' methodological tripod – *empeiria, historia, metabasis* – had not yet been constructed: the Empiricist school was not founded until close to, or shortly after, Herophilus' death. (iii) The claim that Pyrrho's epistemology had a major impact upon Herophilus has been shown to be questionable. (iv) Not until much later did Epicureanism, with its emphasis on induction, or Stoicism seem to have become known in Alexandria. (v) Hippocratic texts were known in Alexandria, and they are rich in causal speculation. But one main authority on method within the Hippocratic tradition (the author of the treatise *On Ancient Medicine*), not unlike the Alexandrian Empiricists, polemicized against physicians who engage in causal hypotheses. The art of medicine, he said, has no need for any (even though the author himself, for all his emphasis on the importance of tradition and experience, offered causal explanations based, for example, on the

---

[16] The authorship is in doubt. *Medicorum Graecorum opera*, vol. 26, pp. 49ff. Sprengel; Deichgräber, 1965: fr. 25. Cf. also Anonymus Londinensis 21.23–6 (*Supplementum Aristotelicum* III.1, ed. H. Diels) = T50a.

[17] Cf. *Metaphysics* A.2.982a28–b2; B.6.1003a13–17, etc.

salty and bitter, sweet and acid, astringent and insipid). Exactness, he said, is difficult to achieve, and small mistakes occur here and there; the healer should simply do his clinical best without resorting to generalizing causal hypotheses. Erasistratus, by contrast, insists that causes can and must be known, and so does Herophilus, although Herophilus adds the crucial qualifier *ex hypothesi*. Some physicians even today might agree with the Hippocratic author that theoretical medicine often has little immediate bearing on clinical medicine.[18] But, for all their clinical interests (see Chapter VIII), the primary efforts of Herophilus and Erasistratus lay precisely in theoretical medicine, and the Hippocratic author therefore could not provide them with more than an anti-model of method.

This leaves us with Aristotle's formulation of the method appropriate to biology as a plausible model for the Alexandrian. Though not adopted wholesale, it does seem to have provided Herophilus with useful ways of reconciling observational activity with the construction of anatomical and physiological theory and hence perhaps helped to make the establishment of scientific medicine possible.

As the chapters which follow illustrate, Herophilus on the whole adhered to his own methodological prescriptions. His sustained, keen observations, especially in dissection, earned him the enduring admiration of most subsequent anatomists of note; at times he was more guarded than Aristotle, Diocles, or Erasistratus in his construction of physiological theory, yet he never abandoned his efforts to build a viable theory on the basis of inference from observation; when certainty seemed out of reach, he seems to have conceded the need to suspend judgment; and he does not seem to have claimed more than a hypothetical status for his causal explanations in physiology and pathology. In short, while the convergence of Herophilus' theory of scientific method with his scientific practice is not perfect, the degree of isomorphism seems to be considerable.

---

[18] On the relation of scientific and clinical medicine in Greek antiquity see Temkin, 1953; Lloyd, 1979: esp. 37–49, 126–69; *id.*, 1983: esp. 58–94, 105–11, 182–200; Viano, 1984: 297ff. Like other Hippocratic works, *On Ancient Medicine* (despite its anti-hypotheticalism) stresses the importance of knowing *aitiai* or 'the things responsible' for illness or health. But such statements tend not to be part of sustained discussions of theories of scientific *method*. Cf., for example, *On Fractures* 25; *On Breaths* 1; *Regimen in Acute Diseases* 11; *On Regimen* 3.70; *On Ancient Medicine* 15, 19–20; *On Sacred Disease* 1, §23.

B · TEXTS

50a P. Londinensis 137 (Anonymus Londinensis, *Iatrica Menonia* 21.18-32; *Supplementum Aristotelicum* III.1, pp. 37–8 Diels)

τοῦ σ]ώματος μ[(ἐν) ο]ῦν τὰ μ(ἐν) (ἐστιν) ἁπλᾶ μέρη, τὰ δὲ
σύνθετα. ἁπλᾶ δὲ καὶ σύνθετα λαμβάνομ(εν) π(ρὸς) αἴσθησιν,
καθὼς καὶ Ἡρόφιλος ἐπισημειοῦται λέγων ο(ὕτως)· 'λεγέσθω
δὲ τὰ φαινόμενα π[ρ]ῶτα, καὶ εἰ μὴ (ἔστιν) πρῶτα.' ὁ μ(ἐν) γὰρ
5 Ἐρασί[στρατ]ος καὶ π[ό]ρρω τοῦ ἰατρικοῦ κανό[νος π]ροῆλθε·
ὑπέλαβεν γ(ὰρ) τὰ πρῶτα [σώμα]τα λόγωι θεωρητὰ (εἶναι),
ὥστε τὴν [αἰσθητ]ὴν φλέβα συνεστάναι ἐγ λόγωι θ[εωρη]τ(ῶν)
σωμάτ(ων), φλεβός, ἀρτηρίας, νεύρο(υ). ἀλλὰ τοῦ[τ]ον παρ-
αιτητέον . . . ἡμῖν δὲ λεκτέον, ὡς τῶν σωμάτ(ων) τὰ μ(ἐν) (εἶναι)
10 ἁπλᾶ τὰ δὲ [σύ]νθετα, π(ρὸς) αἴσθησιν τούτ(ων) λαμβα[νο]-
μέν(ων).

50a Some parts of the body are simple, others compound. But we understand 'simple' and 'compound' with reference to sense-perception, just as Herophilus too observes, saying this: 'Let the appearances be described first even if they are not primary.' Erasistratus went even further in his standard for the physician; for he hypothesized that the primary bodies are perceived by reason, so that the vein perceived by the senses is composed of bodies perceptible by reason, viz. of vein, artery, and nerve. But he must be rejected . . . We, however, should say that some bodies are simple, others compound, so understood with reference to sense-perception.

50b Galenus, *Methodus medendi* 2.5 (x, p. 107K)

καί τις ἐπήνεσεν ἐν τούτῳ τὸν Ἡρόφιλον εἰπόντα κατὰ λέξιν
οὕτως· 'ἔστω ταῦτα εἶναι πρῶτα εἰ καὶ μή ἐστι πρῶτα.'

50b And someone commended Herophilus in this matter for having said literally the following: 'Let these things be first even if they are not primary.'

51 Ioannes Stobaeus, *Eclogae* 4.38.9 (v, p. 901 Hense)

Ἡρόφιλος ἰατρὸς ἐρωτηθεὶς ὑπό τινος, τίς ἂν γένοιτο τέλειος ἰατρός, 'ὁ τὰ δυνατά', ἔφη, 'καὶ τὰ μὴ δυνατὰ δυνάμενος διαγινώσκειν.'

1 Ἡρόφιλος: Roeper (*Philologus* 10, 1895, 569–70), Hense (*cf. autem eius add. et corr. p. XXXVII*): Τρόφιμος codd.   ὑπό τινος: MA corp. Par.: om. S
3 διαγινώσκειν: SM corp. Par.: διαγιγν- ut vid. A

51   When someone asked the physician Herophilus, 'Who would be a perfect physician?' he said: 'He who is capable of knowing the possible from the impossible.'

52   Galenus, *De experientia medica* 13.6 (translated from the Arabic version of the lost Greek original by Richard Walzer, pp. 109–10)

. . . We find, however, that this Herophilus concedes no small importance to experience, nay indeed, to speak the truth (and it is the fittest to be spoken), he makes experience all-important . . . (*See Chapter* vii, *T147 infra.*)

53   Galenus, *De praesagitione ex pulsibus* 2.3 (ix, p. 278K)

ἑξῆς δ' ἐστὶν ἐπί γε τῇ τάξει τοῦ λόγου περὶ ῥυθμῶν διελθεῖν, ὑπὲρ ὧν Ἡροφίλῳ μὲν ἐπὶ πλέον εἴρηται τήρησίν τινα καὶ ἐμπειρίαν ἱστοροῦντι μᾶλλον ἢ λογικὴν μέθοδον ἐκδιδάσκοντι . . . (*Vid. Herophili T176 infra.*)

53   Next in the sequence of the account one can expound upon rhythms, about which Herophilus, who gave an account of some observation and experience rather than teaching a rational method, spoke at greater length . . . (*See Chapter* vii, *T176 infra.*)

54   (Ps.-?) Galenus, *De optima secta ad Thrasybulum* 2 (i, p. 109K)

ὅθεν καταγελᾶν δεῖ τῶν ἰατρῶν, ὅσοι τὴν τῶν φαινομένων κρίσιν οὐχὶ τοῖς αἰσθητηρίοις, ἀλλ' ἀποδείξει τινὶ πειρῶνται ποιεῖσθαι· ὥσπερ ἀμέλει καὶ Ἀσκληπιάδης περὶ τῶν ἐπιπεφυκότων τῇ καρδίᾳ ὑμένων διαλεγόμενος Ἐρασίστρατον πεπλανᾶσθαι

5 φησιν· Ἡρόφιλον γὰρ πολλὰ ἀνατετμηκότα μὴ ἑωρακέναι,
παρὸν αὐτὸν ἐπὶ τὴν τῶν φαινομένων ἐξέτασιν κατὰ τὸ προσῆ-
κον ἐλθόντα ἀποφήνασθαι περὶ τοῦ πράγματος, καὶ μὴ δόξαις
ἠλιθίαις ἀποπιστεῦσαι . . .(Cf. T119 infra.)

54 One must therefore laugh at all the doctors who do not try to
make a judgment of things that appear through sense organs, but
through some logical proof. Just as Asclepiades, arguing about the
membranes attached to the heart, says that Erasistratus erred: for,
Asclepiades says, Herophilus did not see them, although he had made
many dissections and had the opportunity to make a pronouncement
about the matter after proceeding to an examination of the things
that appear, as is proper, without mistakenly putting his trust in
foolish opinions . . . (Cf. Chapter VI, T119 infra.)

55 Galenus, De pulsuum dignotione 1.3 (VIII, pp. 786–7K)

Ἀγαθίνου τοίνυν λέγοντος ἀναίσθητον εἶναι τὴν συστολὴν τῆς
ἀρτηρίας, Ἡροφίλου δὲ διὰ παντὸς ὡς ὑπὲρ αἰσθητῆς διαλεγο-
μένου, χαλεπὸν ὄντως ἦν καὶ ἄπορον ἑτέρῳ πρὸ θατέρου
πιστεῦσαι, τοσαύτην μὲν ἀμφοτέρων σπουδὴν εἰσενηνεγμένων
5 εἴς τε τἄλλα τῆς ἰατρικῆς καὶ τὴν περὶ τοὺς σφυγμοὺς τέχνην
αὐξῆσαι, μακρῷ τε χρόνῳ τόν τε λογισμὸν καὶ τὴν αἴσθησιν
ἱκανῶς γεγυμνασμένων. (Vid. T160 infra.)

55 Now since Agathinus says the contraction (systolē) of the artery is
not perceptible by sense, while Herophilus discusses it throughout as
though he is talking about a contraction perceptible by sense, it was
really difficult, in fact impossible, to believe the one in preference to
the other. For both have contributed such a serious effort especially
towards the growth of the science concerning the pulse and also
towards that of the other branches of medicine, and they trained their
capacity for reasoning as well as their sense-perception sufficiently
over a period of time . . . (See Chapter VII, T160 infra.)

56 Polybius, Historiae 12.25d2–6

ἐχούσης γάρ τι παραπλήσιον τῆς ἱστορίας καὶ τῆς ἰατρικῆς

διὰ τὸ κατὰ τὰς ὁλοσχερεῖς διαφορὰς ἑκατέραν αὐτῶν ὑπάρχειν
τριμερῆ παραπλησίους εἶναι συμβαίνει καὶ τὰς τῶν ἐπιβαλλο-
μένων ἐπ’ αὐτὰς διαθέσεις· οἷον εὐθέως τῆς ἰατρικῆς, ἑνὸς μὲν
5 μέρους αὐτῆς ὑπάρχοντος λογικοῦ, τοῦ δ’ ἑξῆς διαιτητικοῦ,
τοῦ δὲ τρίτου χειρουργικοῦ καὶ φαρμακευτικοῦ γένους, ὁλοσχερῶς . . . τὸ δὲ λογικόν, ὃ δὴ πλεῖστον ἀπὸ τῆς Ἀλεξανδρείας
ἄρχεται παρὰ τῶν Ἡροφιλείων καὶ Καλλιμαχείων ἐκεῖ προσα-
γορευομένων, τοῦτο μέρος μέν τι κατέχει τῆς ἰατρικῆς, κατὰ δὲ
10 τὴν ἐπίφασιν καὶ τὴν ἐπαγγελίαν τοιαύτην ἐφέλκεται φαντασίαν
ὥστε δοκεῖν μηδένα τῶν ἄλλων κρατεῖν τοῦ πράγματος· οὓς
ὅταν ἐπὶ τὴν ἀλήθειαν ἀπαγαγὼν ἄρρωστον ἐγχειρίσῃς,
τοσοῦτον ἀπέχοντες εὑρίσκονται τῆς χρείας ὅσον [καὶ] οἱ μηδὲν
ἀνεγνωκότες ἁπλῶς ἰατρικὸν ὑπόμνημα. οἷς ἤδη τινὲς τῶν
15 ἀρρώστων ἐπιτρέψαντες αὐτοὺς διὰ τὴν ἐν λόγῳ δύναμιν οὐδὲν
ἔχοντες δεινὸν τοῖς ὅλοις πολλάκις ἐκινδύνευσαν. εἰσὶ γὰρ
ἀληθῶς ὅμοιοι τοῖς ἐκ βύβλου κυβερνῶσιν· ἀλλ’ ὅμως οὗτοι
μετὰ φαντασίας ἐπιπορευόμενοι τὰς πόλεις, ἐπειδὰν ἀθροίσωσι
τοὺς ὄχλους, ἐπ’ ὀνόματος τοὺς ἐπ’ αὐτῶν τῶν ἔργων
20 ἀληθινὴν πεῖραν δεδωκότας αὐτῶν εἰς τὴν ἐσχάτην ἄγουσιν
ἀπορίαν καὶ καταφρόνησιν παρὰ τοῖς ἀκούουσι, τῆς τοῦ λόγου
πιθανότητος καταγωνιζομένης πολλάκις τὴν ἐπ’ αὐτῶν τῶν
ἔργων δοκιμασίαν . . .

6 locum post ὁλοσχερῶς valde mutilatum sic restituit Pédech ἐ⟨νίοις⟩ τόλμῃ καὶ
καταψεύδεσθαι τοῦ ἐπιτηδεύματος ⟨συμβαίνει⟩: τις ἐφίεσθαι τολμᾷ τῷ
καταψεύδεσθαι coni. Heyse: και τολμαι και καταψεύδεσθαι leg. Boissevain
13 καὶ M: del. Büttner-Wobst (vid. Fleckeisens Jahrbücher 1889, 681
sq.) 13–14 μηδὲν ἀνεγνωκότες Büttner-Wobst: μηδὲν ἐγνωκότες M: μηδ’
ἀνεγνωκότες Bekker 17 βύβλου M: βυβλίου Büttner-Wobst: βιβλίου
Leutsch 19 ὄχλους Orelli: λόγους M ἐπ’ ὀνόματος M ad posteriora
rett. Hultsch: vulgo cum prioribus coniunctum: ἐπι βήματος Lucht: ⟨τοὺς⟩ ἐπ’
ὀνόματος Cobet: ὑπὸ κομπάσματος E. Schultz: ⟨μόνον οὐ καλοῦντες⟩ ἐπ’
ὀνόματος Büttner-Wobst coll. Polyb. 5.35.2.

56 Since history and medicine have a point of resemblance,
inasmuch as each of the two consists roughly speaking of three parts,
the dispositions of those who apply themselves to history and
medicine also resemble each other. To begin with medicine, for
example, one of its parts is theoretical, the next dietetic, and the third
the surgical and pharmacological kind . . .* The theoretical part,

* The Greek text is badly mutilated and corrupted in the section following this
  tripartite division.

which has its origins mostly from Alexandria – from those who there are called Herophileans and Callimacheans – this theoretical part in some respect has a controlling hold on medical science, and by its ostentation and its claims it gets itself such a reputation that no one else [of those engaged in other branches of medicine] appears to be master of the subject. But when you lead them [sc. these theorists] back to reality and put a patient in their hands, you discover that they fall just as far short in their service as people who have not read a single medical treatise. In fact, some patients who entrusted themselves to these physicians, persuaded by their powers of reasoning, have often thereby endangered their lives, although they had nothing terribly wrong with them at all. For they [sc. 'theoretical' doctors like the Herophileans and Callimacheans] really resemble pilots who steer by the book. But nevertheless they travel to cities with fanfare and, when they have collected the crowds, they reduce, by name, those who have delivered true proof of themselves in their actual deeds, to the most extreme straits and contempt in the view of their audience, because the persuasiveness of speech often contends successfully against the scrutiny of actual deeds.

57 Galenus, *De foetuum formatione* 5 (IV, pp. 678–9K)

ὃ δὲ προσθεῖναι τοῖς προειρημένοις ἀναγκαῖόν ἐστιν, ἀγνοούμε-
νον καὶ αὐτὸ τοῖς γενναίοις φιλοσόφοις, ὥσπερ καὶ τἆλλα τὰ ἐξ
ἀνατομῆς φαινόμενα, καιρὸς ἤδη μοι φράσαι, τὴν ἀρχὴν ἀφ' ὧν
Ἡρόφιλος ἔγραψε ποιησαμένῳ. τὰς γὰρ ἀνατομικὰς διηγήσεις
5 ἀξιοῖ μηδεμίαν ἐκ τοῦ φάναι τόδε τι μόριον ἐκ τοῦδε πεφυκέναι
πρόληψιν ἐργάζεσθαι πρὸς τὰ δόγματα, καθάπερ ἔνιοι κακῶς
ἀκούοντες ποιοῦσιν· ἐξ ἄλλων γὰρ φαινομένων τὰς διοικούσας
ἡμᾶς εὑρίσκεσθαι δυνάμεις, οὐκ ἐξ αὐτῆς ἁπλῶς τῆς θέας τῶν
μορίων.

57 Something must be added to what was said previously, something which, just like the other things that become apparent as a result of dissection, is unknown even to very good philosophers; and now is the right moment for me to mention it, having taken my starting-point from the things Herophilus wrote. For Herophilus does not consider anatomical descriptions fit to produce any general

preconception for the purpose of [formulating] doctrines, just on the basis of saying 'this part has its natural origin in that one', as some people of poor repute do. For [Herophilus thinks] the faculties that control us are discovered on the basis of other things that become apparent, not simply on the basis of the act of looking at the parts.

58 Galenus, *De causis procatarcticis* 13.162–4 (*CMG Suppl.* II, pp. 41–2 Bardong)

quidam enim nil nullius dixerunt existere causam, quidam vero dubitaverunt, si est an non, sicut empirici, quidam autem ex suppositione acceperunt, sicut Erophilus, alii vero quidam, quorum ipse fuit dux, procatarticas causarum removerunt ut
5 male creditas. universi enim hii significatum quod est secundum nomen permutantes occasiones habuerunt argumentorum. si enim ⟨confiterentur⟩ quoniam et utilitatem eorum que fiunt causam dicunt omnes homines et effectivam causam unde principium et cum hiis adhuc materiam et organa, faciliter
10 utique invenirentur quod sophizantur. et enim hoc scilicet omnino non existere aliquid alterius causam, et hoc scilicet nullam procatarticarum nominatarum causarum existere, et alia universa quecunque de natura dictarum causarum dicta sunt male, abhinc dependerunt omnia.

1 nil *om. D*   *vero P*: enim *D*   2 an *P*: aut *D*   2 quidam *P*:
quidem *D*   4 removerunt *coni. Bardong*: moverunt *P*: alias removerunt *D*
5 signati *D*   7 confiterentur *add. Bardong*   10 enim *D*: etiam *P*

58 Some people say nothing exists as a cause of anything, while others, like the Empiricists, dispute whether or not there is a cause, and still others, like Herophilus, accept it on a suppositional basis, and others again – whose leader he was – rejected, among the causes, the 'antecedent initiating causes' (*procatarcticae*) as not very plausible. All these authors got the occasion for their arguments by changing the meaning of this word. For if they grant that everyone also calls the 'usefulness of what happens' a cause, and that they call 'efficient' (*effectiva*) cause that from which the beginning derives and, in addition, matter and organs, they are indeed easily detected to be playing subtle tricks. For clearly, the statement that nothing exists as the cause of something else, and that none of the causes called

'antecedent initiating' (*procatarcticae*) exists, and all the other things said with faulty reasoning about the nature of the aforementioned causes – all of these depend on this . . .

59a Galenus, *De causis procatarcticis* 16.197–204 (*CMG* Suppl. II, pp. 53–5 Bardong)

de Erophilo autem et de ea que circa sermones sapientia magis Erasistrato oportet mirari et increpare eum de timore. dubitans enim de omni causa fortibus et multis rationibus postea ipsemet invenitur utens eis dicendo multis hominibus sic videri. summe
5 enim timidi est dimittendo rationem, ut hominibus videtur, sic existimare.

quid igitur ait? "causa vero, utrum sit vel non, natura quidem non est invenibile, existimatione autem puto infrigidari, estuari, cibo et potibus repleri."
10 que enim argumenta sunt ex significati transpositione posuerunt in dubio Erophilum et cum hiis adhuc ea que de modo generationis uniuscuiusque eorum que qualitercumque fiunt, adhuc autem et hoc scilicet utrum incorporea existens causa incorporei alicuius alterius est factiva ⟨aut corporea existens
15 causa corporis alicuius est factiva⟩ aut corporis factiva alicuius existit incorporea ens aut corpus existens incorporei alicuius est effectiva, et utrum mota moti aut manentis manens ⟨aut mota manentis aut moti manens⟩, et utrum presens presentis vel presens prefacti vel presens futuri.
20 deinde, postquam ita diviserit, probare singula eorum que ex divisione nequit et sic consequenter sillogizat non esse aliquod alicuius causam. ait enim: 'aut corporea corporis aut incorporea incorporei est causa et alia que ex divisione inventa sunt. nullum autem horum apparet existens: manifestum est, quoniam
25 omnino non est causa.'

sed, o sophista, cito omnia que secundum vitam evertes sic argumentans. puta mox in hiis que manifeste apparent, aut veniente aliquo ab hiis que videntur ad oculos nostros aut aliquo a nobis ad singulum illorum aut omnino eo quod a nobis existit
30 id quod ab eis fertur contangente videmus. aut neque enim [illis] ex illis ad nos neque a nobis ad illa lato aliquo sed per

intermedium sicut per baculum sensatio nostra de eis fit. at etiam neque id quod est ·a· neque ·b· neque ·c· neque ·d·; de unoquoque enim horum dubitatum est multiformiter: non ergo
35 videmus.

si vero distinguat aliquis: 'aut est corpus quod videt et quod videtur aut quod videtur est corpus, quod autem videt incorporeum, aut e contrario, aut ambo incorporea', deinde ostendens, quod nullum ipsorum est verum, inferat nichil a nobis videri.
40 rursus secundum alium modum dubitabit sic de proposito iuste distinguens: 'aut manentis manens aut manentis motum ⟨aut moti motum⟩ aut moti manens id quod videt eius quod videtur facit sensum', deinde ostendens, quoniam secundum nullum predictorum est suasibile sentire, interimit videre nos
45 quodcumque.

1 et om. P   circa P: citra D   2 increpere D   3 enim P: autem D
8 puto v: puta PD   10 argumenta P: augmentata D   11 et cum P:
Etenim D   12 fiunt P: fuerit D   14–15 aut corporea . . . est factiva
suppl. Bardong   17 effusiva D   17–18 aut mota . . . moti manens suppl.
Bardong   18 presentis P: presenti D   22–23 incorporea incorporei
Bardong: in corpore incorporei PD: incorporea v   25 omnino D: omnis
P   27 augmentans D   30 videamus D   illis seclusi   30–31 aut
neque ex illis coni. Bardong: neque enim illis aut ex illis P: neque enim illos
D   32 at P: Aut D   34 enim om. D   36 aliquid D   37 aut
quod videtur om. D, qui aut quod videtur est corpus add. post corpus
38 e converso D   41 manentis (sec.) P: moventis D   42 aut moti
motum suppl. Bardong

59a About Herophilus, however, and about the 'wisdom' displayed in his writings, one must be even more amazed than about Erasistratus, and one must chide him for his timidity. For while Herophilus expresses doubt about every cause with many strong arguments, he is himself subsequently detected using them, by saying 'it appears this way to many people'. For it is above all characteristic of a timid person, upon dismissing a rational argument, to think something is 'as it appears to people'.

What, then, does Herophilus say? 'Whether or not cause exists, is by nature undiscoverable, but it is through a supposition that I think I am being chilled, being heated, and being repleted with food and drink.'

For the arguments that are based on a transposition of meaning put

Herophilus in a state of perplexity, as did the arguments that were made about the manner of generation of each thing, in whatever way it was generated, and furthermore, so did the following question: 'Is a cause that is incorporeal the active (*factiva*) cause of some other incorporeal, or is a cause that is corporeal the active cause of some or other body,* or is [a cause], being incorporeal, the active (*factiva*) cause of some body, or is it, being a body, the efficient (*effectiva*) cause of some incorporeal?' Also: 'Is the moved the cause of the moved, or is the stationary the cause of the stationary, or the moved of the stationary, or the stationary of the moved?'† And: 'Is the present [the cause] of the present or is the present [the cause] of the past or the present of the future?'

Then, after setting up these divisions, he could not confirm each of the things in the division singly, and he therefore drew the inference that not anything is the cause of anything. For he says: 'Either a corporeal cause is the cause of a body, or an incorporeal cause is the cause of an incorporeal, and the rest of the things found by this division. But none of these is seen to be the case. So it is evident that cause does not exist at all.'

But, you sophist, you will rapidly overturn everything that is in accordance with the facts of life if you argue that way. Consider, for example, among the things which appear very clearly: we see either because something comes from things that are seen to our eyes, or because something goes from us to each of them, or because what proceeds from us joins up with that which is borne forth from them. Or our sense-perception about them takes place neither because something is carried from them to us nor something from us to them, but through an intermediary, as if through a stick. But neither is *a* the case nor is *b* nor *c* nor *d*. For, concerning each of these there are many kinds of doubts: therefore, we do not see.

If, however, someone were to make this distinction: 'Either it is a body that sees and is seen, or what is seen is a body but what sees is incorporeal, or the reverse, or both are incorporeal', and then showed that none of these is true, he would infer that nothing is seen by us.

Again, he will express doubt in another manner by justly making

---

* 'or whether a cause that is corporeal is the active cause of some or other body' is a plausible supplement suggested by Bardong but not attested by the MSS.
† 'or the moved of the stationary, or the stationary of the moved' is a supplement proposed by Bardong.

the following distinction about the proposition before us: 'That which sees produces sense-perception of that which is seen, either because what sees is stationary, and so is what is seen, or because what sees is in motion and the seen object stationary, or because both are in motion, or because what sees is stationary and the object is in motion.' Then, showing that it is not plausible that sense-perception takes place according to any of the aforementioned, he annuls the fact that we see anything at all.

59b Galenus, *De compositione medicamentorum secundum locos* 3.1 (XII, p. 619K)

... κελεύει διὰ παντὸς ὁ Ἡρόφιλος τί τε καὶ ποῖον καὶ πηλίκον ἐστὶ τὸ τοῦ νοσήματος αἴτιον καὶ κατὰ τί μάλιστα δυναστεῦον ἐπίστασθαι τὸν ἰατρόν, ὅπως καὶ τὴν θεραπείαν ἁρμόττουσαν ἑκάστῳ ποιεῖται. *(Vid. AM.17 infra.)*

59b ... Herophilus throughout prescribes that the physician should know what, and of what kind, and how great the cause of the disease is, and by what it most becomes prevalent, so that he can also make his treatment fitting for each [disease]. *(See Chapter* XXIII, *AM.17 infra.)*

C · COMMENTS

T50a The quotation from Herophilus could also be translated as follows: 'Let appearances be described as [*or:* called] primary things even if they are not primary.' This is the sense of *prōta* attributed to Erasistratus in the next sentence; however, in view of the fact that Herophilus does not identify appearances with primary bodies but insists only on making appearances the starting-point of any investigation (as pointed out in the Introduction to this chapter), 'first' seems preferable to 'primary'.

Simple, compound: By 'simple parts' the Peripatetic author of this papyrus means homogeneous parts (*homoiomerē*) of the body such as sinew, artery, and vein; by 'compound parts', non-homogeneous parts such as leg or head, which cannot be divided into similar parts.

Erasistratus: He believed that the entire body was composed of *triplokiai* or 'three-stranded' braids of primary, invisible nerves, veins, and arteries. Thus even a vein or a nerve would itself consist of such *triplokiai*. Cf. ps.-

Galen, *Introductio sive medicus* 9 (xiv, p. 697K); Galen, *De naturalibus facultatibus* 2.6 (*Scr. min.* iii, p. 171 Helmreich). See also Anonymus Londinensis 22.51.

T51 All the codices read 'Trophimos', not 'Herophilos', but no physician by the name Trophimus is known. Roeper's plausible conjecture ('Herophilos') has therefore found wide acceptance. But cf. Stob. 4.36.24; Photius, *Bibl. cod. 167 (*ii, pp. 156.1, 149n.1, 155n. 2 Henry). Absolute certainty is, of course, impossible. The distinction between 'possible' and 'impossible' is perhaps part of the Hippocratic legacy. Cf. *Prognostic* 1 (i, p. 78Kw): 'To make all those who are ill healthy, is impossible.' See above, Chapter i, n. 48; Plato, *Rep.* 2.360E–361A1; Hp., *On Diseases* 1.1, 6; *id., Art* 3, 8, 11, 13; *id., On Nutriment* 14.

T54 Asclepiades here is criticized for having tried to substantiate his claim (that Erasistratus was mistaken about the existence of the heart-valves) by means of a preposterous 'logical proof', viz. that Herophilus, a superb anatomical observer, had never seen them. For present purposes the main value of this testimonium is its confirmation of Herophilus' reputation as an observer of phenomena, who did not resort easily to unsubstantiated opinions. (On Erasistratus' superior knowledge of the heart-values cf. *infra* Chapter vi.A.6.) On 'observational' claims cf. Lloyd, 1982.

T56 In this passage Polybius writes primarily from an Empiricist viewpoint, and his assessment of the Herophileans is correspondingly polemical and negative. The charge that 'theoretical doctors' are pilots who steer by the book and are inept in practice does not hold up in the case of Herophilus, whose clinical efficacy cannot be shown to have been inferior to that of his contemporaries (cf. *infra*, Chapter viii). Cf. Chapter iv, T49, *supra*.

τὸ λογικόν: see *Comments*, T1, on this use of 'rational' or 'theoretical' medicine. Here it seems to refer specifically to the anatomical and physiological branches of medicine.

T57 On Herophilus' reputation as the earliest systematic dissector of human beings, see Chapter vi.A.1. An important point here is that Herophilus, for all his excellence in descriptive anatomy, did not regard it as the end-all of medicine, but also wanted to proceed to functional questions as a basis for formulating conclusions. It is unclear whether *dogmata* refers only to doctrines (e.g. theoretical 'judgments' about 'the faculties that control us') or also to clinical judgments. Cf. Galen's own view that position (θέσις) – an aspect the descriptive anatomist would record – is not necessarily a reliable guide to function (ἐνέργεια), *De placitis Hippocratis et Platonis* 2.5 (*CMG* v.4.1.2, p. 128 De Lacy).

T58 Procatarcticae: this seems to allude to a Stoic distinction between antecedent 'initiating' or 'occasioning' causes, which Cicero (*De fato* 39–44) also seems to identify with 'proximate' or 'auxiliary' causes (*proximae* or *adiuvantes causae*), and intrinsic capacities, qualities or states that are identified with 'principal and perfect causes' (*perfectae et principales causae*). 'Procatarctic' similarly seems to refer to an external, 'initiating' or 'occasioning' antecedent cause, rather than to an intrinsic or internal 'principal' cause (such as an underlying state), and hence to belong with what Cicero calls the 'proximate' or 'auxiliary' causes. Cicero's famous illustration of the distinction refers to a cylinder which, in order to roll, requires both the intrinsic capacity to roll (*volubilitas*, a 'principal and perfect' cause) and an external agent that will set it in motion by giving it an initial push (a 'proximate', 'auxiliary' – or 'procatarctic'? – cause). See also *SVF* II, 347 (Clement of Alexandria, *Stromata* VIII.9), where a similar distinction is drawn between 'that on account of which' (δι' ὅ) something occurs and 'that which brings something about' (ποιητικόν). On 'procatarctic cause' see especially *SVF* II, 346, 348, 351, 945, 997, and the discussion by Rieth, 1933: 134ff.; Pohlenz, 1940: 106–12; Long, 1971: 181ff.; Frede, 1980: 234ff.; Sorabji, 1980: 272–6. (Later Galen uses 'procatarctic' in the more general sense of an antecedent cause which initiates a sequence of events that leads to an effect that is to be explained – for example, the eating of a given food eventually, after the intervention of additional causes, has led to a given disease; and Caelius Aurelianus seems to use it in the even more general – but fundamentally correct – sense of 'antecedent cause', *Acutae passiones* 1.1.27). For further Stoic causal divisions see *SVF* II, 336–56.

Galen seems to be conflating the Aristotelian and Stoic classifications of cause here: 'procatarctic' or 'initiating antecedent' and 'active' causes belong to the Stoic causal categories, whereas 'the usefulness of what happened', *effectiva*, and 'matter' seem to allude to the Aristotelian final, efficient, and material causes respectively. Galen's vacillation between the Stoic 'active' (*factiva*) and the Aristotelian 'efficient' (*effectiva*) cause is exemplified in T59a; in some parts of his treatise he uses the two terms interchangeably, and they do indeed overlap to some extent.

It seems clear (a) that Herophilus accepted cause only on a hypothetical basis, and (b) that at least some Herophileans did not find the Stoic notion of 'procatarctic' causes very plausible, but it is not clear how much of the remainder of Galen's attack in this testimonium is directed against Herophilus or his followers. (Cf. Chapter XIII, *Cm*.3; Chapter X, T280, *infra*.)

T59a What Galen sees as a contradiction in Herophilus' procedure – expressing doubt about all causal explanation and yet also resorting to the use of 'causes' – can in fact be explained by reference to the provisional status

Herophilus ascribes to causal explanation (see v.A., *supra*), also in the first fragment Galen quotes here ('Whether or not cause exists . . .').

The second fragment in this text ('Either a corporeal cause is the cause of a body . . .'), which ends with the conclusion 'so it is evident that cause does not exist at all', must again be understood in the context of Herophilus' causal hypotheticalism. Proof of the existence of any particular cause, i.e. that *a* is demonstrably and indubitably the cause of *x*, is indeed impossible in Herophilus' view; but Galen here suppresses Herophilus' further conclusion: that cause can therefore only be stated *ex hypothesi*.

The fact that Galen counters with three arguments modelled after Herophilus' but aimed at showing through *reductiones ad absurdum* that visual perception is impossible, is perhaps indirect evidence of the importance Herophilus attached to observation of phenomena as the starting-point of all science (cf. T50, T53, T54). Cf. Chapter XVIII, *Hg.* 3, *infra*; S.E , *M* 9.210, 227–36.

VI

ANATOMY

'*The intimations of higher development among
the subordinate species can be understood only
after the higher development is already known.*'

CHARLES DARWIN

A · INTRODUCTION

At least since Hesiod's pessimistic myth about the degeneration of humanity from a pristine, pre-scientific Golden Age to a scientifically advanced but humanly depraved Iron Age, some forms of scientific progress have prompted value questions and moral ambivalence. Herophilus' striking advances in anatomy and physiology represent a conspicuous instance of indisputable scientific progress which cannot escape from the shadows of such ambivalence. On the one hand, Herophilus has been acclaimed almost universally as the 'father of scientific anatomy' and as a pioneer in the systematic, scientific dissection of human bodies;[1] on the other hand, his revolutionary performance of vivisection on human subjects – condemned criminals – has cast an abiding shadow on his achievements. While fatal drug experiments with humans and vivisectory experiments on animals have been conducted repeatedly in the history of Western

---

[1] Cf., for example, Sarton, 1927–48: vol. I, p. 159: 'The founder of anatomy as a scientific discipline; the greatest anatomist of antiquity; after Hippocrates and Galen the greatest physician of antiquity'; Potter, 1976: 59: 'This one individual made basic discoveries in nearly every system of the body.' (Potter's claim that Herophilus 'had become by Tertullian's time "the anatomist" in the same way Homer was "the poet" ' (p. 46) is, however, perhaps too generous.) Similarly, G. E. R. Lloyd calls Herophilus and Erasistratus 'the two most important biologists' (1973: 75; 'physician' might be more accurate than 'biologist'), and adds 'Herophilus and Erasistratus represent the high-water mark of Alexandrian biology' (1973: 85). P. M. Fraser likewise labels Herophilus 'the unrivalled master of Alexandrian medicine' (1972: vol. I, p. 346), and says 'the medical achievement of Alexandria . . . reached a level never achieved before, or indeed again until the seventeenth century' (vol. I, p. 341).

science from Greek antiquity to our own century, Herophilus and his contemporary Erasistratus stand as isolated, disturbing examples of physicians who – if, as I argue below, the ancient evidence may be trusted – forcibly vivisected other human beings in the name of scientific discovery and of potential benefits that might accrue to future generations of mankind. Some scholars, perhaps unwittingly inspired by an idealization of Greek antiquity that has become entrenched over the last five centuries, have denied the ancient evidence concerning human vivisection any credibility, but, as shown below, a dispassionate re-examination of the relevant ancient texts does not help to disabuse one either of the notion that such vivisections took place or of the impression that they contributed to at least some of Herophilus' remarkable discoveries.

1   *Dissection and vivisection*

Although dissection and vivisectory experiments had been performed before the time of Herophilus, especially by Aristotle, they were performed on animals, not on humans. For their knowledge of human anatomy earlier anatomists without exception seem to have relied mainly on the comparative dissection (and, in some instances, vivisection) of various animals and, like many laymen in cultures with an intimate experience of warfare, on chance observations of wounded or mutilated human bodies. Aristotle, for example, observed in his *Historia animalium*: 'The inner parts [of the body] . . . are unknown, especially those of man; consequently one must refer to the parts of other animals which have a nature similar to the nature humans possess, and examine them' (1.16.494b21-4). There are indications that Diocles (fr. 27 Wellmann, 1901) and Praxagoras (fr. 13 Steckerl), two of the more distinguished physicians of the fourth century B.C., likewise depended on animal anatomy. This was in fact true not only of Herophilus' predecessors but also of most later anatomists of classical antiquity. The illustrious Galen, for example, though writing more than four centuries after Herophilus and though familiar with the human skeleton, relied largely on his dissections of the Barbary ape and perhaps the Rhesus monkey[2] for

---

[2] In his treatise *De anatomicis administrationibus* 1.2 (II, pp. 222-3K) Galen says: 'Choose those apes (sc. for dissection) which most closely resemble humans, with short jaws and small canines. You will find their other parts also resembling those

his anatomical observations. Much of Galen's anatomy, which became canonical for centuries, consequently is a description of the soft parts of the ape – muscles, ligaments, nerves, veins, arteries, alimentary organs, heart, lungs, brain, and so on – superimposed on the human skeleton, and Galen's errors can often be traced to this procedure. Herophilus' anatomy, by contrast, is largely based on human dissection, even though he continued to be interested in comparative anatomy as well.[3] His anatomical descriptions accordingly exhibit striking instances of superior accuracy. Yet, for all the respect Galen and other ancient authors showed Herophilus' anatomical achievements, the Alexandrian physician had to wait until the revival of human dissection in the Renaissance[4] – and the consequent

of the human being, since they can walk and run on two feet . . .' *Ibid*, 6.1 (II, pp. 532–3K) he gives further details concerning the kind of ape he prefers: again, the ones most similar to human beings are preferred, i.e. those with a thumb, a temporal muscle, hair variously hard and soft or long and short, an upright gait, smaller toes than other apes, and a small coccygeal bone, and so on. Since the coccygeal bone is small only in tailless forms such as the Barbary ape, and since the other features also closely fit the Barbary ape, it has been concluded plausibly that Galen relied primarily on the Barbary ape (cf. also *ibid*. 6.14, II, p. 587K on the coccyx). Charles Singer among others has, however, also drawn attention to features which suggest that the Rhesus monkey was used extensively by Galen; cf. Singer, 1956: xix, xxi, and notes 22–4, 36–9, 47–8, 76–7, 95, 102, 31 (on pp. 240ff.). On post-Herophilean human dissection cf. Galen, *De compositione medicamentorum per genera* 3.2 (XIII, p. 604K); Edelstein, 1967: 250–1. See also Chapter X.A; Chapter XVII (Hegetor); Galen, *De anat. adm.* 1.2 (II, pp. 220–1K).

[3] Herophilus more than once compares human organs to those of animals. Cf. Fr60: Herophilus mentions the hare and 'certain other animals' (also, 'not a few other animals'). Galen's statement following Fr61 that Herophilus 'described position, size, and nature of the "testicles" [sc. ovaries] in female creatures (ἐν τοῖς θήλεσι ζῴοις) accurately' might also be a reference to animals, but it is ambiguous and second-hand. (Rufus' reference to a sheep in T105 cannot in itself be construed as proof that comparative reproductive anatomy was undertaken by Herophilus.) The other dissector of human beings in Graeco-Roman antiquity, Herophilus' contemporary Erasistratus, also continued to use comparative anatomy and physiology. Thus Galen reports that Erasistratus used a goat (II, pp. 648–9K) and an ox (*CMG* v.4.1.2, p. 446 De Lacy) for vivisectory experiments, and the Anonymus Londinensis records his use of a bird in a famous experiment designed to verify the hypothesis that invisible emanations from the body take place all the time (Anon. Lond. XXXIII. 44–51; cf. also Anon. Lond., fragment 1). See von Staden, 1975: part I; G. E. R. Lloyd, 1964; von Fritz, 1971a: 75, 138.

[4] See Preface, p. xi. By this I do not mean to suggest that dissection of human cadavers alone ensures anatomical progress. Mondino dei Liucci (or Raimondine dei Liuzzi) dissected humans frequently in the early fourteenth century and

questioning of Galen's deeply entrenched authority – for explicit recognition of his anatomical accuracy.

Religious, moral, and aesthetic considerations, as well as the sheer tenacity of taboos, seem to have inhibited the opening of the human body by the vast majority of physicians in antiquity.[5] Fairly limited surgical incisions and excisions constituted the limit of 'cutting' living human bodies for most ancient physicians, and cutting open a deceased human being was virtually unthinkable. Human corpses admittedly were at times tampered with, but such acts were generally regarded as desecrations and as punishable violations of established norms.[6] That the dissection and vivisection of humans finally became possible – though only briefly – at Alexandria in the early third century B.C. clearly was due only to the exceptional situation which prevailed there. The unusual combination of ambitious Macedonian patrons of science (i.e. the Ptolemies), eager scientists like Herophilus, a new city in which traditional values at first were not considered intrinsically superior, and a cosmopolitan intelligentsia committed not only to literary and political, but also to scientific frontiersmanship, apparently made it possible to overcome traditional inhibitions

his *Anathomia* (1316) enjoyed wide circulation, yet anatomy remained largely dormant until the time of Leonardo da Vinci and Vesalius (sixteenth century). Cf. Sarton, 1927–48: vol. III, part 2, p. 1223: 'The anatomical revival of which Mondino was the protagonist did not develop as one might have expected. On the contrary, the period between Mondino (1316) and the time of Leonardo da Vinci (d. 1517) and Vesalius (1543) saw so little progress that one would almost think of a kind of regression . . .'

[5] Cf. Edelstein, 1932: 50–106; Kudlien, 1969a: 78–94; *id.*, 1968a: cols. 38–48; G. E. R. Lloyd, 1968: 126; also Edelstein, 1935c: 235–48. The theory of Leboucq (1944: 7–40) that Philistion performed dissections on human cadavers in the fourth century B.C. is not substantiated by the evidence. Nor does Praxagoras fr. 67 provide any such evidence (see Steckerl, 1958: 31). I am in fundamental agreement with G. E. R. Lloyd, 1975a.

[6] It has been suggested that these taboos were occasionally contravened, if only surreptitiously, and that religious sanctions would in any case not apply to corpses of criminals, traitors or to bodies found deserted by the wayside. Cf. Pagel, 1898: 77; R. Fuchs, in Neuburger & Pagel, 1902–5: vol. I, pp. 236f.; Neuburger, 1906: vol. I, p. 221; E. Littré, *Hp.* III, pp. 542f. But there is no direct evidence – and only shaky indirect evidence – for this view. Furthermore, as R. von Töply (in Neuburger & Pagel, 1902–5: vol. II, p. 175), Temkin (1928: 28–33), Sigerist (1927: 40), and others (see n. 5) have pointed out, the knowledge of human anatomy in the fifth and fourth centuries B.C. was not based on systematic dissection of humans. Cf. also the discussions in Harris, 1973: 99–103, 24–5; Longrigg, 1981: 158–9, 162–3; Gask, 1940: 387.

against opening the human body. (If P. M. Fraser's contention that
Erasistratus was not active in Alexandria but at the court of
Antiochus in Seleucia is correct, similar circumstances there, as well
as the incentive provided by the acute rivalry of the Seleucids and the
Ptolemies, might have enabled Erasistratus, too, to conduct dissections and perhaps vivisections of the human body; but this remains a
controversial issue.[7])

The ancient reports that Herophilus conducted dissections and,
particularly, vivisections on human subjects have, however, met with
considerable scepticism on the part of some scholars, who point to the
enduring nature of traditional Greek inhibitions and to Herophilus'
failure to make certain observations which, they argue, any vivisector
'inevitably' would have made. But the evidence seems overwhelm-
ingly in favour of the conclusion that he at least *dissected* humans.
Galen's repeated mention of Herophilus as famous for his dissections
(for example, T54, T67–T70, T107) can perhaps not in itself be taken
as proof that these were conducted on human subjects rather than on
animals, but three different ancient sources state unequivocally that
humans were used: Tertullian (T65–T66), who relied heavily on the
writings of a relatively trustworthy physician, Soranus of Ephesus;
Galen (T114), in his discussion of the anatomy of the female organs;
and Vindician, a North African physician who was a contemporary
and acquaintance of St Augustine (fourth century A.D.). Let us
examine the evidence offered by each of these three sources.

Like most patristic authors, Tertullian (*c.* A.D. 200) was strongly
opposed to the scientific research of pagan scientists such as
Herophilus, and did not refrain from disparaging their work. His
hostility has led some scholars to discount his statements about
Herophilus' dissections and vivisections of human subjects as the
product of distorting, sensationalistic polemics.[8] While the equation

---

7   On the life of Erasistratus see Fraser, 1969; Wellmann, 1907a; Harris, 1973: 177–
    8. Julius Beloch and Franz Susemihl (until his palinode) were earlier representa-
    tives of Fraser's view. Much remains inconclusive, however. Cf. also G. E. R.
    Lloyd, 1975b; Longrigg, 1971; *id.*, 1981: 158–60, 177–8.
8   Cf. G. E. R. Lloyd, 1973: 76: 'his [Tertullian's] testimony by itself carries little
    weight. Tertullian was totally opposed to the scientific investigations of pagan
    researchers and did everything he could to defame them and their work.' While
    Tertullian's source, the Methodist Soranus of Ephesus, was opposed to any kind
    of surgical or dissectory intervention, he is a reliable informant. Cf. Waszink,
    1947: 22*–9*. See also Finlayson, 1893: 324: '[Tertullian] uses, as is his wont,
    such violent language, that if it stood alone it might almost be ignored, as it
    carries with it the suggestion of exaggeration and animus.'

of polemics with distortion might normally hold in arenas such as politics, Tertullian's polemics cannot be shown to contain fabrications. On the contrary, the evidence they present is supported independently by other ancient sources. When Tertullian characterizes Herophilus as 'the physician, or rather butcher, who cut up ('exsecuit')[9] innumerable persons in order to examine nature, who hated man in order to gain knowledge, [who] explored the internal parts of man' (T66), there is nothing in the ancient testimonia and fragments that renders any part of this characterization – except the polemical ascription of hatred to Herophilus – questionable. The same is true of his description of Herophilus as a 'dissector even of adults' (T65).

Discussions of Tertullian's veracity have often overlooked the confirmation provided by a non-polemical source: in his *De uteri dissectione* Galen says that Herophilus 'attained the highest degree of accuracy in things which become known by dissection, and he obtained the greater part of his new knowledge not, like the majority [sc. of physicians], from irrational animals, but from human beings themselves' (T114). This is an unequivocal statement by an author who still seems to have had at least three books of Herophilus' *On Anatomy* available to him (Fr 60–2); efforts to discredit this evidence are not likely to succeed.

Finally, Vindician's testimony about Herophilus' dissection of human subjects (T64a, T64b), while perhaps not reliable in every detail (as was suggested in Chapter II (*Comments*, T5)), offers independent confirmation of the claims made by Tertullian and Galen, inasmuch as his enumeration of anatomists is unique and hence does not seem to be derived from either Tertullian or Galen. He admittedly shares with Tertullian a theme common to many Church Fathers – what God has hidden is not intended for human eyes and therefore should not be unveiled artificially in dissection – but his details diverge strikingly from Tertullian's. The cumulative evidence of Galen, Tertullian, and Vindician therefore seems to provide strong support for the view that Herophilus also used human cadavers for dissection.

---

[9] T66 (and particularly 'exsecuit') has been understood to refer only to vivisection (e.g. by Potter, 1976: 46; Fraser, 1972: vol. I, p. 348; Dobson, 1925: 25; Finlayson, 1893), but a careful reading suggests that Tertullian might well be attacking both dissection and vivisection. See *Comments*, T66.

When we turn to the question of vivisection, the most intriguing and disputed authority is our earliest source, Celsus (first century A.D.).[10] In an account of the dissection of human subjects by 'rationalist' physicians, Celsus reports that Herophilus and Erasistratus went even further and performed vivisections on human subjects (T63a). What renders this report particularly plausible is not only the absence of factional polemics on the part of Celsus in this passage[11] – although Celsus himself, while conceding the need for dissecting humans, opposed vivisection as 'cruel and superfluous' – but in particular the vivid details Celsus provides about the unique circumstances, motivations, and justifications which made vivisection possible. (On other ancient evidence of Herophilus' vivisections see *Comments*, T63b–c, T66.)

First, the circumstances: vivisection of humans, according to Celsus, became possible only through royal intervention and patronage – Herophilus obtained imprisoned criminals 'from the kings'. This part of the account seems compatible with the ambitious patronage extended by the first two Ptolemies. Given the tenacious Greek taboos against opening human bodies, the active intervention of ambitious, relatively freethinking Macedonian autocrats (whose 'ancestral' hero – Alexander the Great – had also not shrunk from cruelty in the name of progress[12]) is perhaps exactly what it would have taken to make a vivisectory exploration of human subjects possible. (But see pp. 26–9 *supra* on financial patronage.)

Second, Celsus also reports Herophilus' purpose: to observe in living subjects 'the parts which nature previously has concealed'. Their exact position, shape, size, arrangement, relative density, and so on, are specified as the objects of this observation. It is striking that

---

[10] The other sources are Tertullian, T66; John of Alexandria, T63b; Agnellus (?) of Ravenna, T63c. On the evidence offered by Celsus see Scarborough, 1976, who argues that Celsus' reference to human vivisection represents no more than a reference to a 'rumor'. But see below; cf. n. 13. Gask, 1940: 387, rejects Celsus' account on the grounds that it would be 'embarrassing' to perform human vivisection and 'inconceivable' for Erasistratus to hold that there is air in the arteries if he had vivisected. Cf. *Comments*, T86.

[11] Scarborough, 1976, suggests that polemics against the Ptolemies might have prompted rumours of human vivisection under the Ptolemies. In the absence of evidence, this remains a conjecture, but one worth considering. See below, n. 13.

[12] Alexander's more notorious violent excesses include the Massaga massacre, the murder of Parmenion and Cleitus, and the destruction of Thebes.

these details, too, are identified dispassionately and without any trace of polemical distortion.

Third, Celsus faithfully records the defence of the 'rationalist' or 'dogmatic' vivisectors – of whom Herophilus and Erasistratus are the only known examples – against the charge of inhumanity (without, however, explicitly attributing this classic and notorious justification to either Herophilus or Erasistratus): it is not really 'cruel' to sacrifice a few criminals for the sake of finding cures for the innocent people of all future ages.

It seems unlikely that as discerning and conscientious an author as Celsus would have invented these details about the circumstances, aims, and justification of human vivisection, or would have accepted uncritically the fictions of a polemical source. Celsus was a strongly independent writer, who did not succumb to the temptation to become a mere defender or opponent of any of the schools of medicine about which he wrote. Thus, although it has been suggested that he drew on Empiricist doxography for this part of his *Artes*,[13] he firmly asserts his independence from the Empiricists by endorsing the dissection of human subjects[14] – knowing full well that all dissection was anathema to the Empiricists.[15] None of the traditional school labels – 'Empiricist', 'Methodist', 'Pneumatic', 'Dogmatic' – can be pinned on him successfully. Moreover, even if he did rely on an Empiricist source for this section, Empiricist doxography itself, for all its anti-Herophilean tenor, cannot be shown to have been guilty of distortions so radical as to invent charges of vivisection.[16]

---

13 Wellmann, 1907a: col. 336, and Waszink, 1947: 185, believe that Celsus' account is dependent on an Empiricist source (Heraclides of Tarentum) who was opposed to dissection and vivisection. But see Temkin, 1935a: 249–64. Cf. also Scarborough, 1976; Ferngren, 1982: 272–6; G. E. R. Lloyd, 1982: 144–5; *id.*, 1984: 348; French, 1978: 154, 165 n. 4; Vegetti, 1984: 444; Longrigg, 1981: 158–64.

14 Celsus, *De medicina*, prohoem. 74 (*CML* I, p. 29 Marx): 'Incidere autem vivorum corpora et crudele et supervacuum est, mortuorum discentibus necessarium' – 'To cut open the bodies of living beings is both cruel and superfluous, but [to cut open those] of the dead is necessary for students [of medicine].'

15 Deichgräber, 1965 fr. 24 (especially p. 105.23–9), fr.66–70, fr.14 (especially p. 93.33ff.). One argument the Empiricists used against dissection is that 'aliter pleraque in mortuis se habeant' (fr.14 = Celsus, *De med.*, prohoem, 44, *CML* I, p. 24 Marx); another, indicative of the reassertion of taboos, is that 'mortuorum lacerationem . . . quae etsi non crudelis, tamen *foeda* sit' (*ibid.*).

16 Rejecting and mocking the 'Rationalists' who rush around looking for 'useless' hidden causes is one thing; distorting their practices another. While the

Yet a number of scholars have not only questioned the value of the evidence found in Tertullian, Vindician and Galen, but have attacked Celsus' credibility in particular. Among the arguments advanced against accepting his evidence, three seem particularly prominent.[17]

The first of these one might call the argument from inconceivability: it is inconceivable, it is said, that the Greek inhibitions against cutting open a human body could ever have been overcome. The fact that no Greek physicians are reported to have followed the revolutionary example of Herophilus and Erasistratus either in dissection or in vivisecting humans suggests, it is said, that human subjects were never involved in the first place. But 'inconceivability' is an insidious and capricious criterion for reconstructing the past, as history in general and the history of science in particular amply demonstrate. The unique combination of factors in early Alexandria, to which I referred earlier, might well have made what had been 'inconceivable' in Athens, Cos, or Sicily not only conceivable but also possible in Alexandria. Here I am in full agreement with the observations of G. E. R. Lloyd: 'For all the ancients' respect for the dead, corpses were desecrated often enough by people other than scientists. Moreover, when we reflect that the ancients regularly tortured slaves in public in the law courts in order to extract evidence from them, and that Galen, for example, records cases where new poisons were tried out on convicts to test their effects, it is not too difficult to believe that the

Empiricists enjoyed the former, even at their most polemical they cannot be shown to have committed the latter. Cf. Deichgräber, 1965: 281–8.

[17] See, for example, Simon, 1906: vol. II, pp. xxx ff.; Sigerist, 1924: especially pp. 194–205; Crawfurd, 1919; Allbutt, 1921: 147 n. 3. Dobson (1925: 25–6), and Finlayson (1893: 324–6) are sceptical but do not reject Celsus' evidence outright. Cf. Scarborough, 1976.

The argument that a somewhat similar charge (of inhumane vivisection, referring particularly to abortion) is brought against Archigenes and Galen – of whom it is probably untrue – by Johannes Alexandrinus, and that Celsus' report on Herophilus' vivisectory explorations is therefore equally questionable, is doubly vulnerable. First, Johannes Alexandrinus (seventh century A.D.) cannot be said to be superior to Celsus with regard to accuracy, access to sources, and reliability; second, to conclude that a mistake, because it was made by a seventh-century source concerning author X must also have been made by a first-century source concerning author Y, is not altogether persuasive. Cf. Johannes Alexandrinus' *Commentary on Hippocrates' De natura pueri*, in F. R. Dietz, *Scholia in Hp. et Galenum*, vol. II, p. 216; Finlayson, 1893: 326 n.; Greenhill, 1843: 109 n.; Fraser, 1972: vol. II, pp. 506–7, n. 70.

Ptolemies permitted vivisections to be practised on condemned criminals.'[18] It should also be remembered that, although Herophilus' vivisection of humans might have been revolutionary, vivisectory experiments as such were nothing novel and hence not 'inconceivable'. Thus Aristotle more than once mentions that he mutilated living animals in order to investigate physiological problems experimentally,[19] and Galen later was to conduct many vivisectory experiments on apes and pigs.[20] In an Hippocratic treatise of the Hellenistic period, *On the Heart*, a vivisectory experiment on a pig is also recorded.[21] At issue, therefore, cannot be the 'conceivability' of

[18] G. E. R. Lloyd, 1973: 77. From the earliest recorded occurrences of warfare and ritual violence in Greece (on the latter see, for example, Burkert, 1972: *id.*, 1970) to Roman Imperial times, desecration of the human body recurred in classical antiquity. Cf. also von Staden, 1975: n. 42. Galen, *De antidotis* 1.1 (XIV, p. 2K) reports that Mithridates VI and Attalus III (the last king of Pergamon), who were very interested in toxic substances, used to try out antidotes on criminals under sentence. Fraser, 1972: vol. 1, p. 349, also draws attention to 'the prisoners who were sent [by the Ptolemies] to work in the gold mines of the Eastern desert, and whose misery is so brilliantly depicted by Agatharchides'. See also Temkin, 1962b: 107 n. 69 for a late example of vivisection of a tortured Christian for anatomical purposes; from Theophanes the Confessor's *Chronographia*, ed. Carl de Boor, vol. 1 (Leipzig, 1883), p. 436.

[19] Cf. Aristotle, *De respiratione* 9 (3). 471b19ff.; *De progressu animalium* 8.708b4ff.; *Historia animalium* 3.12.519a25ff.

[20] Cf. Galen, *De facultatibus naturalibus* 3.4 (*Scr. Min.* III, pp. 214–15): vivisection of the peritoneum 'of a still living animal'. Similarly, in *De anatomicis administrationibus* 7.12 (II, pp. 626–32K) Galen describes his vivisection of the heart and lungs to observe the beating of the heart and arteries as well as the consequences of constricting the heart artificially. (In the following chapter of the same work (II, pp. 632–4K) Galen provides an intriguing description of an operation on the slave of a mime-writer, Maryllus; the operation involved excision of the sternum and exposure of the heart, but the slave recovered.) In *De facultatibus naturalibus* 1.13 (*Scr. Min.* III, pp. 127–8) the use of vivisection to demonstrate the function of ureters (i.e. allowing urine to pass from the kidneys to the bladder) is also described, and in *De anatomicis administrationibus* 9.13–14 vivisectory explorations of the nervous system by means of incisions on the spinal cord are described (cf. Duckworth, 1962: 20–6). Cf. also Galen, *De anat. adm.* 8.4, 8.8, 14.7; *De antidotis* 1.1; John of Alexandria, *In Hp. de Natura Pueri Comm.* (II, p. 216 Dietz); Temkin, 1962b: 107 n.69; ps.-Quintilian, *Declamation* 8 (see Ferngren, 1982: 277–89).

[21] *On the Heart* 2 (IX, pp. 80–2L). Cf. also Erasistratus' vivisectory experiment on the arterial pulse, which Galen repeated with contrary results: *On Anatomical Procedures* 7.16 (II, pp. 646–8 K). This experiment is also discussed by Galen, *An in arteriis sanguis contineatur* 8 (pp. 178–80 Furley/Wilkie); Furley & Wilkie, 1972; Amacher, 1964. In *De placitis Hippocratis et Platonis* 7.3 (*CMG* v. 4.1.2. p. 446 De Lacy) Galen also seems to allude to a vivisectory experiment conducted by Erasistratus on oxen. Cf. n. 3.

vivisection in antiquity, but only the use of humans – in this case imprisoned criminals. (Given the extensive medical experimentation with criminals and non-criminals alike in this century, in Western democracies too – and often with fatal consequences – the notion of an 'inconceivable' cruelty to prisoners in a Ptolemaic autocracy surely must be revised.)

Another part of the 'inconceivability' argument points to what is indeed a striking phenomenon: the short-lived history of this revolutionary practice of dissecting and vivisecting human subjects. Ludwig Edelstein's argument that the use of human subjects continued, not only in Alexandria but also elsewhere, until the first century A.D. has been shown to be untenable.[22] The old inhibitions, which had never been vanquished – only momentarily defied – apparently reasserted themselves immediately and powerfully. Furthermore, they now became codified and made theoretically respectable in the Empiricists' theory of scientific method, with its emphasis on passive observation and its censure of the search for hidden causes through dissection, experimentation or any other procedure.[23] Whether or not this is an instance of what E. R. Dodds has characterized as a 'fear of freedom',[24] it clearly represents a regression from the anatomical standards set by Herophilus, as well as a theoretically articulated and 'justified' retreat from the use of both dissection and vivisection.

[22] Kudlien, 1969a. An experiment recorded in On the Heart 10 might refer to human dissection: 'If someone who is skilled at the old way of doing this should remove the heart of one who has died and should push aside one of these heart valves while bending the other upward, neither water nor air, if pushed against [the valves], would pass through the valves into the heart.' While this test successfully demonstrates the irreversibility of the flow of the blood from the heart through the valves (see von Staden, 1975: Part I), the text is ambiguous on several points: first, ἀποθανόντος could refer either to a person or an animal; secondly, the hypothetical formulation, though characteristic of Greek descriptions of experiments (von Staden, 1975: Part II), leaves open the question whether the experiment actually was performed; third, an ad hoc test does not necessarily imply systematic use of dissection; and finally, much of On the Heart suggests that its author used Erasistratus as a source. Cf. Harris, 1973: 84–5, 89.

[23] The Empiricists' censure of dissection as 'etsi non crudelis, tamen foeda sit' (above, n. 15), and of the dissector as 'latrocinans medicus' (Celsus, De medicina, prohoem. 42–3 (CML I, p. 24 Marx); Deichgräber, 1965: 94) are indicative of the fact that religious and moral taboos, too, were at issue in the methodological battle which the Empiricists waged against the Herophileans (see Chapter v).

[24] Cf. Kudlien's remarks, 1969a: p. 93; Dodds, 1951: Chapter VIII: 'The fear of freedom'.

The increasing penetration of Alexandria – also of the Ptolemaic court itself – by indigenous Egyptian views and attitudes[25] may have helped to seal the fate of human dissection and vivisection in antiquity by reinforcing the reassertion of traditional taboos. In his account of Egyptian history, Diodorus of Sicily, a historian of the first century B.C., reports that the *paraschistēs*, i.e. the person responsible for cutting open corpses in preparation for embalming, was usually subjected to active vilification right after performing his task and then had to flee, because the Egyptians 'assumed that every person who applied force to the body of someone of the same race (*homophylos*), and caused wounds in it, was polluted'.[26] While perhaps not an accurate description of Pharaonic practice, this Hellenistic account certainly suggests a native Egyptian attitude which was not conducive to an uninhibited, scientific exploration of the human body.[27] The Egyptian practice of embalming, sanctioned by long centuries of stable religious belief, may have helped a few Greeks in early Alexandria overcome the Greek taboo against opening the human body (as suggested above, Chapter I), but no Egyptian physician ever mistook the accepted tradition of mummification for sanction to dissect, let alone vivisect, any human. Mummification might have had a momentary, indirect, emancipating impact upon enlightened Alexandrian Greeks eager to dissect human cadavers, as some have suggested,[28] but it also seems to have been marked by religious and

[25] Cf. Fraser, 1972: vol. I, pp. 374–6, on the relation of Greek to native Egyptian medicine in later periods. See also *ibid.*, p. 351, and Chapter I (above), pp. 25–6. On the Egyptianization of Alexandria in general see also Fraser, 1972: vol. I, pp. 27, 70–3, 81–92, 115–18, 130–1, 318–19, 715–16.

[26] Diodorus Siculus 1.91.1–4. This part of Diodorus' account, like most of 1.10–98.9, is derived from Hecataeus (*FGrHist* 264F25). Cf. Schwartz, 1903: cols. 670–2, on Hecataeus and Diodorus (= Schwartz, 1959: 45–9). In his elaborate account of embalming, Herodotus (2.86), however, makes no mention of pollution or vilification. Cf. also J. A. Wilson, 1962: 22, who argues that 'it is possible that there was a ceremonial stoning of the individual who made the incision in the side of the corpse, but I believe that it could have been only ritual and did not mean that he was ostracized from his fellow men'. While Diodorus' statement about this is not confirmed by the Egyptian evidence, an argument *ex silentio*, toward which Wilson seems to lean, would be inconclusive at best. Cf. Scarborough, 1976, especially p. 32.

[27] Kudlien, 1969a: 91, makes the interesting suggestion that this Egyptian practice of expelling or ostracizing the embalmer is a reflex of a very ancient rite of purification.

[28] E.g. Harris, 1973: 177.

moral inhibitions not unlike those which had helped to prevent the dissection of humans in Greek societies. Here we seem to have a vivid example of a factor mentioned earlier: that native Egyptian society was no less under the constraints of religious and moral taboos than were Greek societies, and that medical progress, both in Egypt and in the Greek cities, was in part impeded by these taboos.

Moreover, Herodotus' aesthetically unappealing account of the embalming procedures used in Egypt[29] seems to confirm that mummification is as different from scientific dissection as is religion from science: whereas the Egyptian embalmers scraped and drained out the brain piecemeal through the nostrils of the corpse, mangling it beyond anatomic recognition, Herophilus dissected the brain meticulously enough to distinguish its ventricles and to differentiate between several of its other parts with stunning and unprecedented accuracy (see Section 3 *infra*).

When the Egyptian influence grew in Alexandria in the later third and in the second century B.C., not only did these indigenous attitudes, taboos, and procedures become significant forces in Alexandrian society,[30] but some Ptolemies (for example, Ptolemy VIII Euergetes II, also known as Physkon or Kakergētēs) also became explicitly anti-Greek,[31] perhaps in part because some Greeks resisted the Egyptianizing trend.[32] The early Ptolemies by contrast had tried energetically and successfully to lure members of the Greek intelligentsia to Alexandria and had not made strong attempts to fuse Greek and Egyptian scientific culture. One significant consequence of this sharp shift by later Ptolemies seems to have been that the

[29] Herodotus 2.86. Cf. Mokhtar et al., 1973; Cockburn, 1980: 19–20, 55, 93.

[30] Strabo's statements about 'installations suitable for the mummification of corpses' and 'many gardens and tombs' in the Alexandrian suburb Necropolis (*Geography* 795C), and the collocation of Greek and Egyptian systems of burial in this area, which has also been verified by the discovery of mummies, provides, as Fraser (1972: vol. I, p. 27) plausibly concludes, 'a very striking indication of the degree of fusion, both racial and cultural, which some sections at least of the population of Alexandria had undergone' by the time of Strabo (63 B.C. – A.D. 19). Although most of the hypogaea and other tombs in the Necropolis area are of late Ptolemaic and Roman periods, a few are of earlier date; cf. Fraser, 1972: vol. II, pp. 82–3 (n. 186) for the most important evidence.

[31] Cf. Athenaeus, *Deipnosophistae* 4.184b–c, and Chapter III.A above.

[32] Many Greeks remained very hostile, for example, to mummification. Cf. Cumont, 1937: 138–42; Perdrizet, 1934 (discussion of the famous funerary epigram for the son of Epimachus from Hermoupolis Magna; *Sammelb.* 7871 = *Suppl. Epigraph. Graec.* VIII. 621). See also Préaux, 1953: especially p. 206.

enlightened Greek interest in scientific discovery that had been allowed to blossom – and that had made human dissection possible – under the early, pro-Greek Ptolemies now gave way to anxiety, to the Egyptian attitudes exemplified in Diodorus' account, and conceivably in part even to a regressive infusion of the standards of native Egyptian medicine, to which I referred earlier (Chapter 1), into Alexandria.

The Egyptianization of Alexandria, the emergence of the Empiricist school as a dominant force, and the reassertion of traditional taboos need not, however, alone be held accountable for the disappearance of human dissection from ancient science after Herophilus and Erasistratus. Other possible factors are mentioned elsewhere in this study: the periodic eruption of social and political instability, the fact that science did not always enjoy the security within the social order that it had under the first two Ptolemies,[33] and the development of philology and exegesis rather than scientific research as the dominant and most respected brand of learning in Alexandria (see Chapters IX and X). The latter development was, of course, facilitated by the growth of the Alexandrian Library and by the prestige of its scholar-librarians. These factors, along with those explored above, could account adequately for the short-lived history of the dissection and vivisection of human subjects, and the brief duration of this practice is therefore not in itself sufficient or necessary reason to dismiss the testimonies of Celsus and Tertullian.

Another argument which has been advanced against accepting the evidence of Celsus (T63) and Tertullian (T66) is that Galen, who frequently mentions Herophilus' excellence as a dissector (for example, T67–T70, T107, T114) never in his extant treatises alludes to Herophilus' vivisection of humans. But in the very word 'extant' perhaps lurks the answer to this objection: Galen himself refers to a treatise – now lost – in which he dealt with the question of vivisection.[34] More likely than not, this is the place, if any, where he would have discussed vivisections performed on human beings. (He does

---

[33] Cf. Kudlien, 1969a: 91; Fraser, 1972: vol. I, pp. 78, 318–19.

[34] Galen, *De ordine librorum suorum* 2 (*Scr. Min.* II, p. 84 Müller). While Galen's treatise might have dealt primarily with the vivisection of animals, as some have argued, this would surely have been a logical place to mention those vivisectors who had not confined themselves to animals. See also von Töply, 1898: 14–17, on the pseudo-Galenic *De anatomia vivorum*.

refer elsewhere to vivisectory experiments, for example, an experiment concerning the arterial pulse conducted both by Erasistratus and by himself, but he does not state that Erasistratus performed it on a human.[35]) Other lost works of Galen's were also devoted primarily to Herophilus,[36] and he might have dealt with this question in them. But even if Galen never mentioned Herophilus' vivisection of humans, an argument from silence would at best be inconclusive. Celsus, after all, wrote his *Artes* during the reign of the Emperor Tiberius (A.D. 14–37), whereas Galen probably did not complete his main anatomical work until about A.D. 177.[37] Much could have been lost in the roughly hundred and fifty years intervening between them – including Celsus' source or sources. Moreover, the uniqueness of a testimony is, as I argued earlier, never in itself necessary and sufficient ground for rejecting its evidence.

A third class of objection against accepting Celsus' evidence is that Herophilus and Erasistratus would not have made certain mistakes (or neglected to make certain observations), if they had in fact performed vivisection on human subjects.[38] If, however, the psychology of perception or, for that matter, the history of science has taught one lesson forcefully, it is that perceivers in different epochs and cultures do not necessarily always have the same perception when looking at the same object.[39] One does not need to resort to a

---

[35] See above, nn. 20, 21.

[36] See, for example, T176 and the penultimate sentence in T162 (Chapter vii, *infra*).

[37] Singer, 1956: xv; Duckworth, 1962: xi–xii, points out that the work might well have been completed by A.D. 177, but since a fire destroyed Books xii–xv before their publication, Galen had to reconstruct them. Consequently it was not until A.D. 192 that the work as a whole was published.

[38] See above, n. 17. Crawfurd, for example, says (1919: 554, col. 2): 'If Erasistratus had ever dissected a criminal alive, it is difficult to believe that he would have described the arteries as containing only air'; similarly Gask, 1940: 387. But Erasistratus of course acknowledged that blood spurts out when an artery is punctured, and he explained this through the principle of *horror vacui* or, to use a phrase used by Hero of Alexandria about Strato (but not explicitly attested for Erasistratus, though firmly linked to his name by modern scholars), the principle of πρὸς τὸ κενούμενον ἐπακολουθία, 'the following up into the vacated space': as soon as air escapes from a punctured artery, blood rushes in from a vein or veins through *synanastomoseis* or capillary-like connections to fill the potential vacuum. See Harris, 1973: 200–10 for the main sources.

[39] Cf. Arnheim, 1974: especially pp. 47–51, 372ff.; Gombrich, 1961: 3–30 and Chapters 1, 2, 6–10; Kuhn, 1970: especially pp. 111–35.

Heideggerian concept of a pre-structure of understanding[40] or to Gadamer's hermeneutic emphasis on the historicity of understanding and the linguistic boundaries of interpretation[41] or to Michel Foucault's analysis of the varying shifting conceptual and linguistic boundaries of different epochs[42] to recognize that errors have often been made, not only in the inferential process but also in observation itself, and that a modern observer, with a different horizon of perceptual and scientific expectations, is not likely to make the same observational errors as an ancient observer. Moreover, this kind of objection to Celsus' credibility fails to accommodate the fact that many of Herophilus' anatomical observations were in fact superior not only to those of his predecessors but also to those of his successors who no longer used human subjects. As suggested in the next chapter, Herophilus' differentiation of sensory nerves from motor nerves also points to the use of vivisection for heuristic purposes; dissection alone would not have made this discovery possible.

While absolute certainty remains unattainable, no compelling reason for rejecting the evidence of Celsus, Galen, Tertullian, and Vindician concerning Herophilus' practice of dissection and vivisection on human subjects has been found. The thesis advanced at the outset – that Herophilus' extraordinary progress in anatomy might in part be due to his use of human subjects for both dissection and vivisection – accordingly seems tenable.

2 *Herophilus' treatise* On Anatomy

When one turns to the details of Herophilus' anatomy (T60–T129), a relatively rich picture emerges. His anatomical observations on the head (in particular on the brain and the eye), on the nerves, the vascular system, the alimentary organs, and the female and male reproductive organs are especially well represented. Three fragments from his *On Anatomy* are preserved, one each from Book II (Fr60, on the liver), Book III (Fr61, on the female reproductive organs), and

---

[40] Cf. Heidegger, 1963: 310ff., 334–50, 397ff.
[41] Gadamer, 1965: 250ff., 361ff., 477ff.
[42] Foucault, 1966: *passim* (e.g. Chapters 2.iii, 5, 7, 9–10), and 1969. On observational error in later Greek science see Lloyd, 1982.

Book IV (Fr62, on veins). The remainder of the anatomical evidence is arranged as follows:

T63–T74: general evidence on dissection, vivisection, and dissecting technique

T75–T79: anatomy of the brain and skull

T80–T83: the nerves in general

T84–T89: optic nerves and eye

T90–T94: styloid process, hyoid bone

T95–T100: intestinal glands, abdomen, duodenum

T101–T114: reproductive organs (male, female)

T115–T128: vascular system

T129: tibia

T75–T129 are arranged in this sequence not so much because the *a capite ad calcem* principle was widespread in antiquity, but because the three fragments from Books II–IV of Herophilus' *On Anatomy* (Fr60–2) suggest that this sequence might be compatible with his own ordering principles. None of the fragments or testimonia are identified as being from Book I of Herophilus' *On Anatomy*, but given his view that the 'governing principle' of the body is to be sought in the brain, it seems reasonable to suggest that his *On Anatomy* started with a discussion of dissection in general and then dealt with the brain as well as the nerves, whose origin he located in the brain. Fr60 (on the liver) is identified as belonging to Book II, and this suggests that Herophilus' treatment of the alimentary and intestinal organs followed his discussion of the head and the nerves. Next apparently followed his presentation of the generative organs and the foetus, as is suggested by the fact that Fr61, which deals mainly with the ovaries and the uterus, is drawn from Book III of his *On Anatomy*. Finally, Fr62 (on veins) is from Book IV, and this suggests that the anatomy of the vascular system might have followed that of the reproductive organs. How many further books the treatise contained (if any), and what they treated, is not known.

The sequence in which the subject-matter of Fragments 60–2 was treated in Herophilus' *On Anatomy* accordingly seems to indicate that T63–T94 might have been associated with Book I of Herophilus' *On Anatomy*, Fr60 and T95–T100 with Book II, Fr61 and T101–T114 with Book III, and Fr62 as well as T115–T128 with Book IV. But much of this is speculative, and several other ordering principles could in fact have guided Herophilus. Moreover, not all these testimonies necessarily draw on his *On Anatomy*; a few clearly belong to physiological contexts and are included in truncated form in this chapter only because they yield relevant anatomical details. Also, the testimonia concerning the anatomy of the eye and the optic nerves might well be derived from Herophilus' treatise *On Eyes*, from which a therapeutic fragment (Fr260) is preserved by Aëtius of Amida, and some of the ones concerning the female reproductive organs might be from his treatise *On Midwifery*. Others might be derived from his work *Against Common Opinions* (which is, however, only cited in a physiological context; Chapter VII, T203). In the introductory analysis which follows I shall, however, adhere to this provisional sequence; it provides systematic access to his anatomy.

3 *Brain and nerves* (On Anatomy, *Book* I?)

Herophilus' knowledge of the anatomy of the brain is particularly striking when compared to that of his predecessors.[43] The pathophysiological and cognitive significance of the brain was recognized no later than the early fifth century B.C. by Alcmeon of Croton[44] (who perhaps referred to the connection of the brain with the optic nerves[45]). It was reaffirmed in the later fifth century B.C. by the Presocratic philosophers Democritus[46] and Diogenes of Apollonia,[47] perhaps also by Anaxagoras and some Pythagoreans,[48] and then

---

[43] For general background see Woollam, 1958: 5–18; Clarke & O'Malley, 1968: 1–18; 139–53, 260–63, 708–14; Clarke & Dewhurst, 1972: 5–9; Chapter VII.A.2 *infra*.

[44] Alcmeon, 24A5DK (= Theophrastus, *De sensibus*, Chapters 25–6); 24A8DK (= Aëtius, *Placita* 4.17.1; DG, p. 407); cf. also 24A10–11, A13DK, etc.

[45] 24A10DK (= Calcidius, *In Platonis Timaeum comment*, pp. 256–7 Waszink = Herophilus, T86). It is not clear, however, whether 'duas esse angustas semitas quae a cerebri sede, in qua est sita potestas animae summa ac principalis, ad oculorum cavernas meent...' also refers to Alcmeon, or only to Herophilus (or Callisthenes); cf. n. 64 below, *Comments*, T86, and Chapter VII. A.2. For a sound analysis of this passage see G. E. R. Lloyd, 1975a; cf. also Mansfeld, 1975.

[46] Democritus, 68A105DK (= Aëtius, *Placita* 4.5.1; *DG*, p. 391); cf. also 68A135DK, esp. p. 116.15–18 (= Theophrastus, *De sensibus*, Chapter 56), and ps.-Democritus, 68c6DK (p. 227.16).

[47] Diogenes of Apollonia, 64A19DK (= Theophrastus, *op. cit.*, Chapters 39ff.); 64A21DK (= Aëtius, *Placita* 4.16.3; *DG*, p. 406: only hearing).

[48] The evidence is flimsy and problematic. For Anaxagoras see 59A92DK (= Theophrastus, *op. cit.*, Chapter 28), which, however, concerns only auditory

again in the fourth century by Plato[49] and probably Theophrastus.[50] Yet the neuro-anatomical knowledge of the brain remained scanty until Herophilus performed his dissections.

In the Hippocratic Corpus one admittedly also finds numerous excellent observations on the diseases of the brain, and especially on their symptoms; but again, there is little evidence of any direct knowledge on the *anatomy* of the brain. 'The brain of humans, like that of all animals', says the author of the Hippocratic treatise *On the Sacred Disease* (epilepsy), in one of the more complete Hippocratic descriptions, 'is double, being parted down its middle by a thin membrane . . . Veins lead up to it from the entire body, many of which are thin, while two are stout, one coming from the liver [sc. inferior vena cava?] and the other from the spleen [sc. aorta?]'.[51] In the next chapter ('Physiology, pathology') more will be said about the recognition by some Hippocratic authors that the brain is the physiological centre responsible for cognitive activity, emotional states, and certain other functions, but here it suffices to point out that the *anatomical* knowledge displayed by Hippocratic authors tends not to extend beyond the level displayed in the preceding quotation.

perceptions, and 59A108DK (= Censorinus, *De die natali* 6.1; cf. also *DG*, p. 190). For the Pythagorean evidence, cf. 58B1aDK (vol. I, p. 450.17–19DK (= Diogenes Laertius 8.30)), and 44B13DK (Philolaus, quoted by ps.-Nicomachus (= Iamblichus?), *Theologoumena Arithmeticae* (= p. 25.17 Vitt. de Falco)). On the latter see Burkert, 1962: 249ff. (Harris, 1973: 161, erroneously cites the Anonymus Londinensis as the source of Philolaus (44B13DK); perhaps he confused it with 44A27DK (= Anon. Londin. 18.8ff., p. 31 Diels), which deals mainly with Philolaus' views on generation.)

[49] E.g. *Phaedo* 96b; *Timaeus* 44d, 65e, 67b, 70a, 73e. Cf. also Theophrastus, *op. cit.*, Chapters 85 and 6, which seem to be derived from *Timaeus* 67b and 80a–b.

[50] Cf. Theophrastus, *De vertigine* 9 (pp. 402–3 Wimmer) and *De sudore* 3 (pp.405– 6W), 33 (p. 408W). This is, however, flimsy evidence, and neither Priscianus' *Metaphrasis of Theophrastus' On Sense-perception* (ed. I. Bywater, *Supplementum Aristotelicum* I.2 (Berlin, 1886), pp. 1–37) nor Theophrastus' *De sensibus* shows any conclusive sign that Theophrastus moved far from Aristotle's largely negative assessment (see below) of the cognitive significance of the brain. Furthermore, in Priscianus' Neoplatonic metaphrasis, Theophrastus' views are contaminated with those of Plato, Iamblichus, Aristotle, and Priscianus himself. Cf. Rose, 1863: 56ff.; Usener, 1912–14: vol. I, pp. 91–111 (= *RhM* 16 (1861), 259–81); Philippson, 1831: 239ff. (Part 2); Regenbogen, 1940: cols. 1398–9.

[51] *On the Sacred Disease*, Chapter 6 (= 3Gr.). On the vascular anatomy of the brain cf. also *ibid.*, Ch. 6ff., 10; on its pathological importance Ch. 18–19. See also Grensemann, 1968c: 93–4; Harris, 1973: 40ff., 62; and the 'Hippocratic' *On Fleshes* 15.

While the greatest of classical biologists, Aristotle, failed to recognize some major physiological functions of the brain – its main functions, he thought, were to act as a sort of refrigerator which counterbalances the heat of the blood[52] and to produce sleep[53] – his anatomical knowledge does represent an advance over that of his predecessors in several respects. Thus, in his *Historia animalium*, he gives a respectable account of the meninges (dura and pia mater), distinguishes between cerebrum and cerebellum, mentions a cavity in the brain, and discusses three controversial 'ducts' (*poroi*) which lead from the eye: the two larger ones [trigeminal and optic nerve?] to the cerebellum, and the smallest [oculomotor nerve?] to the cerebrum.[54] Furthermore, in his *De somno*, Aristotle comments on the 'slenderness' and narrow bore of what seem to be the vessels of the pia mater (which, he apparently believed, aided the refrigerating function of the brain by spreading material sparsely over a more extensive area).[55] All of this is impressive in its own way.

Yet, when one turns from these earlier anatomical efforts to the suggestive remnants of Herophilus' anatomy of the brain and the nerves, it becomes clear why modern anatomists have typically concluded that Herophilus, and not any of his predecessors, 'may rightfully be regarded as the father . . . of neuroanatomy'.[56] This conclusion is undoubtedly defensible, but unfortunately, as in the rest of Herophilus' anatomy, what has survived most clearly and copiously is Herophilus' innovative anatomical nomenclature rather than his anatomical descriptions or theories. Nevertheless, even the

[52] *De sensu* 5.444a8–15 and 2.438b29–30; *De partibus animalium* 2.7, especially 652a27–9 and 652b16–33; *De somno* 3.457b26–458a10.

[53] *De somno* 3.456b17–28; *De partibus animalium* 2.7.653a10–19.

[54] *Historia animalium* 1.16.494b25–495a18. But cf. also *ibid.*, 3.3.514a15–19; *De partibus animalium* 2.10.656b16–19 ('Ducts run from the eyes into the blood vessels that are around the brain'); *De generatione animalium* 2.6.744a10–11 ('ducts which appear to me to be running from them [the eyes] to the membrane around the brain'). Cf. *De sensu* 2.438b12–16; *De gen. animal.* 4.6.775a1–3. On *poros* see Berg, 1942: 342 n. 3.

[55] Cf. *De somno* 3.458a5–10; cf. *Historia animalium* 1.16.495a7–8: 'The membrane surrounding it [cerebrum] is very venous (*phlebōdes*)', and *De partibus animalium* 2.7.652b30–3: 'With a view to preventing injury occurring through heat, the blood vessels surrounding it [the cerebrum] are not few [and] large but slender and close-packed.'

[56] Woollam, 1958: 11–12, where Erasistratus, too, is granted paternal status. 'Father' is perhaps an appropriately ambiguous metaphor; fathers, too, are not ungenerated.

evidence concerned primarily with nomenclature provides rich
indications of his remarkable advances over his predecessors.

While reiterating a number of Aristotle's correct observations, such
as the distinction (T76–T78) between cerebrum (*enkephalos*, 'brain')
and cerebellum (*parenkephalis*, 'para-brain'), Herophilus also went
further: he seems to have been the first anatomist to distinguish and
describe the main ventricles of the brain. He ascribed great
physiological significance to the fourth ventricle in particular (see
Chapter VII.A.2 *infra*), apparently because of its proximity to the
spinal cord and the motor nerves. He was also the first to describe and
name the 'calamus scriptorius', a cavity in the floor of the fourth
ventricle of the brain (T79), calling it *kalamos*, 'reed pen', because it
resembles the groove of a writing pen.[57]

Another of Herophilus' labels which survives in modern anatomy is
the 'torcular Herophili', the confluence of the four great cranial
venous sinuses – *torcular* being a Latin translation of Herophilus'
label, *lēnos*, 'wine vat' or 'wine press' (T122–T123). No earlier
anatomist seems to have described the confluence of the sinuses, and
the conclusion that Herophilus discovered it therefore seems warranted. Because the junction of right and left transverse sinuses to
form a true torcular is the normal condition in the ox but not in
humans, it has been suggested that Herophilus, like Galen, 'based his
neuroanatomy on the dissection of the brain of this animal'.[58] A 'true'
torcular does, however, also occur in humans, though more rarely.
Moreover, the primary difference between the confluence in humans
and oxen seems to be that the sagittal sinus in the ox divides more or
less equally to form the two lateral sinuses, whereas in humans it tends
to divide unequally.[59] This is not to suggest that Herophilus
completely abandoned comparative anatomy – and the ox was, after
all, a favourite anatomical object not only of Galen but also of
Herophilus' contemporary Erasistratus (cf. nn. 3, 21, 128–9) – but
rather that it has not been shown conclusively that his neuroanatomy
is based only on the dissection of the ox-brain. (Herophilus'
description of a rete mirabile of blood vessels at the base of the brain
(T121) has, with better reason, also been used as evidence that his

[57] For an illustration which makes the aptness of *kalamos* clear, see Fig. 26 (p. 277)
in Singer, 1956. On the ventricles of the brain see Sudhoff, 1913.
[58] Woollam, 1958: 5.
[59] Le Gros Clark, in Woollam, 1958: 18.

neuroanatomy relies on artiodactyls (i.e. an order of ungulate mammals including the ox and the pig); see below, Section 6 on vascular anatomy.)

Perhaps his most spectacular contribution to anatomy was, however, Herophilus' discovery of the nerves. Friedrich Solmsen's careful study of the discovery of the nerves has established beyond reasonable doubt that, although several significant approximations to the discovery of the nerves were made before Herophilus and Erasistratus, Herophilus has to be credited with first discerning the nerves.[60] More will be said in the next chapter ('Physiology') on the questions whether Herophilus, like Erasistratus, distinguished between motor and sensory nerves and whether he consistently used 'nerve' (*neuron*) to refer to nerves, but T80–T85 leave little doubt that he was the first to make a careful *anatomical* study of the nerves. Thus Galen calls Herophilus and his contemporary (cf. T14), the anatomist Eudemus,[61] 'the first persons after Hippocrates to record carefully their dissections of the nerves' (T80). ('After Hippocrates' here is no more than a standard reflex, a genuflection before the putative discoverer of everything a physician might ever wish to know, and it should therefore not be taken at face value.) Furthermore, Rufus of Ephesus reports that Herophilus located the origin of the motor nerves in the brain and in the spine (T81), and Galen seems to ascribe to Herophilus a detailed knowledge of more than seven pairs of cranial nerves, apparently including the optic, oculomotor, trigeminal, motor root of the trigeminal, facial, auditory, and hypoglossal nerves (T82). About the so-called 'sixth pair' of cranial nerves, concerning which Galen claims that Marinus (an anatomist of the second century A.D.) and Herophilus were in complete agreement (T83), Galen says elsewhere: 'In regard to the sixth pair of nerves, neither one of its two units consists of a single nerve springing from either side of the brain, but each of the two consists of three nerves which come off from three roots. We treat it, however, as a single pair, *corresponding to the conception of Marinus* . . . For its three component nerves make their way through a single one only of the

---

[60] Solmsen, 1961: 185: 'Still it seems certain that Herophilus was the actual discoverer of both sensory and motor nerves . . . Thus it was Herophilus who after so many ingenious theories and speculations actually identified the entities . . .' See also Souques, 1934, 1935, 1936a, 1936b: 116–39.

[61] On Eudemus, whom Galen often mentions in the same breath as Herophilus, see Wellmann, 1907b. See also Chapter II, T14, above (with *Comments*), and T67.

foramina of the skull, and, in the dura mater, all these nerves are wrapped up together just as if they were a single nerve.'[62] The 'three nerves which come off from three roots' have been plausibly identified as the glosso-pharyngeal, vagus, and accessory nerves by Duckworth–Lyons–Towers.[63] If Marinus' description indeed coincides with Herophilus', as Galen asserts (both in T83 and in T82), it seems likely that Herophilus also discovered these nerves, or at least that part of them to which Galen refers as 'wrapped up together just as if they were a single nerve'. The facial canal leading from the internal auditory meatus seems to have received particular attention, and Galen records that it was Herophilus who first called it a 'blind' foramen (T82). Not only is his discovery of the nerves therefore a striking achievement, but the detailed nature of his exploration of the nervous system in an age of very limited technology deserves a generous measure of admiration.

Herophilus seems to have been particularly interested in vision and in the structure of the eye, as not only Testimonia 84–9 but also the existence of a separate treatise *On Eyes* (T20, Fr260) suggest. His discovery of the optic nerve is alluded to by Galen in three different treatises: *On Anatomical Procedures* (T82), *On My Own Books* (T84), and *On the Causes of Symptoms* (T85).[64] Herophilus also seems to have been the first to distinguish four 'coats' or membranes of the eye: possibly the sclera-cornea, iris, retina, and the choroid coat (T86–T89; but see *Comments* T86, T87–T89). Again, however, it is primarily his contributions to nomenclature that are singled out for mention by the ancient sources, rather than his anatomical descriptions: *poros* or 'duct' for the optic nerve and tract (already used in a similar sense by Aristotle (see n. 54), 'cobweb-like tunic' and 'net-like coat' for the

[62] Galen, *On Anatomical Procedures* 9.9 (p. 10 Duckworth). A more extensive description is given *ibid.* 14.5 (pp. 197–203 Duckworth).
[63] *Ibid.*, pp. 10, 197–203.
[64] T86, from Calcidius' commentary on Plato's *Timaeus*, confirms T82, T84 and T85, but it is a problematic source inasmuch as it lumps together Alcmeon (fifth century B.C.), Herophilus, and Aristotle's student (?) and relative Callisthenes (*c.* 370–327 B.C.) as the discoverers of the optic nerve, without differentiating between their contributions. The inclusion of the 'Alexander historian' Callisthenes, who was more of an historian than a philosopher or scientist is problematic, although he might have included some second-hand scientific information in one of his numerous digressions. Cf. G. E. R. Lloyd, 1975a and Mansfeld, 1975; cf. also Oppermann, 1925; Waszink's commentary and *Comments*, T86.

retina, 'like the skin of a grape' for the choroid. The only continuous account is Calcidius' (T86), but unfortunately it remains unclear how much of this description is actually derived from Herophilus (see *Comments*, T86).

In what seems to have been his discussion of the vago-glosso-pharyngeal complex, Herophilus bestowed another enduring gift upon anatomical nomenclature: 'styloid process' (T90), a term still used to designate a slender, pointed, bony process from the lower side of the temporal bone. As Galen suggests, Herophilus chose this name because the pointed process resembles the pens (called *styloi*, at least in Alexandria) that were used to write on wax tablets. This again demonstrates his use of a sharp sense of visual similarities to establish an imaginative anatomic nomenclature. Herophilus was, however, not content with just one comparison;[65] he also compared this bony process to the tapering shape of the famous lighthouse on the island of Pharos[66] in the bay of Alexandria – hence 'pharoid process' (T92). The use of 'columnar process' for 'styloid process' in T91 is not a further Herophilean alternative but rather is due to the Arabic translator's inconsistency; the Greek in both T90 and T91 would have been *stylo-eidēs apophysis*, 'styloid process'. Of less enduring influence was Herophilus' designation of the hyoid bone as 'assistant' or 'by-stander' 'because it stands by the tonsils' (T93, 94).[67]

4 On Anatomy, *Book* II *[?]*: *Abdominal cavity*

When we turn from the head to the alimentary organs and other organs of the abdominal cavity – i.e. to what might have been

[65] In the case of the retina, for example, Herophilus also seems to have suggested two names: 'arachnoid' or 'cobweb-like tunic' (T88), and 'net-like coat' (T89). But see Oppermann, 1925: 16–29; Longrigg, 1981: 166–8; G. E. R. Lloyd, 1983: 161.

[66] The lighthouse, of white marble or limestone, was one of the – usually seven – wonders of the ancient world (Schott, 1891) and, in spite of repeated earthquakes, stood until the fourteenth century. It was 'polygonal in shape . . . tapering towards the top' (Fraser, 1972: vol. I, p. 18). Cf. *infra*, p. 207; Strabo, *Geographica* 791–2; Thiersch, 1909; Rostovtzeff, 1953: vol. III, p. 1422; Picard, 1952: 61–95; Bernand, 1966: Ch. 6, pp. 101–11; Reincke, 1938; Letronne, 1842–8: vol. II, pp. 527–33 (DLXII. Phare d'Alexandrie).

[67] παραστάτης (*parastatēs*), literally 'by-stander', but also 'defender', 'comrade', 'assistant', 'helper', was one of Herophilus' favourite anatomical designations. He used it not only of the hyoid bone but also of the seminal vesicles and of the ampullae of the vasa deferentia (see T101–T103 and relevant *Comments*).

covered in Book II of Herophilus' *On Anatomy* – a more meagre account emerges.

The most significant text in this group is the fragment on the liver (Fr60), which with good reason has been called 'the first classic description of the liver'.[68] Strikingly new in this fragment of Herophilus is that the anatomy of the *human* liver is here described accurately for the first time. Although the liver had fascinated Greek authors, both scientific and non-scientific, from Homer to Aristotle, most earlier authors either were not concerned with its anatomy or relied on the anatomy of animal livers for their conclusions about the human liver. Herophilus, by contrast, describes the shape of the human liver as well as its topographical relations to other organs in the abdominal cavity with admirable accuracy. He admittedly remains a 'comparative' anatomist to the extent that he compares the human liver to that of animals (e.g. the hare), but there can be no doubt that his description of the human liver is the product of meticulous autopsy. Another radical departure from previous anatomy is found in Herophilus' view on the blood vessels which are connected with the liver; it is discussed below (Section 6) in the analysis of his anatomy of the vascular system (pp. 180–1).

How much progress Herophilus' description of the liver represents becomes particularly clear when one considers his predecessors' knowledge of the human liver. The inspection of the liver for divinatory purposes – a custom common to Greece, Babylonia, Assyria and Rome – led to a close and repeated scrutiny of the liver from the earliest times, and hence also to a rich 'liver vocabulary' accessible even to laymen such as Aegisthus, but hepatoscopy relied exclusively on the livers of sacrificial animals, and it focused exclusively on surface features of the liver.[69] This is not to suggest that the vital significance of the human liver was ever in doubt in Greek antiquity. Prometheus' vulture-ridden but amazingly recuperative liver might be the best-known liver of Greek antiquity, but there are also reasonably accurate details especially about the topography of the livers of numerous other heroes and humans throughout Greek literature – details perhaps derived both from hepatoscopy and from

---

[68] Mani, 1959–67: pt I, p. 45.

[69] Euripides, *Electra* 826–30. On hepatoscopy see Contenau, 1940; Stengel, 1920: 60ff; Mani, 1959–67: pt. I, pp. 14–17. Cf. also Rufus of Ephesus, *De nominibus partium humani corporis* 180 (p. 158 Daremberg/Ruelle).

observing seriously wounded war casualties. Fictive and philosophical residues of this sense of its importance are found from the Homeric
poems (and the parodistic account of the 'Homeric' frog who, in *The
Battle of Frogs and Mice*, recognized the vital function of the liver and
killed a mouse by piercing its liver) down to late antiquity.[70]

The earlier Hippocratic authors had more of a clinical than an
anatomical interest in the liver, and it is striking that the nomenclature they use for the liver is even simpler and more restricted than that
of Greek hepatoscopy. The fact that the author of the Hippocratic
treatise *On the Nature of Bones* claims that the liver has five lobes also
suggests that Hippocratics relied on the livers of animals, not of
humans, for their knowledge of the anatomy of the liver.[71] This is not
to say that all their anatomical details were incorrect: as will be
pointed out below, they correctly identified some of the blood vessels
connected to the liver. Moreover, like Homer and other Greek
authors, they recognized that it is contiguous with the diaphragm.
But Herophilus' description clearly is an enormous advance on the
Hippocratic Corpus.

Herophilus' anatomy of the liver also does not suffer when
compared to Aristotle's. While Aristotle, too, had recognized the vital
significance of the liver (and while much more evidence about his
pathophysiology of the liver has survived than about Herophilus'),
his *anatomy* of the liver remains fairly limited and is based primarily on
comparative anatomy. He admittedly mentions the *human* liver as

---

[70] Cf., for example, *Iliad* 20.468–72; *Odyssey* 9.299–302; *Batrachomyomachia* 202–3;
Aeschylus (?), *Prometheus* 1021–5; Aeschylus, *Agamemnon* 432, 790–2; *id.*, *Choephori*
271–2; *id.*, *Eumenides* 135; Euripides, *Orestes* 1062–3; Theocritus 13.71; Timaeus
Locrus 100a, 101a (cf. Plato, *Timaeus* 71d, 72c). See also Mani, 1959–67: pt I, pp
20–2; Onians, 1951: 84–9, 152, 505–6.

[71] *On the Nature of Bones* 1 (IX, p. 168L). On the topography of the liver cf. also the
Hippocratic works *On Anatomy* (VIII, pp. 538–9L): 'the liver has two eminences
called gates [portae?]'); *Letter 23* (IX, p. 396: the liver has 'lobes' or, if Ermerins'
reading is accepted, 'varying lobes'); *Epidemics* 2.4.1 (V, pp. 120–4L = *On the
Nature of Bones* 10 (IX, pp. 178ff.)). On the relation of the bloodvessels to the liver
in the Hippocratic Corpus, likewise see *Epidemics* 2.4.1; also *On the Nature of
Humans* 11 (VI, pp. 58–60L) with Galen's comments (*In Hippocratis De natura
hominis comm.* 2.6, *CMG* v.9.1, pp. 68–76 Mewaldt) – but see below, on Polybus
(and n. 93); *On the Sacred Disease* 3 (p. 68 Grensemann); *On the Nature of Bones* 7–9
and 18 (IX, pp. 172–8, 192–4L). Cf. also Gotfredsen, 1942: 321ff.; Mani, 1959–
67: pt I, pp. 25–7, 321ff. As in other details, there is not total agreement among
Hippocratic authors on the topography of the liver.

being 'round like that of an ox'[72] – a plausible comparison which, as Nikolaus Mani has pointed out, still survives in modern handbooks of comparative anatomy[73] – but the rest of Aristotle's observations on the liver tend to be concerned with animal livers. Like Herophilus, he distinguishes between animals with varying numbers of liver lobes, singles out the liver of the hare for special mention, and discusses the blood vessels of the liver.[74] He also took the first incomplete and vague step to hepatic histology by discussing the nature of the 'non-homogeneous parts' or tissues of which the liver is composed, and provided the first scientific description of the hepatic and cystic ducts by which bile is secreted from the liver and the gall bladder respectively into the duodenum.[75] All of this is very impressive, but it remained for Herophilus to provide the first detailed description of the human liver and to describe its size, position, shape, and texture with some accuracy (Fr60). Herophilus' contemporary Erasistratus followed Aristotle's 'histological' example, and perhaps made a more important physiological and pathological contribution than Herophilus to an understanding of the liver (for example, about the role of the liver in the production of bile and the pathogenesis of dropsy),[76] but Herophilus' *anatomical* contribution remained unsurpassed until the second century A.D.

The liver was, however, not the only organ in the abdominal cavity which interested Herophilus. According to Galen (T95), 'some . . . glands (*adenes*) which are located there' were also investigated actively by Herophilus and his younger contemporary Eudemus. Although Galen does not identify these glands, the pancreas seems a good candidate. In this passage (T95), Galen seems to be discussing the secretion of gastric juice, of bile (from the liver), and of a 'glandular' juice, and it is in particular his description of what is secreted from the glands which makes the identification of the latter

---

[72] *Historia animalium* 1.17.496b23–4.

[73] Ellenberger & Baum, 1943: 410; Mani, 1959–67: pt I, p. 38.

[74] *Historia animalium* 1.17.496b15–33; 2.17.507a16–19; 3.4.514a 29–b9 (cf. also 3.3 and the rest of 3.4); *De partibus animalium* 3.12.673b16–18.

[75] *De partibus animalium* 2.1.646b30–647b9. On the formation of the σπλάγχνα ('innards'), among which Aristotle numbers the liver, see *ibid.* 3.10.673a33–b2 and 2.1.647b2–4; 3.4, 7, 12; 4.2. Cf. also Berg, 1942 (especially p. 339).

[76] Galen, *De usu partium* 4.13 (I, p. 223 Helmreich); Fuchs, 1894b: 554; Galen, *De atra bile* 5 (*CMG* v.4.1.1, pp. 80–1 de Boer); id., *De facultatibus naturalibus* 2.2 and 2.4 (*Scr. min.* III, pp. 158, 168–9 Helmreich); ps.-Galen, *In 'Hp.' De humoribus comm.* 3.24 (XVI, p. 447K).

with the pancreas plausible: the 'glandular' secretion, he says, is 'a viscous fluid, similar to saliva'. This characterization seems most compatible with the clear, watery, alkaline juice which the pancreas contributes to the digestive process.

One part of the digestive tract – the first, shortest, and widest part of the small intestine – still owes its name, *duodenum*, to Herophilus: duodenum, 'twelve each', is a mutilated Latin version of Herophilus' Greek name for it, *dōdekadaktylon* or 'twelve fingers [long]'. Galen gives Herophilus credit for this contribution to anatomical nomenclature no less than four times, (T96, T97, T98, T100), and Theophilus Protospatharius, a Byzantine medical author of the seventh or ninth century A.D.,[77] follows suit (T99).

5 On Anatomy, *Book* III *[?]: Reproductive organs*

While the physiology of reproduction interested Greek philosophers and scientists from the earliest times (see next chapter), the anatomy of the reproductive organs remained relatively neglected and primitive until Herophilus' time. Very often anatomy seems to have served as not much more than an ancillary prop for a preconceived theory of generation. Thus the widespread theory that the generation of males is associated with the right-hand side of the body – for example, with the testicle on the right – while that of females has to do with the left side, was supported throughout antiquity, from the Hippocratic Corpus to Aëtius of Amida, often with the concomitant anatomical theory that the uterus has two chambers: the one on the right for male embryos, the one on the left for the female.[78] Even Galen, who was able to build on Herophilus' more accurate and detailed anatomy of both the male and the female reproductive organs, adheres to this classical theory of a *uterus biformis*: 'but in humans and in animals resembling them, just as the whole body is

---

[77] Theophilus' date is uncertain. Deichgräber suggests that he is identical with 'Theophilus' to whom Photius wrote and therefore assigns him to the ninth century A.D. (1934b). But Krumbacher, 1897: 614, 616–17; Temkin, 1932: 46f., and Vogel, 1967: 289 ('During the reign of Heraclius (610–641)'), all agree that Theophilus lived in the seventh century A.D. On *dodekadaktylon* see Benveniste, 1965: 9–10.

[78] Cf. Lesky, 1950: 1263–93 (= pp. 39–69); Diepgen, 1937: 131 ff.; Rousselle, 1980; Manuli, 1980.

double with right and left sides, so too one pocket of the uterus is placed in the right side, another in the left'.[79]

The first more precise description of the genitalia occurs in the third book of Aristotle's *Historia animalium*. He distinguishes the main bloodvessels in the male organ, and describes the ductus deferens, even if not entirely accurately.[80] Inasmuch as his discussion of the anatomy of the uterus is based primarily on a bicameral male model – 'the uterus is bipartite in *all* [females], just as in *all* males there are also two testicles'[81] – and is devoted mostly to birds, fish, oviparous quadrupeds, and snakes, it contributes little to human anatomy.[82] More details might have been provided in Aristotle's lost work *Anatomai* or *Dissections*, to which he refers in his discussion of the uteri of different fishes,[83] but in his extant works the discussion of the physiology of generation is much more detailed and complex than his scanty anatomy of the reproductive organs of humans. Herophilus' contribution here, too, is noteworthy – at least when measured by the standards of his predecessors.

In the male, Herophilus not only recognized, as had some previous authors such as Aristotle, the connection between the testicles and the spermatic duct system by means of which semen is excreted. He also distinguished carefully between various parts of the spermatic duct system itself. First, he seems to have identified and named the epididymis (*lit.* 'on *or* near the testicle' (*didymos*)). It is a narrow, convoluted part of the duct system which lies on the lateral edge of the posterior border of each testis and is composed mostly of efferent tubes. To this day it bears the name Herophilus assigned it. Second, he identified the ampullae or dilations of the two vasa deferentia (i.e. the ducts which carry sperm from each of the two epididymal ducts to the ejaculatory duct). These ampullae he called 'varix-like' or 'varicose assistants' (T101–T103, T105) – 'varix-like' because their dilation resembles that of varicose veins, and 'assistants', as I shall argue in the section on the physiology of reproduction (Chapter

---

[79] Galen, *De usu partium* 14.4 (II, pp. 290–1 Helmreich). Cf. *id.*, *De uteri diss.* 6 (*CMG* v.2.1, p. 44 Nickel).

[80] *Historia animalium* 3.1.510a14–b4; cf. *De generatione animalium* 1.4.717a33f., 1.6.718a10f. See also the diagram in Peck, 1965–: vol. I, p. 236.

[81] *De generatione animalium* 1.3.716b32–3.

[82] Cf. *ibid.*, 1.3.716b32–717a10; 1.8–11.718a35–719a27; *Historia animalium* 3.1.510b6–511a34.

[83] *Historia animalium* 3.1.511a12–13.

VII.A.5), because they 'assist' both in the transportation and, in Herophilus' view, in the production of seed.[84] Third, he also distinguished the two seminal vesicles or vesiculae seminales – two pouches, one on each side of the male reproductive tract, which contribute to the seminal fluid and serve for temporary storage of the sperm – from the vasa deferentia to which they are linked, calling the vesicles 'glandular assistants' (T101, T102). Some scholars have suggested that 'glandular assistants' refers to the prostate gland,[85] but the use of the plural, and the fact that they are identified as 'bordering upon' the vasa deferentia and being 'one on each side' (T101), makes their identification with the seminal vesicles more plausible. That Herophilus' strikingly detailed knowledge of the male reproductive organs is indeed the result of dissection seems to be confirmed by St Augustine's friend Vindician, who in an elaborate account of Herophilus' views on the origin of seed (T191) says that 'tearing open bodies, which the Greeks called "dissection" (anatomē)' according to Herophilus is a witness to his views on spermatogenesis and on reproduction (T104).

Similarly conspicuous advances on his predecessors are found in Herophilus' anatomy of the female reproductive organs (Fr61, T105–114). Yet, though he seems to have abandoned the traditional theory of a two-chambered uterus, he did not always succeed in emancipating himself from the common tendency in antiquity to base explanations of female organs on the analogy of male organs. Even where he seems to have taken some halting steps away from the male model, he remains fundamentally enslaved to it. Thus he expressly denies that the human female has the same 'varix-like' assistants or ampullae of the *vasa deferentia* as the male (Fr61, T105), but when he describes the ovaries and the ducts leading from them, his description

---

[84] Two passages in Galen's De semine (IV, p. 582K; pp. 565–6K = T189 and T190) suggest that both the transportation of sperm and a significant role in the production or refinement of sperm are attributed by Galen to the 'varix-like assistants'.

[85] For example, Duckworth, 1962: 131 (= T101). Potter, 1976: 53, apparently understands the two 'gland-like ducts' mentioned by Galen in T101 to refer to 'the seminal vesicle *and* the prostate gland'. But Galen clearly specifies that these 'two other ducts are found *one on each side*', and while this would be a natural way of referring to the two seminal vesicles, it would be an unlikely way of referring to the prostate gland *and* the two vesicles. Lesky, 1950: 1385, refers to T102 ambiguously: 'Prostata bzw. die Samenblasen' – but *beziehungsweise* concedes more ambiguity and murkiness than T101–T102 demand.

stands squarely in the shadow of the male model. The ovaries are called 'twins' (Fr61 and T109: *didymoi*) – a standard word in Greek medical literature for the testicles – and they are said to '*differ only a little from the testicles of the male*' (Fr61). Similarly, while recognizing that tubes proceed from each of the two ovaries, Herophilus failed to recognize the true course or function of the Fallopian tubes. Calling them 'spermatic ducts', after the male analogy, he concluded that 'the spermatic duct from each testicle [sc. ovary] grows into the fleshy part of the neck of the bladder, *just like the male duct*' (Fr61).[86] The very principle of analogy which might have been heuristically fruitful, inasmuch as it apparently led to the discovery of the ovaries, now misled Herophilus into postulating for the Fallopian tubes a course similar to that of the male spermatic duct. Furthermore, it led to an obstinate entrenchment of this imposition of the male model upon the anatomy of the female: approximately four hundred years later as superb a gynaecologist as Soranus of Ephesus still adhered to the view that the tubes eventually issued into the bladder (T106), and it remained for Rufus and Galen to correct this theory.[87]

Nevertheless, Herophilus' discovery of the ovaries and the tubes, his observations on the cervix of the uterus and the changes it undergoes (T110–T112), his description of the broad ligaments (Fr114), and his careful observations on the blood vessels of the female reproductive organs (Fr61, Fr114) and of the umbilical cord

[86] Potter, 1976: 55–6, argues that Galen – and, I suspect, all subsequent interpreters of Fr61 – misunderstood Herophilus. Although Galen takes the analogy of the female tubes with the male ducts to extend to their issuing into the bladder, Potter makes the interesting suggestion that 'what Herophilus is stressing is that the seminal ducts in both sexes empty *into another vessel*, in the male, the urethra within the prostate gland at the neck of the bladder, in the female, the cavity of the uterus' (p. 56, italics added). Herophilus' Greek does not, however, seem to lend itself conclusively or even readily to this interpretation; ἐμφύω requires either a dative or a prepositional phrase of the object 'into which' the subject is implanted. In this case only εἰς τὸ σαρκῶδες τοῦ αὐχένος τῆς κύστεως 'into the fleshy part of the neck of the bladder', is specified as the object, and there is no mention whatsoever of 'another vessel' (Potter), let alone of 'another vessel' which is *different* in the male and female. Cf. also *Comments*, T61; Lesky, 1950: 1386; Balss, 1936: 12. On the use of the male analogy to explain the female, cf. Rousselle, 1980; Joly, 1966: 111–16.

[87] Galen, *De uteri dissectione* 9 (*CMG* v 2.1, p. 48 Nickel). The suggestion that Rufus of Ephesus, not Galen, discovered the true course of the uterine tubes (Diepgen, 1937: 136) might be correct, but it is based on a passage which refers to 'varix-like vessels growing from the ovary on each side' in female *sheep* (T105), not in women.

(T113) represent an increment of scientific progress no less admirable than the detailed differentiations he introduced into the anatomy of the male reproductive organs.

6 On Anatomy, *Book* IV *[?]: Vascular Anatomy*

There was little agreement in Greek antiquity on the anatomy of the vascular system. As in Greek theories of sensation and cognition, here, too, there was a protracted battle between the head and the heart. In some earlier theories the head had been depicted as the centre from which an increasingly articulated network of blood vessels emanates, whereas in the course of the fourth century with the support of the Sicilian tradition and, to some extent, of Plato, and especially under the influence of Aristotle, the heart became recognized as the source and centre of the vascular network. (Later, however, Galen's view that the liver is the starting point of the vascular system became canonical for more than a millennium.) A brief look at some earlier theories might help us to evaluate the nature and magnitude of Herophilus' contribution.

Aristotle reports in his *Historia animalium* that three scientists of the fifth century B.C. – Hippocrates' putative son-in-law Polybus, the Cypriot physician Syennesis, and the Presocratic philosopher Diogenes of Apollonia – thought that the entire network of blood vessels emanated from the head.[88] According to Syennesis,[89] says Aristotle, the 'thick' or main vessels start from the head and then perform a chiasma in the thorax, passing from left to right and from right to left, the one from the left then proceeding through the liver to the kidney and a testicle, the other to the spleen and then likewise to a kidney and a testicle, and finally into the penis.[90] In this description, the heart is not even mentioned. Diogenes' characterization of the distribution of the blood vessels, which is also preserved by Aristotle, represents an advance over that of Syennesis, in so far as it is far more detailed and includes the vessels of the arms and legs as well as the fruitful notion of vessels 'branching off'. But here, too, the head rather than the heart is

[88] Aristotle, *Historia animalium* 3.2–3.511b24–513a7.
[89] Syennesis' exact date is uncertain. The Hippocratic treatise *On the Nature of Bones* 8 (IX, p. 174L) offers a description remarkably similar to that of Syennesis, but without attributing it to him. (See also Littré's remarks, Hp. I, pp. 419f.L.)
[90] Aristotle, *Historia animalium* 3.2.511b23–30.

depicted not only as the centre of cognition but also as the source from which all the blood vessels emanate.[91] Nevertheless, his description in a limited way foreshadows Aristotle's discovery of the heart as the centre from which (or to which) the vessels proceed, inasmuch as his 'two biggest veins' (vena cava and aorta?) are each said to have 'two very large [branches] leading to the heart'.[92] Polybus' account of the vascular system, which recurs in more elaborate versions in two Hippocratic treatises,[93] depicts only four pairs of blood vessels, all proceeding from the head.[94] As in Syennesis' description, the heart is not even mentioned in this relatively primitive version.

Turning to the fourth century B.C., one might note that many details of Plato's description in the *Timaeus* of the blood vessels as irrigation channels which carry nutrition throughout the body are derived from Diogenes. But Plato, even if only within the framework of a 'likely story',[95] represents a major advance in so far as he explicitly recognizes the heart as a 'knot of veins and a source of the blood which races through all the limbs . . .'[96] Some earlier authors, such as Empedocles, had made the blood or 'the blood around the heart' the physiological centre of sensation and thought,[97] but had

[91] *Ibid.*, 511b31–512b11. In his commentary on Aristotle's *Physics* (*CAG* IX, p. 153.15–16) Simplicius seems to be referring to this account when he mentions an 'accurate anatomy of the bloodvessels' which Diogenes provided in his work *On Nature* (cf. p. 151.28–9: 'in his *On Nature*, which alone of his works has reached me').

[92] *Historia animalium* 3.2.512a1–4.

[93] Hp., *On the Nature of Bones* 9 (IX, pp. 174–8L); *On the Nature of Humans* 11 (VI, pp. 58–60L; *CMG* I.1.3, pp. 192–6 Jouanna).

[94] Aristotle, *Historia animalium* 3.3.512b12–513a7.

[95] εἰκὼς λόγος (Plato, *Timaeus* 30b7, 57c8–d6, 48d2–3); εἰκὼς μῦθος (59c6). Cf. also 56b4, 29c2, 44d1, 40e1–2.

[96] *Timaeus* 70a7–b2; cf. b3–d6.

[97] Empedocles 31B105DK: 'the blood around the heart is men's thought (*noema*)'. Some later doxographers converted Empedocles' αἷμα περικάρδιον ('blood around the heart') into the heart itself: Censorinus, *De die natali* 6 (31A84DK); Theodoretus, *Graecarum affectionum curatio* 5.22 (31A97DK). But see also 31A97DK (Aëtius, *Placita* 4.5.8; *DG*, p. 391): the composition of the *blood* is the source of control according to Empedocles; Galen, *De placitis Hippocratis et Platonis* 2.8 (p. 166 De Lacy): Empedocles and Critias suppose that *blood* is the soul; Tertullian, *De anima* 5: 'Empedocles et Critias ex *sanguine* [sc. animam effingunt]'; Macrobius, *In Somnium Scipionis* 1.14.20: 'Empedocles et Critias *sanguinem* [sc. dixerunt animam]'. Among later sources, Cicero comes closest to preserving the sense of Empedocles' B105: 'Empedocles animum esse censet cordi suffusum sanguinem' (*Tusculan Disputations* 1.9). On the controversial identity of this Critias see Rüsche, 1930: 134 n. 1. Cf. also Onians, 1951: 47f., 63, 481–2.

provided no description of the blood vessels, let alone of their connection with the heart, or of the heart itself. All that seems reasonably clear from the fragments of Empedocles, for example, is that he conceived of the blood as constantly moving to and fro, like ebb and flow, and of the vessels as opening into the pores of the skin (and that he used this as the anatomical basis for his theory of 'poral' or cutaneous respiration, traces of which resurface in Galen's elaborate theory of arterial respiration).[98]

Only with Aristotle and Diocles of Carystus do we reach writers who, though they made the mistake of reasserting the cognitive and sensitive primacy of the heart, tried to give an account both of the heart as the vascular centre and of the blood vessels. Thus Aristotle clearly recognizes the heart as the organ from which all blood vessels arise – a much more definite conception than Empedocles' notion of 'pericardiac blood' as the centre of control or Plato's depiction of the heart as a 'knot of veins'. He also seems to have been the first scientist to recognize that the heart consists of more than one chamber, but he made the peculiar mistake of claiming that the hearts of all large animals, including humans, have three chambers of ventricles. In at least three different treatises – *Historia animalium*, *De partibus animalium*, and *De somno*[99] – Aristotle repeats this theory of three ventricles, and although his descriptions of the connections of the three ventricles with the pulmonary vessels, with the vena cava, and with the aorta are not always consistent, he seems never to have abandoned the three-ventricle theory.

Aristotle conceived of the vascular system 'as a double-trunked tree

---

[98] Empedocles, 31B100DK (= Aristotle, *De respiratione* 7.473b9–474a6); cf. also *De respir.* 474a17–20, 473b1–8. See the divergent interpretations of B100 by Furley, 1957: 31–4 (interprets B100 as a theory of cutaneous breathing; perhaps the most plausible interpretation); Booth, 1960: 10–15 (B100 is a theory of oral, not cutaneous, breathing); O'Brien, 1970: 140–79 (the 'pores' to which Aristotle refers are in the lungs, not on the skin; hence B100 is not a theory of cutaneous breathing). For Galen's perhaps not entirely consistent theory that air is drawn into the heart from the atmosphere through the lungs by way of an artery, cf. *De usu partium* 6.2 and 7.8–9; *De placitis Hippocratis et Platonis* 6.3; *De naturalibus facultatibus* 3.15 (*Scr. Min.* III, pp. 251–7 Helmreich); *De usu respirationis, passim*, esp. 5 (IV, pp. 504–6, 510–11K); *An in arteriis natura sanguis contineatur* 6 (IV, pp. 724–5K). See also Harris, 1973: 338–51, 283–7; Furley/Wilkie, 1984: 40–6; *id.*, 1972.

[99] *Historia animalium* 1.17.496a4–27; *De partibus animalium* 3.4.666b21–667a6; *De somno* 3.458a15–19. Cf. Huxley, 1880: 1–5; Platt, 1921: 521–32.

[100] Harris, 1973: 122.

springing from a common root',[100] i.e. from the heart. His elaborate
though not always accurate treatment of the vena cava, of the aorta,
of the pulmonary artery and pulmonary vein, and of their ramifications never arrives at a general distinction between veins and arteries,
however, and he uses the same word (*phlebs*, 'bloodvessel') for both
veins and arteries.[101] Yet his account not only represents a great
advance over the standard previously set by Diogenes of Apollonia; it
also is the first reasonable approximation of anatomical truth.

If the famous Brussels fragment attributed to Vindician really
provides reliable evidence about Diocles of Carystus, as Max
Wellmann and Werner Jaeger argued,[102] Diocles perhaps corrected
Aristotle's mistake concerning the number of cardiac ventricles.[103]
He also described the two ears or auricles of the heart, but he used this
anatomical advance to reaffirm the erroneous notion of the cognitive
primacy of the heart: the heart is always awake, listening and
understanding, 'quia et aures habet ad audiendum', 'because it also
has ears [auricles] for listening'.[104] Diocles furthermore accepted the
differentiation of vena cava from aorta – a distinction which had
been used by his father Archidamus, by Aristotle, and by some
Hippocratic authors (see below) – but like his predecessors he did not
proceed beyond this differentiation to a general distinction between
veins and arteries.[105]

Although it is therefore clear that more than one earlier physician
and biologist had described both major veins and major arteries,

[101] Cf. *Historia animalium* 1.17.496a4–35, 3.2.511b10–23, 3.3–4.513a16–515a26,
3.19.520b10–521a9; *De partibus animalium* 3.4–5.665b5–668b32. Cf. Harris,
1973: 121–38, 143–55, Fig. 4.
[102] Wellmann, 1901: 2ff.; Jaeger, 1938a: 3, 187–211. But see above, Chapter II.A.2
(with nn. 20–7).
[103] Vindician (?), *Fragmentum Bruxellense* 44 (Wellmann, 1901: 234). Although this
text refers only to the two auricles, not to the cardiac ventricles, the entire
passage suggests a bicameral model not only of the brain but also of the heart. On
Diocles' views concerning the heart cf. also fragments 14, 16, 38, 40, 42, 44, 57,
and 59 in Wellmann, 1901.
[104] Vindician (?), *loc. cit.* This theory that the cardiac auricles have the function of
hearing is rejected in a later Hippocratic treatise, *On the Heart* 8: the heart's 'ears
do not have holes, because they do not listen to shouts and cries but are the
instruments with which nature snatches up air'. Diocles positively modifies the
doctrine of the cognitive primacy of the heart, however, by suggesting that the
right half of the brain provides sensation and the left intelligence, even though
the heart remains the centre which hears and understands.
[105] Wellmann, 1901: fragments 55, 59, 79, and p. 90.

Herophilus' teacher, Praxagoras of Cos, seems to have been the first to make a general, explicit distinction between arteries and veins and to ascribe different functions to them.[106] (It has been argued that Praxagoras claimed that the arteries contained only pneuma, not blood. This is a subject of some controversy, but the view that the arteries carry only pneuma – to whomever it might owe its origin – became very influential and may have inhibited the discovery of the circulation of the blood.[107]) Before Praxagoras, it was especially the aorta and the vena cava that had been distinguished.[108] In a notable occurrence of this distinction – in the Hippocratic treatise *On Fleshes* (*De Carnibus*) – one reads, for example: 'For there are two bloodvessels (*phlebes*) [proceeding] from the heart, the name of one being *artery (artēriē)*, of the other *hollow vein (koilē phlebs)*' – a passage which is especially striking because of its use of the word *artēria*, which was reserved until the time of Aristotle (and in popular usage until late antiquity) as the term for 'windpipe' or 'bronchial tube', not for 'artery'.[109] But it is not until Praxagoras that this distinction is

[106] Steckerl, 1958: fragments 7 ('hollow vein'), 8 ('thick artery'), 9 (arteries), 11 (heart, arteries), 13b ('Cotelydons are the apertures of the *veins and arteries* which lead into the womb'), 26–31 (sphygmology: pulsation as an independent function of the arteries). Some scholars have argued that the distinction between veins and arteries was made much earlier, notably by Euryphon of Cnidus (Wellmann, 1901: 96; Fredrich, 1899: 68). But their only evidence is a text which seems inconclusive inasmuch as it also attributes this distinction to 'Hippocrates', who at best distinguished only vena cava and aorta without recognizing a general distinction between veins and arteries: Caelius Aurelianus, *Tardae passiones* 2.10: 'Differentias etiam fluoris sanguinis veteres quaesierunt. et quidam aiunt unam solam esse vel intelligi, hoc est, vulnerationis, ut Themison libro *Tardarum passionum*. alii vero eruptiones, ut Hippocrates, Euryphon. sed Hippocrates solarum venarum, Euryphon vero etiam arteriarum.'

[107] Steckerl, 1958: fr. 31, 84–5.

[108] For example, by Aristotle (who was probably an older contemporary of Praxagoras'; cf. Chapter II.A.2, with n. 20), perhaps by Diogenes of Apollonia (see n. 91), by Diocles (n. 105), and by the authors of several Hippocratic treatises (which, however, mostly belong to a period after Praxagoras; see below).

[109] *Artēria* is used of the windpipe or bronchial tubes, for example by Plato, *Timaeus* 70d2 and 78c4–5; Aristotle, *Historia animalium* 1.12.493a8; Sophocles, *Trachiniae* 1054; Hippocrates, *Epidemics* 7.12 and 25 (v, pp. 388, 394L). For *artēria* as 'artery' and 'aorta' in other Hippocratic treatises, see below. In the pseudo-Aristotelian treatise *De spiritu* the word *artēria* seems to be used indiscriminately of the windpipe (481a22, 481b13) and of the arteries, which are conceived of as air ducts (484a1); cf. also 484a14. In the Hippocratic work *On the Nature of Bones* 10 (IX, p. 180L), which is identical with *Epidemics* 2.4.1 (v, p. 124), some of the

extended to include a clear recognition of two vascular systems: an arterial–pneumatic and a venous–haematic. The fragmentary remnants of his teachings do not, however, provide any more detailed descriptions of the anatomy of the heart and the bloodvessels (and the relative wealth of pathophysiologic details about the heart and the vessels in his fragments need not concern us here).[110]

If little mention has been made of the Hippocratic Corpus so far, it is because the earlier Hippocratic treatises contain motley and not alwys consistent information on the anatomy of the heart and the bloodvessels, while the more advanced discussions and distinctions almost all occur in Hippocratic treatises which either post-date Herophilus or are of uncertain, but probably late date. The pseudo-Hippocratic essay *On Nutriment*, for example, does distinguish between veins and arteries and recognizes the heart as the centre of the vascular system but, as was pointed out in Chapter III.A.2, it postdates Herophilus, perhaps by as much as two to four centuries.[111] Similarly, the Hippocratic treatise *On the Heart* admittedly provides a detailed and, in part, quite accurate anatomical description of the heart, its auricles, its ventricles, and its valves, but inasmuch as it almost certainly presupposes the careful description of the heart valves by Herophilus' contemporary Erasistratus, it cannot be numbered among Herophilus' predecessors.[112] In another work of

ambiguities of *artēria* are given striking expression when the author uses them of yet another kind of duct, the ureters: 'And *artēriai* [sc. the ureters] grow out from it [the kidney], from here and from there, in the manner of an *artēria* [sc. artery].' Earlier and later in the same passage, *artēria* is used without qualification of the aorta. But cf. Duminil, 1983: 36.

[110] Steckerl, 1958: fragments 50, 62, 65, 69–72, 74–5, 77–9, 84–5, 96; cf. 98.

[111] On the date of *On Nutriment*, cf. Diller, 1936a; Deichgräber, 1973; Kudlien, 1962: 421–2; Duminil, 1983: 54 ('perhaps as early as Praxagoras').

[112] Abel, 1958, in one of the more plausible analyses, argues for a post-Erasistratean date for *On the Heart*. E. Littré (Hp. I, pp. 382–3L) suggested a post-Aristotelian date. Fredrich (1899: 77, 171, 196) in turn dates it to the early fourth century, to what he designates the time of Diocles of Carystus (on whose date see Chapter II above), while Wellmann (1901: 94–107), Hurlbutt (1939), and J. Bidez and G. Leboucq (1944) regard it as belonging to the Sicilian school of Philistion of Locri (fourth century B.C.). Kudlien, 1962: 425–7, argues that it might have been influenced by Posidonius and was written by a member of the Pneumatic school of medicine. Cf. also Lonie, 1973; Unger, 1923, especially 81–94. The accurate knowledge displayed by the author of *On the Heart* of the heart valves seems to point decisively to a period after Erasistratus' celebrated description of the valves, even though the author's failure to accommodate a clear distinction between veins and arteries remains problematic.

the Hippocratic Corpus, *On Joints*, veins (*phlebes*) and arteries (*artēriai*) are twice distinguished from one another,[113] but the date of this work is again uncertain; some modern scholars have even suggested that it was written 'not earlier than Praxagoras'.[114]

Of even less certain date is the longest continuous account of the vascular system in the Hippocratic Corpus, Chapters 2–19 of *On the Nature of Bones* (which, as Galen seems to imply, originally had the more apt title *On Bloodvessels*.)[115] This treatise is an unsystematic, chaotic compilation which includes two passages taken from other Hippocratic works and one from Aristotle. Furthermore, its parts are not all of the same date: Chapter 8 is culled from Aristotle's *Historia animalium*, Book III; Chapter 9 from the relatively early Hippocratic treatise *On the Nature of Man* (probably late fifth century B.C.); Chapter 10 from *Epidemics* II (perhaps the later fourth century B.C.); Chapter 5, in which (as perhaps in Chapter 7) veins and arteries are distinguished, apparently 'cannot . . . be earlier than Praxagoras, and might, of course, be much later';[116] Chapters 6 and 12–19 by contrast offer descriptions of the vascular system which resemble that of the Presocratic philosopher Diogenes of Apollonia (see above) and make no distinction between arteries and veins. But not only does one have to cope with several chronological layers and sources; many of the descriptions are also vague and confused, and the central terms are frequently ambiguous. This treatise accordingly provides a good measure of some of the often insurmountable difficulties confronting the critic who wants to use the Hippocratic Corpus as a standard by which to judge Herophilus' progress.

Two further Hippocratic works of disputed date, *On Diseases* IV and a fragment *On Anatomy*, deserve mention. One states unambiguously

---

[113] *On Joints* 45 and 69 (IV, pp. 190, 286L = II, pp. 171–2, 223 Kuehlewein). But neither passage is entirely unambiguous: *phlebes* could refer to the vascular system, *artēriai* to the tracheal (or to all other 'ducts'). On uses of *artēria* in the Hippocratic Corpus cf. n. 109 above; Duminil, 1983:23–6, 32–45, 50–4, 128f.

[114] Harris, 1973: 53. But Harris contradicts himself, saying on p. 98 that it 'can be placed, with a more than fair degree of probability, in the earliest years of the fourth century B.C.'; Praxagoras' floruit, as I suggested in Chapter II.A, by contrast cannot be placed earlier than the last half or last third of the fourth century B.C.

[115] Hp. IX, pp. 168–96L. Cf. also notes 71, 93, and 109 above. Galen, *Explanatio vocum Hippocratis*, s.v. *parastatas* (XIX, p. 128K): 'in his work *On Bloodvessels*, which precedes *The Reduction of Limbs*'.

[116] Harris, 1973: 57.

that the heart is the source or fount (*pēgē*) of the blood vessels,[117] and
the other seems to distinguish between veins and at least one 'duct':
'From the heart a wide duct (*bronchiē*)[118] goes down into the liver, and
along with the duct a vein (*phlebs*) called 'large', through which the
whole body is nourished.' But, as C. R. S. Harris and others have
suggested, *On Anatomy* belongs to 'a date certainly after Praxagoras',[119] and therefore cannot with certainty be counted among
Herophilus' predecessors. While *On Diseases* IV seems to belong to c.
420–400 B.C. (see Lonie, 1981 : 71), it offers primarily pathophysiological rather than anatomical observations about the vascular system.

Even when one turns to those Hippocratic treatises which can with
reasonable confidence be said to predate Praxagoras and Herophilus,
no uniform theory about the vascular system emerges. Thus, the
author of *On Fleshes* states correctly in an otherwise bizarre and quasi-
philosophical account that the heart is the central source of the blood
vessels, all vessels running into the artery and the hollow vein (vena
cava), both of which proceed from the heart.[120] By contrast, the
author of *On the Nature of Humans* (Polybus?[121]) suggests that the four
major pairs of bloodvessels emanate from the head, and fails even to
mention the heart.[122] He does introduce the interesting notion of
intercommunicating blood-vessels, and this has been used by some
historians to support the erroneous view that 'Hippocrates' was
acquainted with the circulation of the blood. But the passage in
question merely says: 'There are many bloodvessels running from the
belly . . . through which nourishment passes to the body. And they
proceed from the thick vessels . . . and communicate with each other,
those going from the inside outwards and those going from the outside

[117] Cf. *On Diseases* 4.33, cf. 38–40 (VII, pp. 544, 554–62L).
[118] *On Anatomy* (VIII, p. 538L). The author apparently uses *bronchiē* (a *hapax legomenon*;
τὰ βρόγχια is normal usage) since he has already used *artēria* for the windpipe in
the opening sentence of this fragment. Both the use of *bronchiē* and the emphasis
on veins as the vehicles of nutriment seem to suggest that the artery is viewed as
an air-duct, in keeping with the views of, for example, Praxagoras and
Erasistratus, and that this fragment might therefore post-date them.
[119] Harris, 1973: 83; see previous note and Grensemann's caveat, 1968a: 62.
[120] *On Fleshes* 5–6 (VIII, pp. 590–4L). 'Veins' or 'vessels' (*phlebes*) is used of veins and
arteries (other than the aorta) indiscriminately. Among others Rüsche, 1930:
169, Wellmann, 1901: 90, and Harris, 1973: 79, agree that this treatise predates
Diocles of Carystus. Cf. also Deichgräber, 1935: 39–41.
[121] The authorship is disputed. See above, ch. II, n. 46.
[122] *On the Nature of Humans* II (VI, pp. 58–60L) = *On the Nature of Bones* 9 (IX, pp. 174–
8L); cf. Aristotle, *Historia animalium* 3.3.512b8–513a7.

inwards.' Neither capillaries nor circulation seem to be known to the author.

A greater approximation of the truth is achieved by another Hippocratic author who mentions an intercommunication of blood-vessels, the author of *On Places in Humans*. He, too, describes the vascular system in terms of pairs of vessels which proceed from the head, and then adds: 'All the vessels communicate with and run into one another, some of them running into their own branches, and others through the little branch veins that fan out from them and give nourishment to the tissues. In this way they flow into one another.'[123] Though correctly recognizing the free communication of veins with one another, and perhaps even identifying the capillaries, this author (probably writing no later than the mid-fourth century B.C.) still clung to the head as the main source of the vascular system. A similar view is put forward in another pre-Herophilean treatise of the Hippocratic Corpus, *On the Sacred Disease*, whose author maintains that the brain is the centre of the vascular system, and does not seem to distinguish between the tracheal and vascular systems.[124]

This rapid survey of the treatment of the anatomy of the vascular system by some of the more significant pre-Alexandrian biologists and physicians should provide a useful yardstick for assessing Herophilus' contribution, even though the task is enormously complicated by the fragmentary and perfunctory nature of the extant evidence concerning his vascular anatomy.

Although Herophilus – in keeping with the caution advocated in his theory of scientific method (see Chapter v) – said that he did not know what to choose as the starting-point for a description of the vascular system (T115), his discoveries concerning the bloodvessels and the heart were of considerable significance.

At least from the time of Herophilus' teacher Praxagoras vessels emerging from the right ventricle of the heart were called veins (*phlebes*), while those emerging from the left were called arteries (*artēriai*) by authors who accepted the distinction between veins and arteries. Herophilus apparently adhered to this general distinction,

---

[123]   *On Places in Humans* 3 (vi, p. 282L).
[124]   Cf., for example, *On the Sacred Disease* 3, 6 and 10 (pp. 68, 70–2, 76–8 Grensemann). See Duminil, 1983: 83–6.

but he was the first to try to rescue the pulmonary artery – which emerges from the right ventricle – from a mere venous status by calling it 'artery-like vein' (cf. T117, T118 with *Comments*). Furthermore, he established once and for all an *anatomical*, and not only a functional, distinction between veins and arteries: he was the first to observe that the coats of the arteries are thicker than those of the veins (six times as thick, according to T116 and T118).

Herophilus' description of the heart has not survived, but Galen implies that Herophilus had at least some acquaintance with the heart valves (T119–T120), although he apparently did not describe them either as accurately as Erasistratus (T119) or in a manner which Asclepiades, at least, found identifiable with Erasistratus' (T54).[125] Unlike both Erasistratus and Galen, but perhaps like Diocles of Carystus, Herophilus mistakenly regarded the auricles as part of the interior of the heart (T120), and not just as the terminal chambers or processes of the two main veins – i.e. of the vena cava issuing into the right atrium and of the pulmonary vein into the left – through which the blood is then forced into the true interior of the heart: into the right and left ventricles.

Not only the heart, the auricles, the cardiac valves, and the pulmonary vessels were discussed by Herophilus; he also described the subclavian vein, other thoracic vessels (T62), the carotid arteries (which supply blood to the head), as well as various vessels of the head (T121–T125), of the abdominal cavity (T126–T127), and of the reproductive organs (T114). Thus he describes the broad ligaments ('the vessels which nourish the uterus . . . are clothed in membranes . . .', T114) and ovarian vessels (T61), mentioning both an arterial and a venous connection between the uterus and the ovary (T61), i.e. presumably the branch of the ovarian artery which connects with the uterine artery and the communication between the uterine plexus and the ovarian veins. These descriptions of the blood vessels of the female reproductive organs 'must', as one recent

---

[125] Galen's remark (T119) that Herophilus wrote about the heart valves 'in a careless way' has sometimes been misunderstood to mean that Herophilus had no knowledge of the valves. But Galen clearly states that both Herophilus and Erasistratus described the valves – the former carelessly, the latter accurately. More problematic is Asclepiades' claim (T54) that Herophilus 'did not see' the valves ('membranes attached to the heart'). For a discussion of these texts, see *Comments*, T54 (Chapter v) and T119.

historian remarked, 'win our undeserved admiration, especially when we consider the state of knowledge before [Herophilus]'.[126]

Herophilus' description of a *rete mirabile* – the comparison with a net seems to have originated with him – of blood vessels formed at the base of the brain from the internal carotid arteries (T121) received wide acclaim and acceptance in antiquity. It seems to suggest, however, that for all the advances Herophilus made on the basis of *human* dissection, he still relied in part on the dissection of animals. This description cannot readily be reconciled with human anatomy, whereas it is consonant with that of artiodactyls such as the ox, the pig, the sheep, or the goat.[127] 'Ox-brains totally prepared', Galen later observed, '. . . are on sale in the large cities',[128] and though circumstances might not have been quite as propitious in early Hellenistic times, Erasistratus' experiments with goats and oxen (n. 3) and the experiments with a pig by the author of *On the Heart* suggest that artiodactyls were indeed regularly used for medical research in the earlier Hellenistic period.[129]

On the other hand, Herophilus' descriptions of other parts of the vascular system of the head, such as the *torcular Herophili* (T122, T123) and the choroid plexuses (T124, T125), seem compatible with human anatomy.[130] The *torcular*, as pointed out above, is the confluence of the four great cranial venous sinuses (though Herophilus apparently identified only the two transverse or lateral sinuses), i.e. the broad

---

[126] Potter, 1976: 55.

[127] Cf. the anatomist Woollam, 1958: 12: 'The description which he gives of a rete mirabile of blood vessels . . . shows that, at least as far as the brain was concerned, Herophilus was more familiar with the anatomy of artiodactyla than with that of man.' Cf. Le Gros Clark, in Woollam, 1958: 18: 'the rete mirabile which is so characteristic a feature of the base of the ungulate brain'. (The artiodactyl order belongs to the ungulates – i.e. hoofed animals such as horses, cattle, swine, deer.) See also Harris, 1973: 356–8 on various implausible attempts to reconcile Galen's description of the retiform with the anatomy of the human brain; and Sisson & Grossman, 1948: 626, on the rete mirabile in the ox. Cf. Galen, *De placitis Hippocratis et Platonis* 7.3 (*CMG* v.4.1.2, p. 444 De Lacy); id., *De usu partium* 9.4 (II, pp. 1off. Helmreich). Galen seems to have assumed that Herophilus' description of the rete mirabile referred to the human brain, perhaps because of Herophilus' fame as a dissector of humans.

[128] Galen, *On Anatomical Procedures* 9.1 (II, p. 708K).

[129] Already in the fourth century Aristotle had made frequent anatomical and physiological references to oxen, horses, goats, pigs, and other artiodactyls. Cf., for example, *Historia animalium* 2.15.506a8–10, 2.1.499b6–17, and *De partibus animalium* 3.4.666b18–21.

[130] Cf. above, pp. 158–9.

channels which conduct blood from the brain and whose outer coat is formed by the dura mater. To this day the name Herophilus gave it, 'wine vat' or 'wine press', has survived in anatomical nomenclature, albeit in its Latin translation, *torcular*.

The choroid plexuses to which Herophilus refers, and which he was the first to describe, are highly vascular portions of the pia mater that project into the ventricles of the brain (T124). Again, the name Herophilus introduced has endured: 'choroid' because of their resemblance to the foetal membrane, known since Greek antiquity as the *chorion*; 'plexus' or 'something twisted up together' (*systremma*) [131] because they are twisted networks of interlacing or anastomosing vessels. Herophilus not only correctly recognized the vascular nature of these plexuses, saying that they are 'plexuses of veins and arteries held together by thin membranes' (T124) but, Galen seems to imply, also their projection into the ventricles.

Together, these testimonies suggest that Herophilus maintained a high anatomical standard, not only in his anatomy of the nerves, the brain, and the reproductive organs, but also in his exploration of the vessels of the head.

Although Galen in T126 says only that Herophilus 'also wrote about the anatomy of the veins', without specifying the vessels of the abdominal cavity, the context seems to suggest that the abdominal vessels are meant, because in an immediately preceding statement Galen implied that Herophilus gained his knowledge of the *abdominal* cavity by means of dissection. Confirmation of Herophilus' exploration of this part of the vascular system is provided not only by his long fragment on the liver (Fr6o), but also by Galen's perhaps self-serving, perfunctory implication that Herophilus' discussion of the vascular system started with the liver (T115) and by the report that, in Herophilus' view, 'the veins of the mesentery' terminate in the lymphatic glands of the mesentery (T127). The 'veins' to which he refers here would seem to be the lymphatic vessels of the mesentery rather than bloodvessels, but even if Herophilus mistook lymphatic

---

[131] *Systremma* in this use (plexus) is rare, *plegma* (or its plural, *plegmata*) being the more common term. See, for example, Galen's description of the choroid plexus in *De placitis Hippocratis et Platonis* 7.3 (see n. 127). Herophilus had used *plegma* (with the adjective *diktyoeides*, 'net-like') for the rete ('net') mirabile (T121), and therefore perhaps, with his characteristic proclivity for nomenclatural inventiveness, resorted to *systremma* for the choroid plexus. On *chorion* see Kudlien, 1964d. Cf. also 'chorioid', T87–T88.

vessels for veins, this passage indicates an interest in the vessels of the abdominal cavity. Furthermore, the last sentence in the same testimonium ('all other veins proceed upward to the portae' or the transverse fissure on the underside of the liver, T127) points to the first recognition of the function of the hepatic portal vein as the receiving mechanism for all absorptive veins in the intestines, if in fact it represents a view attributable to Herophilus (as Galen seems to imply). One scholar, commenting on Herophilus' discovery of the significance of the hepatic portal system, observed with good reason: 'With [this] discovery . . . Herophilus steered research on the function of the liver on to entirely new courses. Henceforth the views people held on the processes of absorption formed the pivot on which their notions concerning the function of the liver turned. *All subsequent depictions of the physiology of liver started from this basis.*'[132] Galen's remarks on Herophilus' view that in some women 'four . . . vessels branch off from those that go to the kidneys, and enter the uterus' (Fr114) as well as numerous general references to Herophilus made by ancient authors in the context of vascular anatomy (e.g. T69, T70, T128), likewise seem to confirm that his interest in the anatomy of the veins and arteries was comprehensive and not confined to the parts represented more prominently in the fragmentary remains.

Sparse and problematic though the extant remnants of Herophilus' anatomy are, on balance the conclusion that it represents a radical and comprehensive advance on previous anatomy seems reasonable. The careful anatomy of the brain, the distinction of the ventricles of the brain, the discovery of the nerves, the description of the coats of the eye, the classic description of the liver, the identification of duodenum and the investigation of glands, the careful differentiation between various parts of the spermatic duct, the discovery of the ovaries and of at least part of the Fallopian tubes, the first general anatomical distinction of arteries from veins, the discovery and naming of vascular structures such as the *torcular Herophili* and the choroid plexuses – all of this adds up to a remarkable achievement which, had Herophilus' works survived, might long since have allowed Falloppia's perceptive designation of Herophilus as 'the Vesalius of antiquity' to become more entrenched than it is.

[132] Mani, 1959–67: pt I, pp. 46–7 (my translation and italics).

B · TEXTS

1 Fragments ascribed to Herophilus' 'On Anatomy' II–IV

60a Galenus, *De anatomicis administrationibus* 6.8 (II, pp. 570–2K)

60b Oribasius, *Collectiones medicae* 24.25.1–6 (*CMG* VI.2.1 = vol. III, pp. 36–7 Raeder) (Excerpted from Galen)

οὐ μὴν οὐδ' αὐτοῖς τοῖς ἀνθρώποις ὁμοίως ἅπασιν ἔχει κατά τε μέγεθος καὶ πλῆθος λοβῶν (sc. τοῦ ἥπατος). ἀκριβέστατα γοῦν ὑπὲρ αὐτοῦ γράφων Ἡρόφιλος αὐτοῖς ὀνόμασι τάδε φησίν· "ἔστι δ' εὐμέγεθες τὸ τοῦ ἀνθρώπου ἧπαρ, καὶ μεῖζον τοῦ ἔν τισιν
5 ἑτέροις ζῴοις ἰσοπαλέσιν ἀνθρώπῳ. καὶ καθ' ὃ μὲν ταῖς φρεσὶ προσψαύει, κεκύρτωται καὶ λεῖόν ἐστι· καθ' ὃ δὲ τῇ κοιλίᾳ καὶ τῷ κυρτῷ τῆς κοιλίας προσψαύει, ἔνσιμον καὶ ἀνώμαλον. ἀφωμοίωται δὲ κατὰ τοῦτο διασφάγι τινί, καθ' ὃ καὶ τοῖς ἐμβρύοις ἡ ἐκ τοῦ ὀμφαλοῦ φλὲψ εἰς αὐτὸ ἐμπέφυκεν.
10 "οὐχ ὅμοιον δ' ἐστὶν ἐν ἅπασιν, ἀλλὰ καὶ πλάτει καὶ μήκει καὶ πάχει καὶ ὕψει καὶ λοβῶν πλήθει καὶ ἀνωμαλίᾳ τῇ ἐκ τοῦ ἔμπροσθεν, καθ' ὃ παχύτατόν ἐστι, καὶ τοῖς ἄκροις τοῖς κύκλῳ κατὰ τὴν λεπτότητα, ἄλλοις ἀλλοῖον. λοβοὺς γάρ τισι μὲν οὐδ' ἔχει, ἀλλ' ἔστιν ὅλον στρογγύλον καὶ ἄναρθρον, τοῖς δὲ δύο, τοῖς
15 δὲ καὶ πλείους, καὶ πολλοῖς καὶ τέσσαρας ἔχει."
τοῦτ' οὖν ὀρθῶς εἶπεν ὁ Ἡρόφιλος, ἔτι τε καὶ πρὸς τούτοις, ὀλίγων μὲν ἐπ' ἀνθρώπων, οὐκ ὀλίγων δ' ἐπ' ἄλλων ζῴων ἐπιλαμβάνειν αὐτό τι τῶν ἀριστερῶν μερῶν ἀληθῶς ἔγραψεν ἐν τῷ αὐτῷ βιβλίῳ τῷ δευτέρῳ τῷ ἀνατομικῶν, αὐτὸς μὲν μόνου
20 τοῦ λαγωοῦ μνημονεύσας, ἡμῖν δὲ καταλιπὼν ἐπισκέψασθαι καὶ περὶ τῶν ἄλλων ζῴων, ὑπὲρ ὧν ἐπὶ τῇ προηκούσῃ πραγματείᾳ διελθεῖν ἔγνωκα· . . . οὐκ ὀλίγων ἀναγκάζομαι διαφορῶν διαμνημονεύειν, ὥσπερ ἀμέλει καὶ νῦν ἐπὶ τοῦ ἥπατος, οὗ πλείστη μὲν ἐπὶ τοῖς δεξιοῖς ἐστι μοῖρα κατὰ πάντα τὰ ζῷα, προσεπιλαμβά-
25 νει δέ τι καὶ τῶν ἀριστερῶν οὐκ ἴσον ἐν ἅπασιν, ἀλλ', ὥσπερ ὁ μὲν Ἡρόφιλος ἔγραψεν, ἐπὶ λαγωοῦ πλεῖστον . . .

1–2 οὐχ ἅπασιν ἀνθρώποις ὁμοίως ἔχει τὸ ἧπαρ κατά τε μέγεθος *Oribasius*　　4 μεῖζον *Oribasius*: μέγα *Kühn*　　5 ἐντέροις *Oribasii P*
5 ἀνθρώποις *Orib.*　　6 κεκύρτωται *Orib.*: κύρτωται *Kühn*　　6–7 καὶ τῷ κυρτῷ τῆς κοιλίας om. *Orib. fort. recte*　　7 προσψαύσειε σιμὸν *Kühn*

ἀφομοιοῦται *Kühn* 8 διασφαγῇ *Orib.* ἡ *ante* φλέψ *transp.*
Orib. 11 τῇ *Kühn:* τοῦ *Orib.* 12 *post* ἔμπροσθεν *add.* καὶ ὄγκῳ τοῦ ἐκ
τοῦ ἔμπροσθεν *Orib.* 13 λόγους *Orib.* P 14 ἄναρθρον *Singer:*
ἀνορθον *Orib., Kühn* 15 καὶ πολλοῖς *Kühn:* πολλοῖς δὲ *Orib.*
16 ταῦτά τε οὖν *Orib.* ὁ *om. Orib.* καὶ *om. Orib.* 17 ὀλίγον *Orib.*
utroque loco δ' ἐπ' ἄλλων *Gal.:* δὲ πολλῶν *Orib.* P ζῷον *Orib.*
P 18 τι *om. Orib.* 18–19 ἐν τῷ αὐτῷ βιβλίῳ *Singer u.v.:* ἐν αὐτῷ
τούτῳ τῷ βιβλίῳ *Kühn:* ἐν τῷ αὐτῷ *sqq. om. Orib.* qui habet τοῦτο τὸ
σπλάγχνον εἰς τὸ σιμότατον ἑαυτοῦ μέρος ἀνηκούσας ἔχει τὰς ἐκ τοῦ
μεσεντερίου φλέβας (*excerptum e Galeni De anat. admin. 6.11* (II, *p. 575*K))

60a–b Not even in human beings is the liver similar in all with
respect to its size and the number of its lobes. Herophilus writes very
accurately about it, saying the following, in so many words: 'The liver
of humans is of a good size, larger than in certain other animals which
match humans [sc. in size]. And where it touches against the
diaphragm, it is convex and smooth, but where it touches against the
abdominal cavity and against its lump, it is concave and uneven.
Here it may be likened to a certain fissure by which in embryos, too,
the vein from the navel naturally extends into it.

'The liver is not similar in all, but different in different creatures, in
breadth, length, thickness, height, number of lobes, and in the
irregularity both at the front – where it is thickest – and at the
circular parts at the top, where it is thin. In some, it does not even
have lobes, but is completely round and unarticulated, whereas in
others it has two lobes, in still others more, and in many also four
lobes.'

This Herophilus said correctly. Furthermore, in the same Book II of
his *Anatomica* he wrote correctly that in the case of [only] a few human
beings but not a few other animals, the liver occupies some of the left
parts. But he mentioned only the hare, and left it to us to examine the
other animals as well, the details about which I have determined to go
through as my treatise proceeds ... I am compelled to make mention
of not a few differences [between various animals], as, to be sure, now
too in the case of the liver: its largest part is on the right in all animals,
but in addition it occupies some of the left, though not equally in all
creatures but, as Herophilus wrote, most of all in the case of a hare.

61 Galenus, *De semine* 2.1 (IV, pp. 596–8K)

Ἡρόφιλος δὲ οὐκ οἶδ' ὅπως ἐκτὸς ἐκχεῖσθαί φησι τὸ τῶν θηλειῶν

σπέρμα, καίτοι γε περὶ τῶν ὄρχεων ἀκριβῶς ἔγραψε τῶν κατ᾽
αὐτὰς ἐν τῷ τρίτῳ τῆς ἀνατομῆς, ἐν ἀρχῇ μὲν ὧδέ πως εἰπών·
"ἐπιπεφύκασι δὲ τῇ μήτρᾳ καὶ δίδυμοι ἐκ τῶν πλαγίων, ἐξ
5 ἑκατέρου μέρους, ἐπ᾽ ὀλίγον διαφέροντες τῶν τοῦ ἄρρενος."
ἔπειτα ἐν τοῖς ἐφεξῆς οὐ μετὰ πάνυ πολλὰ κατὰ τήνδε τὴν ῥῆσιν·
"δίδυμοι δὲ ταῖς θηλείαις ἐπιπεφύκασι πρὸς ἑκατέρῳ τῷ ὤμῳ
τῆς μήτρας, ὁ μὲν ἐκ τοῦ δεξιοῦ, ὁ δὲ ἐκ τοῦ εὐωνύμου, οὐκ ἐν ἑνὶ
ὀσχέῳ ἀμφότεροι, ἀλλ᾽ ἑκάτεροι χωρίς, λεπτῷ τινι καὶ ὑμενοειδεῖ
10 ὑμένι περιεχόμενοι, μικροὶ καὶ ὑποπλατεῖς, ἀδέσιν ὅμοιοι, κατὰ
μὲν τὸν ἐν κύκλῳ χιτῶνα νευρώδεις, τῇ δὲ σαρκὶ εὔθρυπτοι,
ὥσπερ καὶ οἱ τῶν ἀρρένων, ταῖς δὲ ἵπποις καὶ πάνυ εἰσὶν
εὐμεγέθεις. προσπεφύκασι δὲ ὑμέσι τε οὐκ ὀλίγοις πρὸς τὴν
μήτραν καὶ φλεβὶ καὶ ἀρτηρίᾳ, τῇ ἀπὸ τῆς μήτρας εἰς αὐτοὺς
15 ἐμπεφυκυίᾳ. ἀπὸ γὰρ τῆς φλεβὸς καὶ τῆς ἀρτηρίας τῆς εἰς
ἑκάτερον τῶν διδύμων προσπέφυκε, φλὲψ μὲν ἀπὸ τῆς φλεβός,
ἀρτηρία δὲ ἀπὸ τῆς ἀρτηρίας.
"ὁ δὲ σπερματικὸς πόρος ἀφ᾽ ἑκατέρου οὐ λίαν μὲν φαίνεται,
προσφυὴς δέ ἐστι τῇ μήτρᾳ ἐκ τοῦ ἐκτὸς μέρους, ὁ μὲν ἐκ τοῦ
20 δεξιοῦ, ὁ δὲ ἐκ τοῦ εὐωνύμου. εἵλικταί τε παραπλησίως τῷ τοῦ
ἄρρενος κατὰ τὸ πρόσθεν αὐτοῦ μέρος, καὶ τὸ λοιπὸν κιρσοειδὲς
σχεδὸν ἅπαν ἄχρι τοῦ πέρατος. καὶ ἐμπέφυκεν ἀφ᾽ ἑκατέρου τοῦ
διδύμου ὁμοίως, ὥσπερ τῷ ἄρρενι, εἰς τὸ σαρκῶδες τοῦ αὐχένος
τῆς κύστεως, λεπτός τε ὢν καὶ σκολιὸς ἐν τῷ ἐμπροσθίῳ μέρει
25 καθ᾽ ὃ τὰ τῶν ἰσχίων ὀστᾶ ψαύει, ἐν ᾧπερ καὶ ἀπολήγει, ὡς τὸ
αἰδοῖον ἐξ ἑκατέρου τοῦ μέρους εἰς τὸ ἐντὸς διαπεφυκώς.
παραστάτης δὲ ὁ κιρσοειδὴς οὐχ ἑώραται ἐν τῷ θήλει."
αὕτη μὲν ἡ τοῦ Ἡροφίλου ῥῆσις. ὃ δέ μοι θαυμάζειν παρίστα-
ται μάλιστα, καὶ δὴ φράσω· καὶ θέσιν καὶ μέγεθος καὶ φύσιν
30 ἀκριβῶς γράψας τῶν ἐν τοῖς θήλεσι ζῴοις ὄρχεων, οὐ παρα-
λιπὼν δὲ οὐδὲ περὶ τῆς ἐμβαλλούσης ἑκατέρωθεν φλεβὸς καὶ
ἀρτηρίας οὐδέν, ἀλλ᾽ ἀκριβώσας τὴν διήγησιν, εἶτα ἑξῆς ὑπὲρ
τοῦ σπερματικοῦ πόρου τὸ μὲν ὅτι προσφυής ἐστι ταῖς μήτραις
ἔξωθεν, εἷς ἑκατέρωθεν, ἀληθῶς εἰπών, τὸ δ᾽ ὅτι μὴ λίαν φαίνεται
35 ψευσάμενος (ἀξιόλογον γάρ ἐστι τὸ μέγεθος), ἑξῆς τούτου
πολὺ μεῖζον ἐψεύσατο φάμενος εἰς τὸν αὐχένα τῆς κύστεως
ἐμφύεσθαι τῷ τοῦ ἄρρενος ὁμοίως.

---

2 περὶ *Ald*: πως *P*   2–3 τῶν κατ᾽ αὐτὰς *P*: τῆς κατ᾽ αὐτοὺς *Ald*
5 ὀλίγον *P*: ὀλίγων *Ald*   6 τήνδε τὴν *Ald*: τὴν δ *P*   7 ἑκατέρῳ τῷ

ὤμῳ Ald: ἑκατέρων τῶν ὤμων P   9 ὀσχέῳ Ald: χωρίῳ P   ἑκάτεροι
Ald: ἑκάτερος P   10 περιεχόμενοι Ald: περιεχόμενος P   ὑποπλατεῖς
Ald: ὑπὸ πλαταῖς P   11 ἐν κύκλῳ Ald: κύκλον P   νευρώδεις Ald:
νευρώδη Pˣ (ν- ex λ-?)   εὔθρυπτοι P: ἄθρυπτοι Ald   13 τε P: om.
Ald   ὀλίγοις P: ὀλίγους Ald   15 ἐμπεφυκυίᾳ Charterius: ἐμπεφυκεῖα
P(u.v.): ἐπεφυκίας Ald Bas   16 ἑκάτερον Ald: ἕκαστον P
18 ἀφ' P: ἐφ' Ald.   20 δεξιοῦ ... εὐωνύμῳ Ald: εὐωνύμου ... δεξιοῦ P
εἵλικται Ald Bas: corr. Charterius: ἥλεκται P   τε Ald: δὲ P   τῷ Ald: τὸ
P   21 κατὰ P: καὶ Ald   πρόσθεν Ald: πρὸς P   κιρσοειδὲς Ald:
κυρσοειδὲς P   22 σχεδὸν ἅπαν Ald: ἅπαν σχεδὸν P   22 πέρατος Ald:
σπέρματος P   ἐμπέφυκεν Ald: ἐκπέφυκεν P (-εν e corr.)   23 τῷ ἄρρενι
Ald: τὸ ἄρρεν P   25 καθ' ὃ Ald: καθ' ἣν P   ἰσχίων Ald: ἰσχύων
P   ψαύει Ald: συμψαβει P (voluitne συμψαύει?)   26 διαπεφυκός Ald:
διαπέφυκε P   27 κιρσοειδὴς Ald: κυρσοειδὴς P   31 ἑκατέρωθεν Ald:
ἑκατέρου P   33 ὅτι Ald: ὅταν P   34 εἰς De Lacy (unus Nicolaus): εἷς
P Ald Bas   36 μεῖζον P: μᾶλλον Ald.   37 τῷ Ald: τὸ P

61 Herophilus, however, says that the seed of females is somehow discharged to the outside, even though he wrote with accuracy about the 'testicles' [ovaries] in females in Book III of his *Anatomy*, saying this at the outset:

'Two "testicles" (*didymoi* [ovaries]) are also attached to the uterus on the sides, one on either part, and they differ only a little from the testicles of the male.' Then in what follows, not much later, these are his words:

'In females the two "testicles" [ovaries] are attached to each of the two shoulders of the uterus, one on the right, the other on the left, not both in a single scrotum but each of the two separate, enclosed in a thin, membranous skin. They are small and rather flat, like glands, sinewy at their surrounding covering but easily damageable in their flesh, just like the testicles of males. In mares they are also quite sizable. And they are attached to the uterus with no small number of membranes and with a vein and an artery implanted from the uterus into these "testicles". You see, the attachment is from the vein and the artery that go to each of the two "testicles", a vein from the vein and an artery from the artery.

'The spermatic duct from each "testicle" is not very apparent, but it is attached to the uterus from the outside, one duct from the right, the other from the left. Like the seminal duct of the male, its anterior part is also convoluted, and almost all the rest up to its end looks varicose. And the spermatic duct from each testicle grows into the fleshy part of the neck of the bladder, just like the male duct, being thin and winding in its anterior part where it touches the hip-bones. Here [sc. at the neck of the bladder] it also terminates, like the pudendum penetrating to the interior from either side. But the "varix-like assistant" (*parastatēs kirsoeidēs*) is not observed in the female.'

This is Herophilus' statement. I will mention what especially causes me astonishment: he described position, size, and nature of the 'testicles' in female creatures accurately, not omitting anything, not even about the vein and artery which are attached to them on either side, but rather providing an accurate account of them. But afterwards, although he did mention correctly that the seminal duct is attached to the uterus externally, one on either side, he was mistaken to say it is not very apparent. It is, after all, of quite a considerable size. Subsequently he was much more mistaken than in this matter, when he said that the seminal duct of the female is implanted into the neck of the bladder in a manner similar to the seminal passage of the male. (*Cf. also T105–T114 infra; Chapter* VII, *T193–T202; Chapter* VIII, *T247.*)

62 Galenus, *In Hippocratis Epidemiarum 2.4.1 Commentarius 4* (ad Hippocratis v. 120 sq. L). (From Ḥunain's Arabic translation of the lost original; *CMG* v.10.1, p. 318 Pfaff.)

. . . The veins turn towards the vertebrae and the ribs, the one on the left close to the collar-bone, the one on the right a bit lower, since it is bent toward the back . . . What Hippocrates says about this vein which is a bit lower on the right than on the left, Herophilus, too, already said in Book IV of his treatise *On Anatomy.* Herophilus, you see, first explained that two veins branch off from the thick vein where it reaches the collar-bone, and that one then proceeds to the left side, the other to the right, and that each of these two then is divided again, branching out after four of the ribs of the chest. In this book he then says:

'The vein which proceeds to the right side lies a bit lower than the vein which proceeds to the left.'

What Herophilus says here is in agreement with what appears in dissection and with what Hippocrates said.

2 *Dissection and vivisection*

63a A. Cornelius Celsus, *Medicina* 1 (*Artes* 6), *prohoem.* 23–6
(*CML* 1, p. 21 Marx)

ergo necessarium esse (sc. putant medici rationales) incidere
corpora mortuorum eorumque viscera atque intestina scrutari;
longeque optime fecisse Herophilum et Erasistratum, qui
nocentes homines a regibus ex carcere acceptos vivos inciderint,
5 considerarintque etiamnum spiritu remanente ea, quae natura
ante clausisset, eorumque positum, colorem, figuram, magnitu-
dinem, ordinem, duritiem, mollitiem, levorem, contactum,
processus deinde singulorum et recessus, et sive quid inseritur
alteri, sive quid partem alterius in se recipit ... neque esse
10 crudele, sicut plerique proponunt, hominum nocentium et
horum quoque paucorum suppliciis remedia populis innocenti-
bus saeculorum omnium quaeri.

1 necessarium ergo *J*   4 a regibus ex *FV*: quia regibus *J*
5 etiamnum *FV*²: etiam non *V*: etiam *J*   manente *J*   6 eorumque
VJ: eorum *F*   posituram *J*   7 laevorem *Egnatius*: livorem *vulg.*

63a [According to the 'rationalist' physicians] it is therefore
necessary to dissect the bodies of the dead and to examine their viscera
and intestines. Herophilus and Erasistratus, they say, did this in the
best way by far when they cut open men who were alive, criminals out
of prison, received from kings. And while breath still remained in
these criminals, they inspected those parts which nature previously
had concealed, also their position, colour, shape, size, arrangement,
hardness, softness, smoothness, connection, and the projections and
depressions of each, and whether anything is inserted into another
thing or whether anything receives a part of another into itself
... Nor is it cruel, as most people maintain, that remedies for
innocent people of all times should be sought in the sacrifice of people
guilty of crimes, and of only a few such people at that.

63b Iohannes Alexandrinus, *Commentaria in librum De sectis Galeni* (ad cap.5; I, pp. 78–9K), 5ra35–42 (pp. 57–8 Pritchet)

Iterum instant empirici et dicunt quia, dum anatomiam faciunt dogmatici in vivis, homicidium perpetrare dignoscuntur, cum medicina sit ars in humanis corporibus operans sanitatem. 'vos autem dogmatici econtra homines vivos incidendo interficitis; 5 nos sic non agimus, sed anatomiam in simiam et ursum facimus quia habent aliqua consimilia hominibus.' ad hoc dogmatici, 'hos, qui digni sunt morte et a iudicibus iudicati ut moriantur, occidimus; sic etenim faciebant Erofilus et alii antiqui.'

4 vivos *om. V*   incidendo *om. R*   5 in symeam *B*: insumamus (et insumamus *U*) in simiam *UR*: in simiis *SP*: *corr. Pritchet*   et ursum] in ursum *E*   8 sic] sicut *VECQ*

63b The Empiricists press on again, saying that the Dogmatists are distinguished by committing murder, since they perform dissection on human beings who are alive, although medicine is an art that effects health in human bodies. 'But you Dogmatists, on the contrary, kill living human beings by cutting them open. We do not act in that way; rather, we perform dissection on the ape and the bear, since they have some features entirely similar to human beings'. The Dogmatists, however, [respond]: 'We kill those who deserve death and who have been condemned to die by judges; and indeed, Herophilus and other ancients used to do the same.'

63c Agnellus Ravennas (?), *In Galeni De sectis (cap. 5) comm.* 23 (p. 92, Arethusa Monogr. 8)

Iterum stant imperici et dicent quia 'anathomica male facitis uti in vivis. vos dicitis quia medicina est ars circa humana corpora occupata operans sanitatem, vos econtra agitis homines ut eos occiditis incidendo.' ad hec dicimus quia 'eos incidimus qui 5 digni sunt morti, quia iudicati sunt a iudicibus ut moriantur. hec faciebat Erofilus et alii antiqui ut ratio redderetur.' Nos enim sic non agimus anathomica, sed in simmia aut in urso, qui habent aliqua similia hominibus.

7 urso *A*: sue *P (sed vid. app. crit. ad T63b supra)*

63c The Empiricists stand firm again and say that 'you perform your dissections poorly because you do them on living beings. You say that medicine is an art concerned with human bodies, effecting health. But you, on the contrary, take human beings to kill them by cutting them open.' To this we [sc. the 'Dogmatists'] say that 'we cut open those who deserve death, because they have been condemned to die by judges. Herophilus and other ancients used to do this, in order that an account may be given.' We, to be sure, do not perform dissections in this manner but on apes or on the bear, who have some features similar to human beings.

64a Vindicianus, *Gynaecia*, praef. (vel 2), cod. *L* (K. Sudhoff, *AGM* 8 (1915), pp. 417–18)

maioribus nostris in Alexandria medicinam agentibus, Rufo scilicet et Philippo, Lyco, Erasistrato, Pelope et Erofilo, Ypocrate et Apollonio placuit mortuorum (sc. corpora) scrutari, ut scirent unde et quomodo morirentur, quod ipsa
5 humanitas prohibet facere, eo quod ipsis scrutantibus omnia manifesta atque adaperto essent. (*Vid. T199 infra.*)

64a Our ancestors who practised medicine in Alexandria – Rufus, of course, and Philip, Lycus, Erasistratus, Pelops, Herophilus, Hippocrates, and Apollonius – found it proper to examine the bodies of the dead in order to know for what reason and in what manner they died. Humanity itself prohibits doing this, since all things would be manifest and fully open to those conducting the examination. (*See also Chapter* VII, *T199 infra.*)

64b Vindicianus, *ibid.*, cod. *M*

See Chapter II, *T5b supra.*

65 Tertullianus, *De anima* 25.5 (p. 36 Waszink)

hoc (sc. τὸν ἐμβρυοσφάκτην) et Hippocrates habuit . . . et maiorum quoque prosector Herophilus et mitior ipse Soranus. (*Vid. Herophili T247 infra.*)

65 This [sc. a surgical instrument known as 'foetus slayer']
Hippocrates possessed . . . and so did Herophilus, the dissector even
of adults, and the milder Soranus himself. (*See Chapter* VIII, *T247*
infra.)

66 Tertullianus, *De anima* 10.4 (p. 13 Waszink)

cui vero tantum patuit in dei opera, ut alicui haec (sc. vitalia)
deesse praesumpserit? Herophilus ille medicus aut lanius, qui
sexcentos exsecuit, ut naturam scrutaretur, qui hominem odiit,
ut nosset, nescio an omnia interna eius liquido explorarit, ipsa
5 morte mutante quae vixerant, et morte non simplici, sed ipsa
inter artificia exsectionis errante.

1 haec *om. A*   2 aut *vulg.*: an? *Iun.*   3 septingentos *B*   scutaretur
A corr.   odit *Iun.*: occidit *Diels*   5 simplicis *A*   sed et ipsa
Kellner   6 exectionis *AB Gel.*

66 For by whom has so great an insight into the works of God in fact
been attained, that he could assume that these things [sc. vital
organs] are missing in any creature? The famous Herophilus, the
physician, or rather butcher, who cut up innumerable persons [*lit.*,
'six hundred persons'] in order to examine nature, who hated humans
in order to have knowledge, explored their internal parts – but he
probably did not explore all of them clearly, since death itself changes
what has been alive, especially a death which is not a simple one but
one which is an error in the midst of the artificial processes of
dissection.

67 Galenus, *In Hippocratis De natura hominis commentarius* 2.6 (*CMG*
v.9.1, p. 69 Mewaldt)

ἐγὼ μὲν γὰρ οὐ φεύγω τά τ' ἄλλα τοιαῦτα κριτήρια καὶ τὴν
συμφωνίαν τῶν ἱστορησάντων, καὶ μάλιστα ἂν ἔμπειροι τῆς
ἱστορουμένης ὕλης ὦσιν, ὥσπερ Εὔδημος μὲν καὶ Ἡρόφιλος
ἀνατομῆς, Κρατεύας δὲ καὶ Διοσκορίδης τῶν μεταλλικῶν
5 φαρμάκων.

1 τά τ' ἄλλα τοιαῦτα *Mewaldt*: τά τε τοιαῦτα *L*: τἆλλα *VR*: τὰ παλαιὰ *R²*:

τὰ τῶν παλαιῶν *coni. Müller*   2 ἔμπειρος R^2 3 ὕλης LR^2: ὅλης
VR   ὧσιν *Müller*: εἶεν *codd.*

67 For I do not run away from other such criteria and particularly
not from the agreement between those who have left written records,
especially if they have direct evidence of the material being recorded,
as do Eudemus and Herophilus of dissection, and Crateuas and
Dioscorides of the metallic drugs.

68 Galenus, *De placitis Hippocratis et Platonis* 8.1 (*CMG* v. 4.1.2, p.
480 De Lacy)

πρῶτοι οὖν μακρολογίας αἴτιοι κατέστησαν οἱ καταψευσάμενοι
τῶν φαινομένων, οὐχ Ἱπποκράτης ἢ Ἐρασίστρατος ἢ Εὔδημος
ἢ Ἡρόφιλος ἢ Μαρῖνος ὁ μετὰ τοὺς παλαιοὺς ἐν τῷ μεταξὺ
χρόνῳ τὴν ἀνατομικὴν θεωρίαν ἠμελημένην ἀνακτησάμενος· ὡς,
5 εἴ γε τὸ φαινόμενον ἐκ τῆς ἀνατομῆς εἶπον, οὐκ ἂν ἐμακρολογοῦ-
μεν δι' ἀποδείξεως μιᾶς εὑρημένου τοῦ ζητουμένου.

3-4 οἱ . . . ἀνακτησάμενοι *H* : *corr. DeLacy*

68 The primary culprits responsible for the length of this discussion
are those who have misrepresented [the evidence of] the appearances, and not Hippocrates or Erasistratus or Eudemus or Herophilus
or Marinus, the person who, in the period after the ancients, revived
anatomical theory, which had been in a state of neglect. So, if they [sc.
those who misrepresented evidence] had described what appears in
dissection, we would not need to speak at length, since the matter
under investigation would have been discovered through a single
scientific proof.

69 Galenus, *In Hippocratis De natura hominis* xi *commentarius* 2.6
(*CMG* v.9.1, pp. 69–70 Mewaldt)

οὐδεὶς δ' ἄλλος εἶπεν ἰατρὸς ὀκτὼ φλέβας ἀπὸ ⟨τῆς⟩ κεφαλῆς
ἐπὶ τὰ κάτω τοῦ σώματος ἥκειν, οὔτε τῶν μᾶλλον ἀκριβῶς
ἀνατεμνόντων, οὐ Διοκλῆς, οὐ Πραξαγόρας, οὐκ Ἐρασίστρατος, οὐ Πλειστόνικος, οὐ Φυλότιμος, οὐ Μνησίθεος, οὐ
5 Διεύχης, οὐ Χρύσιππος, οὐκ Ἀριστογένης ἢ Μήδειος ἢ

Εὐρυφῶν, οὔτ' ἄλλος τις ἰατρὸς τῶν ἀρχαίων. τί ⟨δὲ⟩ δεῖ λέγειν
ἔτι περὶ τῶν μετ' αὐτοὺς ἐπὶ πλεῖστον αὐξησάντων τὴν
ἀνατομικὴν θεωρίαν, ὡς Ἡρόφιλός τε καὶ Εὔδημος, οἷς εἰς τὴν
μέθοδον οὐκέτι οὐδεὶς προσεξεῦρεν οὐδὲν ἄχρι Μαρίνου τε καὶ
10 Νομισιανοῦ, οὐδ' Ἡρακλειανός, ᾧ συνεγενόμην ἐπὶ τῆς Ἀλεξανδρείας οὐκ ἐν παρέργῳ;

1 ἰατρὸς εἶπεν VR   τῆς add. Mewaldt cf. pp. 70.16 et 69.8 (CMG
v.9.1)   5 διευχὴς R (-ῆς L)   ἀντιγένης codd.: corr. Rosenbaum
6 οὔτ' coni. DeLacy: οὐκ codd.   δὲ add. Mewaldt: autem Rasarius   7 ἔτι
om. L   9 τε om. L

69 No other physician said that eight veins proceed from the head
to the lower parts of the body; neither any of those who conducted
dissections more accurately – i.e., not Diocles, Praxagoras, Erasistratus, Plistonicus, Phylotimus, Mnesitheus, Dieuches, Chrysippus,
Aristogenes, Medius, or Euryphon – or any other physician among
the ancients. Why is it then necessary to speak further about those
who, after them, advanced anatomical theory most, like Herophilus
and Eudemus? With respect to this inquiry no one – not even
Heraclianus, whom I consulted in Alexandria in no casual manner –
made any further discovery, i.e. in addition to those of Herophilus
and Eudemus, until Marinus and Numisianus.

70 Galenus, De usu partium 6.13 (1, p. 341 Helmreich)

ὁ γὰρ ἔσωθεν χιτὼν (sc. τῆς ἀρτηρίας) ὁ παχὺς καὶ σκληρός, ὁ
τὰς ἐγκαρσίας ἔχων ἶνας, οὐδ' ὅλως ἔστι ταῖς φλεψί. σὺ (sc. ὧ
Ἀσκληπιάδη) δ' εἴτ' ἐστὶν εἴτ' οὐκ ἔστι, μὴ πολυπραγμονήσας,
ὑπὲρ ὧν οὐδὲν οἶσθα σαφές, ἀποφαίνεσθαι τολμᾷς ὡς εἰδώς, ὁ
5 τὰς Ἡροφίλου διαπτύων ἀνατομάς, ὁ κατεγνωκὼς Ἐρασιστράτου καὶ μικρὸν φροντίζων Ἱπποκράτους. ἆρ' ἀγνοεῖς
ὄντως οὐκ ἐχούσας τὸν ἔσωθεν χιτῶνα τὸν σκληρὸν τὰς φλέβας
τοῦ πνεύμονος;

2 οὐδ' ὅλως ἔστι ACDNPU: ὁ αὐτὸς οὐκ ἔστιν B: οὐκ ἔστιν ὁ αὐτὸς L
2-3 σὺ δ' αὐτὸ DL   3 μὴ om. BU   5 ἀναπτύων διατομὰς D
6 μικρόν τι B

70 The thick, hard inner tunic [the tunica media of the artery] with transverse fibres does not exist at all in veins. But you [Asclepiades], who are not inquisitive about whether it is present or not, have the audacity to make statements about things of which you know nothing clearly, as though you knew them – you who spit on the dissections of Herophilus, have contempt for Erasistratus, and pay little attention to Hippocrates. Are you really ignorant of the fact that the veins of the lung do not have the hard inner tunic?

71 Galenus, *De anatomicis administrationibus* 10.4 (II, p. 43 Simon; translated from Ḥunain's Arabic translation of the lost original by Duckworth, pp. 47–8)

As regards the clarity of expression at which we are aiming in our account of the dissection, there is nothing to prevent us from saying of one and the same part at one time that it is the natural beginning of the structure whose description is being summarized here, and at another time that it is not the beginning but rather the end, adopting the custom of Herophilus in the use of words.

72 Galenus, *De anatomicis administrationibus* 3.2 (II, p. 349K)

ὅταν οὖν ἀκριβῶς ἴδῃς τοῦτό σοι κατωρθωμένον, ἀνατείνας ἀγκίστροις ἑκάτερον τῆς τομῆς τὸ χεῖλος, ὑπὸ τὸ δέρμα πειρῶ τέμνειν ἀποχωρίζων αὐτοῦ τὸν ὑμένα. μόνοις δὲ οὐ χρὴ τοῖς δακτύλοις ἄνευ σμίλης ἐπιτρέπειν τοὔργον, ὥσπερ ὅταν
5 ἐκδέρωμέν τι ζῷον. ὁ γὰρ ὑμὴν τῶν ὑποκειμένων σωμάτων ἑαυτῷ ἀπολύεται κατὰ δάρσιν, ὡς Ἡρόφιλος ὠνόμαζεν ἀπὸ τοῦ δέρω ῥήματος ὄνομα ποιήσας, τῆς ἐνεργείας τε καὶ τοῦ πάθους κοινόν, ὥσπερ γε καὶ ἀπὸ τοῦ τέμνω τὸ τῆς τομῆς ὄνομα γέγονεν, ἐνέργειαν μὲν σημαῖνον τοῦ τέμνοντος ἀνθρώ-
5 που, πάθος δὲ τοῦ τεμνομένου σώματος.

72 Whenever, therefore, you see that you have succeeded accurately in this [sc. removing the skin correctly], having stretched each 'lip' of the incision upward with surgical hooks, try to make an incision under the skin, severing the [underlying] tissue from it. But

you should not entrust this task to your fingers alone, without a surgical lancet, as we do whenever we flay an animal. For the membrane of the bodies lying underneath it is loosened by 'flaying' (*darsis*), as Herophilus named it. He derived this noun from the verb 'I flay' (*dero*), the noun being common both to the activity and to the 'being acted upon', just as the noun 'incision', which arose from 'I incise', on the one hand signifies the activity of the human being making the incision, and on the other the 'being acted upon' of the body which is cut.

73 Galenus, *De anatomicis administrationibus* 12.2 (II, p. 103 Simon; translated from Ḥunain's Arabic translation of the lost original by Duckworth, p. 112)

But if you detach and remove from it [sc. the uterus] the membrane enveloping it from all sides, there show themselves to you two cavities, of which the one allows itself to be separated from the other with the minimum of effort without the knife, by means of the process which Herophilus calls 'flaying, excoriating', in the way in which the skin that envelops the whole body comes to be separated from that which lies beneath it. For the bodies which one frees from one another by means of 'flaying, excoriating', are bound together only by means of arachnoid-like ligaments.

74 Galenus, *In Hippocratis Epidemiarum 2. commentarius 4* (ad Hippocratis v.120 sq. L) (From Ḥunain's Arabic translation of the lost original; *CMG* v.10.1, p. 322 Pfaff)

By saying that the attachment of the diaphragm to the liver is an attachment in which separation is not easy, Hippocrates has shown that he uses the designation 'attachment' of those organs of which, ever since Herophilus, we say that their separation is achieved through 'skinning' and 'flaying', like the separation of the skin from what lies underneath it. This, too, is after all a kind of attachment, even if it is only weak. For this attachment consists of thin strands, similar to the threads of a spider's web.

3 *Head, brain, nerves ('On Anatomy' 1?)*

75 Vindicianus, *Gynaecia* 3 (Karl Sudhoff, *AGM* 8 (1915), p. 418; pp. 430–1 Rose; pp. 13–14 Schipperges)

caput nostrum commissuras habet quinque angulosas, alterutrum se continentes, femina vero in circuiti tantum, sicut scripsit Synanchus et Erophilus anathomici, calvaria id est galea supposita est, quam Greci mecanen appellabant, que coheret
5 membrano, cui superposita est cutis, que habet capillos, non causa decoris, sed ut ab estu et frigore cerebrum nostrum custodiat; hinc ergo calvaria subiacent timpora, que continentur spiritualibus venis cerebri, quibus superposita sunt supercilia, pilis vestita, ut si copiosus sudor venerit opposita pilorum
10 stacione contineatur, donec abstergatur, ne oculis obesse possit.

3 Erophilus anathomici *L*: summus auctor Erophilus *F*: summus anathomicus Herophilus *B*: anathomicus filius *C*: Erophilus *om. M*.
4 mecanen *conieci*: mecan *L*: mecanem *D*: mecani *C*: merhanon *B*: non vadena *G*: metanem *F*: micharin *P*   7 timpora *coni.* Sudhoff: tipora *codd.*

75 Our head has five angular sutures, one bordering on the next; and only in the female is it, in fact, all the way around, as the anatomists Synanchus and Herophilus wrote. The skull, i.e., the 'helmet', which the Greeks used to call 'crane' [*mēchanē*?], is placed underneath and it coheres with a membrane, on which is placed the skin. The skin has hair, not for the sake of ornament, but to protect our brain against heat and cold. The temples then lie below the skull and are adjacent to the pneumatic veins of the brain. And above them the eyebrows are placed, adorned with hair, so that if copious perspiration came [down], it would be contained by this 'checkpoint' of hair placed in its way until it is wiped off, so that it could not obstruct the eyes.

76 Theophilus Protospatharius, *De corporis humani fabrica* 4.5.4–5 (p. 135 Greenhill)

μήνιγγες δὲ αἱ περιέχουσαι τὸν ἐγκέφαλον, ὥσπερ τινὰ ἐνδύματα ἢ σκεπάσματα αὐτοῦ, εἰσι δύο, ἡ μὲν ἐκτὸς τοῦ κρανίου, ἡ δὲ ἐντός, ἐκτὸς δὲ τῆς ἑτέρας μήνιγγος, σκληρὰ καὶ παχεῖα

οὖσα κατὰ τὴν σύστασιν· παχυτέρα δὲ γίνεται κατὰ τὴν μέσην
5 ῥαφὴν καὶ κατὰ τὴν λαβδοειδῆ παρὰ τὸ ἄλλο αὐτῆς μέρος ὅσον
τετραπλάσιον, ὥστε τῇ ἐπαναδιπλώσει αὐτῆς τῇ κατὰ τὰς
ῥαφὰς γινομένῃ σωλῆνί τινι ἐοικέναι. τοῦτον τὸν σωλῆνα
ὠνόμασαν οἱ περὶ τὸν Ἡρόφιλον πύελόν τε καὶ χώνην· ὡς ἡ μὲν
ὑποδεχομένη τοὺς πόρους κοιλότης ἀπὸ τοῦ σχήματος πύελος
10 ὀνομάζεται, ἀπὸ δὲ τῆς χρείας χώνη, τέτρηται γὰρ εἰς τὸ
κάταντες αἰσθητῷ πόρῳ ὡς χώνην μιμεῖσθαι.

1 δὲ EC: δέ εἰσιν vulg.   post τινὰ add. οὖσαι τούτου vulg.: om. E   ἢ E:
καὶ cett.   2 αὐτοῦ EC: om. cett.   εἴσι C: εἴσι δὲ cett.   ἡ δὲ ἐντὸς om.
E   3 ἐκτὸς ... μήνιγγος E: om. cett.   5 παρὰ E: περὶ vulg.
6 κατὰ vulg.: περὶ F   7 σωλῆνα (pr.) τινὰ E   8 χώνη vulg.: χοάνην
(ὀνομάζουσιν) Galeni De usu partium 9.3 (II p. 8.14 Helmreich)

76 There are two membranes which envelop the brain like
garments or coverings, one outside the skull, the other inside the skull.
And the one which is outside the other membrane is hard and thick in
its composition. But it becomes as much as four times thicker
compared to its other parts at the middle of the suture of the skull, i.e.
at the Λ-shaped suture. Consequently its double fold, which occurs at
the sutures, resembles a 'channel' This channel the followers of
Herophilus called 'tub' as well as 'funnel' [*infundibulum cerebri*]. As the
cavity which receives the [nerve] passages, it is called 'tub' on the
basis of its shape, but 'funnel' on the basis of its function; for it is
pierced downward by a perceptible passage, and consequently
represents a funnel.

77a Galenus, *De usu partium* 8.11 (I, pp. 482–3 Helmreich)

ἀλλ' ἐπεὶ πάντα τὰ κατὰ τὸ σῶμα νεῦρα τὰ κάτω τῆς κεφαλῆς ἢ
ἐκ τῆς παρεγκεφαλίδος ἢ ἐκ τοῦ νωτιαίου πέφυκεν, ἐχρῆν καὶ τὴν
ταύτης κοιλίαν ἀξιόλογόν τ' εἶναι τὸ μέγεθος καὶ τὸ προκατειρ-
γασμένον ἐν ταῖς προσθίοις ψυχικὸν πνεῦμα μεταλαμβάνειν.
5 ὥστ' ἀναγκαῖον ἦν γενέσθαι τινὰ πόρον ἐξ ἐκείνων εἰς ταύτην,
ἀτὰρ οὖν καὶ φαίνεται μεγάλη μὲν αὕτη, μέγιστος δὲ καὶ ὁ ἀπὸ
τῶν ἔμπροσθεν κοιλιῶν εἰς αὐτὴν ἐμβάλλων πόρος. καὶ κατὰ
τοῦτόν γε μόνον ἡ σύμφυσίς ἐστι τῇ παρεγκεφαλίδι πρὸς τὸν
ἐγκέφαλον. οὕτω γὰρ ἑκατέραν τὴν μοῖραν αὐτοῦ καλεῖν ἔθος
10 ἐστὶ τοῖς περὶ τὸν Ἡρόφιλον, τὴν μὲν ἔμπροσθεν τῷ τοῦ παντὸς

ὀνόματι διὰ τὸ μέγεθος· ὄντος γὰρ αὐτοῦ διφυοῦς, ὡς εἴρηται,
τῶν μορίων ἑκάτερον πολὺ μεῖζόν ἐστιν ὅλης τῆς παρεγκεφαλί-
δος· τὴν δ' ὄπισθεν, ὅτι τῆς πρόσθεν φθασάσης τὸ τοῦ παντὸς
ὄνομα σφετερίσασθαι δικαιότερον οὐκέτ' ἦν εὑρεῖν ἕτερον ὄνομα
15 τῇ παρεγκεφαλίδι τοῦ νῦν ὄντος ... διειργόμενος οὖν ἀπὸ τῆς
παρεγκεφαλίδος ὁ ἐγκέφαλος, ὡς καὶ πρόσθεν εἴρηται, τῇ τῆς
παχείας μήνιγγος διπλώσει, δεόμενος δὲ κἂν καθ' ἕν τι συναφθῆ-
ναι μέρος ἕνεκα τῆς τοῦ προειρημένου πόρου γενέσεως, εἰς μίαν
πρότερον χώραν τὰς κοιλίας ἀμφοτέρας ἐπεράτωσεν, ἣν δὴ
20 τετάρτην ἔνιοι τῶν ἀνατομικῶν ἀριθμοῦσι τοῦ παντὸς ἐγκεφάλου κοιλίαν.

1 ἐπεὶ BL: οὐ D   2 πεφυκέναι χρὴ D   2–3 τὴν ταύτης κοιλίαν BLU:
τὴν ταύτην κοιλίαν D   3 τ' om. D   4 ταῖς προσθίοις DU: τοῖς
προσθίοις BL   5 γενέσθαι L: γίνεσθαι cett.   τινὰ L: τὸν cett.   7 εἰς
αὐτὴν ἐμβάλλων L: ἐμβάλλων εἰς αὐτὴν cett.   8 σύμφυσις L: ἔμφυσις
cett.   9 ἑκατέρω ἂν BU   13 πρόσθεν BLU: πρώτης D   15 οὖν
codd.: νῦν Charterius   17 δὲ L: om. cett.   17 συναχθῆναι Oribasius

77a Now since all the nerves of the body below the head grow either
from the cerebellum (*parenkephalis*) or from the spinal marrow, the
ventricle of the cerebellum had to be of quite a considerable size and
had to get a share of the psychic pneuma which was previously
prepared in the front ventricles [sc. lateral ventricles of the brain].
Consequently there must be a passage from those ventricles into the
ventricle of the cerebellum. The latter [ventricle], then, also appears
large, and the passage entering into it from the anterior ventricles is
very large indeed; by it alone does a connection between the
'cerebellum' (*parenkephalis*) and 'cerebrum' (*enkephalos*) exist. These,
you see, are the names Herophilus and his followers are in the habit of
giving its two parts. The anterior part was called by this name of the
whole [sc. *enkephalos*, 'brain'] on account of its size. For, although it is
double in nature, as was mentioned, each of its two parts is much
bigger than the entire cerebellum. The posterior part [sc. cerebel-
lum], by contrast, got its name because the anterior part had been the
first to expropriate the name of the whole [sc. *enkephalos*] for itself, and
therefore it was no longer possible to find a different, more just name
for the cerebellum (*par-enkephalis* ('para-brain')) than it now has
... Since, then, the cerebrum is separated from the cerebellum by the
fold of the thick membrane [*tentorium cerebelli*], as was also said

previously, but needs to be attached – even if only at one part – for the sake of forming the aforementioned passage, the cerebrum has caused both its ventricles [sc. laterals] to terminate first in one space, which some anatomists count as a fourth ventricle of the entire brain.

77b Oribasius, *Collectiones medicae* 24.1.18–20 (*CMG* VI.2.1; vol. III, p. 6 Raeder). Excerpted from Galen, *De usu partium* 8.11

μία δ' (sc. κοιλία) ἡ ἐν τῇ παρεγκεφαλίδι, τὸ κατειργασμένον ἐν ταῖς προσθίοις ψυχικὸν πνεῦμα μεταλαμβάνουσα· διὸ καὶ ἀναγκαῖον ἦν γενέσθαι τινὰ πόρον ἐξ ἐκείνων εἰς ταύτην. ἀτὰρ οὖν καὶ φαίνεται μέγιστος ὁ ἀπὸ τῶν ἔμπροσθεν κοιλιῶν εἰς
5　αὐτὴν ἐμβάλλων πόρος, καὶ κατὰ τοῦτό γε μόνον ἡ σύμφυσίς ἐστι τῇ παρεγκεφαλίδι πρὸς τὸν ἐγκέφαλον· οὕτως γὰρ ἑκατέραν αὐτοῦ τὴν μοῖραν ἔθος ἐστὶ καλεῖν τοῖς περὶ τὸν Ἡρόφιλον, τὴν δ' ὄπισθεν παρεγκεφαλίδα. διειργόμενος οὖν ἀπὸ τῆς παρεγκεφαλίδος, ὡς καὶ πρόσθεν εἴρηται, τῇ τῆς
10　παχείας μήνιγγος διπλώσει . . .

1 κατεργασμένον *E*　　6 οὕτω *L*, *C e corr.*　　ἑκατέρων *AE*　　10 *post* διπλώσει, δεόμενος *et sqq. ut in Galeni De usu partium libro usque ad* ἐγκεφάλου κοιλίαν (*vid. Herophili T77a*)

77b And there is one ventricle in the cerebellum (*parenkephalis*) which gets a share of the psychic pneuma which has been prepared in the front [sc. lateral] ventricles. There must, therefore, be a passage from these front ventricles into the ventricle of the cerebellum. The passage from the anterior ventricles into it accordingly also appears to be very large indeed, and by it alone is there a connection between cerebellum (*parenkephalis*) and cerebrum (*enkephalos*). For these are the names Herophilus and his followers are in the habit of giving its two parts, and the posterior one [they called] *parenkephalis*. Since, then, it [sc. the cerebrum] is separated from the cerebellum, as was mentioned previously, by the fold of the thick membrane . . .*

---

* The text that follows is identical with the Galenic text in T77a, from which it was excerpted by Oribasius.

78 Galenus, *De usu partium* 8.11 (1, p. 484 Helmreich)

καὶ οἷς γε τετάρτη τις αὕτη κοιλία (sc. τὸ ὑπὲρ τὴν κοινὴν
κοιλότητα μόριον ἐγκεφάλου ἢ καμάριον) νενόμισται, κυριωτάτην εἶναί φασιν αὐτὴν ἁπασῶν τῶν καθ' ὅλον τὸν ἐγκέφαλον.
Ἡρόφιλος μὴν οὐ ταύτην, ἀλλὰ τὴν ἐν τῇ παρεγκεφαλίδι
5 κυριωτέραν ἔοικεν ὑπολαμβάνειν.

4 μὴν *L²U*: μὲν *cett.*

78 Those who hold the view that this cavity [sc. the fornix] is a
fourth ventricle, say that, of all the ventricles in the entire brain, it
exercises most control. Herophilus, however, seems to assume that
not this ventricle, but the one in the cerebellum (*parenkephalis*),
exercises more control.

79 Galenus, *De anatomicis administrationibus* 9.5 (11, p. 731K)

εἶτα πρόσεχε τὸν νοῦν, ὅπως ἀνακλωμένου μὲν αὐτοῦ (sc. τοῦ
πέρατος σκωληκοειδοῦς) πρόσω γυμνοῦσθαι συμβαίνει τὴν
ὀπίσω κοιλίαν τὴν τετάρτην (sc. τοῦ ἐγκεφάλου), ἔμπαλιν δὲ
κινουμένου κατακαλύπτεσθαι μὲν αὐτῆς τὸ πλεῖστον μέρος,
5 ἐκεῖνο δὲ φαίνεσθαι μόνον, ὅπερ Ἡρόφιλος εἴκαζεν ἀναγλυφῇ
καλάμου, ᾧ διαγράφομεν. ὄντως γάρ ἐστι τοιοῦτον, ἐν μὲν τῷ
μέσῳ κοιλότητά τινα κεκτημένον οἷον τομήν, ἑκατέρωθεν δ'
αὐτῆς τοσοῦτον εἰς ὕψος ἀνατεινόμενον ἑκάτερον τῶν πλαγίων
μερῶν, ὅσον ἐν τοῖς καλάμοις ἀπὸ τῆς μέσης ὑψοῦται γραμμῆς.
10 καὶ μάλιστά γε κατὰ τὴν Ἀλεξάνδρειαν οὕτω γλύφουσι τοὺς
καλάμους οἷς γράφομεν, ἔνθα διατρίβοντα τὸν Ἡρόφιλον ἡνίκ'
ἀνέτεμνεν εἰκὸς δήπου τῇ τῆς εἰκόνος ὁμοιότητι προσαχθέντα
τοὔνομα θέσθαι.

79 Next pay attention to how, when it [the vermiform process, sc.
the woodworm-shaped process lying on the *aqueductus cerebri*] is bent
forward, the result is that the posterior ventricle [of the brain], the
fourth, is exposed, and, when it is moved backwards, that the larger
part of the ventricle is covered and only that part is visible which
Herophilus likened to the carved out groove of a pen [*kalamos*] with
which we write. You see, it really is like a pen, since it has a hollow,

like an incision [*posterior median sulcus*], in the middle, and on either side of this each of the two lateral parts [*eminentia facialis*] extends up to as great a height as they rise in pens from the line in the middle. Particularly in Alexandria they carve out the pens with which we write in this way, and since Herophilus lived there, it is likely that, when he was dissecting, he applied this name [sc. 'pen', *kalamos*], being induced to do so by the similarity of the image.

80 Galenus, *De locis affectis* 3.14 (VIII, p. 212K)

ἐπιστάμενος οὖν τις ἐξ ἀνατομῆς ἀρχὰς τῶν εἰς ἕκαστον μόριον ἀφικνουμένων νεύρων, ἄμεινον ἰάσεται τὰς ἀναισθησίας καὶ ἀκινησίας ἑκάστου μέρους. ἀδιόριστον δὲ τοῦτο καταλειφθὲν ὑφ' Ἡροφίλου τε καὶ Εὐδήμου, τῶν πρώτων μεθ' Ἱπποκράτην
5 νεύρων ἀνατομὴν ἐπιμελῶς γραψάντων, οὐ σμικρὰν ζήτησιν παρέσχε τοῖς ἰατροῖς, ὅπως ἔνιαι μὲν τῶν παραλύσεων αἴσθησιν μόνην, ἔνιαι δὲ τὴν προαιρετικὴν κίνησιν, ἔνιαι δὲ ἀμφοτέρας διαφθείρουσι.

80 If, therefore, on the basis of dissection a person has gained knowledge of the beginnings of the nerves that reach each part, he will more successfully treat the loss of sensation and movement in each part. Since this [sc. the beginning of each nerve?] was left undefined by Herophilus and Eudemus, the first persons after Hippocrates to record carefully their dissection of the nerves, it provided physicians with no small investigation into why some paralyses destroy only sensation, while others destroy voluntary motion, and others again destroy both.

81 Rufus Ephesius (?), *De anatomia partium hominis* 71–5 (pp. 184–5 Daremberg/Ruelle)

νεῦρόν ἐστιν ἁπλοῦν σῶμα καὶ πεπυκνωμένον, προαιρετικῆς κινήσεως αἴτιον, δυσαίσθητον κατὰ τὴν διαίρεσιν. κατὰ μὲν οὖν τὸν Ἐρασίστρατον καὶ Ἡρόφιλον αἰσθητικὰ νεῦρά ἐστιν· κατὰ δὲ Ἀσκληπιάδην οὐδὲ ὅλως. κατὰ μὲν οὖν τὸν Ἐρασίστρατον
5 δισσῶν ὄντων τῶν νεύρων αἰσθητικῶν καὶ κινητικῶν, τῶν μὲν

αἰσθητικῶν ἃ κεκοίλανται ἀρχὰς εὕροις ἂν ἐν μήνιγξι, τῶν δὲ
κινητικῶν ἐν ἐγκεφάλῳ καὶ παρεγκεφαλίδι. κατὰ δὲ τὸν Ἡρόφιλον ἃ μέν ἐστι προαιρετικά, ἃ καὶ ἔχει τὴν ἔκφυσιν ἀπὸ τοῦ
ἐγκεφάλου καὶ νωτιαίου μυελοῦ, καὶ ἃ μὲν ἀπὸ ὀστοῦ εἰς ὀστοῦν
10 ἐμφύεται, ἃ δὲ ἀπὸ μυὸς εἰς μῦν, ἃ καὶ συνδεῖ τὰ ἄρθρα . . .

2 αἴτιον om. A.   καὶ add. ante κατὰ A   6 ἃ vulg.: οὐ A

81 Nerve (neuron) is a simple, solid body, the cause of voluntary
motion, but difficult to perceive in dissection. According to Erasistratus and Herophilus there are nerves capable of sensation, but
according to Asclepiades not at all. According to Erasistratus there
are two kinds of nerves, sensory and motor nerves; the beginnings of
the sensory nerves, which are hollow, you could find in the meninges
[sc. of the brain], and those of the motor nerves in the cerebrum
(enkephalos) and in the cerebellum (parenkephalis). According to
Herophilus, on the other hand, the neura that make voluntary
[motion] possible have their origin in the cerebrum (enkephalos) and
the spinal marrow, and some grow from bone to bone, others from
muscle to muscle, and some also bind together the joints.

82 Galenus, De anatomicis administrationibus 9.9 (II, pp. 8–9 Simon;
translated by Duckworth, pp. 9–10, from Ḥunain's Arabic
translation of the lost original)

After these pairs [sc. of cranial nerves, viz. optic, oculomotor,
trigeminal and motor root of trigeminal] you find, following in
succession, if you go backwards with your dissection, another
pair of nerves of which each unit consists of two component
parts. But as the origin of each nerve of the two components of
that unit lies close to the place of origin of the others, Marinus
came to reckon these four nerves as a single pair, although we
clearly see that two nerves come to both sides of the head, the
right and the left, opposite the ears, and enter into two foramina,
one anterior, that is the auditory canal, and the other in the
petrous bone. Of these two pairs the one which lies at the back is
the auditory pair. But concerning the other [facial nerve], that
one which enters into the blind foramen, it was believed
previously that it did not reach through to the exterior. And the

same opinion was held of the foramen itself. Consequently
Herophilus and his supporters named this foramen the 'blind'
one . . . But for the present do you restrict yourself for your part
to designating both these pairs [facial and auditory] as a fifth
pair, in agreement with the method of nomenclature of the
modern surgeons, counting both these pairs as one . . . For
many surgeons do not know that in his work on the roots of the
nerves Marinus has enumerated only those same roots which
Herophilus specifies, but Marinus has concluded that there are
seven pairs, whereas Herophilus says there are more than seven,
regardless of the others.

83 Galenus, *In Hippocratis Epidemiarum 2.4.2 commentarius 4* (ad
Hippocratis v. 124 sq. L). (From Ḥunain's Arabic translation
of the lost original; *CMG* v.10.1, p. 330 Pfaff)

. . . I say this nerve, of which Hippocrates speaks here [v, 124.9–
11 L], branches off from the brain near the start of the spinal
marrow. In addition to this pair of nerves only one other pair
proceeds from the brain, running through the beginning of the
spine . . . This is the pair which Marinus, after Hippocrates,
designated the sixth pair of nerves proceeding from the brain.
People believe that Marinus and Herophilus disagreed on this.
But I do not need to tell you anything about the disagreement
here, since the discussion of this pair – i.e. whether one should
count it as the sixth, seventh, eighth, ninth, or still another pair
of the nerves proceeding from the brain – has to do* with
another road, which is long.

84 Galenus, *De libris propriis* 3 (*Scr. Min.* II, p. 108 Mueller)

ἐν δὲ τῷ ἐνάτῳ καὶ δεκάτῳ (sc. τῶν τοῦ Μαρίνου βιβλίων
ἀνατομικῶν εἴκοσι) περὶ τῶν ἀπ' ἐγκεφάλου πεφυκότων νεύρων
καὶ περὶ ὀσφρήσεως καὶ πόθεν ἄρχεται τὸ αἰσθητήριον αὐτῆς

---

* sich . . . beziehen *Pfaff pro* sich . . . bezieht (sc. die Erörterung darüber . . .) *u.v.*

καὶ περὶ τῶν ἐπὶ τοὺς ὀφθαλμοὺς νεύρων, ἃ καλοῦσιν Ἡρόφιλός
5 τε καὶ Εὔδημος πόρους.

2 τῶν om. Ald spatio 3 litt. relicto   3 περὶ τῶν ῥήσεων Q: περὶ τῶν ῥύσεων
edd.: corr. Mueller

84 In Book 19 [sc. of his twenty anatomical books, Marinus writes]
about the nerves that grow from the brain [cerebrum?], about smell
and from what source its perceptual organ begins, and about the
nerves that go to the eyes, which Herophilus as well as Eudemus call
'passages' (poroi).

85 Galenus, De symptomatum causis 1.2 (VII, pp. 88–9K)

δοκεῖ δέ μοι τὸ ἀπ' ἐγκεφάλου καταφερόμενον ἐπὶ τὸν ὀφθαλμὸν
νεῦρον, ὃ δὴ καὶ πόρον ὀνομάζουσιν οἱ περὶ τὸν Ἡρόφιλον, ὅτι
τούτου μόνον φανερόν ἐστι τὸ τρῆμα, πνεύματος ὑπάρχειν ὁδὸς
αἰσθητικοῦ. (Vid. Herophili T140 infra.)

3 τούτου Solmsen: τοῦτο Kühn

85 The nerve which proceeds down from the brain to the eye –
which Herophilus and his followers in fact also call a 'passage'
(poros), because its perforation [lumen?] alone [sc. unlike that of other
nerves] is clearly visible – seems to me to exist as a pathway for
sensory pneuma. (See also Chapter VII, T140 infra.)

86 Calcidius, In Platonis Timaeum comment. 246, pp. 256.22-257.15
Waszink (Corpus Platonicum Medii Aevi: Plato Latinus IV)

demonstranda igitur oculi natura est, de qua cum plerique alii
tum Alcmaeo Crotoniensis, in physicis exercitatus quique
primus exectionem aggredi est ausus, et Callisthenes, Aristotelis
auditor, et Herophilus multa et praeclara in lucem protulerunt:
5 duas esse angustas semitas quae a cerebri sede, in qua est sita
potestas animae summa et principalis, ad oculorum cavernas
meent naturalem spiritum continentes; quae cum ex uno initio
eademque radice progressae aliquantisper coniunctae sint in
frontis intimis, separatae bivii specie perveniant ad oculorum
10 concavas sedes, qua superciliorum oblique tramites porrigun-

tur, sinuataeque illic tunicarum gremio naturalem humorem
recipiente globos complent munitos tegmine palpebrarum, ex
quo appelantur orbes.

    porro quod ex una sede progrediantur luciferae semitae,
15 docet quidem sectio principaliter, nihilo minus tamen intellegi-
tur ex eo quoque, quod uterque oculus moveatur una nec alter
sine altero moveri queat.

    oculi porro ipsius continentiam in quattuor membranis seu
tunicis notaverunt disparili soliditate; quarum differentiam
20 proprietatemque si quis persequi velit, maiorem proposita
materia suscipiet laborem.

2 tum *plurimi*: tamen *A Val (corr. Val²) Col Cam* τ: tam *Ba (corr. Ba²)*:
tan *N*   5 duas dicunt Π   7 meant *Ba (corr. Ba²) Reg₈*¹
11 humorum *Υ* (humores *Ba, corr. Ba.²) La*   19 disperili Λ *(corr. Val²)*
Lu Ba (corr. Ba²)   20 prosequi ΛΣΖΠ

86 The nature of the eye therefore must be demonstrated. About
this very many others have brought many things to light very clearly,
especially Alcmeon of Croton, who, well versed in natural philosophy, first dared to proceed to dissection [?*exectio*], and Callisthenes,
Aristotle's pupil, and Herophilus: namely, that there are two narrow
ducts containing natural pneuma (*spiritus naturalis* (*pneuma physikon*))
and that these ducts proceed from the seat of the brain, in which the
highest, principal power of the soul is located, to the cavities of the
eyes. And although these two ducts proceed for a while from a single
starting-point and from the same root and are united in the deep
internal part of the forehead, yet, when they reach the concave seats
of the eyes where the slanting cross-ways of the eyebrows extend, they
are separate, like two roads. There the two ducts curve and, where the
'lap' [sinus] of the tunics receives natural moisture, they fill [with
pneuma?] the eyeballs, which are protected by the covering of the
eyelids and therefore are called 'circles' (*orbes*).

    Furthermore, dissection is, to be sure, the primary teacher of the
fact that the light-bearing ducts proceed from one location, yet this
fact is understood no less [by reason] from the fact that each eye
moves together with [the other] and neither could move without the
other.

    They also recorded that the area adjacent to the eye itself consists of
four membranes or tunics of unequal thickness. If someone wished to

pursue the differences and individual qualities of these tunics, he will undertake a labour greater than the subject-matter proposed here.

87 Rufus Ephesius (?), *De anatomia partium hominis* 12–13 (p. 171 Daremberg/Ruelle)

τὸ δὲ τετρημένον σῶμα (sc. τοῦ ὀφθαλμοῦ) λεῖον μέν ἐστιν ἔξωθεν, κατὰ ὃ προσπίπτει τῷ κερατοειδεῖ, δασὺ δὲ ἀπὸ τῶν ἀπεστραμμένων, ὡς φησιν Ἡρόφιλος, δορᾷ ῥαγὸς σταφυλῆς ὅμοιον, καταπεπλεγμένον ἀγγείοις. καλεῖται δὲ δεύτερος (sc. χιτὼν) μὲν
5 τῇ τάξει, τετρημένος δὲ ἀπὸ τῆς κατασκευῆς, καὶ ῥαγοειδὴς ἀπὸ τῆς ἐμφερείας, καὶ χοριοειδὴς, ὡς ὁμοίως χορίῳ κατηγγειωμένος.

3 ῥαγὸς σταφυλῆς δορᾷ *Clinch*   3–4 ὅμοιος καταπεπλεγμένος *A Clinch*   4–5 δεύτερος *usque ad* κατασκευῆς *codd.*: οὗτος δεύτερος τῇ τάξει, καὶ τετρήμενος τῇ κατασκευῇ *Clinch*   6 ὡς *om. Clinch*

87 The perforated body [sc. of the eye; *iris?*] is smooth on the outside where it meets with the horn-like [coat of the eye; *cornea?*], but rough on the side that is turned away, as Herophilus says, resembling the skin of a grape, being interwoven with blood-vessels. This coat [sc. pars iridica retinae?] is called the 'second' on account of its position, 'perforated' on the basis of its structure, 'grape-like' on the basis of the resemblance, and 'chorioid' on the ground that it is interlaced with blood-vessels like the foetal membrane (*chorion*).

88 A. Cornelius Celsus, *Medicina* 7 (*Artes* 12).7.13B (*CML* I, p. 319 Marx)

hae duae tunicae cum interiora oculi cingant, rursus sub his (sc. ceratoidi et chorioidi) coeunt, extenuataeque et in unum coactae ⟨per⟩ foramen, quod inter ossa est, ad membranam cerebri perveniunt eique inhaerescunt. sub his autem, qua parte
5 pupilla est, locus vacuus est; deinde infra rursus tenuissima tunica, quam Herophilus arachnoidem nominavit.

1 haec *F*   sub his *J*: ubi *FV*¹: sub ubi *V*²   3 per *J*: om. *FV*   3 ad *J*: et *FV*   4 eoque *J*   sub *F*²*J*: sum *FV*   6 qua *V*   hero pilus *FV*   araconide *J*   *ad* nominavit *sqq. vid.* Oppermann, *1925: 28–30*

88 These two coats [sc. the 'ceratoid coat' – i.e. cornea and sclerotic coat – and the 'chorioid' coat] enclose the interior parts of the eye, but they coalesce again behind them; and after becoming thinned out and joined into one, they go to the membrane of the brain through the aperture which is between the bones, and stick to the membrane. Under these two coats, however, at the part where the pupil is, is an empty space. Then underneath this again is the thinnest coat, to which Herophilus gave the name 'cobweb-like' (*arachnoeides* (*retina*)).

89 Rufus Ephesius, *De nominatione partium hominis* 153 (p. 154 Daremberg/Ruelle)

ὁ δὲ τρίτος (sc. χιτὼν τοῦ ὀφθαλμοῦ) περιέχει μὲν ὑαλοειδὲς ὑγρόν· καλεῖται δὲ ἀρχαῖον ὄνομα ἀραχνοειδὴς διὰ λεπτότητα. ἐπειδὴ δὲ Ἡρόφιλος εἰκάζει αὐτὸν ἀμφιβλήστρῳ ἀνασπωμένῳ, ἔνιοι καὶ ἀμφιβληστροειδῆ καλοῦσιν· ἄλλοι δὲ καὶ ὑαλοειδῆ ἀπὸ
5 τοῦ ὑγροῦ.

3 ἀνεσπασμένῳ *Clinch*   4 καλοῦσιν ἀπὸ τοῦ ὑγροῦ αὐτόν, ἄλλον καὶ ὑαλοειδῆ *Clinch*

89 The third [coat of the eye; retina?] encloses vitreous liquid. The ancient name by which it is called is 'cobweb-like', on account of its fineness. But since Herophilus likens it to a casting-net that is drawn up, some also call it 'net-like'. Others call it 'vitreous', too, on the basis of the liquid.

90 Galenus, *De anatomicis administrationibus* 14.5 (II, p. 183 Simon; translated from Ḥunain's Arabic translation of the lost original by Duckworth, p. 201)

I have already said previously that Herophilus calls the process of the skull which others call 'awl-pointed' or 'needle-pointed', and which is a slender cartilaginous process, 'styloid'. This is because many people in Alexandria, and many others besides them among the peoples inhabiting the regions of the Orient, who speak bad Greek, call the pens with which one writes upon waxed tablets 'styloi'.

91 Galenus, *De anatomicis administrationibus* 11.1 (ii, pp. 61–2
Simon; translated from Ḥunain's Arabic translation by
Duckworth, pp. 67–8)

After this flesh [sc. submandibular salivary gland], when it has
been removed, and all the fascial coverings reflected which
clothe and veil the entire laryngeal region, there appears the
muscle of the mandible which one rightly calls 'tendinous', since
its intermediate part is tendinous and fleshless [*M. digastri-
cus?*] . . . The state of this muscle I have already demonstrated
above. And here, in connection with it, I will explain this further
point, that its root [origin] adjoins the root of that part of the
skull which Herophilus calls the 'columnar' process [*processus
styloideus*] and which we call 'awl-like' or 'needle-like'.

92 Galenus, *De anatomicis administrationibus* 10.7 (ii, p. 51 Simon;
translated from Ḥunain's Arabic translation of the lost
original by Duckworth, p. 56)

But in regard to what lies outside the mouth, you find where the
bone which is called 'that which resembles the letter Λ in the
Greek script' (*lambdoid* (=*hyoid*)), there this bone stands in
relation with the tongue through the muscles, and in many
animals, as for instance in apes, with the skull also. In these
[latter] animals on each of the two sides there runs up in the
direction of the tongue a muscle which springs from the cranium
near the process which Herophilus calls the 'pharoid' ('light-
house-like', i.e., the styloid process). *Cf. Gal.* xviiiB. *957–9K.*

93 Rufus Ephesius, *De nominatione partium hominis* 155 (p. 155
Daremberg/Ruelle)

τὸ δὲ ὑπὸ ταῖς ἀντιάσιν ὀστοῦν, τὸ περιειληφὸς τὴν κεφαλὴν
τοῦ βρόγχου, οἱ μὲν ὑοειδὲς διὰ τὸ σχῆμα ὀνομάζουσιν, ὅτι
ἔοικεν τῷ Υ γράμματι· Ἡρόφιλος δὲ παραστάτην καλεῖ, ὅτι
παρέστηκε ταῖς ἀντιάσιν.

2 ὑψηλοειδὲς *Clinch*

93 Some people call the bone below the tonsils, surrounding the
head of the windpipe, 'Y-shaped' (*hyo-eides* (hyoid bone)) on account
of its shape, because it resembles the letter *Υ*[psilon]. But Herophilus
calls it 'assistant' (*parastatēs*), because it 'stands by' (*parestēke*) the
tonsils. (*Os hyoideum; not larynx.*)

94 Pollux, *Onomasticon* 2.202 (*Lexicographi Graeci* IX. I, p. 145
Bethe)

ταῖς γε μὴν ἀντιάσιν ὀστοῦν ὑπόκειται περιειληφὸς τὴν τοῦ
βρόγχου κεφαλήν, καλούμενον ὑπ᾽ ἐνίων ὑοειδές, ὅτι προσέοικε
τῷ τοῦ γράμματος σχήματι· Ἡρόφιλος δ᾽ αὐτό, διὰ τὸ
παρεστηκέναι ταῖς ἀντιάσι, παραστάτην ὠνόμαζεν.

2 καλούμενος *A*   ὑοειδές II   3 γράμματος *plurimi*: πράγματος *A*
Ἡρόδοτος αὐτὸ *C*

94 A bone lies under the tonsils, surrounding the head of the
windpipe, and some people call it 'Y-shaped', because it resembles the
shape of the letter. But Herophilus gave it the name 'assistant'
(*parastatēs*) on account of the fact that it 'stands by' (*parestēkenai*) the
tonsils.

4 Abdominal cavity ('On Anatomy' II?)

95 Galenus, *De semine* 2.6 (IV p. 646K)

εἰς ἔντερα δὲ τά τ᾽ ἐκ τῆς γαστρὸς ἥκει, καὶ τὸ χολῶδες ὑγρὸν ἐξ
ἥπατος, ἐξ ἀδένων τέ τινων ἑτέρων αὖ πάλιν ἐνταῦθα τεταγμένων ὑγρὸν γλίσχρον ὅμοιον σιέλῳ, περὶ ὧν ἀδένων οὐ σμικρὰ
ζήτησις γέγονε τοῖς ἀνατομικοῖς, ἀπὸ Ἡροφίλου τὲ καὶ
5 Εὐδήμου τὴν ἀρχὴν λαβοῦσα.

2 τεταγμένων *Ald*: τετάγμενον *P*   3 σιάλῳ *P*   4 ἀπὸ *Ald*: ἐπ᾽ *P*

95 The substances [secreted] from the stomach come into the
intestines, and so does the bilious humour from the liver and a viscous
fluid, similar to saliva, from some other glands which are located
there. About these glands no small investigation arose among
anatomists, an investigation that received its first impetus from
Herophilus and Eudemus.

96 Galenus, *De venarum arteriarumque dissectione* 1 (II, pp. 780–81 K)

ἐντεῦθεν (sc. ἀπὸ τῶν τοῦ ἥπατος πυλῶν) γὰρ ἐκφυομένη
μεγάλη τις φλὲψ ἀποτείνεται λοξὴ πρός τε τὰ κάτω καὶ ἄλλα
τοῦ 3ῴου μόρια, κατὰ μέσην πως μάλιστα τὴν δωδεκαδάκτυλον
ὑπὸ Ἡροφίλου καλουμένην ἔκφυσιν. ὀνομά3ει δ᾽ οὕτως ἐκεῖνος
5 τὴν ἀρχὴν τοῦ ἐντέρου, πρὶν εἰς ἕλικας ἐλίττεσθαι.

96 From the portal veins of the liver a large vein grows out and
extends obliquely both to the lower parts and to other parts of a living
being, especially along the middle of the growth called 'twelve fingers
long' [sc. *duodenum*] by Herophilus. And he gives this name to the
beginning of the intestine, before it twists into convolutions.

97a Galenus, *De anatomicis administrationibus* 6.9 (II, p. 572K)

97b Oribasius, *Collectiones medicae* 24.19.10 (*CMG* VI.2.1; vol. III, p.
33 Raeder)

μετὰ δὲ ταύτην δωδεκαδάκτυλον οὖσαν τὸ μῆκος, ὡς Ἡρόφιλος
ἀληθῶς ἔφη, κατακάμπτεται πολυειδῶς εἰς ἕλικας, ἀγγείων
παμπόλλων πλῆθος ἔχουσαν, ὅπερ ὀνομά3ουσι νῆστιν, ὅτι
κενὸν ἀεὶ τροφῆς εὑρίσκεται.

1 δωδεκαδάκτυλος οὖσα *Orib.*   2 ἕλικα *Kühn*   3 ἔχουσα πλῆθος *Orib.*

97a–b After this [sc. first part of the intestine], which is twelve
fingers long [sc. *duodenum*], as Herophilus said correctly, the intestine
bends downward into convolutions in many folds with a host of very
many bloodvessels. This part they call the 'fasting' intestine [sc.
jejunum] because it is always found to be deprived of food.

98a Galenus, *De locis affectis* 6.3 (VIII, p. 396K)

ἐδείχθησαν δὲ καὶ οἱ νεφροὶ τὸ ὑδατῶδες ἐν αἵματι ἕλκειν, μὴ
μέντοι τὴν κύστιν ἕλκειν ἐκ τῶν νεφρῶν, ὥσπερ μηδ᾽ ἐκ τῆς
κοιλίας τὰ ἔντερα· πέμπειν δ᾽ ἐκκρίνοντας, εἰς μὲν τὴν κύστιν
τοὺς νεφροὺς διὰ τῶν οὐρητήρων, εἰς δὲ τὴν νῆστιν τὴν κοιλίαν
5 διὰ τῆς ἐκφύσεως, ἣν Ἡρόφιλος ὠνόμασε δωδεκαδάκτυλον ἀπὸ
τοῦ μήκους αὐτῇ τὴν ἐπωνυμίαν θέμενος.

98a It was also shown that the kidneys draw to themselves the watery substance in the blood, but not that the bladder draws it from the kidneys, just as the intestines do not draw it from the abdominal cavity. Rather, the kidneys secrete it and send it into the bladder through the urinal ducts (*urēteres*), while the abdominal cavity sends it to the 'fasting' intestine [sc. *jejunum*] through the process which Herophilus named 'twelve fingers long' [sc. *duodenum*], giving it its name from its length.

98b Theophilus Protaspatharius, *De corporis humani fabrica* 2.7.10 (p. 68 Greenhill)

ὑπέρκειται δὲ τῇ νήστει ἡ δωδεκαδάκτυλος ἔκφυσις, ἔντερον οὖσα καὶ αὐτὴ τῶν λεπτῶν, δώδεκα δακτύλων τὸ μέγεθος ἐπιτείνουσα· διὰ τοῦτο οὖν αὐτὴν Ἡρόφιλος ὠνόμασε δωδεκα-δάκτυλον.

1 τῇ νήστει *E*: τῆς νήστεως *vulg.*   2 δώδεκα δακτύλων *E*:
δωδεκαδάκτυλον *vulg.*   3 ἐπιτείνουσα *E*: ἔχουσα *vulg.*

98b Above the 'fasting part' [sc. *jejunum*] lies the duodenal process, which is a part of the bowels, that is, it is itself part of the small intestines, extending for the size of twelve fingers. For this reason Herophilus gave it the name 'twelve fingers long'.

99 Galenus, *De anatomicis administrationibus* 13.1 (II, p. 126 Simon; translated from Ḥunain's Arabic translation of the lost original by Duckworth, p. 138)

All these structures are clad and ensheathed in a delicate covering [*lesser omentum*], as are other structures which come after them in the region of the organ known as the pancreas. There is also similarly covered the first outgrowth of the intestine for which there is no name at all. For that reason the anatomists have simply called it 'outgrowth', but some speak of it also as 'the outgrowth measuring twelve fingers' [*duodenum*], because Herophilus has said that this is its length.

100a Theo Smyrnaeus, *Expositio rerum mathematicarum ad legendum Platonem utilium* 46 (p. 172 Dupuis; p. 104 Hiller)

Ἡρόφιλος δὲ "τὸ τῶν ἀνθρώπων ἔντερον πηχῶν", εἶναί φησι, "κη'", ὅ ἐστι τέσσαρες ἑβδομάδες.

1 ἡρόφιλος: η *in ras. A*

100a And Herophilus says, 'The intestines of human beings are twenty-eight cubits long', i.e., four hebdomads.

100b Anatolius, *De decade* (p. 36 Heiberg)

Ἡρόφιλος δὲ "τὸ τοῦ ἀνθρώπου ἔντερον πηχῶν" εἶναί φησι "κα'", ὅπερ εἰσὶ τρεῖς ἑβδομάδες.

100b And Herophilus says, 'The intestines of a human being are twenty-one cubits long', which is precisely three hebdomads.

5 *Reproductive organs ('On Anatomy' III?)*

101 Galenus, *De anatomicis administrationibus* 12.8 (II, p. 120 Simon; translated from Ḥunain's Arabic translation of the lost original by Duckworth, p. 131)

For the seminal vessels or ducts join this part [sc. sphincter muscle] of the neck of the bladder after they have dilated and enlarged themselves, in the same way in which the veins dilate on which the disease named *kirsos* breaks out, and from here [this resemblance] Herophilus has named them 'varix-like parastates'* [*ampullae* of *vasa deferentia*?]. We give them the same name, as we follow old custom in the application of names. Herophilus, then, has named 'varix-like' both these two ducts or vessels. He gave them this name, deriving it from what happens to them, that is, the fact that near the place of their attachment and coalescence with the neck of the urinary bladder they dilate

---

* Duckworth reads 'prostates', but see, for example, T102, which confirms that Herophilus' term was *para-statēs* (plural *para-statai*); Simon's reads 'parastates'.

and enlarge themselves, just as the veins which are affected by
the disease named *kirsos* [sc. enlargement of a vein; *varicocele*].

Bordering upon these two, two other ducts are found, one on
each side, and these two ducts Herophilus has called the 'gland-
like' – 'glands' being that 'spongy flesh' [*vesiculae seminales*]. He
gave them that name simply because they originate from the
spongy flesh which just at this place joins the neck of the urinary
bladder at the very same point as that to which those two vessels
or ducts are attached.

102 Galenus, *De usu partium* 14.11 (ii, p. 321 Helmreich)

καὶ τοὺς ἐκ τούτων τῶν σωμάτων (sc. τῶν ἀδενοειδῶν)
ὁρμωμένους πόρους οὐκ ὀκνοῦσιν (sc. οἱ πρότεροι) ὀνομάζειν
ἀγγεῖα σπερματικά, καὶ πρῶτός γε Ἡρόφιλος ἀδενοειδεῖς
παραστάτας ἐκάλεσεν, ὅτι καὶ τὰ τῶν ὄρχεων ἐκφυόμενα
5 κιρσοειδεῖς ἔφθανεν ὀνομάζειν παραστάτας.

3 ἀγγεῖα] αἴτια *AU*   γε] τε *ABLU*   4 παραστάτας *ABLU*:
προστάτας *D*   ὅτι *om. B*   καὶ τὰ] κατὰ *D*

102 Earlier authors do not hesitate to name the passages starting
from these bodies [sc. 'the glandular bodies': seminal vesicles]
'seminal vessels'. Herophilus was in fact the first to call them
'glandular assistants' (*parastatai adenoeideis*), because he had also been
the first to call the vessels that grow from the testicles 'varix-like
assistants' (*parastatai kirsoeideis*).

103 Galenus, *De semine* 1.16 (iv, p. 582K)

καὶ τὸ κατὰ τὴν ἐπιδιδυμίδα περιεχόμενον (sc. ὑγρὸν) ἐκ τούτου
(sc. τοῦ ὄρχεως) μετείληπται πρὸς αὐτήν, ὥσπερ ἐκ ταύτης εἰς
τὸ σπερματικὸν ἀγγεῖον, οὗ παραστάτην κιρσοειδῆ τὸ πρὸς τῷ
καυλῷ μέρος Ἡρόφιλος ὠνόμασεν. (*Vid. T189 sqq.*)

1 ἐπιδιδυμίδα *P Ald*: διδυμίδα *M*   3 κιρσοειδῆ *MP Ald*: *corr. Kühn*
3-4 τὸ πρὸς τ.κ. μέρος *P Ald*: τῷ πρὸς τ.κ. μέρει *M*

103 And the seminal fluid contained in the epididymis is transferred
from the testicle to the epididymis just as it is from there into the

seminal vessel. To the part of the seminal vessel bordering on the shaft [penis] Herophilus gave the name 'varicose assistant' (*parastatēs kirsoeidēs*). (*See Chapter* VII, *T189ff. infra.*)

104 Vindicianus (?), *Fragmentum Bruxellense de semine* I, e codice Bruxellensi 1348–59, fol. 48r (Wellmann, 1901: 208; Werner Jaeger, *Diokles von Karystos* (Berlin, 1938; ²1963), pp. 191–2)

Erasistratus et Herofilus essentiam seminis dicunt sanguinem ... primo igitur, ut Herofilus ait, abruptio corporum hoc testatur quam Graeci ἀνατομήν vocant. etenim seminalium vasculorum interiora atque secretius remota sanguinulenta 5 videntur, sequentia vero sive secunda plurimum a praescriptis demutata sunt, inferiora ac proxima seminis colorem habent. (*Vid. Herophili T191 infra.*)

1–2 erofilus *B (utroque loco)*   2 abruptio *B Neu Wellmann*: aper:io *coni. Jaeger fort. recte*   6 habentia *B Neu: corr. Wellmann*

104 Erasistratus and Herophilis say that the essence of seed is blood ... First, then, as Herophilus says, tearing open bodies, which the Greeks called 'dissection' (*anatomē*), is a witness to this. For, the internal parts of those seminal vessels that are also at a more remote distance [sc. from the genitalia] appear full of blood, whereas the ones that follow next [sc. somewhat closer to the genitalia] are changed very much compared to the aforementioned ones, and the lower, more accessible ones have the colour of seed ... (*See Chapter* VII, *T191 infra.*)

105 Rufus Ephesius, *De nominatione partium hominis* 184–6 (pp. 158–9 Daremberg/Ruelle)

τὰ δὲ σπερματικὰ ἀγγεῖα ἔστι μὲν τέσσαρα, δύο μὲν κιρσοειδῆ, δύο δὲ ἀδενοειδῆ· ἐκαλοῦντο δὲ καὶ γόνιμοι φλέβες. καὶ τῶν κιρσοειδῶν τὰ πρὸς τοῖς διδύμοις, παραστάται· ἐνίοις δὲ καὶ πάντα παραστάτας καλεῖν διαφέρει οὐδέν. σκεπτέον δὲ καὶ εἰ 5 τοῖς θήλεσι τὰ αὐτὰ πεποίηται, ὥσπερ καὶ τοῖς ἄρρεσιν· Ἡροφίλῳ μὲν γὰρ οὐ δοκεῖ τὸ θῆλυ κιρσοειδεῖς ἔχειν παραστάτας. ἐν δὲ προβάτου ὑστέρᾳ εἴδομεν ἐκ τῶν διδύμων πεφυκότα τὰ

ἀγγεῖα κεκιρσωμένα ἑκατέρωθεν. συνετέτρητο δὲ ταῦτα εἰς τὸ
κοίλωμα τῆς ὑστέρας, ἀπὸ ὧν ὑπόμυξον ὑγρὸν πιεζούντων
10 ἀπεκρίνετο· καὶ ἦν πολλὴ δόκησις σπερματικὰ ταῦτα εἶναι, καὶ
τοῦ γένους τῶν κιρσοειδῶν. τοῦτο μὲν δὴ οἷόν ἐστιν, αἱ ἀνατομαὶ
τάχα δείξουσιν.

2 ἀδενοειδῆ *plurimi*: ἐλαειδῆ *L*   3 τοὺς διδύμους *Clinch*   προστάται
ἐνίοι *L*   9 ὑπὸ *Clinch*   πιεζόντων *Clinch*   10–11 ἀπεκρίνετο . . . τοῦ
γένους τῶν *om. L*   12 τάχα *codd.*: δίχα *Clinch*

105   The seminal vessels are four in number, two being varix-like
[*vasa deferentia*], two glandular [seminal vesicles]. They also used to be
called 'reproductive veins'. And the parts of the varicose ones that are
adjacent to the testicles are [called] 'assistants' (*parastatai*). But to
some people it makes no difference to call all the seminal vessels
'assistants'. One must examine whether in females, too, the same
vessels have been constructed [by nature] as in males. For, while
Herophilus thinks that the female does not have the 'varix-like
assistants' (*kirsoeideis parastatai*), we have seen that vessels which have
become varicose grow out of the 'testicles' [sc. ovaries] in the womb of
a sheep, [one] on either side. These opened directly into the cavity of
the uterus, and when they were compressed, a somewhat mucous
liquid was excreted from them. And there was a widespread belief
that these vessels are seminal, and belong to the varix-like kind.
Dissections will perhaps show of what nature this is.

106   Soranus, *Gynaecia* 1.12.2–3 (*CMG* iv, p. 9 Ilberg)

ὁ σπερματικὸς δὲ πόρος ἀπὸ τῆς ὑστέρας δι' ἑκατέρου φέρεται
διδύμου καὶ τοῖς πλευροῖς παραταθεὶς μέχρι τῆς κύστεως εἰς
τὸν ταύτης ἐμφύεται τράχηλον. ἔνθεν δὲ δοκεῖ τὸ τοῦ θήλεος
σπέρμα πρὸς ζῳογονίαν μὴ συλλαμβάνεσθαι τῷ εἰς τὸ ἐκτὸς
5   ἐκχεῖσθαι, περὶ οὗ διελάβομεν ἐν τῷ περὶ σπέρματος λόγῳ· ἔνιοι
δέ, καθὼς βούλεται καὶ Ἡρόφιλος, καὶ ἀνὰ ἕνα κρεμαστῆρά
φασιν αὐτοῖς ἐμπεφυκέναι. καὶ ἡμεῖς δὲ τοῦτο ἐπὶ τῆς αὐτοψίας
ἱστορήκαμεν ἐπί τινος ἐντεροκηλικῆς γυναικός . . .

6 καὶ Ἡρόφιλος *coni. Ilberg cf. Galeni De semine 2.1* (iv p. 596 K = Fr 61): καὶ
ὁ χῖος *P*: καὶ χῖος *Oribasius* (*qui Soranum excerpsit*), *Coll. medic. 24.31.20*
(*CMG* vi.2.1. = vol. iii *p. 43 Raeder*): καὶ Βακχεῖος *Rose*: ὁ Καλχηδόνιος

conieci   ἀνὰ ἕνα κρεμαστῆρά *Reinhold*: ἀνακρεμαστῆρά *Oribasius l.c.*:
ἀνακρεμαστῆρας *P et u.v. archet.* ΑΝᾹ   7 αὐταῖς *Oribasius Pal.*
ἐμπεφυκέναι *Oribasius*: ἐκπεφυκέναι *P*

106 The spermatic duct goes from the uterus through each of the two
'testicles' [ovaries] and, extending along the sides of the uterus up to
the urinary bladder, it grows into its neck. The seed of the female,
therefore, does not seem to contribute to reproduction, since it is
excreted to the outside. With this I dealt separately in my treatise *On
Seed*. And some people say, as Herophilus, too, would have it, that a
suspender (*krēmastēr* (cremasteric muscle?)) is attached to them, one
to each. I, too, have observed this upon personal visual inspection in
the case of a woman suffering from an intestinal hernia.

107 Galenus, *De uteri dissectione* 9 (*CMG* v.2.1, pp. 48–50 Nickel)

καὶ μὴν καὶ τὰ ἀποφυόμενα τῶν ὄρχεων (sc. θηλείων) ἀγγεῖα τὰ
σπερματικὰ πάλιν ὁμοίως φαίνεται περιέχοντα σπέρμα ὡς καὶ
ἐπὶ τῶν ἀρρένων, ἐγγὺς μὲν αὐτῶν τῶν ὄρχεων εὐρέα τε ὄντα καὶ
αἰσθητὴν ἔχοντα τὴν κοιλότητα, στενότερα δὲ καὶ οἷον ἀκοίλια
5 γινόμενα μικρὸν ἀπωτέρω, εἶτα πάλιν εὐρυνόμενα παρὰ ταῖς
κεραίαις, ἔνθα καὶ εἰς τὴν μήτραν καταφύονται. ταύτας δὲ τὰς
ἐμφύσεις οὔτε Ἀριστοτέλης οὔτε Ἡρόφιλος οὔτε Εὐρυφῶν
οἶδεν· ἐμνημόνευσα δὲ τούτων οὐχ ὡς μόνον οὐκ εἰδότων, ἀλλ'
ὡς κάλλιστα ἀνατεμόντων ... οὔτε γὰρ καταγινώσκειν τούτων
10 τολμῶ διὰ τὴν ἐν τοῖς ἄλλοις ἀκρίβειαν, οὔτε μικρὰ οὕτως ἐστὶν
ταῦτα τὰ ἀγγεῖα, ὥστε ἄν τινα λαθεῖν. ἀλλὰ περὶ μὲν τῶν εἰς τὸν
τράχηλον τῆς κύστεως ἐμφυομένων ἀκριβῶς εἴρηται αὐτοῖς,
ὅτι τε εἰς τὸν αὐτὸν τόπον ἐμβάλλει, εἰς ὃν καὶ ἐπὶ τῶν ἀρρένων,
καὶ ὅτι ἀδενοειδῆ ἐστι τὰ ἀγγεῖα ταῦτα καὶ ὅτι ἀπὸ τῶν διδύμων
15 ἐκτείνεται, τῇ μήτρᾳ παραφυόμενα. περὶ δὲ τῶν κατὰ τὰς
κεραίας οὐδὲν εἰρήκασιν.

3 αὐτῶν *om. Nicolaus*   7 Εὐρυφῶν *codd.*: eudimus (-amus *Nic.ᵃ*) *Nicolaus*

107 And indeed the seminal vessels which grow from the [female]
'testicles' [ovaries] are observed to contain seed, again in a similar
manner as in males: close to the 'testicles' [ovaries] themselves these
vessels are wide and have a perceptible hollow, but a little further
away [from the ovaries] they become narrower and, as it were, not

hollow; then they become wider again at the horn-like projections (*keraiai* (tubes)) where they also grow into the uterus. Of these insertions neither Aristotle nor Herophilus nor Euryphon knows. I mentioned these authors not only because they do not know them, but because they dissected most excellently . . . For neither do I dare condemn these authors, because of their accuracy in all other matters, nor are these vessels so small that they could escape one's notice. On the other hand, concerning the [vessels] which grow into the neck of the urinary bladder, they accurately said both that these enter into the same place as in males and that these vessels are gland-like and extend from the 'testicles' [sc. ovaries], growing along the uterus. But concerning the vessels at the horns they said nothing.

108a Galenus, *De uteri dissectione* 3 (*CMG* v.2.1, p. 38 Nickel)

108b Oribasius, *Collectiones medicae* 24.29.6–8 (*CMG* vi.2.1, vol. iii, p. 40 Raeder) (Excerpted from Galen)

108c Aëtius Amidenus, *Libri medicinales* 16.1 (p. 2 Zervos) (Excerpted from Galen)

τὸ δὲ σχῆμα αὐτῆς (sc. τῆς μήτρας) τὸ μὲν ἄλλο πᾶν σῶμα καὶ μάλιστα ὁ πυθμὴν κύστει ἔοικεν· καθ' ὅσον δὲ ἐπὶ τῶν πλαγίων ἀποφύσεις ἔχει μαστοειδεῖς, πρὸς τὰς λαγόνας ἀνανευούσας, ταύτῃ οὐκέτι ἔοικεν. αὐτῶν δὲ τούτων τὸ σχῆμα ὁ μὲν Ἡρόφιλος 5 ἡμιτόμῳ κύκλου ἕλικι εἰκάζει, Διοκλῆς δὲ κέρασι φυομένοις, διὰ ταῦτα καὶ ὠνόμασε κεραίας παρωνύμως ἀπὸ τοῦ κέρατος.

1–6 *Aetii excerptum valde mutilatum*   1 σῶμα *non habet Oribasius*   2 ἐπὶ *codd.*: ἐκ F (*Orib.*): καὶ P(*Orib.*)   3 ἐπιφύσεις *Orib.*   λαγόνας *codd.*: femora *Nic.*   ἀνανεζούσας V   4 ταύτην F (*Orib.*)   5 ἡμιτόμῳ] ἡμιτόμου P²F(*Orib.*), semi inscisi *Nic.*   κύκλου *e* κύκλω *corr.* V.   ἕλεκον F (*Orib.*)   ἀπεικάζει *Orib. plur.*: ἀπεικάζεται F (*Orib.*)

108a–c As far as the shape [sc. of the uterus] is concerned, its entire body, and particularly its base, resembles the urinary bladder. But in so far as it has breast-like offshoots on the sides which tilt upward towards the flanks, it no longer resembles the bladder. The shape of these very offshoots Herophilus likens to a half-curve of a circle, whereas Diocles likens them to horns that grow out, and on account of this also gave them the name 'horn-like [projections]' (*keraiai*), deriving it from 'horn' (*keras*).

109 Galenus, *De usu partium* 14.11 (II, p. 323 Helmreich)

εἰς δὲ τὰ παρὰ τῶν ἰδίων ὄρχεων (sc. ἀγγεῖα?) αἱ κεραῖαι καὶ διὰ
τοῦθ' ὡς πρὸς τὰς λαγόνας ἀνανενεύκασιν ἄνω καὶ κατὰ βραχὺ
γιγνόμεναι στενότεραι τελευτῶσιν εἰς ἀκριβῶς στενὰ πέρατα,
συναπτόμενον ἑκάτερον αὐτῶν τῷ καθ' ἑαυτὰ διδύμῳ. καλεῖ γὰρ
5 Ἡρόφιλος οὕτω τὸν ὄρχιν.

1 τὰ *coni. De Lacy:* τὸ *codd.:* τὸν *Bas.* 4 συναπτόμενον ἑκάτερον *AL²U:*
συναπτομένων ἑκατέρων *cett.:* συναπτομένης ἑκατέρας *Helmreich* ἑαυτὰ
codd.: ἑαυτὴν *Helmreich*

109 The 'horn-like projections' [go] to the [ducts/vessels] that come
from the [female's] own 'testicles' (*orcheis* (ovaries)), and for this
reason they tilt upward toward the flanks and, gradually becoming
narrower, terminate in extremely narrow ends [sc. in the ducts], each
of which is attached to the 'twin' on its own side; for 'twin' (*didymos*) is
what Herophilus calls the 'testicle' [ovary].

110 Galenus, *De uteri dissectione* 7 (*CMG* v.2.1, p. 46 Nickel)

εἰκάζει δὲ αὐτοῦ (sc. τοῦ τῆς μήτρας αὐχένος) τὴν φύσιν ὁ
Ἡρόφιλος βρόγχου τῷ ἄκρῳ.

1 αὐτῆς *V: corr. Corn. Kühn* 2 βρόγχου τῷ ἄκρῳ *codd.:* bronchio duro
Nic.

110 Herophilus likens the nature of the neck of the uterus [cervix?] to
the upper part of the windpipe.

111a Soranus, *Gynaecia* 1.10.3 (*CMG* IV, p. 8 Ilberg)

111b Oribasius, *Collectiones medicae* 24.31.13 (*CMG* VI.2.1; vol. III,
p. 43 Raeder; excerpted from Soranus)

κατὰ μέντοι τὴν φύσιν τρυφερόν ἐστιν (sc. τὸ τοῦ γυναικείου
αἰδοίου στόμιον) καὶ σαρκῶδες ἐπὶ τῶν ἀδιακορεύτων, σομ-
φότητι πνεύμονος ἢ τρυφερίᾳ γλώττης ἐοικός, ἐπὶ δὲ τῶν
ἀποκεκυηκυιῶν τυλωδέστερον γίνεται, κεφαλῇ πολύποδος ἢ

5 ἄκρῳ βρόγχου, καθώς φησιν Ἡρόφιλος, ὅμοιον, τυλούμενον τῇ
παρόδῳ τῶν ἀποκρινομένων καὶ ἀποτικτομένων.

2-3 σοφότητι *P*   3 πλεύμονος *Oribasius (F exc.)*   4 κεφαλῇ *P (Orib.)*:
ὡς κεφαλὴ *P*: κεφαλὴ *F (Orib.)*

111a–b [The mouth of the female pudendum] by nature is delicate
and fleshy in the case of undeflowered women, resembling the
sponginess of the lung or the tenderness of the tongue, but in the case
of women who have given birth it becomes more callous, similar to the
head of an octopus or to the upper part of the windpipe, just as
Herophilus says, since it is made callous by the passage of what is
excreted and of what is brought to birth. *(Cf. Chapter* vii, *T201 infra.)*

112 Galenus, *De usu partium* 14.3 (ii, p. 290 Helmreich)

μὴ τοίνυν ἔτι θαυμάζειν ἢ ἐν ταῖς τῶν ζῴων διαιρέσεσι θεώμενος
ἢ παρ' Ἡροφίλῳ γεγραμμένον ἢ ἄλλῳ τινὶ τῶν ἀνατομικῶν
εὑρίσκων, ὡς ὁ τῶν ὑστερῶν αὐχὴν διέστραπταί τε καὶ σκολιός
ἐστι κατὰ τὸν λοιπὸν ἅπαντα χρόνον, ἐν ᾧ μήτ' εἴσω φέρεται τὸ
5 σπέρμα μήτ' ἔξω τὸ ἔμβρυον· ἕπεται γὰρ τοῦτο τῇ προειρημένῃ
κατασκευῇ συμμέτρως ἐχούσῃ μαλακότητός τε καὶ σκληρότη-
τος.

1 θαυμάζεις *B*: θαύμαζε *Ch*   5 τῇ *plurimi*: ἡ *U*: om. *A*

112 No longer be surprised, therefore, if you either see in dissections
of animals or find in the writings of Herophilus or some other
anatomist that the neck of uteri [i.e., the cervix?] is both twisted and
crooked at all other times, i.e., when neither seed is passing to the
inside nor the foetus to the outside. For this follows from the
aforementioned construction [sc. of the 'neck' of the uterus], which
has a due proportion of both softness and hardness.

113 Soranus, *Gynaecia* 1.57.3–4 (*CMG* iv, p. 42 Ilberg)

καὶ αὐτὸ δὲ τὸ ἐμβρύων ἐμφυόμενον εἰς σῶμα καλοῦμεν ὀμφαλόν.
συγκέκριται δὲ ⟨ἐκ τεσσάρων⟩ τὸν ἀριθμὸν ἀγγείων, δύο
φλεβωδῶν καὶ δύο ἀρτηριωδῶν, δι' ὧν εἰς θρέψιν ὕλη αἱματική
καὶ πνευματικὴ παρακομίζεται τοῖς ἐμβρύοις ... οἱ δὲ πολλοὶ

5 τὰς φλέβας μὲν εἰς τὸ ἧπαρ (sc. ἐμφύεσθαι) οἴονται, τὰς ἀρτηρίας δὲ εἰς τὴν καρδίαν. Ἡρόφιλος δὲ τὰς φλέβας μὲν εἰς τὴν κοίλην φλέβα, ⟨τὰς⟩ ἀρτηρίας δὲ εἰς τὴν παχεῖαν ἀρτηρίαν τὴν παρατείνουσαν τοῖς σπονδύλοις, πρὸ δὲ τῆς εἰς αὐτὴν ἐμφύσεως παρὰ τὴν κύστιν αὐτὰς πλαγιοφορεῖσθαι παρ' 10 ἑκατέρας πλευράς.

1 ἐμβρύων *Ilberg*: ἔμβρυον *P*: ⟨τῷ⟩ ἐμβρύῳ *Ermerins*   εἰς *Ilberg*: ὡς *P*   2 ἐκ τεττάρων *add. Ermerins* (τεσσάρων *Ilberg*)   ἀγγείῳ *P*: *corr. Dietz*   3 ἀρτηριωδῶν *Schöne*: ἀρτηριῶν *P*   5 ὁρῶνται *P*: *corr. Ermerins*   7 φλέβαν *P*: τὰς *add. Ermerins*   παχεῖαν *Ermerins*: τραχίαν *P*   8 σφονδύλοις *Rose*

113 That which grows into the body of foetuses is itself called umbilical cord (*omphalos*). For it is a combination of vessels, four in number, two of them being venous and two arterial. Through these vessels blood-like and pneumatic matter is conveyed to the foetuses for nourishment ... Most people think the veins grow into the liver, and the arteries into the heart. Herophilus, however, thinks the veins enter the hollow vein [*vena cava*], while the arteries enter the thick artery [*aorta*] which extends along the vertebrae, but before they grow into it they move transversely across the urinary bladder along either side.

114 Galenus, *De uteri dissectione* 5 (*CMG* v.2.1, pp. 42–4 Nickel)

"ἕτερα δὲ τέτταρα (sc. ἀγγεῖα) οὐκ ἐπὶ πασῶν γυναικῶν, ἀλλ' ἔστιν ἐφ' ὧν", φησὶν Ἡρόφιλος, "τῶν ἐπὶ τοὺς νεφροὺς ἰόντων ἀποφυόμενα εἰς τὴν μήτραν ἐμβάλλει", ὅπερ ἐπὶ μὲν τῶν ἄλλων ζῴων οὐχ εὗρον πλὴν σπανίως ἐν πιθήκοις. οὐ μὴν ἀπιστῶ τὸ 5 πολλάκις εὑρεῖν αὐτὰ ἐπὶ γυναικῶν τὸν Ἡρόφιλον· ἱκανὸς γὰρ ἦν τά τε ἄλλα τῆς τέχνης καὶ τῶν δι' ἀνατομῆς γινωσκομένων ἐπὶ τὸ ἀκριβέστατον ἥκων καὶ τὴν πλείστην ἐπίγνωσιν οὐκ ἐπὶ ἀλόγων ζῴων, καθάπερ οἱ πολλοί, ἀλλ' ἐπ' αὐτῶν τῶν ἀνθρώπων πεποιημένος. οὕτως δὲ καὶ ὑμέσιν ἠμφιέσθαι τὰ 10 τρέφοντα τὴν μήτραν ἀγγεῖά φησιν, ὧν ἐλέγομεν ἐξηρτῆσθαι αὐτήν, καὶ γίνεσθαι τοὺς ὑμένας ἀεὶ παχυτέρους τε καὶ σκληροτέρους καὶ τυλωδεστέρους ταῖς πλείονα κυησάσαις.

3 ὅπερ *codd.*: que (sc. vasa) *Nicolaus*   5 πολλάκις *om. Nicolaus*   6 τῆς τέχνης *om. Nicolaus*   9 πεποιημένοι *V*: *corr. C et sec. Nicolaum*

(erophilum . . . facientem) *P²* οὕτως *codd.*: iste *Nicolaus*, οὗτος *P²*
ἡμφιέσθαι *codd.*: ἐμφύεσθαι *Kühn* 10 λέγομεν *V: sec. Nicolaum*
(dicebamus) *corr. Nickel* 11 αὐτήν *codd.*: vesicam *Nicolaus*: κύστιν
Kühn 12 πλείονα *codd.*: πλείω *Kühn*

114 'Not in the case of all women but in some', says Herophilus, 'four other vessels branch off from those that go to the kidneys, and enter the uterus.' This I did not find in other living beings, except occasionally in apes. I do not, however, disbelieve the fact that Herophilus often found them in women. For he was not only competent in other branches of the art [of medicine], but he attained the highest degree of accuracy in things which become known by dissection and he obtained the greater part of his new knowledge not, like the majority [of physicians], from irrational animals but from human beings themselves. Thus he also says that the vessels which nourish the uterus, and from which I said it is suspended, are clothed in membranes, and that these membranes again and again become thicker, harder, and more callous in women who have become pregnant several times.

6 Vascular anatomy ('On Anatomy' IV?)

115 Galenus, *De placitis Hippocratis et Platonis* 6.5.22 (*CMG* v.4.1.2, p. 392 De Lacy)

οὐδεὶς τῶν ἀνατομικῶν ἀνδρῶν ἐπὶ τὸ γράφειν ἀφικόμενος
ἀνατομὴν φλεβῶν ἑτέραν ἀρχὴν τῆς διδασκαλίας ἐπιτήδειον
ἠδυνήθη ποιήσασθαι παρελὼν τὸ ἧπαρ, ἀλλ' εἴτ' ἀπορεῖν ὑπὲρ
ἀρχῆς ἔφησεν, ὡς Ἡρόφιλος, εἴτ' εὐπορεῖν, ὡς ἄλλοι πολλοὶ καὶ
5 ὁ ἡμέτερος Πέλοψ, ὅμως τήν γε διδασκαλίαν ὀλίγου δεῖν
ἅπαντες ἀφ' ἥπατος ἐποιήσαντο.

6 ἐφ' *H: corr. Kalbfleisch (1892)*

115 No anatomist, when he has come to record the anatomy of the veins, could pass over the liver and establish a different, but still appropriate, starting-point for his instruction. Rather, whether he said that he was at a loss concerning a starting-point, as did Herophilus, or that he had a clear resolution, as did many others, including my [teacher] Pelops, practically all of them nevertheless established their instruction, at least, starting from the liver.

116 Galenus, *De usu partium* 6.10 (I, p. 325 Helmreich)

ἐν μὲν γὰρ τοῖς ἄλλοις ἅπασι μορίοις τῆς ἴσης ἀρτηρίας τῇ
φλεβί, τὸ πάχος τῶν χιτώνων οὐκ ἴσον, ἀλλ' εἰς τοσοῦτον ἄρα
διενήνοχεν, ὥσθ' Ἡρόφιλος ὀρθῶς ἐστοχάσθαι δοκεῖ, τὴν
ἀρτηρίαν τῆς φλεβὸς ἐξαπλασίαν ἀποφηνάμενος εἶναι τῷ
5 πάχει.

2 ἄρα *om. B*   3 ὥστ' *B²U:* ὡς *D¹*

116 In all the other parts [of the body, as opposed to the artery that
goes to the lungs], when an artery is equal [in size] to a vein, the
thickness of their coats is not equal. Rather, it is different to such a
degree that Herophilus seems to have conjectured correctly when he
stated that the artery is six times as thick as the vein.

117 Rufus Ephesius, *De nominatione partium hominis* 203–4 (p. 162
Daremberg/Ruelle)

Ἡρόφιλος δὲ ἀρτηριώδη φλέβα τὴν παχυτάτην καὶ μεγίστην
τὴν ἀπὸ τῆς καρδίας καλεῖ φερομένην ἐπὶ τὸν πλεύμονα· ἔχει
γὰρ ὑπεναντίως τῷ πλεύμονι πρὸς τὰ ἄλλα. αἱ μὲν φλέβες
ἐνταῦθα ἐρρωμέναι καὶ ἐγγυτάτω τὴν φύσιν ἀρτηριῶν, αἱ δὲ
5 ἀρτηρίαι ἀσθενεῖς καὶ ἐγγυτάτω τὴν φύσιν φλεβῶν.

2 τῶν ἀπὸ *L*

117 Herophilus calls the thickest and largest vein that proceeds from
the heart to the lung 'artery-like' (sc. the pulmonary artery); for, in
the lung the situation is the opposite of the other parts, inasmuch as
the veins there are strong and very close in nature to arteries, whereas
the arteries are weak and very close in nature to veins.

118 Scholium F in Oribasii *Collectionum medicarum* librum incertum
15.19 (XXII). (*CMG* VI.2.2, vol. IV, p. 105 Raeder)

(*Ad* ἀρτηρίας δ' ἐξαπλάσιον ἢ κατὰ φλέβα πάχος ἐχούσης.) τὸ
περὶ ἀρτηρίας τοῦτο ἐν τῷ ις' κεφαλαίῳ ἐμνημόνευσεν (sc. ὁ
Γαληνὸς) ἐν τῷ περὶ χρείας μορίων, ἀποδεχόμενος τὸν Ἡρόφιλον ὀρθῶς περὶ τούτου, καί φησιν ὅτι κατὰ τὸν πνεύμονα μόνον,

5 διὰ τὸ ἀνάπαλιν ἡμῖν πρὸς ἀρτηρίας καὶ φλεβός, ἡ δὲ φλὲψ ἀρτηρίας ἔχει πάχος· καὶ τούτου τὴν αἰτίαν ἐπεξέρχεται.

5 ἡ μὲν ἀρτηρία add. post καὶ Daremberg

118 [*A scholiast's comment on* 'the artery having a thickness six times as great as that of the vein'; *from Galen, De semine, 1.13 (IV, p. 560K)*] Galen mentions this about the artery in Chapter 16 of his *On the Usefulness of the Parts*, correctly accepting Herophilus' view concerning this. He says that only in the lung, on account of the inverse relationship of the vein to our arteries there, the vein has the thickness of an artery. He gives a full account of the cause of this, too.

119 Galenus, *De placitis Hippocratis et Platonis* 1.10.3–4 (*CMG* v.4.1.2, p. 96 De Lacy)

ἐμοὶ μὲν δοκεῖ (sc. ᾽Αριστοτέλης) τὰς ὑπὸ ῾Ηροφίλου νευρώδεις διαφύσεις ὠνομασμένας αὐτὸς οὐ νευρώδεις ἀλλ᾽ ἄντικρυς εἰρηκέναι νεῦρα. πέρατα δ᾽ ἐστὶ ταῦτα τῶν ἐπὶ τοῖς στόμασι τῆς καρδίας ὑμένων, ὑπὲρ ὧν ᾽Ερασίστρατος μὲν ἀκριβῶς ἔγραψεν,
5 ῾Ηρόφιλος δὲ ἀμελῶς. (*Cf. T54 supra.*)

1 ἡροφίλου C¹ (ο¹ *ex* ρ *u.v.*)   2 αὐτὰς C: *corr. Herbst (1911)*: ταύτας
Schöne (*vid. De Lacy p. 37, §4*)

119 It seems to me that what Herophilus called 'nerve-like strands' Aristotle did not call 'nerve-like' but simply 'nerves'. These are the terminal points of the membranes [sc. valves] at the openings of the heart, about which Erasistratus wrote accurately, Herophilus, however, carelessly. (*Cf. Chapter v, T54 supra.*)

120 Galenus, *De anatomicis administrationibus* 7.11 (II, pp. 624–5K)

εἰρήσεται δὲ καὶ ὅτι τὰ τῆς καρδίας ὦτα τῶν κοιλιῶν αὐτῆς ἐκτός ἐστιν. εἰ δέ τις αὐτὰ μέρη τοῦ σπλάγχνου θέμενος, ὥσπερ ῾Ηρόφιλος, ἐπὶ πλέον ἐξέτεινε τὸν ἀριθμὸν τῶν στομάτων, καὶ ταύτῃ δόξει διαφωνεῖν ᾽Ερασιστράτῳ τε καὶ ἡμῖν εἰρηκόσι δ᾽ τὰ
5 πάντα εἶναι στόματα τῶν κατὰ τὴν καρδίαν ἀγγείων τεττάρων.

120 It will also be explained that the auricles of the heart are outside its ventricles. But if anyone were to postulate that the auricles are

parts of the interior, as does Herophilus, and thus to increase the number of orifices, then in this, too, he will seem to differ both from Erasistratus and from myself, since we have said that the total number of orifices is four, for the four vessels of the heart.*

121 Galenus, *De pulsuum usu* 2 (v, p. 155K; p. 200 Furley/Wilkie)

ἀλλὰ καὶ αὐτοῦ τούτου (sc. δαπανωμένου τοῦ ψυχικοῦ πνεύματος, ἐπεί τις μέχρι πολλοῦ καλῶς ἔτρεχε) τὸ δικτυοειδὲς πλέγμα
πρὸς τῶν ἀμφὶ τὸν Ἡρόφιλον κληθὲν ἐδόκει τὴν αἰτίαν ἔχειν. ἐκεῖ
γὰρ αἱ ἐπὶ τὸν ἐγκέφαλον ἀνιοῦσαι καρωτίδες ἀρτηρίαι, πρὶν
5 διελθεῖν τὴν σκληρὰν μήνιγγα, σχίζονται πολυειδῶς ὑπ' αὐτῆς,
περιπλεκόμεναι κατὰ πολλοὺς στίχους, ὡς εἰ νοήσαις ἀλλήλοις
ἐπικείμενα δίκτυα πλείω, καὶ χώραν παμπόλλην ἣν καλοῦσιν
ἐγκεφάλου βάσιν καταλαμβάνουσιν, ἐνὸν αὐταῖς εὐθὺς μὲν
διεκπεσεῖν τὰς μήνιγγας, ἐμφῦναι δὲ εἰς τὸν ἐγκέφαλον, οὗπερ ἐξ
10 ἀρχῆς ἴενται.

10 ἴενται *S Ald*: ἰέναι *Kühn*

121 But the 'net-like plexus' [*rete mirabile*], as it is called by those around Herophilus, seemed to be the cause of just this [sc. that the psychic pneuma becomes exhausted when someone runs hard and far]. For when the carotid arteries ascend toward the brain, this is where they are divided in many ways by the dura mater, before they go through it. They twist around in many rows, as they would if you were to conceive of several nets lying on each other, and they occupy a very great area, which they call the 'base' (*basis*) of the brain. They have the capacity to escape into the meninges right away, and to root themselves in the brain, to which, in fact, they are proceeding from the outset.

122a Galenus, *De anatomicis administrationibus* 9.1 (II, p. 712K)

122b Oribasius, *Collectiones medicae* 24.1.7–8 (*CMG* VI.2.1, vol. III, pp. 4–5 Raeder; excerpted from Galen)

---

* I.e., for pulmonary vein, vena cava, pulmonary artery, aorta.

ἐν αὐτῷ μὲν οὖν τῷ γυμνοῦσθαι τῶν περικειμένων ὀστῶν τὰς
διπλόας τῆς μήνιγγος πολλάκις ἀπορρήγνυταί τι καὶ διασπᾶ-
ται. καὶ τοῦτ' ἀρχή σοι γενήσεται τοῦ καθιέναι τι τῶν εἰρημένων
ὀργάνων εἰς τὴν κοιλίαν τοῦ αἵματος. εἰ δὲ καὶ μὴ διασπασθείη,
5 τέμνων ὀξείᾳ σμίλῃ τὴν πλευρὰν ἑκατέραν τῆς διπλῆς μήνιγγος
ἐν τοῖς κάτω μέρεσιν, ἔνθα πρῶτον ἐμπίπτει τῷ κρανίῳ, κᾆπειτα
καὶ ἐκεῖ ἐμβαλὼν διὰ τῆς τομῆς τὴν σμίλην, ἄνω βιάζεσθαι πειρῶ
μέχρι τῆς κορυφῆς, ἔνθα συμβάλλουσιν ἀλλήλαις αἱ δύο φλέβες,
ἥντινα χώραν Ἡρόφιλος ὀνομάζει ληνόν. ἔστι δ' αὕτη μὲν ἥν
10 ἐκεῖνος οὕτως ὀνομάζει διὰ βάθους μᾶλλον, ἐπιπολῆς δ' ἑτέρα
συμβολὴ φλεβῶν μικρῶν ἐπικειμένων τῇ ληνῷ κατὰ τὴν παχεῖαν
ὡσαύτως μήνιγγα γεγενημένη.

1–8 ἐν αὐτῷ . . . κορυφῆς non habet Oribasius   8 ἔνθα δὲ Oribasius   9 ὁ
Ἡρόφιλος Oribasius   αὐτὴ Oribasii C   10 οὕτως om. Oribasius
11 ἐπικειμένη Oribasius

122a–b In the act itself of stripping the surrounding bones from the
folds of the meninx, some part of the meninx often is torn and
detached. This will be the place for you to insert one of the
instruments mentioned [*dipyrēnon, smilē, spathomēlē*] into the cavity
containing blood [sinus]. But if it is not detached, make an incision
with a sharp scalpel on either side of the fold of the meninx in the
lower parts where it first reaches the skull, and then, also inserting the
scalpel there through the incision, try to force it up to the top where
the two veins meet, the area which Herophilus calls a 'wine vat' [sc.
torcular Herophili]. But while the area to which he gives this name lies a
little deeper, there is on the top a different junction of small veins
which lie on the 'torcular', having arisen in like manner at the thick
meninx.

123 Galenus, *De usu partium* 9.6 (II, p. 19 Helmreich)

συμβάλλουσι δὲ κατὰ τὴν κορυφὴν τῆς κεφαλῆς αἱ παράγουσαι
τὸ αἷμα διπλώσεις τῆς μήνιγγος εἰς χώραν τινὰ κοινὴν οἷον
δεξαμενήν, ἣν δὴ καὶ δι' αὐτὸ τοῦτο προσαγορεύειν ἔθος ἐστὶν
Ἡροφίλῳ ληνόν· ἐντεῦθεν δ' οἷον ἐξ ἀκροπόλεώς τινος ἅπασι
5 τοῖς ὑποκειμένοις μορίοις ὀχετοὺς ἐπιπέμπουσιν.

1 συμβάλλουσαι BDL¹U: -ουσι L²   2 κοινὴν codd.: κενὴν Ald Kühn

123 At the crown of the head the folds of the membrane [*sinus transversus*] that conduct the blood come together into a common space like a cistern, and for this very reason it was Herophilus' custom to call it 'wine vat' (*lēnos* (*torcular Herophili*)). From this point, as from some acropolis, they [sc. the sinuses] send forth canals to all the parts lying below them.

124 Galenus, *De anatomicis administrationibus* 9.3 (II, pp. 719–20K)

ὄψει δὲ καὶ τὰ καλούμενα χοροειδῆ πλέγματα κατὰ ταύτας (sc. κοιλίας τοῦ ἐγκεφάλου). ὀνομάζουσι δ' οἱ περὶ τὸν Ἡρόφιλον αὐτὰ χοροειδῆ συστρέμματα, παρονομάσαντες δηλονότι τῶν χορίων, ἃ τοῖς κυουμένοις ἔξωθεν ἐν κύκλῳ περιβέβληται,
5 φλεβῶν ὄντα καί ἀρτηριῶν πλέγματα, λεπτοῖς ὑμέσι συνεχο-
μένων.

124 You will also see in the ventricles [of the brain] what is called the 'choroid plexuses'. Those around Herophilus call them 'choroid twisted clusters', obviously naming them after the membranes (*choria*) which are wrapped in a circle around the outside of foetuses, since these choroids are plexuses of veins and arteries held together by thin membranes.

125 Rufus Ephesius, *De nominatione partium hominis* 149–50 (p. 153 Daremberg/Ruelle)

ὁ δὲ καλύπτων τὰς κοιλίας ἔνδοθεν χιτὼν χοριοειδής· Ἡρόφιλος δὲ καὶ μήνιγγα χοριοειδῆ καλεῖ. τὰ δὲ ἀπὸ τοῦ ἐγκεφάλου
βλαστήματα, νεῦρα αἰσθητικὰ καὶ προαιρετικά, διὰ ὧν αἴσθησις
καὶ προαιρετικὴ κίνησις καὶ πᾶσα σώματος πρᾶξις συντελεῖται.

1 χοροειδής L Clinch

125 The tunic covering the ventricles [of the brain] on the inside is chorioid. Herophilus also calls it 'chorioid meninx'. And the offshoots from the brain [he calls? are?] the sensory and voluntary motor nerves, through which sensation and voluntary motion and all action of the body are accomplished.

126 Galenus, *In Hippocratis Epidemiarum 2.4.1 comment. 4* (ad
Hippocratis v. 120 sq. L). (Translated from Ḥunain's Arabic
translation of the lost original; *CMG* v.10.1, p.312 Pfaff)

Just as Hippocrates recognized these things [sc. the anatomy of
the abdomen] only by making an incision in the skin and
observing what lies beneath it, so, too, Herophilus later gained
knowledge of it. He did not confine himself to learning this from
5 Hippocrates, but made an effort to learn things from nature
itself – through which you, too, could recognize what he
recognized. Like Hippocrates, he also wrote about the anatomy
of the veins. Many physicians have also exposed these veins in
the bodies of human beings and have seen them and have
10 written the same about them as did Hippocrates and Herophilus.

5 Herophilus *Pfaff (pro* Hippocrates *u.v.)*

127 Galenus, *De usu partium* 4.19 (I, pp. 246–7 Helmreich)

πρῶτον μὲν γὰρ παντὶ τῷ μεσεντερίῳ φλέβας ἐποίησεν (sc. ἡ
φύσις) ἰδίας, ἀνακειμένας αὐτῶν τῇ θρέψει τῶν ἐντέρων, μὴ
περαιουμένας εἰς τὸ ἧπαρ. ὡς γὰρ καὶ Ἡρόφιλος ἔλεγεν, εἰς
ἀδενώδη τινὰ σώματα τελευτῶσιν αἱ φλέβες αὗται, τῶν ἄλλων
5 ἁπασῶν ἐπὶ τὰς πύλας ἀναφερομένων.

1 ἐν παντὶ *BLU*   2 αὐτῶν *L²*: αὐτῷ *BDU*   4 αὗται αἱ φλέβες *D*

127 First, throughout the mesentery [nature] created special veins
[lymphatic vessels] which are devoted to the nourishment of the
intestines themselves but which do not pass on into the liver. For as
Herophilus, too, says, these veins terminate in certain glandular
bodies [sc. lymphatic glands of the mesentery], although all the other
veins proceed upward to the porta.

128 Galenus, *De anatomicis administrationibus* 13.10 (II, p. 161
Simon; translated by Duckworth, p. 177, from Ḥunain's
Arabic translation of the lost original)

As regards the other things that you see in the arteries and the veins, there is no difference between mature and foetal bodies. But now, since Erasistratus and Herophilus, and other anatomists who lived after them, when they had completed their discussion of the dissection of the veins and of the arteries which have no veins alongside them, wanted to enumerate these in a single list, but never included them all, I think that I should supplement here my description . . .

7 Bones

129 Rufus Ephesius, *De nominatione partium hominis* 123 (p. 149 Daremberg/Ruelle)

τῶν δὲ ὀστῶν τὸ μὲν ἔσω, κνήμη, καὶ τούτου τὸ ἔμπροσθεν, ἀντικνήμιον [τὸ δὲ ἔξω, κερκίς]· Ἡρόφιλος δὲ καὶ τὴν κνήμην κερκίδα ὀνομάζει.

2 τὸ . . . κερκίς *del. Daremberg*

129 One of the bones [sc. of the lower leg], the inner one, is called *knēmē* [tibia], and the part in front of it *antiknēmion* [shin]. Herophilus, however, also calls the tibia *kerkis* [*lit.*, 'weaver's shuttle; taper rod'].

C · COMMENTS

T60 Since Oribasius copied this passage from Galen, Galen remains the primary source for T60, which contains one of the more substantial fragments in this collection. But significant textual variants occur in Oribasius' text, and these are recorded in the apparatus. *Orib.*, without further specification, refers to *P*, which Raeder has identified as the source of all other MSS containing Book xxiv of Oribasius' *Collectiones medicae*.

On the earlier anatomical treatments of the liver, see above, pp. 162–4 and nn. 68–76 (cf. also *Comments*, T127). A measure of the anatomical advance represented by this fragment is the fact that Galen, about four and a half centuries later, still accepted Herophilus' account as correct in all essential respects: 'This Herophilus said correctly' and 'Herophilus writes very accurately [*or*: most accurately] about it' (T60).

The number of its lobes: the number of hepatic lobes had been a long-standing problem in Greek antiquity, in part because of the dependence of earlier anatomists upon the examination of animal livers. In the Hippocratic treatise *On the Nature of Bones* 1 (IX, p. 168L) the liver is said to have five lobes or *loboi* (on the fourth of which, it is said, the gallbladder lies), whereas only one lobe (*lobos*) is mentioned in *Epidemics* 2.4.1 (V, pp. 120ff.L) and in Plato's *Timaeus* 71C1. The analysis of pre-Aristotelian uses of λοβός (*lobos*) with reference to the liver is complicated by the fact that *lobos* does not always clearly refer to the hepatic lobe or lobes rather than to the processus pyramidalis or processus caudatus or to the liver in general. Plato, *Timaeus* 71C1; Hp., *Epidemics* 6.8.28 (V, p. 354L); and Euripides, *Electra* 827 provide examples of such ambiguous uses of *lobos*; in Aeschylus *Eumenides* 159 it seems to be used of the liver itself. Herophilus' text is, however, unambiguous in this respect, and it is the first to describe a two-lobed human liver. Aristotle, as I mentioned earlier, correctly observes that the liver does not have the same number of lobes or the same structure in all living beings: τό τε γὰρ ἧπαρ τοῖς μὲν πολυσχιδές ἐστι, τοῖς δὲ μονοφυέστερον (*De partibus animalium* 3.12.673b16–18); cf. *Historia animalium* 2.17.507a11–14: some have an 'undivided liver' (ἀσχιδὲς ἧπαρ), others a liver which is 'divided from the start' (ἐσχισμένον ἀπ' ἀρχῆς). But Aristotle never identified the human liver as having four (or two) lobes, and it remained for Herophilus to establish this point. Herophilus' description, though later praised as exceptionally accurate by Galen (T60), was not accepted by all subsequent physicians. Celsus, for example, describes only a liver with four lobes (*Medicinae* 4.1.5, *CML* I, p. 150 Marx), and in ps.-Rufus, *On the Anatomy of the Parts of the Body* 28 (p. 175 Daremberg/Ruelle), the liver is described as having four *or* five lobes. Cf. also Galen, *De usu partium* 4.8 (I, p. 208 Helmreich): 'All animals do not have the same number of lobes', and May, 1968: vol. I, p. 214 n. 24 on Galen's reversion to animal livers.

Where it [the liver] touches against the diaphragm: a topographical detail which occurs in Greek literature as early as the time of Homer: *Iliad* 11.579 (ἧπαρ ὑπὸ πραπίδων). Cf. also Hp., *On the Nature of Bones* 10 (IX, p. 180L): φρένες δὲ προσπεφύκασι τῷ ἧπατι; so too, *Epidemics* 2.4.1. (V, p. 122L; *vid.* n. 71); Aristotle, *Historia Animalium* 1.17.496b15ff.; Galen, *De usu partium* 4.13 and 14 (I, pp. 221, 231 Helmreich); Rufus of Ephesus, *On Naming the Parts of Humans* 177 (p. 158 Daremberg/Ruelle).

Convex (κεκύρτωται) . . . concave (ἔνσιμον): The description of the liver by Rufus of Ephesus, *On Naming the Parts of Humans* 177 (p. 158 Daremberg/Ruelle), provides the same details: the liver is convex (κυρτός) where it touches the diaphragm, concave (σιμός) where it touches the stomach. This part of Rufus' account is probably dependent, either directly or indirectly, on Fr60 of Herophilus but, in accordance with the principles developed above (see *Note on text, arrangement, and translation*), it is not included among the testimonia. The description of the liver in Celsus (*Medicina* 4.1.5, *CML* I, p. 150 Marx; cf., e.g., *cavum . . . gibbum*) also displays several affinities with Herophilus' (concave/convex, the topographical relation of liver to abdomen, etc.), and might likewise depend in part on Herophilus. Most other post-Alexandrian authors, including Galen and Pollux (*Onomasticon* 2.213), also seem to have adopted Herophilus' terminology – convex (κυρτός) and concave (σιμός) – to distinguish the two sides of the liver. For Galen, see, e.g., *De usu partium*, 4.13 and 14 (I, pp. 221, 231 Helmreich), 15.4 (II, p. 351 Helmreich); *De anatomicis administrationibus* 6.12 (II, p. 578K), 13.1 ('hollow aspect'; p. 138 Duckworth); *De constitutione artis medicae ad Patrophilum* 16 (I, p. 285K); *De locis affectis* 5.7 (VIII, pp. 351f.K); *Ad Glauconem de medendi methodo* 2.4 (XI, p. 93K). The concavity to which Herophilus was apparently the first to refer actually consists of depressions caused by the organs behind and below it pushing in its surface; as soon as the living liver is taken out of its position, as in surgery, these depressions disappear.

Here it may be likened to a certain fissure . . . : Herophilus, still talking about the 'concave' side, seems to be referring to the postero-inferior or dorso-caudal surface of the liver, where indeed there is a 'fissure': the porta, a deep and broad depression through which the portal vein (see T127 and pp. 180–81 above) enters the liver.

Vein from the navel: the umbilical vein, which in antiquity was widely believed to enter directly into the foetal liver. Cf., for example, Empedocles 31A79 DK (=Soranus, *Gynaecia* 1.57, *CMG* IV, p. 42 Ilberg); Aristotle, *Historia animalium* 7.8.586b18–20; Galen, *De usu partium* 15.4 (II, p. 351 Helmreich). Closer to the truth is, however, a view attributed to Phaedrus by Soranus, *loc. cit.*: that the vessels which supply embryos with nourishment proceed into the heart. (The vitelline vein, coming from the yolk sac, and the umbilical vein in fact join just behind the foetal *heart* and enter it together, as modern anatomy has established. The foetal liver is only formed subsequently, when endoderm and mesoderm cells migrate into the spaces between the vitelline-umbilical capillaries, surround these capillaries, and become liver cells.)

Completely round and unarticulated: perhaps an Aristotelian echo; see n. 72, pp. 163–4 above, and the comment (above) on 'the number of its lobes'.

Some of the left parts: the question whether the liver lies on the right or left prompted comment by a number of ancient writers, perhaps not only as a result of the influence of hepatoscopy but also because of the general physiological significance attached to right and left (cf., for example, Lesky, 1950: 1263–93). Aristotle had introduced one of his discussions of the liver as follows: 'Below the diaphragm on the *right* side is the liver, on the *left* the spleen' (*Historia animalium* 1.17.496b15ff.; but cf. *De partibus animalium*

3.7.669b30ff.). Herophilus perhaps recorded his more complex – and accurate – view of the locus of the liver in response to this misleading Aristotelian generalization. The conclusion Galen seems to share with Herophilus – that 'its largest part is on the right . . .' – is essentially correct, inasmuch as the largest of the four hepatic lobes lies to the right of the midline.

The hare: in the comparative anatomy of the liver, the hare had an unusually prominent place, also before Herophilus. Aristotle, for example, twice refers to 'a certain kind of hare, especially near lake Bolbe in the so-called Fig Country (Sykinē), of which one might well hold the opinion that they had two livers . . .' (*Historia animalium* 2.17.507a16–19; and, geographically more vague, *De partibus animalium* 3.7.669b34–5, where some fish, too – especially sharks – are said to have two livers). The author of the pseudo-Aristotelian *De mirabilibus auscultationibus* 122 similarly states: 'They say that in Crastonia . . . the hares which are caught have two livers . . .' (842a15–16). Galen clearly implies that he also examined the liver of hares, stating his agreement with Herophilus' view that it extends into the left hypochondrium.

T61 The seed in females is discharged: Herophilus here follows a long tradition, dating back to the Presocratics, that the female – like the male – secretes seed. Alcmeon (24A14DK), Parmenides (28B18DK), Empedocles (31B63DK), and Democritus (68A142DK) are among the Presocratics who seem to have held this view. While Diocles of Carystus (fr. 172 Wellmann) followed their example, Aristotle firmly rejected it (cf. *De generatione animalium* 1.20.727b33–728a9), only for Herophilus to return to the earlier view. Lesky, 1950: 73, has cast doubt on the value of Aëtius' testimonium concerning Democritus (68A142DK = Aëtius, *Placita* 5.5.1; *DG*, p. 418), arguing that it smells of Herophilean influence and hence of anachronism. Aëtius attributes to Pythagoras, Democritus, and Epicurus (cf. Lucretius, *De rerum natura* 4.1209–1259) the view that a woman contributes seed to reproduction 'because she possesses παραστάτας ἀπεστραμμένους [sc. 'assistants' which are turned to the sides]'. Lesky argues that Aëtius' mention of 'assistants (*parastatai*) presupposes discoveries made by the Alexandrians, in particular, Herophilus' discovery of the ovaries, and that the testimony hence can concern only Epicurus, not Democritus. If these *parastatai* do indeed refer to the ovaries (or Fallopian tubes), Lesky's suggestion of an anachronistic Herophilean colouring would have considerable merit. But as far as we know, Herophilus never used *parastatai* of any part of the female reproductive organs – only of the male (e.g. T101–T103, T105: Herophilus used *parastatai*, with different qualifiers, of the seminal vesicles and the ampullae of the vasa deferentia respectively). Furthermore, there is nothing uniquely Herophilean about the use of *parastatai* to designate genital parts (although Herophilus' usage is innovative to the extent that it is applied to previously unknown parts of the spermatic duct system). It had been used of genital parts as early as the fifth century B.C. (see *Comments*, T101–T103), also in non-scientific literature, and Aëtius' use of the word therefore does not necessarily point to the influence of Herophilus. What is unusual in Aëtius' report is the attribution of seed-producing or -transporting *parastatai* to *women*. But Herophilus in fact denied that women had what he called *parastatai*, and it remained for Galen and Rufus of Ephesus – both of whom post-date Aëtius – to attribute either something analogous to *parastatai* or *parastatai* themselves to females (see below, p. 233, on varix-like assistant, and T105). Aëtius' testimony, instead of being an example of the distorting impact on Herophilus' discoveries of philosophical doxography, or of the use of anachronistic terminology by Aëtius or his sources (e.g. the *Vetusta placita*), might therefore be an accurate report of an early instance of the Greek tendency to depict female anatomy and physiology as analogous to that of the dominant model: the male. Cf., for example, Aristotle, *De generatione animalium* 1.19.727a3–4: 'It is evident that the menstrual fluid is something *analogous* in females to the seed in males'; 1.3.716b32–3: 'The uterus is double in all [females], *just* as there are also two testicles in all males.' See also *ibid.*, 1.20.728b21ff; 4.8.776b10–28; Lesky, 1950: 130–3, 162; Herophilus, Fr61 and T109.

δίδυμοι (**didymoi**), 'twins': Herophilus was apparently the first (cf. T109) to use it of the testicles and of the ovaries. Perhaps under his influence it soon made its way into the Septuagint; cf. Deuteronomy 25.1:, a text apparently translated into Greek (perhaps in Alexandria) as early as Herophilus' own lifetime: '. . . if a woman stretches out her hand and grabs him [sc. her husband's opponent] by his 'twins' (*didymoi*, testicles), you will chop off her hand'. Subsequently Herophilus' innovation – using δίδυμοι interchangeably with ὄρχεις, especially when referring to the female 'testicles' or ovaries – found acceptance among medical authors (e.g. Galen in T61, T107, T109, and *De uteri dissectione* 4 and 9 (*CMG* v.2.1, pp. 42, 48–50 Nickel); Soranus in T106) and even among poets (e.g. in the first century B.C., Philodemus in an erotic epigram of the Palatine Anthology, 5.125: 'Either I have absolutely no senses [left] or it is his "twins" [*didymoi*] that must be removed right now – with an axe'). Galen's description of the ovaries and tubes in *De uteri dissectione* 9 (an earlier work) seems to be dependent on Herophilus in other respects as well, although he disavows Herophilus as a model (T107); cf. Nickel's judicious comments *ad loc.* (*CMG* v.2.1, pp. 86ff.; also pp. 76ff.). See also Galen, *De venarum et arteriarum dissectione* 8 (II, p. 810K). (The Herophilean Andreas may have transmitted Herophilus' neologism to the Septuagint translators; see Chapter XI, n. 11 *infra.*)

They differ only a little from ... the male: Although the use of argument by analogy has its limits and can be misleading (cf. VI.A, above), this sentence as well as the subsequent phrase 'just like the testicles of the male' indicate that the principle of analogy, which had been used extensively by Aristotle in his biological works, here was applied to medicine with remarkably positive consequences: the discovery of the ovaries and parts of the tubes (cf. Lesky, 1950: 162–3). The widespread view that Diocles of Carystus, and not Herophilus, was responsible for the discovery of the ovaries and the Fallopian tubes, rests on an ambiguous and misleading statement by Wellmann (1901: 97). None of the texts (usually Diocles, fr. 25–9 Wellmann) cited by those who, like Wellmann and Balss, attribute this discovery to Diocles conclusively supports their argument (cf. Balss, 1936: 5). In fact, in Diocles' fr. 25 Galen states unequivocally that Diocles must be numbered among those who were *ignorant* of the Fallopian tubes and of their attachment to the uterus (a point belatedly conceded by Wellmann in a note on p. 127). Furthermore, Diocles' use of 'horns' (T108 above; Diocles, fr. 27 Wellmann) in connection with 'offshoots' of the uterus is no proof that he knew the tubes; rather, the 'horn-like projections' mentioned by Diocles are fictitious formations which he thought of as existing *inside* the hollow of the uterus; see *Comments*, T108 (below). Galen's lavish praise for the accuracy of Herophilus' description of the ovaries – the kind of praise traditionally reserved for a πρῶτος εὑρετής – is perhaps a further indication that Herophilus, and not Diocles, was the discoverer of the ovaries.

It has been suggested that Aristotle already recognised the ovaries. Cf., e.g., LSJ, s.v. πόρος, 1.6b, with reference to certain 'uterine passages' (*porous hysterikous*), of which Aristotle says that eels do not possess them (*Historia animalium* 6.16.570a5). The text is so unspecific, however, that one cannot claim with confidence that it implies knowledge of the Fallopian tubes or ovaries. Oviducts – also called uteri (*hysterai*) – are known to Aristotle, but only in certain animals, e.g. fish, invertebrates, and sauropsids. He likewise knew of the gonads of sea urchins and oysters (*De partibus animalium* 4.5.680a11–15, b3–9). Of greater relevance appears to be his description of the excision of a small part of the *kapria* (sg.) of sows in order to still their sexual appetites and to fatten them rapidly (*Historia animalium* 9.50.632a21ff.). It is not impossible that *kapria* refers to an ovary, especially in light of Aristotle's report that 'they cut the lower belly [of the sow] where, in the males, the testicles mostly grow, for that is where the *kapria* is attached to the *mētrai*' (i.e. to the uterine 'horns'?). *Ibid.* 6.18.572a21, 573b2 *kapria* refers to a coveted pharmacologial substance secreted by all mature sows after copulation (perhaps a mucous substance thought to be produced in the sow's *kapria*?). Aristotle never refers to the *kapria* of any other species, however, and it therefore would be wrong to imply that he discovered the ovaries as a general phenomenon of mammalian, let alone human, female anatomy.

εὔθρυπτοι, 'easily damageable': Although the Aldine edition reads ἄθρυπτοι ('firm, immune to damage') and, in general, represents a better MS tradition (see Ph. De Lacy's forthcoming edition (*CMG*) of Galen's *De semine*), the reading in the Parisinus seems to be supported by at least two considerations. First, Herophilus is explicitly comparing the ovaries to the testicles and, shortly after this quotation, Galen – perhaps with Herophilus' text still at hand or in mind – specifically observes that the epididymis protects the *soft flesh* of the male's testicles (IV, pp. 590–1 K). Secondly, in the pseudo-Galenic *Definitiones medicae*, an eclectic work which probably pre-dates Galen, εὔθρυπτος is put to similar use (*Def.* 58; XIX, p. 362K).

mares: like the mention of the hare in Fr60, this confirms that Herophilus continued using comparative anatomy even though he is best remembered for having initiated the systematic dissection of humans.

And they [the ovaries] are attached to the uterus: The 'membranes' to which Herophilus refers here and in T114 are probably the so-called broad ligaments, two bilaminate lateral ligaments of the uterus passing from the side of the uterus to the walls of the pelvis, but also giving passage between the two layers of each ligament to the Fallopian tubes and to blood vessels – Herophilus, too, mentions a vein and an artery in this context – and bearing the ovary suspended from the dorsal or posterior surface.

A vein from the vein: on a possible identification of these vessels, see above (*Introduction*, p. 178).

The spermatic duct: Fallopian tube (tuba uterina).

Just like the male duct: see nn. 86–7 above and pp. 167–8 on Herophilus' error concerning the course of the uterine tubes.

varix-like assistant: In T105, too, Herophilus denies that the female has this 'assistant'. In *On Anatomical Procedures* 12.7 (p. 123 Duckworth *et al.*; II, p. 113 Simon) Galen agrees with the view here attributed to Herophilus – that the 'varix-like assistant' has never been observed in females – but in *De usu partium* 14.11 (II, pp. 323–4 Helmreich) he says the uterine tube 'is *analogous* to those called varix-like assistants (*kirsoeideis parastatai*) in males'.(Helmreich with good reason athetizes the passage (*ibid.*, II, p. 321) in which *parastatai adenoeideis*, 'glandular assistants' or seminal vesicles, are attributed to females by Galen; it is absent both in the best MSS of *De us. part.* and in Niccolò da Reggio's fourteenth-century Latin translation.) Rufus of Ephesus went a step further, implying that women also have 'varix-like assistants', apparently referring to the Fallopian tubes, although he concedes that he has only observed them in the womb of a sheep and that only dissections will provide certainty (T105). On the 'varix-like assistants' in the male, see Chapter VII, T101–T105 with *Comments*. Cf. also T189.

Subsequently he was much more mistaken: In T107 (*De uteri dissectione* 9 (*CMG* v.2.1, p. 48 Nickel) Galen likewise expresses his astonishment that as excellent an anatomist as Herophilus (or Aristotle or Euryphon) could have failed to observe the entrance of the 'spermatic ducts' (Fallopian tubes), which grow from the ovaries, into the uterus. On Potter's attempt to rescue Herophilus from Galen's charge, see n. 86. Cf. also the comments made by Rufus of Ephesus in T105, on vessels which 'grow out of the "testicles" [sc. ovaries] . . . on either side of the womb of a sheep and open directly into the cavity of the uterus', which might be taken as an indication that Rufus was the first to correct Herophilus' error. Less certain is Daremberg/Ruelle's identification of the *plektanai* ('tentacles') mentioned by Rufus with the tubes (*De nominatione partium hominis* 194, p. 160 D/R); so too Diepgen, 1937: 136. On *plektanai* see *Comments*, T108.

T62 Galen here is commenting on the following passage from Hp., *Epidemics* 2.4.1. (v, pp. 120–2L): 'From here [sc. the collar-bone] some veins branch off [from the liver vein or *hepatitis*] to the neck and some to the shoulder-blades, and some are bent back downwards and turn off along the vertebrae and the ribs.' The same passage recurs in Hp., *On the Nature of Bones* 10 (ix, p. 178L). The 'liver vein' here is what was later identified as 'hollow vein' or 'thick vein' (see below), and was regarded as one of the two main veins, the other being the 'spleen vein'. See also Galen, *De plac. Hp. Plat.* 6.8.56–67 (*CMG* v. 4.1.2, pp. 418–20 De Lacy).

This vein which is a bit lower on the right: Hp., *Epidemics, ibid.*, p. 122: 'One vein bends back on either side [of the vertebrae?], and another bends back a little lower down [than] the place whence the first left it behind and supplies the ribs until, bending back to the left, it meets the vein [coming] out of the heart itself.' On this Hippocratic description cf. Harris, 1973: 60–2.

Thick vein: vena cava. Cf. Galen, *In Hp. De nat. hom.* 2.6 (*CMG* v.9.1, pp. 68–75).

T63a medici rationales: cf. *Comments*, T1 (Chapter II *supra*). The contrast here is with the medical Empiricists who, as Celsus reports a few paragraphs later (*prohoem.* 40–4; *CML* I, pp. 23–4 Marx) rejected not only dissection but also vivisection; the latter, they said, was both cruel and scientifically useless on account of the changes induced in the body by vivisection. Similarly, the changes caused by death render dissection an illusory method of discovery. For a similar argument in a patristic author see T66.

regibus: see pp. 27–30, 141–4, 150–1 *supra*.

spiritu: i.e. *pneuma*, regarded by many Greek physicians and biologists, including Herophilus and Erasistratus, as a substance necessary to life that was present not only in the lungs but also in the arteries. See next chapter ('Physiology'). (On the controversy concerning the value of Celsus' testimonium, see the *Introduction* to this chapter, pp. 144–53, and nn. 10,13.)

T63b–c The two recently edited commentaries on Galen's *De sectis ad introducendos*, ascribed respectively to Agnellus of Ravenna (codex Ambrosianus C 108 inf. of the ninth century) and to the elusive John of Alexandria (extant in at least seven MSS of the thirteenth and fourteenth centuries), display elements of identity, convergence, and divergence that have not been adequately accounted for. Here, however, both testimonia (T63b–c) seem at least indirectly dependent on Celsus' *De medicina* (T63a): among their possible sources Celsus is unique in reporting unambiguously (see *Comments*, T66, on Tertullian's account) (a) that Herophilus practised vivisection; (b) that he did so on condemned criminals. In *De sectis* itself no mention is made either of Herophilus or of vivisection practised on criminals (indeed, throughout the treatise Galen is remarkably reticent about identifying individual adherents of the medical 'schools' he discusses; Erasistratus and Asclepiades, ch.5, 1 p.75K, are rare exceptions). On cod. Ambros. C 108 inf. and its relation to Alexandrian commentaries on Galen's *De sectis* see above, Ch. iv, *Comments* on T46–T47; also Beccaria, 1959–71 (especially 1971).

T64 See *Comments*, T5a and T5b, on the question of the accuracy of this testimonium and on the identity of the physicians enumerated by Vindician.

T65 On the ἐμβρυοσφάκτης, used to kill the embryo, see below, T247.

   maiorum, 'adults': The contrast is apparently between Herophilus' dissection of adults and the slightly more 'acceptable' – though, to a physician of the Methodist school, such as Tertullian's source Soranus, still problematic – abortion of a foetus.

   prosector: a *hapax legomenon*. (Although *anatomicus* and verbal phrases with *secare* and its compounds are the usual forms of referring to a dissector, the basic meaning here is not in doubt.)

   milder Soranus: This probably is intended to imply that Soranus, although he possessed the same 'foetus slaying' instrument as Herophilus and Hippocrates, used it only for compelling surgical reasons and, faithful to his Methodist school of medicine, rejected dissection. But see G. E. R. Lloyd, 1983: 188–9, 192–3; Frede, 1982: 14.

T66 sexcentos ('six hundred') has been interpreted literally by a number of scholars (e.g. Schneider, 1967–9: vol. ii, p. 411), but it is of course a metonym for 'innumerable', 'an immense number' – similar to our 'hundreds' or 'thousands'.

   exsecuit ('cut up'): Some critics (n. 9) have argued that Tertullian is attacking Herophilus' use of vivisection, but dissection might well be a target

as well. 'Exsecuit', 'he cut up', does not necessarily refer to the cutting of
living humans, and 'odiit', 'he hated', could refer to Herophilus' putative
disrespect and irreverence toward the living as well as the dead, i.e. also to his
violation of the taboo about desecrating corpses – a taboo that was shared by
pagans and Christians alike. Soranus, Tertullian's (pagan) source, was an
adversary not only of anatomy, but even of some forms of surgery (cf. Caelius
Aurelianus, *Passiones acutae* 2.38.219, against venesection; Kind, 1927c: col.
1128). See Karpp, 1934, and Waszink, 1947: 25*–29* and 185–6. The most
conclusive evidence that vivisection is, however, at least part of the target of
Tertullian's attack is the reference to 'morte non simplici sed ipsa inter
artificia exsectionis errante', 'not a simple death but one in the midst of the
artificial processes of cutting – [a death] which is an error'. Tertullian
suggests that Herophilus' 'cutting' was not only sacrilegious and cruel but
also scientifically useless, because death – and especially an artificial death
such as that caused by vivisection – changes the body, with the consequence
that the corpse does not yield reliable information about the constitution and
functions of a living body. A similar objection had been raised by the medical
Empiricists; see *Comments*, T63a. On *exectionem* cf. also T86 with *Comments*.

   In Chapter 10 Tertullian is trying to refute the view that *spiritus* [*pneuma*,
'life-breath'; see next chapter] is a substance responsible only for respiration,
and separable from the soul [*anima*], which is responsible for life. Anatomy,
he argues in 10.4, is not capable of furnishing conclusive data concerning this
question – and especially not when the anatomist, like Herophilus, practises
vivisection.

   On the value of Tertullian's polemical report, see *Introduction*, pp. 142–
143. For a further example of Christian polemics against Alexandrian
vivisection see St Augustine, *De anima et eius origine* 4.ii.3–4.vi.7 (*PL* 44, pp.
525–9). See also Fulgentius, *Mitologiae* 1.16 (p. 9 Helm); Aelian, *Variae
Historiae* 12.1 (p. 124.7–13 Dilts); Pliny, *Nat. Hist.* 29.6.12ff., 29.8.18; St
Augustine, *Civitas Dei* 22.24.

T67 Eudemus. A contemporary of Phylotimus, and hence of Herophilus;
see Chapter II.A.2 and *Comments*, T14 (with n. 43).

   ἱστορησάντων and ἱστορουμένης probably refer to *historia* as used by the
Empiricists: the reporting and transmission of what has been established
'empirically' through observation, etc. Cf. the phrase περὶ κρίσεως ἱστορίας
in Galen, *CMG* v.9.1., p. 69.12 Mewaldt, and Deichgräber, 1965: 95.19,
127.9–10, etc.

T68 Marinus: Frequently mentioned by Galen as one of the greatest
anatomists since Herophilus (e.g. in a passage immediately following upon
Herophilus' T126, *In Hp. Epidemiarum 2.4.1 Comment.4* (*CMG* v.10.1, p. 312),
where Marinus is also said to have lived at the time of Galen's grandparents).

Likewise mentioned with Herophilus in T69. Cf. also Galen's extensive account of his own summary in four books of Marinus' treatise in twenty books *On Anatomy: De libris propriis* 3 (*Scr. Min.* II, pp. 104–8 Mueller). Further details in Deichgräber, 1930.

T71 Galen seems to suggest that Herophilus, like himself, squarely faced the problem of the relativistic and ambiguous nature of 'beginning' and 'end' when used in the description of insertions or origins of some anatomical structures. This represents an advance on the confidence with which 'beginning' and 'terminal point' had been used in previous anatomical descriptions. Cf. T115.

T84–T89 These testimonia might belong to Herophilus' *On Eyes* (see ch. VIII, Fr 260); they are included here because of their anatomical significance.

T85 This is one of two passages used by Solmsen (1961: 186ff.) as evidence for the conclusion that Herophilus took over the pneumatic theory of motion and sensation from Aristotle (and others), but Galen here is attributing to Herophilus only the name *poros* for the optic nerve and the description of its lumen as visible, apparently claiming for himself the view that this nerve serves as a pathway for pneuma. T140 (below, Chapter VII) does, however, support Solmsen's conclusion.

   Poros, a word meaning 'duct', 'passage', or 'strait', had often been used by Greek writers before Herophilus of the sensory channels such as the optic tract. In the introduction to this chapter it was pointed out, for example, that Aristotle used this term of the optic tract (see also n. 54), and in the early fifth century B.C. the Presocratic Alcmeon of Croton is reported to have said: 'All the senses [sense-organs?] are connected with the brain. Consequently they are mutilated if the brain is moved or changes its position; for it blocks the ducts (*poroi*) through which sensations [take place]' (24A5DK(see n. 44)). Plato, too – or whoever wrote the dialogue *Axiochus* – used *poros* in this manner (366a).

   If then, *poros* had such a rich tradition as a term for sensory (and especially optic) ducts, why does Galen bother to single out Herophilus' use of *poros* of the optic nerve for explicit and pointed mention in no less than three different treatises (T84, T85, T140)? The answer would seem to lie in Herophilus' reservation of *poros* not for all sensory ducts or all sensory nerves, but specifically for the optic nerve, and with explicit – and correct – reference to its unique lumen. In dissection he had perhaps seen that the central artery and vein of the retina run through the substance of that centimetre of the optic nerve which is closest to the eyeball. Perhaps never having seen another nerve with such a lumen, he might have introduced 'duct' or 'passage' (*poros*) rather than simply *neuron* for the optic nerve. For a slightly different view see Kollesch, 1973: 106–7. Cf. also Berg, 1942: 342 n. 3.

T86 The most judicious recent discussions of this testimonium are by G. E. R. Lloyd, 1975a, and Mansfeld, 1975. Both conclude that the detailed description of the eye in this passage, as well as the implication of dissection, is attributable to Herophilus rather than to Alcmeon and Callisthenes, although Alcmeon may have 'cut out' the eye and observed a passage behind it. Lloyd's comments on *exectionem* (1975a: 117ff.) are very useful. But the use of the corresponding verb, *exsecare*, by Tertullian (T66, 'exsecuit') to refer to what appears to be Herophilus' dissecting activity gives one pause about accepting the view that *exectio* and its cognates are unlikely to refer to dissection. See also *Comments*, T66. While *exectio* remains fraught with ambiguity, there cannot be much doubt that Herophilus – and not Alcmeon – initiated dissection of humans as a scientific method. Cf. also ps.–Quintilian, *Declamation* 8, proem. (p. 151.8 Håkanson): *execuit*, apparently of vivisection; see also French, 1978: 165 n. 12.

T87–T89 Opperman's (1925) argument that Herophilus was the first to advance a 'four-coat' version of the anatomy of the eye, and that Callimachus (*Hymn to Artemis* 53) was influenced by it, is persuasive. Nevertheless, in accordance with the editorial principles discussed above (pp. xvi–xvii), these three testimonia are presented in such a way as to emphasize that Celsus, Rufus, and the author ('ps.-Rufus') of *On the anatomy of the parts of human beings*, all of whom adopted the four-coat theory, explicitly report only the following about Herophilus: (1) that he commented on the rough and smooth sides of the second 'coat' or membrane of the eye (under the cornea), comparing them to a grape skin; (2) that he called the third coat 'cobweb-like' or 'arachnoid'; (3) that he compared this third coat to a casting net that has been drawn up (Latin: *rete*→retina). Only Calcidius (T86) explicitly ascribes a four-coat theory to Herophilus (and apparently to Alcmeon and Callisthenes as well: *notaverunt*, plur.; cf. *Comments*, T86) but he offers neither Herophilus' nomenclature nor any anatomical details concerning the coats. Many *details* of ophthalmological nomenclature and anatomy ascribed to Herophilus by Opperman and others therefore are no more than plausible – and inviting – inferences. It is striking that Galen, who elsewhere is not reluctant to record Herophilus' nomenclative innovations and anatomical discoveries, fails to mention Herophilus at all in his anatomy of the eye: *On anatomical procedures* x.2–3 (pp. 33–4 Duckworth).

In addition to Celsus, Galen, Rufus, and the Anonymus (ps.-Rufus), the following are among those influenced by the four-coat anatomy which originated with Herophilus: ps.-Galen, *Introductio sive medicus* 11 (xiv, pp. 711–12K); ps.-Galen, *Definitiones medicae* 41 (xix, p. 358K); Pollux,

Onomasticon 2.70–1 (I, pp. 104–5 Bethe); Aëtius of Amida, *Libri medicinales* 7.1 (*CMG* VIII.2, pp. 253–4 Olivieri). Cf. also Oribasius, *Collectiones medicae* 24.4 (*CMG* VI.2.1; vol. III, pp. 12–16 Raeder), where much of the same terminology recurs, drawn in part from Galen's *De usu partium* 10.1–4, 6 (II, pp. 54ff. Helmreich). See also pp. 72–4, 155, 160–1, 252–4; *Comments*, T86; Longrigg, 1981: 166–8; Lloyd, 1983: 158, 161. On 'chor(i)oid' see also T124–T125; on *chorion* Kudlien, 1964d.

T101–T103 parastatai ('assistants'): See above, *Comments* on T61. The comedian Plato (*c.* 460–385 B.C.) had already used *parastatai* of the testicles (fr. 174.13 Kock: 'for Conisalus [a Priapic demon; penis] and his two assistants [*parastatai*: testes], a little platter of myrtleberries [clitoris] plucked by hand . . .'), and the author of the Hippocratic compilation known as *On the Nature of Bones*, 14 (IX, p. 188L), used it of a part of the male genitalia which is not clearly specified (and which Galen, perhaps anachronistically, identifies as the epididymis).

T107 Cf. Nickel *ad loc.* (CMG V.2.1, pp. 89–90; cf. *id.*, pp. 100–3).

T108 Breast-like offshoots on the sides: Galen here seems to be describing the Fallopian tubes, as Nickel (*CMG* V.2.1, pp. 69–71) has suggested. Herophilus' comparison of these 'offshoots' with the 'half-curve of a circle' or the 'halved spiral of a circle' is perfectly compatible with the form and course of the tubes. More problematic is Galen's assumption that Diocles' 'horn-like projections' (*keraiai*) are identical with Herophilus' tubes. While Galen more than once used 'horns' or 'horn-like projections' of the tubes (e.g. *De usu partium* 14.11 (II, p. 323 Helmreich)), the word had also been used to refer to certain extremities of the uterus (cf. Hp., *Superfetation* 1, VIII, p. 476L) or to fictitious formations *inside* the uterus. Soranus of Ephesus, for example, reports: 'Diocles says there are teats for sucking (*kotyledones*) and tentacles and horn-like projections (*keraiai*) in the wide area of the uterus, and these are breast-like outgrowths . . . made with forethought by nature, for the sake of giving the embryo preliminary exercise in sucking the nipples of the breasts' (*Gynaecia* 1.14.2, *CMG* IV, p. 10 Ilberg = Diocles, fr. 27 Wellmann). Diocles' use of 'horn-like projections' to refer to intra-uterine nipple-like growths – in whose existence several Presocratics, e.g. Democritus (68A144DK) and Diogenes (64A25; cf. 38A17DK) also believed – clearly is remote both from Galen's use of 'horns' and from Herophilus' description of tubes resembling 'half-curves of a circle' that are *external* to the uterus (see also Galen, *De symptomatum causis* 3.11 (VII, p. 266K); and Herophilus, Fr61 and T106). Galen therefore seems to have overlooked the homonymy that lurks in *keras* and *keraia* and consequently to have conflated, in a misleading manner, the Herophilean-Galenic view with Diocles' bizarre but more traditional account. In a similarly questionable doxographic conflation, Galen adds (*CMG* v.2.1, p. 38) that Praxagoras and Phylotimus called the same offshoots *kolpoi* ('bosoms; bays'), while Euenor named them *plektanai* ('tentacles'). Cf. Nickel, *CMG* v.2.1, pp. 69–71, 100–3.

T117 Most modern scholars believe that Herophilus is the culprit who first called the pulmonary artery 'artery-like vein' and the pulmonary vein 'vein-like artery' (e.g. Gossen, 1912: 1106; Dobson, 1925: 21; L. G. Wilson, 1959: 295; Lonie, 1973: 7; Harris, 1973: 179; Longrigg, 1981: 170). Galen adopted this nomenclature, which prevailed well into the Renaissance (Latin: *vena arterialis* and *arteria venalis*); cf. Bylebyl and Pagel, 1971. Furley/Wilkie (1984: 25) and Longrigg (1985b), however, conclude from T117 that Herophilus departed from the Praxagorean and Erasistratean practice of calling *all* vessels originating from the left side of the heart 'arteries' and *all* vessels attached to the right side of the heart 'veins'. Furley/Wilkie claim that Rufus 'quite plainly says he called the big vein ἀρτηρίαν ['artery'] and not ἀρτηριώδη ['artery-like', 'arterial']', but Daremberg and Ruelle (Rufus, p. 162) offer no MS variants for ἀρτηριώδη. Longrigg, 1985b, reads ἀρτηριώδη but speculates that Rufus falsely attributes an Erasistratean invention (i.e. 'arterial vein' for pulmonary artery) to Herophilus, in order to rescue Herophilus from inconsistency. The history of science is replete, however, with retrospectively recognizable – and retrospectively puzzling – inconsistencies, contradictions, and 'inconceivabilities' perpetrated by the most esteemed of scientists. The evidence is explicit on one point only: that Herophilus used 'artery-like vein' to refer to the vessel we call 'pulmonary artery'. Of 'vein-like artery' (for pulmonary vein) there is no explicit mention in the extant Herophilean testimonia and fragments, nor of the view that *all* arteries and veins are characterized by the left–right distinction. Nevertheless Herophilus' use of 'artery-like vein' and his apprenticeship with Praxagoras render plausible the suggestion that he accepted at least the left-right arterial-venous distinction. See also vi.a.6 *supra*; Tallmadge, 1939: 443.

T118 chapter 16: A reference to Galen, *De usu partium* 6.10 (1, p. 325 Helmreich) = T116.

T119 'nerve-like strands': Herophilus did not always distinguish nerves from ligaments, tendons, muscles, and similar fibrous tissues, and 'nerve-like' seems to be a generic concept under which several kinds of fibrous tissues can be subsumed. It is unclear exactly to what part of the valve attachments 'nerve-like strands' refer. C. R. S. Harris suggests 'papillary muscles, or chordae tendineae, or perhaps the tendon of the infundibulum?' (1973: 179), and all three indeed seem to be reasonable possibilities. For a somewhat different use of 'nerve-like' by Herophilus see T141 and the discussion of the motor nerves in Chapter VII (A. 2). It seems reasonably clear that Herophilus here uses νευρώδεις διαφύσεις (nerve-like strands) because he has discovered the nerves and reserved for them the name *neura*; hence he does not call the attachments of the cardiac valves *neura* – as Aristotle had done – but only 'nerve-*like*'. Perhaps the older sense of *neuron* ('sinew') continues to lurk in Herophilus' use of the adjective. For διάφυσις, 'strand', see Galen, *De usu partium* 10.2 (II, p. 57 Helmreich) and *De motu musculorum* 1.1 (IV, p. 371K). Herophilus seems to have initiated this particular use of the word.

νεῦρα **(nerves)**. What Aristotle meant when he called the attachment of the cardiac valves *neura* was not 'nerves' – as Galen implies – but 'sinews' or 'ligaments'. Upon dissecting larger animals Aristotle, as Harris (1973: 161) plausibly suggests, 'may have been struck by the sinew-like attachments of the valves, the musculi papillares and the chordae tendineae'. Cf. Aristotle's definition of *neuron* in *Generation of Animals* 2.3737a36–b4 as the sticky or tough structure that holds parts together; see also *History of Animals* 3.5 (especially 515a27–b18) on the heart as the starting-point (ἀρχή) of the sinews (*neura*).

Erasistratus. Galen's judgment that Herophilus' anatomy of the heart was not as advanced as Erasistratus' seems correct: *De placitis Hp. et Platonis* 6.6, for example, gives an indication of how detailed Erasistratus' knowledge of the tricuspid and bicuspid valves was. See von Staden, 1975: 183–4, and Harris, 1973: 197–8. In *De usu pulsuum* 5 (V, p. 166K) Galen even says that it would be superfluous for him to describe the valves, since Erasistratus' discussion is perfectly adequate (αὐτάρκως). (Cf. also *De plac.* 1.6, where Erasistratus' and Chrysippus' knowledge of the heart is compared.)

T120 Galen apparently wishes to state that Herophilus viewed the auricles as part of the heart – rather than viewing them as the terminal processes of the pulmonary vein and the vena cava – and that this erroneously adds two to the number of the heart's valves. While he might well have viewed the lowest valve of the vena cava as another 'orifice', there is, as Harris (1973: 180) points out, no similar structure in the pulmonary vein.

T127 On the topography of the liver cf. also Fr60. A description similar to Herophilus' is also given by Galen in another treatise: *De venarum arteriarumque dissectione* 1 (II, p. 785K). Mani (1959–67: pt I) has made the suggestion (p. 46) that the discovery of the lymphatic vessels of the mesentery and of the lymphatic glands might have been made in the course of vivisection, but nothing in this description necessitates such a conclusion. On the significance of this text as a witness to Herophilus' discovery of the function of the hepatic portal system, see above pp. 180–1. Cf. also Mani, 1959–67: pt I, pp. 63, 72.

VII · PHYSIOLOGY
AND PATHOLOGY

'Give me your hand,
and let me feel your pulse.'
SHAKESPEARE, *The Comedie of Errors*

A · INTRODUCTION

Spectacular discoveries and descriptions of the form, position, and structure of numerous parts of the human body may have provided Herophilus with his most enduring claim to scientific fame, but he was no less interested in the causes and nature of the functions and dysfunctions of these parts, i.e. in physiology and pathology. His dissections provided him with a more accurate knowledge of the brain, the nerves, the heart, the bloodvessels, and the reproductive organs than any of his predecessors had possessed, and he did not hesitate to exploit this anatomical knowledge for the construction of pathophysiological theories.

Modern discussions of Herophilus' pathophysiology naturally have tended to focus on the best documented aspect, namely his theory of the pulse – a theory of great interest to ancient physicians too, not only because it concerned a vital function but also because of the considerable diagnostic significance the pulse assumed in antiquity in the absence of many modern diagnostic tools. But before I turn to an analysis of Herophilus' pulse-lore, more fundamental questions concerning the general basis of his physiology and pathology must be considered.

1 *Humours, faculties*

The most fundamental question is whether Herophilus, like earlier physicians,[1] attributed normal functions and abnormal conditions of the body to balance and imbalance, respectively, in the four humours, or whether he succeeded – as did his illustrious contemporary Erasistratus[2] – in breaking the tenacious spell of the humoral theory. Was his approach to the entrenched humoral tradition marked by the same audacious frontiermanship, by the same radical innovation that characterized much of his anatomy? The author of a pseudo-Galenic treatise, *Introductio sive medicus* (perhaps first century A.D.) seems to suggest exactly the opposite: 'Some people', he says, 'attributed *both* the constitution of things that are in accordance with nature *and* the cause of things that are contrary to nature *to the humours* (χυμοῖς) *alone*, as did Praxagoras and Herophilus.'[3] A more cryptic remark by Galen – Herophilus said there are 'four faculties (*dynameis*) which administer living beings'[4] – appears to confirm the report in the *Introductio*. In another work Galen becomes more explicit: Plato, Aristotle, and their pupils 'tried to emulate Hippocrates' theory of the humours (χυμῶν), and so did the most reputable of the ancient physicians, viz. Diocles, ... Praxagoras, ... and Herophilus'.[5] While 'emulation' leaves some room for a revisionary process, it does not suggest a radical rejection of the traditional humoral theory.

Despite this apparently unequivocal evidence that Herophilus, for all his remarkable departures from the Hippocratic tradition,

---

[1] Humoral theory was, of course, neither a monolithic nor a static doctrine in earlier medicine. For the numerous forms it assumed cf. Schöner, 1964.

[2] Erasistratus, says Galen (v, p. 123K), never mentioned black bile, but he did not completely abandon the notion of morbid bodily juices (ὑγρασίαι) In general, he considered *plethora* of blood or hyperaemia, which causes blood to pass from the veins into the arteries, as the main cause of disease. Cf. Galen, *De plenitudine* 6 (vii, pp. 537–9K); Caelius Aurelianus, *Tardae passiones* 3.8.111, 3.8.124, and 2.1.15; Galen, *In Hp. De officina medic. comment.* 3.24 (xviiib, pp. 867–8K). Cf. also Fuchs, 1892b.

[3] T130. For Praxagoras see fr. 46 Steckerl. Cf. also Praxagoras, fr. 51: he called the phlegmatic humour 'vitreous humour'.

[4] T131. This is a problematic reference to 'faculty', because it occurs in the context of pulse-lore. But the only 'faculty' to which Herophilus otherwise refers in sphygmological contexts is the pulsating faculty which flows to the arteries through the arterial walls from the heart (T144). The only fourfold division in his pulse-lore is that of the differentiae specificae of pulses into vehemence or strength, speed, size, and rhythm (T162); these are, however, certainly not 'faculties' (*dynameis*), but attributes used to differentiate one pulse from another. I have therefore tentatively concluded that 'four faculties' might refer to Herophilus' acceptance of the four humours. But cf. Index s.v. 'faculty'.

[5] T132. See *Comments* on T132 for further details.

remained a traditionalist in his affirmation of a humoral basis for his pathophysiology, it has been argued by a respected scholar that Herophilus' attitude to the traditional theory was marked by scepticism.[6] This argument is based on two texts. In the first, the author of the pseudo-Galenic work *Medical Definitions* (perhaps first century A.D.) states: 'The Herophileans say [a chronic disease] is an affection which is difficult to resolve and to change, and its cause lies in *moistures* (ὑγροῖς).'[7] The second passage, from Celsus, attributes to Herophilus the view that *in umidis omne vitium est*, 'every defect lies in the *moistures*'.[8] Fridolf Kudlien maintains that Herophilus, too sceptical to accept the traditional humoral theory, established his distance from it by resorting to a more comprehensive and less specific term, 'moistures' (*in umidis*, ἐν ὑγροῖς), for 'humours' (*humores*, χυμοί). Kudlien moreover suggests that Herophilus used his 'moisture-based' pathology only in practice, i.e. for therapeutic purposes, and, at the level of generalizable theory, completley abandoned the formulation of general pathological principles[9] – an ingenious and appealing interpretation, especially in the light of Herophilus' views on causal explanation and his innovative spirit. But does it stand up to scrutiny?

While Herophilus apparently believed that all causal explanation remains hypothetical or provisional, and in that sense was indeed 'sceptical', as I argued earlier,[10] a number of factors seem to militate against the conclusion that he abandoned traditional humoral pathology. First, and most significant, there are the texts I mentioned at the outset, which testify unequivocally that Herophilus resorted to the same humoral theory as Diocles, Praxagoras and others among his medical predecessors.[11] Even if one disregards, as one probably should, the statement in a pseudo-Galenic commentary (on Hippocrates' *On Nutrition*) that Herophilus held the same traditional view as Plato, Diocles, and others on black bile or melancholy[12] – the commentary is probably a Renaissance forgery[13] – there remain the

⁶ Kudlien, 1964a: 7–8.   ⁷ T205(a).   ⁸ T133.
⁹ Kudlien, 1964c: 8: 'Vielleicht hat Herophilos für die Theorie von einer verbindlichen Pathologie ganz abgesehen und nur in der Praxis mit einer solchen Hygropathologie operiert.'
¹⁰ Chapter v.A.   ¹¹ T130–T132.
¹² T134. On theories of melancholy in Greek antiquity see Flashar, 1966. Cf. also Starobinski, 1960.
¹³ Ernst Nachmanson, who had undertaken to provide a critical edition of this work, discovered that it is a compilatory forgery produced in the Renaissance; cf. Diels, 1914: 128–9: Nelson, vs. Schubring in Gal. xxK (repr. 1965), p. XLVIII.

unambiguous statements by Galen and by the author of the pseudo-Galenic *Introductio* that Herophilus attributed both the functions and the dysfunctions of the human body to the humours. I see no intrinsic reason to grant this evidence less credence than the two texts cited by Kudlien.

Secondly, in the pseudo-Galenic *Definitions*, to which Kudlien appeals for his 'moisture' hypothesis, the reference is not to Herophilus but to the 'Herophileans'. It is striking that none of the eighteen Herophilean physicians presented in Part 2 of this volume seems to have subscribed to the humoral theory, and that the only possible reference to the humours in Chapters XI–XXVIII is an oblique attribution of causal status to 'decay and excess of liquid (*liquoris*)' in a discussion of hydrophobia by Aristoxenus,[14] a Herophilean physican of the first century A.D. It is accordingly conceivable, though by no means certain, that the scepticism – or at any rate the discomfort with the humoral theory – which Kudlien wants to attribute to Herophilus, in fact only developed among his successors, who in general had a much more limited propensity to develop theories.[15] (Against an emphasis on 'Herophileans' in the passage from *Definitions* it could, of course, be pointed out (a) that 'Herophileans' often means 'Herophilus *and* the Herophileans' – a point readily conceded – and (b) that a later Latin version of this passage actually substitutes 'Herophilus' for 'Herophileans'; this second point self-destructs, however, because the Latin version then also proceeds to substitute *in humoribus*, 'in the humours', for 'in moistures', ἐν ὑγροῖς,[16] perhaps revealing the interchangeability of 'humour' and 'moisture'.)

What remains in favour of the view that Herophilus abandoned humoral pathology is Celsus' statement that, in Herophilus' opinion, *in umidis omne vitium est*.[17] Very striking in this context is, however, another passage from Celsus, which seems to caution against drawing a sharp and highly significant distinction between 'humour' (*umor* or χυμός) and 'moisture' (*umidum* or ὑγρόν, ὑγρότης). In his discussion of the correlation between seasons and diseases, Celsus says that infants and young children are likely to suffer from 'thrush, vomiting,

---

[14] See *infra*, Chapter XXV, Ar. 6: 'corruptionem atque abundantiam liquoris'.
[15] Cf. the discussion of this later Herophilean movement away from theoretical medicine below, Chapter X.A.
[16] T205b, from the pseudo-Soranian *Medical Questions*.
[17] T133.

insomnia, *umor* from the ears, and inflammation around the navel' in summer.[18] What makes this use of *umor* interesting is that Celsus is simply providing a truncated translation of a Hippocratic *Aphorism* (3.24), where the corresponding term is not 'humour' (χυμός) but 'moistures' (ὑγρότητες).[19] Celsus, in other words, seems to regard 'humour' and 'moisture' as interchangeable terms, and in all likelihood no special significance should be attached to his attribution of pathology based on 'moistures', rather than 'humours', to Herophilus.

Finally, and perhaps most significantly, 'moisture' and 'humour', *hygron* and *chymos*, are used interchangeably not only by Celsus but as early as the Hippocratic Corpus itself. Thus the author of *On Seed* or *On Generation* (περὶ γονῆς) enumerates four innate humours – blood, bile, water, and phlegm – which are responsible for all diseases, and introduces them not as 'humours' but as 'moistures': εἰσὶ δὲ τέσσαρες ἰδέαι τοῦ ὑγροῦ, αἷμα, χολή, ὕδωρ καὶ φλέγμα, τοσαύτας γὰρ ἰδέας ἔχει ξυμφυέας ὁ ἄνθρωπος ἐν ἑωυτῷ, καὶ ἀπὸ τουτέων αἱ νοῦσοι γίνονται (VII, p. 474L). Similarly, the Hippocratic author of *On Diseases* IV says man and woman are both constituted of four humours – phlegm, blood, bile, and aqueous humour (hydrops) – from which all diseases that do not result from violence arise, and again he introduces them as forms of 'moisture' (ὑγρόν), not as 'humours' (χυμοί): ἔχει δὲ καὶ ἡ γυνὴ καὶ ὁ ἀνὴρ τέσσαρας ἰδέας ὑγροῦ ἐν τῷ σώματι, ἀφ'ὧν αἱ νοῦσοι γίνονται, ὁκόσα μὴ ἀπὸ βίης νουσήματα γίνεται. αὗται δὲ αἱ ἰδέαι εἰσὶ φλέγμα, αἷμα, χολὴ καὶ ὕδρωψ (VII, p. 542L). 'Moisture' and 'humour' are, therefore, used in identical ways as early as the Hippocratic Corpus, and the argument that the use of 'moisture' for 'humour' signals Herophilus' sceptical retreat from Hippocratic humoral theory seems less enticing.

Within the limits of his insistence on the hypothetical and provisional nature of causal explanation, Herophilus therefore seems to have accepted the traditional humoral theory – a striking instance of the persistence of tradition within an innovative scientific commu-

[18] Celsus, *Medicinae* 2.1.18 (*CML* I, p. 49 Marx): ' . . . infantes tenerosque adhuc pueros serpentia ulcera oris, quae ἄφθας Graeci nominant, vomitus, nocturnae vigiliae, *aurium umor*, circa umbilicum inflammationes exerceant.'
[19] Hp., IV. p. 496L: 'At different stages of life the following [affections] occur: in small and new-born children, thrush, vomiting, coughing, sleeplessness, fears, inflammation of the navel, moistures [discharges] from the ears (ὤτων ὑγρότητες)'.

nity. No matter how hard or how fast we run, Nietzsche said, the chain of the past runs with us, and the Alexandrian physician seems to have been no exception. But despite the chain, Herophilus went considerably beyond his predecessors in some aspects of his pathophysiology. Galen, who was often quick to criticize Hellenistic physicians, in fact puts Herophilus on the same pedestal as Aristotle, describing him as an author who 'wrote much – and wrote well – about the usefulness of the parts'.[20] An examination of the fragmentary remains presented in this chapter appear to substantiate this characterization.

2 *Control centre, nerves*

A question discussed by many Greek philosophers, namely the location of the controlling faculty or 'command centre' within the body, was also treated by Herophilus. Whereas previous authors had developed fairly general solutions – the head, the brain, the chest, the heart, the blood around the heart, the pneuma around the heart, and so on[21] – Herophilus, like his contemporary Erasistratus, tried to apply his more accurate anatomical knowledge to answering this question. Having accepted Aristotle's distinction between cerebrum and cerebellum, as pointed out in the previous chapter,[22] Herophilus – unlike Aristotle – now assigned major pathophysiological significance to the brain. He also proceeded to differentiate the ventricles, and among them he attributed greatest significance to what is identified, first, as 'that ventricle of the brain which is also its base *(basis)*'[23] – not to be confused with the modern sense of 'brain stem' – and, secondly, as 'the ventricle in the cerebellum *(parenkephalis)*'.[24] These two statements seem to assign a major controlling function to the hindbrain, and, more specifically, either to what today is known as the fourth ventricle (in the hindbrain), or to the roof portion of the hindbrain which we call cerebellum. The proximity of the hindbrain to the spinal cord and hence to the nerve tracts, and conceivably, the vivisectory discovery that the cerebellum is the centre responsible for the muscular activity and for maintaining the equilibrium of the body, may have led Herophilus to the conclusion

---

[20] T136.   [21] See T137; Ch. VI.A.3 *supra*; and cf. Solmsen, 1961.
[22] Cf. Chapter VI.A. 3; Aristotle, *Historia animalium* 1.16.494b32 and 495a12 (where Herophilus' – and all later authors' – word for cerebellum, παρεγκεφαλίς, makes its first appearance).
[23] T137.   [24] T138.

that this part of the brain exercises the most significant control over
the body. This conclusion became one of Herophilus' more influential
physiological theories, because Galen accepted it as valid (on the
basis of his experiments with animals).

The standard of precision at which Herophilus' location of the
'command centre' aims is novel, and his firm rejection of Aristotle's
notion that the brain is nothing but a cooling agent which tempers the
heat of the blood and helps us sleep[25] is a major step forward. But the
pathophysiological significance of the brain had, of course, been
recognized in general terms as early as the Presocratics and
Hippocratics. Sensory and cognitive activity, in particular, was
attributed to it relatively consistently. Thus, in the fifth century B.C.,
Alcmeon of Croton pointed out that sensory activity is impaired
'when the brain is moved and changes its place'.[26] Diogenes of
Apollonia, too, made the brain the centre of all sensory activity,[27]
and Democritus, especially in his explanation of hearing,[28] also
assigns the brain a major role. In the fourth century Plato followed
this Presocratic example, locating the cognitive part of the psyche in
the head and actively using the term 'brain' in his explanations of
sensation and perception.[29] But Herophilus' most significant predecessor is Hippocratic: the author of On Sacred Disease, who went
beyond the recognition of the sensory and cognitive function of the
brain and attributed a more comprehensive pathophysiological role
to the brain (and to the humours and bloodvessels connected with it).
'The brain is in fact responsible', he said, 'for this disease [sc. the
'sacred disease' or epilepsy], just as it is for the rest of the more serious
diseases.'[30] Furthermore, he affirms that the brain is a key to

[25] Aristotle, De somno 3.457b20-458a10, and De partibus animalium 2.7.652b31-6.
[26] Alcmeon, 24A5 (I, p. 212DK) = Theophrastus, De sensibus 25-6: all the senses are
connected with the brain, διὸ καὶ πηροῦσθαι κινουμένου καὶ μεταλλάττοντος
τὴν χώραν. Cf. also Calcidius in 24A10DK and Aëtius, Placita 4.17.1; DG, p.
407, who is more straightforward, but also more schematized, making use of
anachronistic terminology. Cf. Ch. VI.A.3 supra.
[27] Cf. Diogenes, 64A19DK (= Theophrastus, De sensibus 39ff.); 64A21 DK
(= Aëtius, Placita 4.16.3; DG, p. 406).
[28] Democritus, 68A135DK, especially II, p. 116.15-18 DK (= Theophrastus, op. cit.,
chapter 56); 68A105 (= Aëtius, op. cit., 4.5.1; DG, p. 391; T137a infra).
[29] Cf. Plato, Phaedo 96A-B (where Socrates' assessment of this view of brain function
is, however, characteristically elusive). See also Timaeus 44D, 65E, 70A, 67B,
73D-E, 76A, 76C.
[30] Hp., On the Sacred Disease 6 (= 3.1, p. 68 Grensemann).

understanding not only abnormal conditions but also the normal functions of the body: 'I think the brain has the greatest power in humans, for when it is healthy it is our interpreter [*hermeneus*] of things caused by air (air, you see, provides intelligence), . . . and the brain is the interpreter of understanding . . .'[31] In the Hippocratic treatise *On Fleshes* the brain is likewise granted this traditional cognitive role.[32] The author of *On Sacred Disease*, moreover, makes the brain the centre of all emotions, of our aesthetic activity, and of our moral judgment: 'People should know that our pleasures, joys, laughter, and jests arise from no other source than this [sc. from the brain]; and so do our pains, griefs, anxieties and tears. Through it . . . we also discern ugly and beautiful, bad and good, pleasant and unpleasant . . .'[33]

Impressive though this sustained pre-Alexandrian concern with the physiological and pathological function of the brain is, Herophilus' isolation of the cerebellum or fourth ventricle as being of particular importance represents a new attempt at precision, and so does his theory concerning the connection of the nerves with the brain (more on this below). What remains unanswered by the ancient sources is, however, the relation of this view of the brain and the nerves to Herophilus' humoral theory. It is unclear, for example, whether Herophilus would have agreed with the Hippocratic author of *On Sacred Disease* that the 'corruption' of the brain is caused by humours, above all by phlegm and bile.[34] But if Herophilus was indeed a humoral pathologist, he would probably have been inclined to agree with some version of such an explanation. The Hippocratic author had also used the concept of pneuma – which Herophilus perhaps thought of as flowing through the nerves (see below) – and attributed aphasia, for example, to the inability of air or pneuma to reach the brain when phlegm blocks the vessels which serve as air ducts.[35] Herophilus' view of the relation of the humours to motor or sensory functions and dysfunctions almost certainly was more sophisticated, as a brief examination of his view of the nerves will

[31] *Ibid.*, 19 (= 16.1–2 and 16.6, pp. 84–6 Grensemann).
[32] Hp., *On Fleshes* 16–17 (Deichgräber, 1935: 16, 49–51).
[33] *On the Sacred Disease* 17 (= 14.1–2, p. 82 Grensemann). For further historical background see Woollam, 1958; Clarke & O'Malley, 1968: 1–18, 140–53, 260–3, 708–13; Clarke & Dewhurst, 1972: 5–9.
[34] Hp., *On the Sacred Disease* 18 (= 15.1–2, p. 84 Grensemann).
[35] *Ibid.*, 10 (= 7.1–15, pp. 72–4 Grensemann).

show, but the exact relation of the humours to the rest of his physiology remains shrouded in silence.

Herophilus' remarkably detailed anatomy of one of his major discoveries, the nerves, was discussed in the preceding chapter (see pp. 159–60); here, drawing on many of the same texts and a few additional ones, we turn to the physiology of the nervous system. While Herophilus' contemporary Erasistratus achieved a more detailed understanding of the nervous system, as Friedrich Solmsen recognized in his pioneering study on the discovery of the nerves,[36] Herophilus' own contribution to the study of the nerves was not confined to detailed anatomical observations, as the following points will illustrate.

First, the question 'what agencies or faculties are responsible (a) for voluntary bodily movements and (b) for sense perception?' had preoccupied numerous philosophers and physicians prior to Herophilus, as Solmsen has shown in detail,[37] but no one before Herophilus, not even Aristotle – who made a brilliant attempt to explain both activities by the same psychophysical principles[38] – had discovered that the same organs, i.e. the nervous system, are responsible for both activities. The claim that Herophilus not only discovered the nerves but succeeded in differentiating between motor and sensory nerves has understandably met with scepticism, but Rufus of Ephesus, among others, seems to make clear beyond reasonable doubt that Herophilus actually did make the distinction: 'According to Erasistratus and Herophilus there are nerves capable of sensation ... (αἰσθητικά). But according to Herophilus ... the nerves that make voluntary things possible (προαιρετικά) have their origin in the cerebrum and spinal marrow, and some grow from bone to bone, others from muscle to muscle, and some also bind together the joints'.[39] While the last phrase suggests that Herophilus was not always successful in differentiating nerves from ligaments and tendons, the rest of the passage indicates that he knew of two kinds of nerves, *aisthētika* (or sensory) and *prohairetika* (or motor) nerves. For

[36] Solmsen, 1961: 184–97. Cf. also Souques, 1934; 1935; 1936b: 116–39.
[37] Solmsen, 1961: 150–84. Cf. Souques, 1936b: 11–115.
[38] Cf. Solmsen, 1961: 169–78.
[39] Cf. *supra*, Chapter VI, T81. (Potter, 1976: 51 makes the plausible suggestion that this text is marred by an omission.)

motor nerves Erasistratus used the expression *kinētika neura* instead, but Herophilus' term is no less felicitous, in so far as *prohairetika* ('capable of choosing, purposive') stresses the fact that Herophilus is resorting to the motor nerves to explain only voluntary motions, not involuntary functions such as the pulse. *Prohairetikos* does not seem to have been used before Aristotle, and Herophilus might well have chosen it under the influence of the prominent role it, and the noun from which it is derived, *prohairesis* or 'choice', play in Aristotle's theory of action.[40]

One ancient passage has been used to cast doubt on Herophilus' discovery: although Galen in one work credits the Alexandrian with discovering the roots of more than seven pairs of cranial nerves,[41] in another work he complains that Herophilus and Eudemus, 'the first persons after Hippocrates to record carefully their dissection of the nerves', did not trace all motor and sensory nerves from their terminal points to their beginnings, and hence left 'physicians with no small investigation into why some paralyses destroy only sensation, while others destroy voluntary motion, and others again destroy both'.[42] But this complaint about a task left incomplete clearly does not need to be interpreted as evidence of Herophilus' failure to distinguish sensory nerves from motor nerves; it is the task of tracing the nerve paths, not the fundamental distinction between motor and sensory nerves, that is at issue in Galen's criticism.

A further testimonium is tantalizing but more ambiguous. Rufus of Ephesus, reporting that 'Herophilus calls the tunic covering the ventricles of the brain chorioid meninx', immediately adds 'and the offshoots from the brain, the sensory (*aisthētika*) and voluntary nerves (*prohairetika neura*), through which sensation and voluntary motion (*prohairetikē kinēsis*) and all action of the body are accomplished.'[43] It is unclear whether Rufus intends to say 'and the offshoots from the brain [*Herophilus calls*] sensory and voluntary motor nerves . . .' or simply 'and the offshoots from the brain [*are*] sensory and voluntary motor nerves . . .'.[44] Rufus' use of an expression associated above all

---

[40] Cf. especially Aristotle, *Nicomachean Ethics*, Book 3, Chapters 4–7. For προαιρε-τικός see also *ibid.*, 2.6.1106b36; 5.14.1137b35; Hp., *Aphorisms* 4.52, 7.83.

[41] Cf. Chapter VI, T82.   [42] Chapter VI, T80.   [43] Chapter VI, T125.

[44] The ellipsis in Rufus' text could be understood either as 'he [sc. Herophilus] calls', 'he says that', preceding βλαστήματα, and followed by an accusative (αἰσθητικά, etc.) with a further ellipsis of εἶναι, or as a simple ellipsis of ἐστι between βλαστήματα and αἰσθητικὰ νεῦρα.

with Herophilus' description of the motor nerves, namely *prohairetika neura*, is, however, very striking, and it is possible – though by no means certain – that Rufus intended also to attribute the statement concerning the nerves to Herophilus.

A second important point which illustrates Herophilus' interest in physiology is that he was not content just to ascribe voluntary motor functions to some nerves and sensory functions to others, but apparently also tried to explain how they work. The only relatively unambiguous evidence we have is unfortunately limited to the optic nerves. From the preceding chapter[45] it already is clear that Herophilus and the Hellenistic anatomist Eudemus 'called the nerves which proceed [down from the brain] to the eyes "passages" (*poroi*).'[46] In two different treatises Galen elaborates on Herophilus' reasons for calling the optic nerves *poroi* ('passages' or 'ducts' or channels'). First, in *On the Usefulness of Parts* Galen says about 'the sensory nerves (*aisthētika neura*) which descend to the eyes from the brain' that 'Herophilus also calls them *poroi*, since they alone have clear, perceptible paths for the pneuma.'[47] In a second passage, in *On the Causes of Symptoms*, a similar – but far from identical – explanation is attributed more ambiguously to οἱ περὶ τὸν Ἡρόφιλον [lit. 'those around Herophilus'], i.e. either 'the followers of Herophilus' or 'Herophilus and his followers' (οἱ περί is notoriously ambiguous and permits of both interpretations): 'The nerve which proceeds down from the brain to the eye – which those around Herophilus in fact also call a "passage" (*poros*), because its perforation [lumen?] alone is clearly visible – seems *to me* [i.e. to Galen] to exist as a pathway for sensory pneuma.'[48] The shift in the second passage is significant: while both passages attribute recognition of the unusual (in fact, unique) lumen of the optic nerve to Herophileans or their leader, Galen attributes the view that the optic nerves are 'paths for pneuma' to Herophilus only in the first passage, acknowledging this as his own view – but not as Herophilus' – in the second.

Fortunately, a third text seems to confirm that Herophilus himself thought of the optic nerves as containing pneuma. Calcidius, who

---

[45] Cf. Chapter VI. A.3, and T84–T85.
[46] T140(c) (= Chapter VI, T84).
[47] T140(a). On earlier uses of *poroi* cf. G.E.R. Lloyd, 1975a.
[48] T140(b) (= Chapter VI, T85).

translated Plato's *Timaeus* into Latin shortly after A.D. 400, reports in his commentary that, in Herophilus' view,

duas esse angustas semitas quae a cerebri sede, in qua est sita potestas animae summa et principalis, ad oculorum cavernas meent naturalem spiritum continentes . . .

there are two narrow ducts containing natural pneuma (*naturalem spiritum*) which go from the seat [base] of the brain, in which the highest, principal power of the soul is located, to the cavities of the eyes . . . [49]

Although Calcidius lumps together Alcmeon, the Peripatetic Callisthenes, and Herophilus as the authors of this view, the elaborate anatomy of the eye which follows has been widely recognized as being Herophilean. The uniquely Herophilean emphasis on 'the seat of the brain' (i.e. the cerebellum or fourth ventricle – similarly identified as *basis* or 'base' of the brain in a testimonium mentioned earlier) as the locus of the psychophysical command centre of the body, clearly points to Herophilus. In the absence of further evidence it is unclear whether Herophilus qualified his use of 'pneuma' either with 'sensory' (αἰσθητικόν), as does Galen,[50] or with 'natural' (*naturalis*, φυσικόν), as does Calcidius. The concept 'sensory pneuma' 'was in the air', as Solmsen put it,[51] and so was 'natural pneuma'. But 'natural pneuma' would be a more problematic usage in this context: if, as some ancient sources imply,[52] the distinction between 'natural pneuma' (as that which nourishes living beings) and 'psychic pneuma' (as the pneuma responsible for all sensory and motor activity) had become widely accepted by the early Hellenistic period, one would have expected Herophilus to use 'psychic pneuma' – or its

---

[49] See above, Chapter VI, T86, with *Comments*; cf. also Chapter VI, nn. 45, 64.

[50] T140(b) (= Chapter VI, T85).

[51] Solmsen, 1961: 188. Potter, 1976: 52, by contrast argues that 'Galen has applied his own theory anachronistically to Herophilus', but adduces no convincing arguments in refutation of Solmsen's conclusions.

[52] Cf. *SVF* II, 716, from ps.-Galen, *Introductio sive medicus* 9 (XIV, p. 697K). (The source, however, simply says this division existed κατὰ τοὺς παλαιούς, without specifying who these 'ancients' were. But since Stoics – unfortunately of undetermined date – are said to have 'introduced a third kind of pneuma' – that which holds it all together, τὸ ἑκτικόν (cf. Chapter X, T280) – ps.-Galen seems to imply that the division of pneuma into 'psychic' and 'natural' antedates the Stoic introduction of a third kind.) Aristotle's concept of σύμφυτον πνεῦμα or 'connate pneuma' might be part of the pneuma theory ps.-Galen here ascribes to 'the ancients'. But the identity of these 'ancients' remains highly problematic.

subordinate concept[53] 'sensory pneuma' – but not 'natural pneuma' to refer to the content of the optic nerves.

It is not clear whether these texts concerning the optic nerve allow the generalization that, in Herophilus' view, *all* sensory nerves contain pneuma. Solmsen makes the reasonable observation that Galen 'does not say that Herophilus found ὁδοί [passages, ducts] of the πνεῦμα [pneuma] only in the optic nerves but that here only were these "ways" visible and clearly present (αἰσθηταί, σαφεῖς) and that here only was the perforation (*lumen*, τρῆμα) to be seen'.[54] Since Herophilus, like most physicists and physicians, accepted the notion that 'one kind of motion is perceptible by reason, the other by sense', Solmsen suggests that Herophilus extended this distinction between two kinds of motion to the problem of sensory pneuma in the nerves: whereas the pneuma-path is visible in the case of the optic nerve, 'the most natural and methodical inference from Galen's statements is that the pneuma in the other sensory nerves was for Herophilus a λόγῳ θεωρητόν, something whose presence was to be inferred by reason'[55] but was not visible. Given the prominence the concept *pneuma* had been gaining in psychophysiology, especially from Aristotle onward,[56] Solmsen's inference has a great deal of historical plausibility. Yet the ancient sources' silence – especially Galen's – concerning the question whether, in Herophilus' view, *all* sensory nerves contain sensory pneuma and communicate with the 'command centre' in the cerebellum (or fourth ventricle) by means of this pneuma, remains troubling. Whatever doubt about the extent of Herophilus' use of pneuma in his explanation of the nervous system

---

[53] In ps.-Galen, *op. cit.*, 13 (XIV, p. 726K) 'natural pneuma' is described as that which nourishes living beings and plants, while 'psychic pneuma' is subdivided into sensory and motor pneuma; von Arnim (*SVF* II, 716) seems to think that this subdivision dates back at least to Chrysippus, and this seems plausible. If Herophilus in fact used both 'sensory pneuma' and 'motor pneuma' to explain the functions of the nerves, the Stoic subdivision might have been inspired by the Alexandrian physician. It is unclear whether this development was also influenced by Erasistratus' distinction between 'vital pneuma' (πνεῦμα ζωτικόν), which exists in the heart and in the arteries, and 'psychic pneuma' which is located in the brain (cf. Galen, *De placitis Hippocratis et Platonis* 1.6.3; 7.3.23–8; 2.8.38). See also n. 56 *infra*.

[54] Solmsen, 1961: 187.   [55] *Ibid.*

[56] Cf. Solmsen, 1961: 169ff.; Verbeke, 1945: especially pp. 11ff. and 175ff. (on psychic pneuma: pp. 518–28); Jaeger, 1913; De Lacy, *CMG* v.4.1.2, pp. 617, 676.

this massive silence might inspire unfortunately is reinforced when one turns to the evidence concerning his view of the way the motor nerves function.

In his treatise *De tremore, palpitatione, convulsione et rigore* Galen first criticizes Herophilus 'for having the ambition to demonstrate that tremor always arises in connection with the nerve-like class [sc. of bodily parts; τὸ νευρῶδες] . . . [and for thus] attributing the affection of the faculty to its organs', but subsequently he gives Herophilus full credit for 'recognizing correctly that the nerve-like class (τὸ νευρῶδες γένος) – and not the arterial class – serves the voluntary motions (ταῖς κατὰ προαίρεσιν κινήσεσιν)'.[57] Although the 'nerve-like class' or 'nervous genus of bodily parts' may include tendons and ligaments, as the evidence discussed above indicates,[58] it almost certainly refers to the nerves themselves too. This is made particularly clear not only by the choice of 'nerve-like' – rather than 'muscle' or 'fibre' or another word for 'ligament' or 'sinew' (for example, σύνδεσμος, μῦς, τένων, ἴς)[59] – but also by Galen's statement that Herophilus attributes 'motions by *prohairesis*', i.e. voluntary motions, to the 'nerve-like genus' of parts; the related verbal adjective *prohairetikos* is, of course, exactly the term Herophilus used to refer to motor *nerves* (see above).

Furthermore, in a subsequent reiteration of his criticism, Galen twice switches from 'nerve-like genus' to a straightforward use of 'nerves': Herophilus failed to recognize, says Galen, 'that the body of the nerves (τὸ σῶμα τῶν νεύρων) is not itself the cause of motion but

---

[57] T141.

[58] See especially Chapter VI, T81.

[59] All of these terms were used in pre-Alexandrian science. Cf. Aristotle, *De partibus animalium* 2.6.652a16 (σύνδεσμος; cf. also 652a19: νευρώδης of 'sinewy' marrow); Euripides, *Hippolytus* 199 (μελέων σύνδεσμα); Hp., *On the Art* 10 (the flesh surrounding cavities that is called 'muscle', μῦς). τένων is common for 'sinew' or 'tendon' as early as the Homeric poems: cf. *Iliad* 5.307, 4.521, 20.478, 22.396; *Odyssey* 3.449. It remained in use in medical and biological literature: Hp., *On Fractures* 11 (II, p. 63Kw; of the 'back tendon' or 'Achilles' tendon'); Aristotle, *Historia animalium* 3.5.515b9: the tendon, τένων, is a double-sinew, νεῦρον διπτυχές (cf. Galen, *De ossibus ad tirones*, praef. [II, p. 739K]: there are three types of *neura*: *prohairetika*, which proceed from the brain and the spinal cord; *syndetika neura* or *syndesmoi* which proceed from bones; τένοντες, 'tendons' which proceed from a muscle). Ἴς (usually plural, ἶνες), 'sinew', 'tendon', or 'fibrous vessel', likewise has a history reaching from Homer to later scientific authors: cf. *Iliad* 17.522, 23.191; *Odyssey* 11.219; Plato, *Timaeus* 82c8, 84A2; Aristotle, *Historia animalium* 3.6.515b27 (ἶνες are intermediate between sinew (νεῦρον) and bloodvessel (φλέψ)) – but see also *De partibus animalium* 2.4.650b14.

rather its instrument (*organon*)', and, similarly, 'in the case of the dead neither the nerves (τὰ νεῦρα) nor the muscles (οἱ μύες) are in the state of suffering all those affections which Herophilus . . . thinks they suffer; all motion is absent from them immediately with [the departure of] the soul, for muscles (μύες) and nerves (νεῦρα) are just the instruments of the soul'.[60]

At the very least the first of these two Galenic uses of 'nerves' indicates that he understood Herophilus to have said that nerves are responsible for voluntary motion, while the second suggests that 'nerve-like genus' might include muscles. This impression is reinforced by another testimonium concerning Herophilus' view of 'tremor' (τρόμος), i.e. of the very affection he is here said to have attributed to the 'nerve-like genus' of bodily parts. This passage is from a treatise on pulse-lore attributed to Rufus of Ephesus (but of disputed authorship): 'Herophilus says . . . pulse occurs only in the arteries and the heart, whereas palpitation and spasm and tremor occur in *muscles* as well as *nerves* . . . And the pulse at all times attends us involuntarily (ἀπροαιρέτως) . . . whereas the others are within our power to choose (ἐν τῇ ἡμετέρᾳ προαιρέσει), mainly by pressing out and depressing the parts [sc. muscles and nerves?] frequently.'[61] Here the association of nerves *and* muscles with voluntary motion is attributed unequivocally to Herophilus. Whereas Praxagoras[62] still assigned all of these motions – pulse, spasm, tremor, palpitation – to the arteries, Herophilus' discovery of the nervous system now allows him to differentiate between (a) the arteries as the vehicles of the involuntary motion in the vascular system, i.e. of pulsation, and (b) the nerves and muscles as the vehicles of voluntary motions. (But among the affections of the voluntary motor organs he specifically includes tremor, palpitation, and spasm – all of which we would, of course, classify as involuntary motions.)

It therefore seems likely that Herophilus' explanation of voluntary motions included not only the motor nerves, extending from the cerebellum or fourth ventricle of the brain to various parts of the body, but also tendons, ligaments, and muscles, all of which he viewed as species of 'the genus of nerve-like parts'.[63] But exactly how does motion actually take place? Did Herophilus conceive of the

---

[60] T141.   [61] T149.   [62] Praxagoras, fr. 27 Steckerl.
[63] T141: τὸ νευρῶδες γένος.

motor nerves – and perhaps of the tendons, ligaments, and muscles – as 'pathways for motor pneuma', just as he apparently conceived of the optic nerves as pathways for sensory pneuma?

Galen's criticism of Herophilus' theory of voluntary motion does not provide an encouraging answer. Herophilus, says Galen, did not recognize 'that the body of the nerves is not itself the cause of motion but rather its instruments (*organon*), whereas its moving cause is the faculty (*dynamis*) which extends through the nerves. Here I reproach Herophilus for not having distinguished faculty from instrument.'[64] If Galen's criticism is accepted as valid, Herophilus attributed voluntary motion to the motor nerves, ligaments, tendons, and muscles (all of which presumably were ultimately controlled by the command centre in the hindbrain), but did not introduce an additional faculty or medium such as motor pneuma through which the hindbrain could communicate with them. Solmsen, who correctly emphasizes pneuma as a strong element of continuity in Greek theories of motion and sensation, extrapolates from the evidence concerning the presence of pneuma in the optic nerve that it is 'practically certain that Herophilus throught of the pneuma as operating also in the motor nerves'.[65] While arguments from conceivability, internal consistency, and historical probability all point to Solmsen's conclusion, it is a conclusion which renders Galen's criticism of Herophilus incomprehensible. Though Galen was quick to polemicize, the texts presented in this volume do not reveal him to have been guilty of such radical distortion or misunderstanding of Herophilus' views. Perhaps more significantly, Galen's unqualified willingness to give Herophilus credit for attributing voluntary motion to the 'class of nerve-like parts' lends his immediately following claim, namely that Herophilus thought of 'the *body* of the nerves' – rather than of some 'faculty' or medium, such as psychic or kinetic pneuma – as the cause of motion, an air of credibility.

Herophilus' view on the question whether a foetus is a living being provides further evidence, but it is no more conclusive than the texts examined up to this point. According to the doxographer Aëtius (c. A.D. 100) – and according to the pseudo-Galenic *De historia philosopha* (c. A.D. 500), which depends on Aëtius (or perhaps on Aëtius' source) – Herophilus grants foetuses 'natural motion' but not

---

[64] T141.   [65] Solmsen, 1961: 186; Potter, 1976: 52, is sceptical.

'pneumatic motion' (T202). If this text preserves Herophilus' terminology, 'natural motion' probably refers to involuntary motions such as pulsation and respiration. 'Pneumatic motion', being distinct from 'natural motion', would accordingly have to be voluntary motion (and possibly sensation), i.e. the kind of motion Herophilus ascribes to the nerves or to the 'nerve-like class' of organs. And indeed, Aëtius adds: 'But the nerves are the cause of [or: responsible for] the motion', presumably referring to 'pneumatic motion', since the nerves are certainly not responsible for the 'natural tendency' of the lungs to dilate or for the 'natural motion' of arterial pulsation. If 'pneumatic motion' is not Aëtius' anachronistic substitution – perhaps under Stoic or Pneumatic influence – for Herophilus' 'voluntary motion' or 'motion by choice' (κίνησις κατὰ προαίρεσιν), this testimonium would therefore provide strong evidence that Herophilus conceived of the motor nerves as containing pneuma and operating by means of pneuma. Aëtius' terminology is however, often notoriously anachronistic, and it is not inconceivable that 'pneumatic motion' (qua 'motion of air') refers to respiration, as Dobson (1925: 24) maintains, while 'natural motion' – an expression Herophilus himself would have rejected – refers to all other motions, including those controlled by the motor nerve system. (That Herophilus might have granted foetuses 'voluntary motion' does not seem inconceivable, since the kicking and similar movements of a foetus probably would have been observed by as active a gynaecologist as Herophilus.) In that case, Aëtius' account would not support the view that Herophilus thought of motor nerves as containing pneuma, since he would merely be denying the foetus a respiratory, 'pneumatic' motion. Because of the fundamental uncertainty concerning the provenance and meaning of Aëtius' terminology, it would be inadvisable to build too ambitious an edifice on this single occurrence, in a doxographic source, of the expression 'pneumatic motion', especially in the light of Galen's criticism of Herophilus' theory of voluntary motion.

It therefore remains possible that Herophilus put the concept of pneuma to fairly limited use and failed to provide a satisfactory account of the mechanisms by which the command centre in the hindbrain transmits its decisions to the nerves and to other organs of voluntary motion. It is, moreover, unclear whether Herophilus attributed impairments of our motor activity simply to lesions of the motor nerves, of the muscles, and so on, or whether he had recourse to his humoral theory to explain them (for example, by having humours block the nerve paths, as the author of *On the Sacred Disease* attributes aphasia and similar affections to the blockage by humours of the passages leading to the brain). The limitations of his theory of the nervous system and the fragmentary nature of the extant evidence should not be allowed, however, to obscure the monumental breakthrough that Herophilus' discovery of the nerves and his attempt to explain their functions represent.

3 Respiration

With the help of the nervous system Herophilus could approximate an explanation of how sensation and voluntary motor activity take place. But, as we have seen, he was also acutely aware of the existence of natural, involuntary motions in the body – notably respiration, digestion, and the pulsating motions of the vascular system – which could not be explained by a theory of the nerves, and he attempted to give physiological accounts of these as well.

Many of Herophilus' predecessors and contemporaries thought there was a close connection between breathing and heart-beat or between the respiratory and vascular systems.[66] Since the air surrounding us is the ultimate source of all pneuma, and since Herophilus seems to have thought of pneuma as present not only in the lungs but also in the arteries – and, of course, in at least some nerves – there would appear to be a prima facie case for assuming that Herophilus followed the traditional pattern of explaining respiration in terms of the vascular system. Yet the extant evidence, which is admittedly sparse, does not suggest that he insisted on this link.

While Plato, Aristotle and others had emphasized the cooling function of respiration, which helps to keep down the temperature of the blood and the heart, and hence stressed the initiatory role of the heart or the blood in their theories of respiration, Herophilus seems to have resorted to a different explanation for respiration – one which did not grant the blood or the heart a central role.

According to Aristotle, respiration takes place when the heat in the

---

[66] For a compilation of the relevant material see Rüsche, 1930: 115–27, 208–39, 249. See also Wellmann, 1901: 82–5, 71, 100; Furley & Wilkie, 1984: 3–39.

heart is increased and the heart's contents are expanded; the
expanded heart is raised up, and hence the organ surrounding it – i.e.
the lungs – must also expand. When the lungs expand, they draw in
cold air from the outside, which cancels the excessive heat of the
heart. Consequently both the heart and the lungs subside again, and
the air is expelled – but now the air breathed out is hot because it has
absorbed heat from the heart in the lungs.[67] The heart, in other
words, plays a central role in Aristotle's theory of respiration; both the
origin and the central function of respiration – tempering the heat –
for Aristotle would be inexplicable except in terms of the heart.

A firm link between the respiratory functions and the vascular
system was a prominent feature of most other ancient explanations of
respiration too. Plato, for example, begins his explanation of the
origin of the double process of inhalation (ἀναπνοή) and exhalation
(ἐκπνοή) by saying: 'One must suppose the cause of the origin of this
movement to be the following: every animal has heat in his interior
around the blood and the vessels, like a fountain of fire existing in
him . . .'[68] And Herophilus' distinguished contemporary, Erasistratus, though breaking new ground, reasserts an essential connection
between the respiratory and vascular systems: the arteries contain
only pneuma, and this pneuma is pumped into the arteries by the left
ventricle of the heart, to which it has in turn been drawn from the
outer atmosphere via the throat, the windpipe, the bronchi or 'first
arteries', and the pulmonary vein.[69] Later Galen was to adapt this
view to the purposes of his own pneumatology.[70]

The evidence concerning Herophilus' theory of respiration is

---

[67] Aristotle, De respiratione 20–1 (479b17–480b30). This passage is open to different
interpretations, but the summary provided here is faithful to what I gather
Aristotle's principal intentions to have been.

[68] Plato, Timaeus 79C7–D2; cf. also 79A5ff. Diocles of Carystus adopted a similar
explanation; cf. Wellmann, 1901: 82ff.

[69] Cf. Galen, De usu respirationis 2 (IV, pp. 473–84K); An in arteriis natura sanguis
contineatur 2 (IV, pp. 706–9K); De usu partium 7.8 (I, pp. 389–92 Helmreich); De
locis affectis 5.3 (VIII, pp. 314–16K). One decisive difference between Aristotle
and Erasistratus is, however, that Erasistratus does not accept Aristotle's notion
of 'connate pneuma'; all pneuma in the lungs, the arteries (vital pneuma), the
brain (psychic pneuma), and the muscles is ultimately derived from the outside.
Cf. also Galen, De usu respirationis 1 (IV, p. 471K): 'Or . . . do we breathe for the
sake of refilling the arteries, as Erasistratus thinks?' See Furley/Wilkie, 1984: 26–
37.

[70] Cf. Temkin, 1951; Harris, 1973: 283–7, 336–54, 363–6; Furley/Wilkie, 1984:
40ff.

limited, but it clearly suggests that he tried to counter this general tradition of explaining respiration in terms of the movement or nature of the heart. His resistance appears to have been radical: he did not grant the heart any role at all in initiating or maintaining respiration (even though he too thought of the arteries as containing at least some pneuma). Instead of referring the movement of the lungs to the movement and heat of the heart, Herophilus ascribed to the lungs themselves and to the thorax a natural tendency to dilate and contract.[71] 'The drawing in of pneuma from outside accordingly is the activity of the lung alone', he said, not of the heart.[72]

Having established this general principle, Herophilus explained breathing as a continuous process involving four stages in each of its cycles of inhalation and exhalation – and in none of these four stages does the heart play any role whatsoever. First, on account of a repletion of air occurring outside and on account of the lung's natural tendency to dilate and contract, the lung, when it dilates, draws in air or pneuma from the external atmosphere. Secondly, when the lung contracts, the thorax simultaneously dilates and the inhaled pneuma is diverted from the contracting lung to the dilating thorax. Third, when the thorax 'is filled and no longer capable of drawing this pneuma in, it lets the excess flow back again into the lung'.[73] In this stage the thorax is contracting while the lung is again simultaneously dilating; the third motion hence is also described as the one 'by which the lung receives again into itself the *contracted* pneuma from the thorax'. It is unclear whether 'the excess' (τὸ περιττόν) simply means (a) the pneuma which the thorax, when completely filled, cannot contain, or (b) the pneuma which is 'excessive' in so far as it is not required for distribution to the arteries and nerves (if indeed all nerves contain pneuma in Herophilus' view [see above]); but in this context the latter is perhaps the more obvious and plausible interpretation. The fourth and final motion is the next contraction of the lung, by which pneuma is expelled into the external air. A cycle of inhaling and exhaling is now completed, and with the immediately ensuing natural dilation of the lung a new cycle begins as air or pneuma once again is drawn in from the outside. In each cycle of

---

[71] T143a–b: τὸν οὖν πνεύμονα νομίζει μόνον ὀρέγεσθαι διαστολῆς καὶ συστολῆς φυσικῶς.

[72] *Ibid.*: ἐνέργειαν . . . τοῦ πνεύμονος τὴν ἔξωθεν τοῦ πνεύματος ὁλκήν.

[73] T143a–b.

inhalation and exhalation the lung accordingly dilates and contracts twice, while the thorax dilates and contracts only once.

Very striking in this theory of respiration, at least when measured by the the theories of Herophilus' predecessors and contemporaries, is not only the absence of any reference to the heart and to the blood, but also to cooling or heating. Other theories had, of course, also stressed the dilation and contraction of the lungs, but had explained these movements in terms of the expansion and contraction caused by changes in temperature attributed directly to the heat of the heart or the blood. Herophilus' explanation is therefore novel in so far as it introduces, instead of systolic or diastolic change due to temperatures, the concept of a *natural* tendency to dilate and contract. This is not a voluntary motion, and hence not explicable in terms of the motor nerves and their command centre in the hindbrain, but rather one of the involuntary motions, calling for an entirely different kind of explanation. When the ancient sources report that 'Herophilus admits a motor faculty for bodies in the nerves, arteries, and muscles', they are quick to recognize this and to add that he also introduced another, distinct motor capacity, namely the natural tendency of the lungs to dilate and contract.[74] The nerves and muscles serve voluntary movements, as we have seen, and the arteries are the vehicle of involuntary pulsation (see below), but distinct from – and independent of – all these motions are, in Herophilus' novel approach, the natural, involuntary motions of the lungs.

4 Vascular physiology; pulse-lore ('On Pulses')

A further involuntary motion interested Herophilus even more: the dilation and contraction of the arteries.[75] Herophilus' anatomy of the vascular system was dealt with in the preceding chapter, and the analysis which follows is therefore confined to its pathophysiological aspects.

Central to Herophilus' theory is the notion that the arteries contain

---

[74] T143a–c. But whether Herophilus shared Erasistratus' view that all pneuma is 'acquired', i.e. drawn in from the outside, or Aristotle's view that some pneuma is acquired while some is connate, remains unclear. What is clear, however, is that his theory of respiration itself does not insist on the traditional link between respiratory and vascular activity.

[75] Cf. T144–T188.

pneuma (whether this is all they contain is discussed *infra*)while the veins contain blood. His teacher Praxagoras was the first to introduce this distinction,[76] and it became widely accepted in antiquity, among others by Herophilus' contemporary Erasistratus.[77] How the pneuma (whose movement from the external atmosphere through the lungs into the thorax, and back out again, was traced above) actually reaches the heart and the arteries, is, however, not explained satisfactorily in any of the testimonia or fragments concerning Herophilus, and this remains one of the more serious gaps in our knowledge of his physiology. It has admittedly been argued that 'Herophilus . . . seems to have adopted the theory of Empedocles that both heart and arteries draw in *pneuma*, not only through the lungs but also through the pores from the surface of the skin.'[78] But the Galenic passage on which this interpretation apparently rests is highly problematic, because it conflates a number of fairly distinct views:

The pneuma is not 'sent' [sc. by the heart into the arteries] but 'drawn', and not from the heart alone but from everywhere, as Herophilus and, before him, Praxagoras, Phylotimus, Diocles, Plistonicus, Hippocrates, and countless others thought.[79]

Empedocles' theory of cutaneous breathing (if indeed that is how fragment B100DK should be interpreted) cannot be shown to have been accepted by all the physicians enumerated in this passage, and it is striking that Herophilus makes no mention of cutaneous breathing in his reasonably elaborate explanation of respiration.[80] Furthermore, Herophilus has a fairly accurate knowledge of the heart, its valves, and the arterial system – even if not as precise a knowledge as Erasistratus' – and he refers to these parts repeatedly, yet there is no suggestion in any other testimonium concerning Herophilus that pneuma in the arteries could come from any proximate source but the

---

[76] Praxagoras, fr. 28–9, 31 Steckerl. According to fr. 85 (Steckerl), Praxagoras' father, Nicarchus, also 'does not give the arteries a share in blood' (= Galen, *De plenitudine* 11 (VII, pp. 573–4K)). Cf. n. 102 *infra*.

[77] Cf., for example, Galen, *De venae sectione adversus Erasistratum* 3 (XI, p. 153K); *De placitis Hippocratis et Platonis* 7.5; *An in arteriis natura sanguis contineatur* 8 (IV, pp. 731–6K = pp. 18ff. Albrecht = pp. 176–82 Furley/Wilkie). See also Lonie, 1964: 426–43; Wilson, 1959; Temkin, 1951; Lammert, 1940–41: 125–31.

[78] Harris, 1973: 181. A further possibility would be that Herophilus adopted Aristotle's theory of 'connate pneuma', but there is no evidence to this effect.

[79] T145a.   [80] T143a–c.

heart. The phrase 'but from everywhere' could, of course, be interpreted to mean that pneuma, having been 'drawn from everywhere', is then first channelled into the heart before it is actually drawn or attracted into the arteries. But in that case the statement that pneuma is drawn into the arteries 'not from the heart alone but from everywhere' would seem to lose much of its point. Instead, Galen seems to be conflating several authors' views in a misleading manner, and the extent of Herophilus' agreement with most other physicians in the enumeration seems limited to the notion that the heart does not 'send' or pump pneuma into the arteries (as Erasistratus maintains) but that the pneuma instead is 'drawn' or attracted into the arteries from the heart. (That this 'drawing in' of pneuma in Herophilus' view is accomplished by the dilation or diastole of the arteries – just as pneuma is 'drawn into' the lungs from the external atmosphere through the dilation of the lungs – becomes clear in texts considered below).

The same Galenic passage has been used by C. R. S. Harris to argue that Herophilus 'definitely repudiated the conception of his master Praxagoras and his . . . contemporary Erasistratus that the arteries contained only *pneuma*';[81] instead, in Harris' view, Herophilus thought of the arteries as containing both pneuma and blood. What Galen says seems to be considerably less conclusive:

When the followers of Erasistratus are at a loss to explain how pneuma will be carried from the heart to the entire body if the arteries are filled with blood, it is not difficult to solve their problem by saying that the pneuma is not 'sent' but 'drawn', and not from the heart alone but from everywhere, as Herophilus and, before him Praxagoras . . . and countless others thought . . . [82]

Galen is not attributing the view that the arteries contain blood to all these authors – Praxagoras seems to have denied that the arteries contained any blood, as Galen himself suggests more than once[83] – but again only the view that the pneuma is not pumped into the arteries by the heart (as Erasistratus had claimed); instead these

---

[81] Harris, 1973: 180. Cf. Viano, 1984: 302, 307–8, 330–1.
[82] T145a.
[83] See n. 76 and Praxagoras, fr. 84 = Galen, *De pulsuum dignotione* 4.2 (VIII, p. 941 K; χυμοί must include blood).

physicians all agreed that pneuma is drawn or attracted into the arteries.[84]

A papyrus in the British Museum offers better – though unique, and hence not independently confirmed – support for the argument that Herophilus conceived of the arteries as containing not only pneuma but also blood.[85] According to the anonymous author of this papyrus (best known as Anonymus Londinensis) Herophilus thought the arteries and veins have an equal desire for nourishment and hence and equal power to absorb nutriment. But because the arteries dilate and contract, whereas the veins do not, greater absorption in fact takes place into the arteries than into the veins, and the arteries therefore are the main distributors of nutriment to the tissues. This part of the papyrus is remarkably free of lacunae and indecipherable readings, and there can therefore be little doubt that the author of the papyrus – who himself argues the converse, namely that the absorption in the veins is greater than the absorption in the arteries – actually attributes to Herophilus the view that the arteries bear the major responsibility for distributing nourishment throughout the body.

What, then, is the form in which nutriment is absorbed into the arteries? In most Greek theories of digestion food is changed into blood (for example, by concoction)[86] and blood, as a refined form of nutriment, is then absorbed into, and distributed by, the vascular system. The author of the papyrus leaves no doubt that this is his own view too. He argues that veins and arteries both contain blood as well as pneuma, but that the veins contain more blood and less pneuma than the arteries; and 'since in an artery the pneuma is more, but in a vein the reverse is the case, it is more likely that the distribution taking

---

[84] Cf. Praxagoras, fr. 29 Steckerl; Diocles, fr. 16 Wellmann (cf. also fr. 18). (Plistonicus and Phylotimus were members of Praxagoras' 'school'; cf. Steckerl, 1958: 108ff, 124ff.) See also Wellmann, 1901: 77ff., on Diocles' general views concerning the distribution of pneuma from the heart.

[85] T146; cf. Furley & Wilkie, 1984: 25–6; Longrigg, 1981: 170ff; id., 1985b: 169–70.

[86] Cf., for example, Empedocles, 31B81DK, 31A76–77DK; Plato, Timaeus 80D1ff. (τέμνοντος μὲν τὰ σιτία τοῦ πυρός . . .); Diocles, in: 'Vindician', Fragmentum Bruxellense, Chapter 42 (Wellmann, 1901: 233; cf. pp. 85ff.), and fr. 43 Wellmann; Hp., On Fleshes 13 (pp. 12–14 in Deichgräber's edition). Aristotle mentions or alludes to this process numerous times; cf., e.g., Parts of Animals 4.4.678a6–11; 2.3.650a2–b13. (But also see Aristotle's account of nutrition of the embryo in Generation of Animals 2.7.)

place in the vein is greater than in the artery'.[87] But does Herophilus, too, mean 'distribution of blood' when he refers to the 'distribution of nutriment' in the arteries and veins? There is no explicit evidence either to confirm or to deny this, but the Anonymus seems to leave no doubt that this is exactly what he understood Herophilus – like most authors who wrote on 'distribution' through the arteries and veins – to have meant.

Yet the possibility that Herophilus conceived of 'absorption' or distribution (ἀνάδοσις) by the arteries as the distribution of pneuma, or of both pneuma and blood, cannot be excluded a priori. Aristotle already had depicted liquid derivatives of food both as being 'pneumatized' or 'vaporized' by connate heat in the heart (see *infra*) and as being turned into blood, the 'ultimate nourishment' for the whole body. With reference to Aristotle, A. L. Peck has argued plausibly that 'an important part of this process [sc. of forming blood] was the "pneumatization" of the blood, i.e. the charging of it with σύμφυτον πνεῦμα and with the special "movement" requisite to enable it (a) to maintain the "being" of the animal, and (b) to supply its growth.'[88] It is conceivable that Herophilus, without accepting the details of Aristotle's scheme, similarly thought of a mixture of blood and pneuma, and not only of blood, as being absorbed in the arteries. A more radical, but less likely, possibility is that 'distribution of nutriment' through arteries means distribution of pneuma only. Herophilus would not have been the only Hellenistic physician to hold such a view. Praxagoras and Phylotimus apparently said we 'breathe only for the sake of *nourishing* the psychic pneuma' in the arteries, and, according to the pseudo-Aristotelian *De spiritu*,[89] a certain Aristogenes also regarded breath or pneuma not just as life-sustaining in general but specifically as nutriment. A major function of respiration, in Aristogenes' view, is therefore to nourish the body: air is first digested or 'concocted' in the lungs and then is distributed

---

[87] Anonymus Londinensis 28.40–5.   [88] Peck, 1943: lxiv.

[89] Praxagoras and Phylotimus: Praxagoras: fr. 32 Steckerl (= Galen, *De usu respirationis* 2 (IV, p. 483K); cf. also *ibid.*, 1.2 (IV, p. 471.4; p. 80 Furley/Wilkie: θρέψις for ῥῶσις)). Ps.-Aristotle, *De spiritu* 2.481a28ff. One might be tempted to include Erasistratus in this group, but in *De usu respirationis* 1 (IV, p. 471K) Galen specifically differentiates Praxagoras' view of the purpose of respiration (i.e. 'strengthening' or 'nourishing' the soul, or the psychic pneuma) from Erasistratus' view (i.e. that we breathe for the sake of refilling – or keeping full – the arteries). See also Furley/Wilkie, 1984: 28–9.

through the vascular system, while waste or excess is discharged (presumably through exhalation). There are, however, no reasonable indications that Herophilus shared Aristogenes' theory, and in all likelihood he followed the example of most of his predecessors, understanding 'distribution' to refer to the distribution of blood.

Two further considerations seem to support this interpretation. First, Herophilus grants the distribution of nutriment not only by the arteries but also by the veins (saying only that in the veins it is less than in the arteries);[90] since there is no evidence that he thought of the veins as containing anything but blood, it seems likely that the distribution in both veins and arteries is understood to be distribution of blood. If this is so, Herophilus accepts the presence of blood as well as pneuma in the arteries, anticipating the view not only of the Anonymus and of the Pneumatic school but also of Galen himself.

Second, if Herophilus indeed anticipated Galen's view that the arteries contain both blood and pneuma, this might explain why Galen in his numerous physiological treatises (and most notably in *An in arteriis natura sanguis contineatur*) criticizes Erasistratus, but never once Herophilus, for adopting Praxagoras' view that the arteries are bloodless and that they contain only pneuma. This argument from Galen's silence is as insidious as all *argumenta e silentio*, but, if correct, it would provide further support for the hypothesis that Herophilus thought of the veins as containing only blood but of arteries as having both blood and pneuma.

The exact relation between these two substances, blood and pneuma, in the arteries remains a mystery, because Herophilus apparently focused mainly in the pulse at the expense of the content of the arteries (at least if one may generalize on the basis of the more than fifty extant testimonia and fragments concerning his theory of the vascular system[91]).

The magnitude of Herophilus' contribution to pulse theory might be measured more accurately if an analysis of the relevant testimonia and fragments is prefaced by a brief survey of pre-Alexandrian Greek pulse-lore.

Well before Praxagoras' distinction between veins and arteries the beat of the heart and the throbbing motion of certain blood vessels

---

[90] T146: ἀμφότεραι (sc. αἱ ἀρτηρίαι καὶ αἱ φλέβες) ὀρεκτικῶς ἔχουσι τῆς τροφῆς.
[91] T144–T188 and Chapter VI, T115–T128.

had been commented upon by Greek writers. In the *Iliad*, for example, Andromache's heart leaps up as far as her mouth when she anticipates Hector's death,[92] and in Plato's *Phaedrus* an anguished soul, separated from a youth's beauty, throbs like a pulse in fever.[93] But in these older usages 'pulse' (σφυγμός) and 'to pulsate' (σφύζειν) were used primarily of violent motions and pathological symptoms associated with, for example, fear and fever, not of the normal vital function of the pulse. Even Praxagoras' distinction between veins and arteries, and his discovery that only arteries pulsate, were not enough to relieve pulsation of its pathological associations. Thus Erasistratus still used 'pulse' in the old pathological sense,[94] and as late as the *Rhetoric* of Cassius Longinus (third century A.D.) 'pulsate' still refers to a violent throbbing motion.[95]

Herophilus was, however, not the first to recognize the pulse as a normal and constant physiological function. Although the Hippocratic author of *On Places in Humans* thought of the vascular system as emanating from the head, and although he failed to recognize that pulsation is a constant in all arteries, he explicitly acknowledged that some blood vessels always pulsate, i.e. not only in abnormal conditions. A pair of 'veins' running along the temples 'press close to the eyes and are always pulsating (σφύζουσιν ἀεί)', he says, 'because these alone among the veins do not irrigate, for the blood is turned away from them; and the blood which is turned away wishes to run away, while the blood which flows in from above wishes to run downward, so they [sc. the two streams of blood] push and pour against each other and by moving round create the pulsation (τὸν σφυγμόν) in the blood vessels.'[96] Although pulsation is here divested of pathological significance, this text reveals recognition only of limited, local throbbing of bloodvessels, and hence is far from a general pulse theory.

---

[92] Homer, *Iliad* 22.452.   [93] Plato, *Phaedrus* 251d.

[94] Cf. T153 (= Galen, *De placitis Hippocratis et Platonis* 6.1); Galen, *De pulsuum differentiis* 4.2 (VIII, p. 716K). But elsewhere Galen implies that Erasistratus also used 'pulse' in the Herophilean, i.e. more modern, sense; cf. Galen, *ibid.*, 4.2 (VIII, p. 714K): 'Erasistratus says the pulse is a movement of the arteries arising by dilation and contraction through the agency of a vital and psychic faculty, and it occurs for the sake of keeping full the arteries, which have vital pneuma in themselves'. Cf. Hp., *Prog.* 7; *Epid.* VII.2,3,5; *Morb.* III.1.

[95] Cassius Longinus, *Rhetorikē Technē*, p. 201 Hammer (in L. Spengel, Rhetores Graeci, vol. 1.2, 2nd edn. (Leipzig, 1894)).

[96] Hp., *On Places in Humans* 3 (cf. Hp., VI, p. 280L, n. 9); 13 (VI, p. 302.10L).

Aristotle was apparently the first to depict pulsation as a constant in *all* blood vessels and to suggest its connection with the heart, even though the distinction between two vascular systems, the venous and arterial, was not worked out until the generation after Aristotle. In his *Historia animalium*, for example, Aristotle says: 'The blood in animals pulsates (σφύζει) in *all* the blood vessels *throughout* [the body] at once.'⁹⁷ And in *On Respiration* he attempts to explain how the pulse, once again viewed as a physiological constant, arises:

The pulsation (σφύξις) accompanying the heart, which the heart appears to be producing continuously, is similar to [the throbbing of?] abscesses [*or* bubbles?] . . . And in the heart the heat-produced increase in the bulk of the moisture – which constantly comes to it from the nutriment – causes a pulsation (σφυγμός), namely when the increased bulk [of moisture] is raised to the furthest coat [wall] of the heart. And this occurs continuously, for moisture flows to the heart continuously [sc. from nutriment], and from it the nature of blood arises; you see, it is in the heart that the blood is first created . . . And all the blood vessels pulsate (σφύζουσι), and they do so simultaneously with each other, because they are hung from the heart. The heart is always in motion, consequently they always are too – and simultaneously with each other – when it is in motion . . . Pulsation (σφύξις), then, is the evaporation [volatilization; pneumatization] of the heated moisture.⁹⁸

Both heart-beat and pulse are, therefore, in Aristotle's view normal and constant bodily functions, and they both result from the pneumatization or vaporization of food derivates which are in liquid form. This 'pneumatization' of the moisture is effected through the agency of the connate heat which, as he explains elsewhere, is primarily resident in the right ventricle of the heart.⁹⁹ When heat converts a moisture into air or vapour, an increase in volume results, as Aristotle tries to show in *De caelo*,¹⁰⁰ because vapour occupies more space. This heat-produced increase in the volume of the nutriment results in a push of hot moisture against the 'coat' or wall of the heart which causes the heart to swell, and this in turn causes the lung to expand. It thus sets respiration in motion (see Section 3 above). The cold air drawn into the heart now causes the swelling of the heart to subside again. In this way dilations and contractions of the heart are

⁹⁷ *Historia animalium* 3.19.521a6–7.
⁹⁸ Aristotle, *On Respiration* 20.479b26–480a15.
⁹⁹ Cf. Aristotle, *On Youth and Old Age* 4.469b6–20, 6.470a19ff.; *Parts of Animals* 3.4.667a1–6.
¹⁰⁰ Aristotle, *De caelo* 3.7.305b11–16.

produced continuously. The resulting pulsation in the bloodvessels therefore has to be traced not only to the heart but also to digestion and respiration – a remarkable and influential attempt to link digestion, pulsation, and respiration, and to explain all three by means of a single, coherent theory.

Praxagoras' discovery of a generalizable distinction between artery and pulse and his recognition that pulsation occurs only in the arteries, not in the veins,[101] represent a significant advance, but in other respects his theory of the pulse does not constitute an improvement on Aristotle's conception. First Praxagoras' influential insistence that the arteries are bloodless,[102] containing only pneuma, for centuries wreaked havoc with Greek physiology. Secondly, although Praxagoras recognized that the heart dilates and contracts, he believed that the arteries' capacity to pulsate is completely autonomous – i.e. independent even of the heart. He tried to verify this assertion by means of an experiment: 'If a person were to cut some flesh out of a living being and put it on the ground while it is quivering [palpitating], he would clearly see the movement of the arteries.'[103] Praxagoras' conception of an independent pulsation of the arteries does not represent progress and when we turn to Herophilus we find that he firmly rejects this part of his teacher's theory and reverts instead to more promising aspects of the Aristotelian model.

Herophilus reasserts the continuity of the arteries with the heart, but he does not believe that the arteries have an innate faculty to pulsate; instead, the faculty (*dynamis*) which enables them to dilate and contract flows to them from the heart through the arterial coats.[104] The heart, therefore, is 'like a fountain of the faculty which dilates the arteries',[105] and Praxagoras' theory of independent arterial pulsation in Herophilus' view must be wrong. When the transmitted or received faculty in the arterial coats causes the arteries

---

[101] Cf. Galen, *De placitis Hippocratis et Platonis* 6.7; *id.*, *De pulsuum differentiis* 4.2 (VIII, p. 702K); *id.*, *De tremore, palpitatione, convulsione et rigore* 5 (VII, p. 598K). [= Praxagoras, fr. 27–8 Steckerl.]

[102] See above, n. 76. Cf. also Harris, 1973: 109: '[The doctrine] of the air-filled arteries was really one of the tragical mistakes in the history of Greek medicine, a mistake which more almost than any other prevented the discovery of the circulation'. See also De Martini, 1964; Lammert, 1940–41: 125–31.

[103] Galen, *De placitis Hippocratis et Platonis* 6.7 = Praxagoras, fr. 28 Steckerl.

[104] T155; T144.

[105] T145a.

to dilate, they draw in 'that which will fill their dilation', as Galen cautiously phrases it[106] (i.e. if the suggestion developed above is correct, they attract pneuma and blood from the heart – and, perhaps, pneuma 'from everywhere they can' via the heart – by means of their dilation), and then pass it on through contraction. All the arteries dilate and contract in unison with the heart, as in Aristotle's theory of pulsating bloodvessels. (For diagnostic and prognostic purposes, however, one only needs to examine the arterial pulse without having recourse to an examination of the pulsation (σφυγμός) of the heart, according to Herophilus.[107])

A further significant and positive revision Herophilus made in the pulse theory of his teacher Praxagoras concerns the differentiation of pulse from tremor (τρόμος), spasm (σπασμός), and palpitation (παλμός). Praxagoras regarded all four of these motions as essentially similar arterial motions, claiming that they differ only quantitatively, i.e. in the 'size' of their motions: pulse is natural, spasm is due to a slight increase in motion, tremor is due to a greater increase, and palpitation is the most agitated of these 'arterial motions'.[108] While Herophilus agrees with Praxagoras that 'all the motion of the arteries that we see existing in us ... is pulse',[109] we saw earlier that he regards 'tremor' as a pathological affection of the 'nerve-like class' of organs, i.e. of nerves, muscles, and perhaps tendons and ligaments, and not of the arteries. Similarly, Herophilus removes palpitation from the arterial context to which Praxagoras had assigned it, and instead views it as an affection of the muscles.[110] No explicit information about Herophilus' explanation of 'spasm' has survived, but he left no doubt that it, too, should be classified as an affection of organs of the voluntary motor system, such as muscles and nerves.[111] It was perhaps only with Herophilus' discovery of the nervous system, and in particular of the motor nerves, that a clear differentiation between an involuntary vascular motion (pulse) and pathological affections of the voluntary motor system – tremor, spasm, palpitation – became possible. As we saw earlier, Herophilus went even further and also differentiated the involuntary vascular motion, or pulse, from the involuntary pulmonary motion (i.e. respiration),

[106] T144. On Galen's own views see Amacher, 1964; Furley/Wilkie, 1984: 40ff.
[107] T148.
[108] Cf. T149–T150; see Praxagoras, fr. 27 Steckerl, for further evidence.
[109] T148; cf. T151.   [110] T152.   [111] T149.

thereby establishing at least three different systems of bodily motion.

The pulse itself according to Herophilus consists of two phases or parts: contraction (*systolē*) is the activity or *energeia* of the arteries, while dilation (*diastolē*) is 'the return to the proper and natural condition of their body'.[112] If Galen may be believed, Herophilus' reason for characterizing the dilated state of the artery as its 'natural condition' and the contracting movement as its 'activity' is his observation that arteries in dead bodies still have a perceptible lumen or, as Galen says, 'the coat [wall] of the artery is seen to be distended'; consequently, 'in those who are alive, too, it must be distended as much as possible' in its natural condition.[113] Analogy can, of course, be a fruitful heuristic tool. But it can also be a very deceptive form of reasoning, and Herophilus may have recognized this only after he had used the analogy between the dead and the living, because Galen in another part of *On Differences Between Pulses*[114] attributes two divergent – and inconsistent – views on this question of the 'activity' vs. the 'natural condition' of the arteries to Herophilus: sometimes, says Galen, Herophilus considered both the dilation and the contraction of the artery an activity or *energeia*, but at other times – in fact, most often – only the contraction. Unfortunately, however, the rest of the Galenic text in question is uninformative on this question, and no clear statement of Herophilus' reasons for vacillating has survived.

Herophilus' emphasis on the contraction rather than dilation of the arterial wall as the 'activity' of the artery may have given rise to a question which baffled Galen (and which was explicitly faced in a number of pulse definitions produced by followers of Herophilus), namely whether the contraction or systole is perceptible. Galen says he himself in the course of many years had not developed the ability to discern any part of the contraction or systole, but only the dilation, and yet he finds that Herophilus, for whom he has the highest respect in these matters, 'discourses throughout as though [he is talking] about a *perceptible* contraction'.[115] Certainly the followers of Herophilus, though often opposed to each other's views, seem to have agreed with rare unanimity that the systole is a perceptible motion[116] and

---

[112] T157.   [113] *Ibid.*   [114] T158.   [115] T159–T160.

[116] Cf. *infra* Chapter xx, *Cr.* 1; Chapter xxii, *AP.* 3; Chapter xxviii, *DP.* 1. See also Chapter x.a and Chapter xxv.a on the internecine polemics within the Herophilean school in its last known generation.

hence to have accepted the founding master's characterization of the systole as perceptible. But the Herophileans were the only ones who could achieve unanimity on this issue: neither the followers of Erasistratus nor the members of the Pneumatic school of medicine, says Galen,[117] agreed among themselves about the perceptibility or imperceptibility of the arterial contractions. Herophilus himself not only talks about the contraction 'as though it is perceptible'; he left no doubt that he regarded it as being just as perceptible to one's touch as the diastole. Although he conceded that some bodily motions are perceptible (κίνησις αἰσθητή), while others can only be inferred by reason (κίνησις θεωρητή), more than one testimonium confirms that Herophilus called all *perceptible* motions of the arteries 'pulse'[118] – and 'pulse', he says, after all consists of dilation *and* contraction. While the notion that all perceptible arterial motions are pulse does not allow the conclusion that all pulse motions are perceptible, it is not incompatible with the theory of the perceptibility of the systole.

The generic description of the pulse developed by Herophilus, and his discussion of its motions in terms of *diastolē* and *systolē* of the arteries, were pioneering achievements which have had an enduring impact not only on medical nomenclature. But he went beyond the 'genus' pulse and also developed an elaborate classification of different 'species' of pulse, first by general differentiae and, secondly, by age or stages of life (ἡλικίαι).[119]

The key to his differentiation between various pulse types is provided in an invaluable fragment from Book 1 of his treatise *On Pulses* (quoted in Galen's *On Differentiating between Pulses*), in which Herophilus twice enumerates the primary differentiae of pulse 'species':

In general, then, pulse seems to differ from pulse in volume [mass], in size, in speed, in vehemence [strength], and in rhythm. From the fact that they differ in these respects, the pulse clearly at times becomes 'fitting' [*oikeios*, 'conforming to its true nature'] at times not 'fitting'. One pulse appears to differ from another, and in general to be recognized [as different], in

---

[117] Cf. T160.
[118] Cf. T148, T151, T159, T160. (See also T142 on 'sensually perceptible motion' and 'motion perceptible by reason'.)
[119] In T162 Galen seems to suggest that Herophilus first developed the four primary differentiae of pulse types (at the beginning of Book 1 of his treatise *On Pulses*), and then turned to 'pulse differences according to stages of life'. Cf. T162, line 95: πῶς δ' ἐφεξῆς τὰς καθ' ἡλικίαν διαφορὰς ἐκτιθέμενος . . .

rhythm, size, speed, and vehemence [strength], as was said. But if, in the same rhythm, one pulse appears to differ from another, then in speed, size, and vehemence.[120]

Galen is quick to point out (T162) that one of the differentiae listed in Herophilus' first enumeration, namely 'mass' or 'volume' (πλῆθος), is missing in the second, and indeed 'volume' does not play a prominent role in his classificatory scheme. None of the texts presented in this chapter confirms that Herophilus used 'volume' to describe or classify any pulse, and 'volume' might therefore be a later interpolation. If this is so, there are four basic differentiae. But the Pneumatic physician Archigenes (early first century A.D.) reports that Herophilus not only classified pulses 'by size, speed, vehemence [or: strength], and rhythm', but by further subdivisions involving 'regularity and irregularity, evenness and unevenness',[121] and, as shown below, these subdivisions were indeed used by Herophilus to describe certain kinds of pulse. That all these distinctions were actively used in practice, and not merely set up as a theoretical model, seems to follow from Galen's comment, in the context of the diagnostic uses of pulse-lore, that 'primary genuses and primary differences . . . were mentioned countless times by Herophilus and almost all Herophileans'.[122] Not all the differentiae are discussed extensively in the extant evidence, but all four primary differentiae are introduced in ways which merit further comment.

First, the 'vehemence' (σφοδρότης) or strength of a pulse, according to Herophilus, is due to the strength (ῥώμη) of the vital faculty (3ωτικὴ δύναμις) in the artery.[123] If Galen, to whom we owe this information, is not making anachronistic use of his own concept of 'vital faculty' or 'vital pneuma', this represents the only evidence that Herophilus used the notion 'vital faculty'. Aristotle had spoken of 'vital heat' (and possibly of 'vital moisture')[124] – i.e. 'vital', in the

---

[120] Fr162, lines 80–6.
[121] T163a, T163b. (These two testimonia are culled from Book II of Galen's *On Differences Between Pulses*, but the relevant parts of the texts are Galen's direct quotations from Archigenes.)
[122] T165. For other manifestations of Herophilus' strong taxonomic instinct see above, Chapter IV (and below, T226).
[123] T164. σφοδρός is usually translated 'strong' (e.g. by Harris, 1973: *passim*), but I prefer 'vehement' since this is closer to the usual meaning of the word, which has an overtone of 'excess'.
[124] Aristotle, *On the Generation of Animals* 2.4.739b23 (seed, like rennet, contains 'vital

sense of making life possible and hence also being necessary to maintenance of life – and in Herophilus' own time Erasistratus was applying the concept 'vital' to the pneuma in the arteries (as opposed to the more refined 'psychic pneuma' in the meninges of the brain); it has also been suggested that some Stoics were using the notions of 'vital pneuma' and 'vital *tonos*'.[125] It is therefore not inconceivable that Herophilus used the concept 'vital' and became the first to apply it to a faculty or *dynamis*. But what could he have meant by 'vital faculty'? Nowhere in the extant evidence does Herophilus refer to it again, and not until at least two hundred years later is there any mention again of a 'vital faculty' within the Herophilean school: in the mid-first century B.C. a follower of Herophilus, Chrysermus, defined the pulse generally – and not just the 'vehement' pulse – as 'a distention and contraction of arteries, when the arterial coat, through the agency of a *psychic* and *vital* faculty, rises on all sides and then again shrinks together . . .'.[126] But there is no evidence that Herophilus himself used Chrysermus' distinction between 'psychic' and 'vital', and the only 'faculty' (*dynamis*) to which he ever refers elsewhere in sphygmological contexts is the above-mentioned faculty which flows to the arteries from the heart through the arterial coats and enables the arteries to contract and dilate; it is, therefore, perhaps to this faculty that 'vital faculty' refers. The relative strength of this involuntary faculty, which is born with us and dies with us – and which Herophilus therefore may well have described as 'vital' or 'life-sustaining' – would then be what determines the 'vehemence' of a pulse and would hence provide one of the differentiae specificae of pulses. (Whether excessive strength, producing a 'vehement' pulse, or deficient strength, producing a weak pulse, were ultimately explained or explicable in humoral terms, is again a question to which the available evidence provides no answer.)

---

heat'). The reference to 'vital moisture' (see below) might, however, be an interpolation, as Jaeger suggested; cf. Aristotle, *On the Movement of Animals* 11.703b23, with E. S. Forster's note (1937: 478–9). Cf. Nussbaum, 1978: 384.

[125] For possible examples of the Stoics' uses of 'vital' see *SVF* II, fr. 879, 889, and 945. None of these texts establishes conclusively, however, that the Stoics in fact used the concept 'vital', and I am inclined to question von Arnim's inclusion of at least some of these texts. For Erasistratus cf. Galen, *De pulsuum differentiis* 4.2 (VIII, p. 714K); *id.*, *Plac. Hp. Plat.* 1.6. 3 (p. 78 De Lacy).

[126] Chapter xx, *Cr.* 1.

About another differentia specifica of pulses, rhythm, we are more generously informed. 'Rhythm', says Herophilus, 'is a motion which has a defined regulation in time',[127] and it is this temporal rhythm which he tried to analyse in an elaborate system which became famous throughout antiquity especially for its use of musical and metrical analogies. As late as Censorinus' treatise on time and the divisions of time (*De die natali*, third century A.D.) and Remigius of Auxerre's Carolingian commentary on Martianus Capella, Herophilus was still renowned for his theory that 'the pulsations of the bloodvessels move in musical rhythms'.[128]

Not all ancient authors found Herophilus' concept of rhythm and his use of musical analogies to explain pulse rhythms comprehensible. 'Just what he means by "rhythm"', complains Galen in *On Differentiating between Pulses*, 'is very difficult to discover: is it the ratio of the time of dilation to the time of contraction only, or does he also attribute to "rhythm" the time of the pause [quiescence] which follows each of these two motions? . . . Not even among those who are named "Herophileans" after him is there agreement concerning just what Herophilus really thought about rhythms.'[129] And in *On Prediction based on Pulses*, Galen again complains that Herophilus 'is confused and does not clearly articulate the distinction between contraction and rest [pause]'.[130] While Galen's discomfort with Herophilus' theory of rhythm is understandable in the light of his own emphasis on the pauses or inactive intervals between the contracting and dilating motions, Herophilus' silence about the pauses or periods of inactivity is not due to any ambiguity on his part: rhythm is defined purely in terms of systole and diastole, and the pauses or quiescent intervals therefore are not made part of his mechanism for differentiating between rhythms. 'Just as musicians establish rhythms according to certain defined sequences of time-units, comparing up-beat (*arsis*) and down-beat (*thesis*) with each other, so, too', says Galen in another work (*Synopsis of my Books on the Pulse*), 'Herophilus supposes that the dilation of the artery is analogous to the up-beat, while the contraction is analogous to the down-beat.'[131] And just as

---

[127] T172. Cf. also Chapter XIV *infra*, Ba.3.
[128] T187, T188b. See below, n. 136; cf. Kümmel, 1977: 23 ff., on the influence of Herophilus' analogies.
[129] T173.
[130] T176. See also *Comments* on T176.   [131] T183.

most musical theory up to the time of Herophilus views up-beat and down-beat as contiguous in time, and hence recognizes no pause between them, so Herophilus – unlike later writers on music and pulse-lore – regards the contracting and dilating motions of the artery as immediately adjacent in time and hence finds no need to elaborate on the intervals of inactivity between contraction and dilation. Archigenes, Galen, Rufus, and others, by contrast, were at pains to accommodate these pauses within their theories of the pulse,[132] and in some cases their analysis of the quiescent intervals (ἠρεμίαι, διαλείμματα) between 'up-beat' and 'down-beat' usurped the analysis of dilation and contraction.

Up-beat and down-beat, *arsis* and *thesis*, were therefore the general units Herophilus used to establish a basic analogy between musical rhythm and pulse rhythm, but he also developed the analogy in intricate detail. First, Herophilus established what he apparently called a 'primary perceptible time unit' (πρῶτος χρόνος αἰσθητός), defining it as the interval of time in which he usually found the artery

---

[132] On Archigenes see Wellmann, 1895a: 186–7. For Galen, see, e.g., T178, T183, and *On Differences Between Pulses* 1.6 (VIII, pp. 509–11K). [Ps.-?] Rufus' usage is probably derived from Archigenes; cf. *Synopsis on Pulses*, p. 232 (Daremberg/Ruelle). Cf. also Harris, 1973: 402–3. Wellmann (1895a: 187) and Harris (1973: 192) attribute a theory of intervals to Herophilus (Harris: 'between these two movements [sc. contraction and expansion of the arteries] there were two perceptible intervals, during which the coats of the arteries remained motionless'), but this attribution has no firm foundation in the ancient evidence. Galen in fact complains several times – as Harris concedes – that Herophilus did not put the notion of intervals to use (e.g. T183: 'not making any distinctions at all concerning either of the moments of rest' following contraction and dilation respectively). It should be noted that T178 merely attributes the establishment of 'primary time units' to Herophilus; the rest of the statement, with its reference to intervals, is not attributed to Herophilus by Galen. In T174 'either the motions only or also the pauses' reflects Galen's uncertainty (a product of his own preoccupation with 'pause'), and again not an attribution of a theory of pause to Herophilus. Furthermore, in T157 Galen seems to imply that Aristoxenus' use of 'rest' (ἠρεμία) was a deviation from Herophilus' teaching (cf. Chapter XXV *infra*, Ar. 2). The only texts to which Wellmann and Harris seem to be able to appeal in support of their view are in the same category as T183, lines 12ff., or as Galen, *De pulsuum differentiis* 1.7 (VIII, p. 512K): 'Those who say they perceive the contraction' also use the concept of 'pause' or 'interval'. But Herophilus is not explicitly included in this group – apparently because, as Galen suggests elsewhere, he failed to put the concept of 'pause' to any use in his pulse-lore. Herophilus' implicit rejection of the notion of interval or quiescence or pause (διάλειμμα, ἡσυχία, ἠρεμία) of course corresponds more closely to the modern understanding of 'pulse'. See also n. 162 *infra*).

of a new-born child dilating.[133] This 'primary perceptible time unit'
is characterized as analogous to the *breve* or short unit used in the feet
of musical metres, and it becomes the basic unit (a) by which the
length of each contraction and each dilation is measured (each can
consist of one, two, etc. 'primary perceptible time units'), and (b) by
which the rhythm, i.e. the relation of the duration of contraction to
the duration of dilation, is established. It has often been argued that
Herophilus derived this conception of rhythm from the metrical
theory of his contemporary Aristoxenus of Tarentum, a Peripatetic
philosopher and musical theorist who proposed a theory of metrical
'feet' (*podes*) composed of long and short syllables. Aristoxenus'
famous concepts *chronos prōtos* (see *Comments*, T183) and *alogoi podes*
('irrational feet'; see *Comments*, T177) might well have inspired
Herophilus' uses of *prōtos chronos* and *alogos sphygmos* ('irrational pulse';
see below), and Herophilus might also have found Aristoxenus'
analogy between *harmonia* in the body and musical harmony
(*Comments*, T187) suggestive. Yet the musical theorists' extensive
attention to pauses or quiescent intervals between units of rhythm did
not find a sympathetic ear in Herophilus (as opposed to Galen and
other medical writers), and Aristoxenus' least ambiguously attested
definition of rhythm – 'time divided in each of the faculties that are
capable of being moved in measures' (sc. the faculties *lexis*, *melos*, and
bodily movement) – along with his verdict that 'not every order or
defined regulation (*taxis*) of time possesses rhythm' seems to warn us
against exaggerating the extent and depth of Aristoxenus'
influence.[134] Furthermore, while Herophilus in his pulse lore put to

[133] T183. Cf. T174 ('Herophilus was the first to establish a time unit in relation to
sense-perception'). See *Comments* on T183.
[134] On Aristoxenus as Herophilus' source see, e.g., Wellmann, 1895a: 188–91;
Harris, 1973: 187–8; Pigeaud, 1978: 262–3; Longrigg, 1981: 173–5 (but what for
Wellmann was still mere *Vermutung* for the others is a certainty). For
Aristoxenus' definition of rhythm see Westphal, 1883–93: vol. II, p. 75 (*Rhythmica*
I, Fragm. ap. Bacchium Ger. p. 23 Morelli; *Musici Scriptores Graeci* p. 313 Jan). A
second definition cited by Westphal (*ibid.*) is ascribed not only to Aristoxenus
but also to Hephaestion, and it corresponds to Herophilus' (T172) and to those
of the Herophileans Bacchius (ch. XIV, *Ba.* 3) and Zeno (ch. XV, *Zn.* 2, with some
modification; see ch. X.A and von Staden, 1982: 86–7). But this second definition
seems less reliable than the first, in part because of (a) Aristoxenus' analysis of
rhythm in terms of the *rhythmizomena* (*Rhythmica* 2.6, 2.9, etc.; Westphal, 1883–
93: vol. I, 5–13, vol. II, 78–9, 91), which the first – but not the second – definition
explicitly accommodates, and (b) his statement that 'not every *taxis* of time-
units possesses rhythm' (*Rhythmica* 2.7; cf. 2.8; Westphal, 1883–93: vol. II, 78),

use three elementary types of metre also recognized by Aristoxenus –
trochee, spondee, iamb (see below) – the range of rhythms and
musical analogies the physician deployed violates Aristoxenus'
taxonomy. Since arguments from silence almost always invite
scholarly suspicion, let it merely be mentioned that none of the
numerous ancient sources which acknowledge Herophilus' debt to
musical theory or metrics[135] characterize it as a debt to Aristoxenus.
Whatever the provenance of Herophilus' theory of pulse rhythms
might be, its impact was enormous, and his general analogy between
metrical-musical rhythm and pulse rhythm became a topos of both
medical and musical literature until the Renaissance.[136]

The next step after establishing a notion of rhythm based on
'primary perceptible time units' was apparently to apply this theory

which does not necessarily contradict the second definition but reflects the same
characteristic desire for precision which Aristoxenus also displays in the first
definition. (The second definition, *pace* Westphal, does not appear to be reported
by the musical theorist Bacchius Geron but by an anonymous scholiast on
Hermogenes' *De ideis* 1.20; cf. *Rhetores Graeci* VII.2 p. 892 (Waltz); Hephaestion,
fr. 1 (p. 76 Consbruch; I, p. xi Gaisford). For Bacchius Geron see *Musici Scriptores
Graeci*, pp. 285–316 Jan. Pighi's edition of Aristoxenus' *Rhythmica* regrettably
was not available to me.) See also nn. 140, 147 *infra*; Pöhlmann, 1960: 32–40;
Jaeger, 1960: vol. II, pp. 441–53 (on Aristotle's methodological influence on both
Aristoxenus and medicine).

[135] Cf. the references to Herophilus's debt to 'the musicians' in the general in T183
('just as musicians'); T184, lines 37–8 ('what a person worthy of the art of
medicine should have learnt from musicians'); T185 ('Herophilus . . . divided
the pulse . . . into musical feet'); T186 (Herophilus divided the pulse 'into
definite measures and metrical laws'); T187 ('the pulsations of the bloodvessels
move in musical rhythms'); T188b ('if the pulse . . . is in accordance with
natural metrical feet'); T177 (one can adapt the proportions of pulses 'to a
demonstration based on scansion' – but how much of this particular testimonium is drawn directly from Herophilus remains problematic). Cf. also the
musical analogy in T171 ('just as when very thin web-like [covers] have been
placed around the holes in flutes and a musician then breathes into the
flutes . . .'). Cf. Kümmel, 1977: 23–7.

[136] Galen, for example, in T178 ('as Herophilus used to measure the pulse'). But see
also T174. Cf. Aristides Quintilianus, *De musica* 2.15, 3.8 (pp. 82, 106
Winnington-Ingram); Achilles, *Isagoge in Arati Phaenomena* 16 (p. 43 Maass);
Daremberg/Ruelle, *Rufus*, p. 634, on Avicenna, Savonarola, Fernel, and
Marquet; Vitruvius 1.1.15; Varro in Gellius, *Noctes Atticae* 3.10.13. A somewhat
different analogy (between harmony in the body and musical harmony) also
remained popular: cf. Lactantius, *Institutiones divinae* 7.13 and *De opificio Dei*
16.13–17 (Aristoxenus fr. 120c–d Wehrli).Cf. Aristides Quintil. 1.13 (p. 31.18–
20 Winnington-Ingram). See Kümmel, 1977.

of rhythm to a classification of pulses according to stages of life.[137] While Aristotle had already observed what modern science has confirmed, namely that the pulse rate of new-born infants is far more rapid than that of adults,[138] Herophilus was the first to produce an elaborate theory of four stages in the development of human pulse rhythms. According to Herophilus, as we saw, the dilation in most new-born children consists of one primary time unit and so does the contraction.[139] The normal pulse rhythm of infancy is, therefore, analogous to the metrical foot known as pyrrhic (∪∪).[140] The pulse rhythm of infants is, however, also described as *alogos*, 'irrational' or 'without definable ratios', 'for it has neither a double ratio nor a ratio of one and a half to one nor any other proportion (*logos*), but instead is completely short . . . like the prick of a needle'.[141] That Herophilus would call a 1:1 ratio of his primary time units *alogos* at first seems puzzling, especially (a) since all other intervals of time are measured by the primary time unit – which must, therefore, be clearly and exactly definable, and which in fact is defined precisely as the time of the dilation of an infant's pulse – and (b) since a subsequent 1:1 ratio (namely a spondee; see below) is not characterized as *alogos*. If our source (Rufus or pseudo-Rufus) is suggesting that the infant's pulse is 'irrational' or *alogos* because each of its two 'pinprick' movements is so small as to be only an indeterminate fraction of the 'primary time unit', then he is not only contradicting his own characterization of the infant pulse as 'a short-syllabled metrical foot' or pyrrhic (∪∪), i.e. consisting of the two equal – and complete – 'primary time units', but he is also undermining the basis of Herophilus' whole theory of rhythms, namely the definition of the 'primary time unit' as the duration of dilation in an *infant's* pulse. Recourse to later conceptions of 'irrational pulse', such as that of the Pneumatics, is not of much help in this context, but there might well be a connection between Aristoxenus' refusal to recognize the pyrrhic as a metrical unit and

---

[137] Cf. T176–T186; *Comments*, T175.

[138] Cf. Aristotle, *De respiratione* 20.480a9–10.

[139] T177 ('consisting of two [short] quantities'); T183. See also *Comments* on T177, T187.

[140] T177, T183 ('the pulse in the newborn infant occurs with a rhythm that is equal' in diastole and systole, and each of these two movements equals one 'primary perceptible time unit', i.e. equals a metrical *breve*). This would seem to be an example of a metre – pyrrhic – not accommodated in Aristoxenus' *Rhythmics*.

[141] T177; line 11 (τῷ μεγέθει βελόνης κεντήματι ὁμοίως).

Herophilus' statement that the pyrrhic is *alogos*.[142] The reason for both positions might be that there is no operation of real measurement against minima – no *logos* – in a sequence of two minima.

As the body comes into full growth the 'ratio' in the pulse also increases, and in 'growing children' and adolescents the natural pulse rhythm has become trochaic (– ⏑).[143] Each cycle of diastole and systole now consists of three primary units, the dilation lasting for two units, the contraction for one.

By the prime of life, the normal pulse rhythm consists of four primary time units equally divided between contraction and dilation, and hence this is a spondaic stage of life (– –).[144] Herophilus also called the pulse rhythm of this state *dia isou* or a pulse 'in equal quantity', according to the *Synopsis on Pulses* widely (but not unanimously) attributed to Rufus of Ephesus.[145] 'Up-beat' and 'down-beat' now last equally long, as they did in infancy, but Herophilus does not call this pulse rhythm *alogos* or 'without definable ratio' (as he had called the infant rhythm). This might be because the longer duration in his view renders the ratio more determinate or definable, or less 'like the prick of a needle', as one source implies, but in that case Herophilus' use of the 'prick of the needle' as a 'primary, perceptible time unit' by which to measure all other units – and hence to determine all ratios –would seem open to objection, as suggested above. The available evidence does not seem to permit a clear resolution of this problem.

Finally, those who are beyond their prime and, as Rufus (or pseudo-Rufus) puts it, 'almost already old people', have entered an iambic (⏑ –) stage of life.[146] Their pulse again consists of three primary time units, as in adolescence, but in an inverse ratio: the dilation (*diastolē*) lasts for the duration of one unit, the contraction (*systolē*) twice as long (or even longer[147]).

---

[142] Cf. Wellmann, 1895a: 188ff. See also Westphal., 1883–93: vol. I, pp. 151–7; vol. II, pp. 82–3. Cf. *Comments*, T177.

[143] T177, lines 20–1.   [144] *Ibid.*, lines 23–6.

[145] *Ibid.*, line 27 ('equal', of course, refers to a contraction and dilation of equal duration).

[146] *Ibid.*, lines 28–30.

[147] While the dilation in those beyond their prime apparently lasts only a single 'primary time unit', the contraction in Herophilus' view can last anywhere from two (T177: τὴν συστολὴν τῆς διαστολῆς διπλῆν) to ten primary time units; cf. T176, T183. T178 also seems to allude to Herophilus' suggestion that the

Nature's music in our arteries therefore assumes pyrrhic, trochaic, spondaic, and iambic forms in four successive stages of our lives; these are the 'natural' or normal pulse rhythms in our arteries. But Herophilus was also acutely interested in deviations from the natural rhythms. Pulse-lore interested him not only as an intriguing and challenging exercise in theoretical speculation and observational verification; for him it also had immense clinical relevance, since it provided a major diagnostic and prognostic tool. Galen, in his treatise *On Differentiating between Pulses*, confirms that 'Herophilus himself in many places mentions rhythms with a view to *prognoses*',[148] and Herophilus' descriptions of several deviant pulse conditions have been transmitted both by Galen and by other ancient sources (see below).

The most vivid evidence of Herophilus' clinical interest in the pulse is his unique construction of a portable water-clock or clepsydra which he apparently used on his medical rounds to take the pulse of his patients. According to Marcellinus,[149] an author probably of the second century A.D.,[150] this water-clock could be calibrated to suit the age of the patient, a feature which strikingly demonstrates Herophilus' desire to bridge the gap between theory and practice. Just as he emphasized in his *theory* of rhythms that normal pulse rhythms differ according to age, so in his *practice* he used a timing device adaptable to his patients' ages. Herophilus, Marcellinus says explicitly, 'constructed a water-clock capable of containing a specified amount [sc. of water] for the natural pulse-beats of each age'. The only example of his use of the clepsydra is intriguing, because it demonstrates that he used this device not only as an adaptable timer

contraction of an older person's pulse can last ten primary time units. The fact that the ratio in old age can range from 1:2 (iambic) to 1:10 again seems to reveal the limited applicability of Aristoxenus' *Rhythmics* to Herophilus' theory of pulse rhythm. (1:2 might, however, be the normal ratio, and 1:10 a pathological ratio.)

[148] T173.

[149] T182. See also *Comments* on T182.

[150] The latest author mentioned by Marcellinus in his *On Pulses* is a leader of the Pneumatic school, Archigenes, who was at his prime in the early second century A.D. during the reign of Trajan (cf. *Suda*, s.v. Archigenes = α. 4107 Adler). Since Galen's extensive pulse-lore, presented in at least eight different treatises, is not mentioned even once in Marcellinus' work, the latter was probably written in the mid–second century A.D. – a conclusion which is also compatible with Marcellinus' style. (See my forthcoming edition, *CMG*.)

but also as a thermometer. Because Herophilus thought the frequency of the pulse is a correlate of body temperature – the greater the frequency, the higher the temperature – he would use his water-clock also when feeling the pulse of feverish patients, and, after adjusting the water-clock to the patient's age, 'by as much as the movements of the pulse exceeded the number that is natural for filling up the [adjusted] clock, by that much he also declared the pulse too frequent – i.e. that [the patient] had either more or less of a fever'.[151]

Here the pulse rhythms of different ages are not at issue – they could hardly be measured by a clepsydra, if indeed the *breve* or 'primary time unit' is only as long as the 'pinprick' duration of the dilation of an infant's pulse – but the frequencies with which these rhythms occur. Herophilus' application of a theory of four stages of life to pulse-lore accordingly is based not only on those different rhythmic patterns within a *single* pulse-beat that were discussed above (trochee, spondee, etc.), but also on differences in the frequency with which these 'rhythmic' beats occur over a longer span of time.

Exactly how Herophilus' water-clock worked is not reported, but there seem to be several feasible constructions (e.g. a set of four perforated 'sinking bowls' of different sizes, one for each age group, or a single traditional overflowing or draining container with four receptacles of different sizes, or a draining or receiving container with a 'dipstick' marked for different ages).[152] The recent argument that 'from the technical point of view it can hardly fail to arouse some suspicions'[153] is therefore not compelling, and Marcellinus' account of Herophilus' clinical application of his theory concerning the four stages of life (and of a rare attempt, at least in medicine up to this period, to introduce an exact quantifying procedure) may be accepted as plausible – as indeed it has been by Hermann Diels and other historians of ancient technology.[154]

So far we have examined two of the primary differentiae Herophilus used to distinguish pulse from pulse – vehemence and rhythm –

---

[151] T182, lines 13–16.
[152] I am indebted to the late Derek de Solla Price for some of these suggestions. Cf. also Zervos, 1909. For other early models of Greek clepsydrae cf. *The Athenian Agora. A Guide*, 3rd edn (1976): 17, 21, 59, 168–9, 248–9; H. A. Thompson, 1954: 37–8; Brumbaugh, 1966: 68–73; Diels, 1915; Usher, 1954: 142–6; West, 1973.
[153] Harris, 1973: 191.
[154] Diels, 1920: 27. See also M. C. P. Schmidt, 1912: vol. II, pp. 44–5, 102 n. 2; Fraser, 1972: vol. II p. 518 n. 113; Gotfredsen, 1942: 191–2. Cf. n. 152.

and the second, rhythm, emerged as a concept of unusual theoretical and clinical consequence in so far as it also serves as a cornerstone of Herophilus' theory of four stages of life.

A further element of Herophilus' theory of stages is, as his use of the water-clock demonstrated, the differentiation of pulses of different ages by reference to the *frequency* of pulse-beats. His use of frequency as a criterion is puzzling, because 'speed' rather than 'frequency' was mentioned in Book I of Herophilus' *On Pulses*[155] as one of the four primary criteria by which one can distinguish one pulse from another. The extant evidence is too scanty to establish conclusively whether Herophilus thought of 'speed' and 'frequency' as different characteristics of the pulse, but later physicians such as Archigenes, Marcellinus, and Galen certainly drew a sharp distinction between pulse 'speed' and pulse 'frequency'.[156] Whatever the exact relation of 'speed' to 'frequency' in Herophilus' pulse-lore might be, it is clear from more than one ancient text that 'speed' – and not only 'frequency' – was actively used by Herophilus to define certain kinds of pulse, i.e. that he did not merely develop 'speed' as a hypothetical differentia which in practice was abandoned in favour of 'frequency'. Thus the pulse known as *formicans* or 'ant-like' (μυρμηκίζων, 'moving like an ant') is described by Herophilus as not being 'fast',[157] i.e. as not having much speed. And Pliny confirms in his *Natural History* that

[155] T162.
[156] According to Wellmann's plausible reconstruction (1895a: 185-8) all of Book v of Archigenes' *On Pulses* was devoted to pulse speed vs. pulse frequency. The pulse divisions used in Galen's *De pulsibus ad tirones* (VIII, p. 453–92) and in his *De pulsuum differentiis* (VIII, pp. 493ff.) are based on the tenfold classification Archigenes used in his *On Pulses* (as Wellmann, 1895a: 175ff., showed), and it is therefore not surprising that the distinction between pulse frequency and pulse speed plays a prominent role in the Galenic treatises. (Galen's approach to pulse-lore was, however, not merely one of slavish imitation; cf. Deichgräber, 1956.) The pulse division in the pseudo-Galenic *De pulsibus ad Antonium* (XIX, pp. 629–42K) is likewise dependent on Archigenes. Cf. also Marcellinus, *On Pulses*, Chapter 6 (pp. 460–1 Schöne), entitled 'In what respect speed differs from frequency'; Rufus (?), *Synopsis on Pulses*, pp. 231–2 (Daremberg/Ruelle), and Daremberg's comments in the Appendix, Section VIII (pp. 610–43) – *ibid.*, p. 642, the second pulse type refers to speed, and the fifth, relying on the notion of interval, to frequency. All later authors based their concept of pulse 'frequency' on the theory of periods of quiescence following each systole and disastole; Herophilus' silence regarding these intervals (see n. 132 *supra*) might indicate that – if he did in fact use frequency as a criterion – his concept of frequency was not based on the interval or pause. See also *Comments*, T182.
[157] T180.

Herophilus made use of speed as a differentia in his theory of stages of life: Herophilus, he says, 'divided the pulsation of the arteries into definite measures and metrical laws according to age: regular (*stabilis*) or fast or slow'.[158] Exactly how speed is determined – and in particular how a 'regular' or 'normal' speed, to which 'fast' and 'slow' could be referred, is defined – is, however, not revealed by the extant evidence.

'Size', the fourth and remaining primary differentia of pulse kinds, was also used in Herophilus' theory of stages of life. The information ancient sources provide about this differentia again is sparse, but it is more revealing than in the case of 'speed' and 'vehemence'. Galen, in his *Synopsis* of his own sphygmological treatises, agrees with Herophilus that the normal pulse of children is 'good-sized' or 'adequate in size' – rather than 'small', as Archigenes and others had claimed.[159] The reason Galen cites for not calling it 'small' reveals much about Herophilus' (and Galen's) conception of pulse size: unlike the 'primary perceptible time unit', which is an absolute measuring device, 'size' (μέγεθος) is a relative concept, because the 'size' of a pulse always has to be defined in relation to the circumference of its artery. Compared to the pulse of an adult, the child's pulse might be small, but relatively speaking, i.e. in relation to the circumference of a child's artery, it is as 'adequate in size' or 'good-sized' as the adult's pulse. Within this relativistic framework, 'adequacy' of size appar-

---

[158] T186. Pliny adds that by his time this Herophilean classification of pulse according to age and to pulse speed had been abandoned 'on account of its excessive subtlety', while the observation of pulse frequency and pulse strength still served as 'a pilot in life'. The statement that the strength and frequency of the pulse were still being used as diagnostic criteria, but that its speed had been abandoned – about rhythm and size, Herophilus' two other primary criteria, Pliny says nothing – can only mean that Pliny was not well informed about the efflorescence of pulse-lore in the Pneumatic school of medicine. The 'Pneumatics' not only took over Herophilus' four primary criteria (size, vehemence or strength, speed, and rhythm) and four of his subsidiary criteria (regularity and irregularity, evenness and unevenness); they added at least two more: frequency and fullness. Wilamowitz and Wellmann (1895a: 172 n. 8) argued that these aspects of Pneumatic pulse-lore first took definitive shape in the work of Pliny's contemporary Agathinus – although the pulse-lore of Agathinus' pupil, Archigenes, is much better documented – and if this is so, all the specific differentiae introduced by Herophilus, including 'speed', were far from extinct in Pliny's own day. Cf. also T185.

[159] T179–T181, T184. Cf. also the reference to size in T182: the pulse of a patient who has a fever is not only more frequent (πυκνότερος) and more vehement (σφοδρότερος), but also bigger (μείζων).

ently was thought of as characteristic of normal or healthy pulses at all ages, and deviations from the 'adequate' size of a given age group would consequently be viewed as a pathological symptom. Just how Herophilus thought that this kind of 'adequacy', or 'being good-sized', could be determined, is however, unfortunately not spelled out in the extant evidence.

Glancing back, we see that each of the four primary differentiae Herophilus introduced to distinguish different 'species' of pulse – size, speed, vehemence or strength, rhythm – is given significant application in his pulse-lore. Furthermore, in the extant evidence two of these differentiating devices also are made an integral part of his theory that there are four stages of life (infancy, adolescence, adulthood, old age), each with its own sphygmological character-istics. The two subsidiary differentiae – regularity and irregularity, evenness and unevenness – by contrast are not prominent in his stage theory. But the claim of Archigenes that Herophilus did in fact 'mention regularity and irregularity, also evenness and unevenness by specific kind',[160] is borne out by some of Herophilus' descriptions of abnormal pulses – descriptions which became renowned primarily because of his nomenclatural inventiveness: for example, the gazelle-like pulse (δορκαδίʒων, famous in Latin pulse-lore as *caprizans*) of a certain eunuch, the ant-like pulse (μυρμηκίʒων or *formicans*), and the quivering pulse (τρομώδης or *tremulus*).[161]

Numerous other pulse distinctions have also been attributed to Herophilus by modern scholars – for example, the classification of pulse by rational and irrational, by 'eurhythmic' and 'arhythmic', by 'pararhythmic' and 'ecrhythmic'[162] – but, with the exception of the

---

[160] T163a, T163b.

[161] Cf. T169 – T170, T180. The terms 'ant-like' pulse and 'gazelle-like' pulse appear to have been introduced by Herophilus. Later they were joined by the 'worm-like' pulse, *pulsus vermiculans*, or ὁ σκωληκίʒων σφυγμός (cf. for example, Marcellinus, *On Pulses* 33 (p. 469 Schöne); Galen, *De pulsuum differentiis* 1.26 (VIII, p. 553K)) and by a host of other pulse-types. Harris' implication (1973: 191) that the 'worming' pulse also received its name from Herophilus has no basis in the ancient evidence. For a survey see Schadewald, 1866; cf. Wellmann, 1895a: 199–200.

[162] For example, by Wellmann, 1895a: 189ff. But the main text on which this claim appears to rest is Galen, *De pulsuum differentiis* 1.7–8 (VIII, pp. 512–17K), and neither Herophilus nor 'the Herophileans' are mentioned in this passage. As I pointed out above (n. 132), not every occurrence of the phrase 'those who say they can perceive the contraction [of the arteries]' – the phrase with which this

single problematic reference to the pulse of a new-born infant as 'irrational' (see above), none of these distinctions is explicitly attributed to Herophilus by ancient sources, and they probably originated much later in the Pneumatic school, either with Agathinus (first century A.D.) or with Archigenes (c. A.D. 100). Archigenes' pulse-lore in particular appears to have been heavily indebted to Herophilus' theory, as Wellmann argued,[163] but the debt of the later physician should not be allowed to be misconstrued or distorted into an identity between the later and the earlier theories.[164]

The basic errors Herophilus made in his theory of the pulse are obvious (for example, the assumption that the pulmonary artery is a vein, the belief that the dilation of the arteries coincides with the expansion of the cardiac ventricles, the notion of an arterial 'faculty' of pulsation and the concomitant failure to recognize that the heart is a pump), and modern scholars naturally have tended to argue about which of these errors was most responsible for Herophilus' failure to discover the circulation of the blood. But Herophilus' own perspective was, of course, not that of Harvey; his perspective was largely determined by the views of the pulse that had been developed by Praxagoras, Aristotle, some Hippocratic authors, and his other predecessors. Historically, his advance on these predecessors was a stunning achievement. Galen recognized as much and devoted an entire treatise – unfortunately not extant – to Herophilus' pulse-lore,[165] in addition to citing him numerous times in his other works on pulse-lore. 'Herophilus', Galen says in On Medical Experience, 'is a man who is known by everybody to have surpassed the great majority of the ancients, not only in width of knowledge but in intellect, and to

Galenic discussion of eurhythmic, arhythmic, etc. is introduced – must necessarily be read as a reference to Herophilus; many ancient physicians (including Galen's own source, Archigenes) shared Herophilus' view that the systole or contraction of the artery is perceptible (cf. T159, T160), and it is quite possible that Galen is referring here to his immediate source, Archigenes, and to other Pneumatics who held Archigenes' view. See Comments, T175, for further texts.

[163] Wellmann, 1895a: 169–200.

[164] Wellmann's pioneering analysis (ibid.) – inspired by Archigenes' obvious debt to the Alexandrian – is unfortunately marred by the tendency to attribute many of Archigenes' apparent innovations to Herophilus too. The same tendency has coloured Harris' approach (1973: 181–95) to Herophilean pulse-lore.

[165] T162.103–6. Cf. also T176: 'what I shall write separately about Herophilus' art concerning the pulse'; whether this refers to the same work on Herophilus depicted in T162 as already completed is unclear.

have advanced the art of medicine in many ways; as, for instance, by his logos of the pulsation of arteries, which one needs more now and finds more useful than any other logos, for deriving benefit therefrom . . .'[166] While Erasistratus' understanding of the heart, and in particular of its intake and outlet valves, was superior to Herophilus', it was Herophilus' theory of how the music in our arteries is made that became a model for almost all subsequent ancient writers on pulse-lore.

5 Male reproductive physiology; spermatogenesis

Herophilus' remarkably detailed anatomy of the male and female reproductive organs has become well known (see Chapter VI. A.5 and T101–T114), but less attention has focused on the fact that he also tried to account for the generation of male 'seed'. In pre-Alexandrian philosophy and medicine there had been a rich tradition of speculating about the origin of human 'seed', and a brief glance at these theories might help us to assess the historical role of Herophilus' contribution.

In the fifth and fourth centuries B.C. there were several models of seed (sperma) formation. First, there is a theory, perhaps of Persian provenance,[167] according to which seed either originates in or is part of the brain, i.e. the so-called encephalogenetic theory of seed. 'Sperma,' a Pythagorean says, 'is a drop dripping from the brain.'[168] The mechanism by which seed was thought to be transported from the brain to the penis seems to have been bloodvessels; as I pointed out above (Chapter VI), a prominent theory at the time was that the vascular system emanates from the head and proceeds past the ears and neck down the spinal column to the loins, the genitalia, and so on. The Hippocratic author of Airs, Waters, Places seems to refer to this

---

[166] T147. Cf. also T166: 'He alone understands and the shades flit around' (see Comments on T166).

[167] Cf. Lesky, 1950: 10–11 (= 1234–5). Whether the Persian influence Lesky discusses actually extends to spermatology seems uncertain.

[168] D.L. 8.28 (= 58B1aDK): τὸ δὲ σπέρμα εἶναι σταγόνα ἐγκεφάλου, and 'it contains warm breath'. Diogenes Laertius here is excerpting Alexander Polyhistor (FGrHist 273F93). On the date see Wiersma, 1942; Wellmann, 1919. Because the Presocratic Alcmeon of Croton (24A13) also subscribed to the encephalogenetic view of seed formation, it is possible that this theory entered the Greek world through the Pythagorean – or at least a Western Greek – school of philosophy. Cf. Lesky, 1950: 10–11 (= 1234–5); Geurts, 1941: 24ff., 56, 73ff.; Lonie, 1981: 101–2.

link between the vascular system and the generative system when he says with reference to the impotence of Scythians: 'For, by the side of the ear are vessels and if someone cuts them [i.e for the purpose of bloodletting], those so cut become impotent.'[169] Similarly, the author of the Hippocratic treatise *On Seed* attributes the infertility of eunuchs to bloodletting behind the ears, for 'the greatest amount of seed comes from the head along the ears into the spinal marrow. This duct is, however, hardened as a result of the formation of a scar after the cut has been made.'[170] This encephalogenetic theory, which appears also in a myelogenetic version (i.e. with the spinal marrow instead of the brain as the ultimate source of seed),[171] was perhaps originally inspired by the conviction of the supremacy of the brain in all vital functions (or by the related conviction of the 'divine' nature of the head and the 'divine' origin of seed). Strong echoes of the theory can be found in the fourth century B.C. too, for example in Plato's *Timaeus*[172] and in Diocles' physiology.[173]

A second theory of seed formation seems to have started usurping the encephalogenetic or myeologenetic model no later than the late fifth century B.C. Apparently of atomistic provenance, this theory states that seed originates not in the brain but in all parts of the body (or at least in all its moist parts); the theory hence is known as the 'pangenesis' theory or the 'panspermatic' model – a model which is, of course, more compatible with contemporary genetic theory. The author of the Hippocratic treatise *On Sacred Disease* is an adherent of this theory, claiming that 'seed comes from everywhere in the body – sound seed from the sound parts, diseased seed from the diseased parts'.[174] It is, however, characteristic of the agon between the old and the new, also within the Hippocratic Corpus, that both the

---

[169] Hp., *Airs, Waters, and Places* 22. On bloodletting behind the ear see also Hp., *Epidemics* 6.5.15 (with Galen's commentary *ad loc.*, *CMG* v. 10.2.2, pp. 300f. Wenkebach).

[170] Hp., *On Seed* (or: *On Generation*) 2 (VII, p. 472L; p. 1 Lonie).

[171] Cf. the Presocratic Hippo, 38A12DK (= Censorinus, *De die natali* 5.2). See also Hp., *On Seed/Generation* 1 (VII, p. 470L; p. 1 Lonie), where the spinal marrow is likewise stressed as crucial to the formation and transportation of seed. See below, n. 177.

[172] Plato, *Timaeus* 73B1–D2.

[173] Diocles, fr. 170 Wellmann (= ps.-Galen, *Definitiones medicae* 439 (XIX, p. 449K)); 'Vindician', *Fragmentum Bruxellense*, Chapter 5 (p. 211 Wellmann, 1901): 'viae seminales a cerebro . . .'.

[174] Hp., *On the Sacred Disease*, Chapter 5 (= Chapter 2.5, p. 68 Grensemann).

archaic, encephalogenetic view and the newer, pangenetic view of
seed are found in one and the same Hippocratic work: in *On Airs,
Waters, and Places* there is not only the allusion to the encephalogenetic
view[175] mentioned earlier, but also the following 'panspermatic'
statement: 'For the seed comes from all parts of the body, healthy seed
from healthy parts, diseased seed from diseased parts . . . Bald
parents, therefore, for the most part have bald children, grey-eyed
parents grey-eyed children, squinting parents squinting children, and
so on . . .'[176] The author of this treatise does not even try to reconcile
these two spermatological theories with each other (whereas there is
an inchoate but unsuccessful attempt at harmonizing them in *On
Seed*[177]). In general, however, the pangenetic theory dominates the
Hippocratic Corpus, and it is represented both in so-called 'Coan'
treatises (e.g. *Airs, Waters, Places; On Sacred Disease*) and in treatises
traditionally known as 'Cnidian' (for example, the 'trilogy' *On Seed,
On the Nature of the Child, On Diseases* IV).

A third influential theory concerning the generation of human
seed, is that it is formed in the blood through a process of concoction,
i.e. that it is a residue or a more fully concocted form of blood (and
hence ultimately derived from nourishment), reaching the genitalia
through the vascular system. Although a less elaborate formulation of
this haematogenous theory of seed formation is attributed to the
Presocratic philosopher Diogenes of Apollonia,[178] its most famous
proponent is, of course, Aristotle. In *On the Generation of Animals*[179]
Aristotle depicts a process by which food after mastication passes into
the stomach, where it is 'concocted' or 'ripened' by means of natural
or vital heat. Next it is passed on to the heart in liquid form as we saw

---

[175] See n. 169.

[176] Ch. 14 (*CMG* I.I.2, p. 58 Diller). Cf. also Aristotle's account of the arguments
used in favour of pangenesis, *On Generation of Animals* 1.17.721b7–722a1 (but
Aristotle himself of course rejects this theory). See Lonie, 1981: 64–7, 115–17.

[177] Hp., *On Seed/Generation* I (VII, p. 470L): seed comes from all the moisture in the
body, and then gathers in the spinal marrow. See Lonie, 1981: 99–110.

[178] Diogenes of Apollonia, 64B6DK; the fragment quoted by DK from Aristotle's
Historia animalium 3.2.512b8–11 is somewhat ambiguous, but 'Vindician'
(Wellmann, 1901: 208) leaves no doubt: 'spumam sanguinis eius [sc. seminis]
essentiam . . .' Cf. also 64A24DK. On other Presocratic views see Lesky, 1950:
1233ff., 1263ff., 1294ff., 1255ff., 1344ff.; Longrigg, 1985a.

[179] Aristotle, *Generation of Animals* 1.16–19.721a26–727b30. See also *Part. An.*
2.6.651b20f., 4.10.689a9. For a useful general summary see Peck, 1943: lxiii–
lxvii.

above, and there it is turned into blood through a further process of concoction. In the heart the blood is also charged with connate pneuma, and then it is distributed through the blood vessels. But since more blood is produced than is necessary for maintaining life and supplying growth, there is a surplus which may undergo a further process of concoction. Among the useful kinds of surplus or 'residue' are seed in the male, and menstrual 'moisture' and mother's milk in the female; among the useless are the excrements. Seed, then, is surplus blood which, like menstrual blood, has undergone a further stage of concoction and thereby has become a useful generative residue in the male. It is also a vehicle of soul, containing connate pneuma and already potentially possessing the principle of the sentient soul (whereas menstrual blood possesses only nutritive soul potentially).

The formation of seed, in Aristotle's view, is largely completed in the bloodvessels before they reach the genitalia. The testicles are not an integral part of the spermatic duct system, and the ductus deferens mainly provides a kind of transit lounge or passage for the discharge of seed; the testicles do not contribute in any way to seed formation itself. This does not mean that Aristotle relaxes his usual teleological approach to bodily organs: the testes, which are likened to the stone weights which women hang on their looms when weaving,[180] keep the spermatic duct hanging down from the rest of the body and thus, by virtue of making the journey of sperm longer and more convoluted, 'make the movement of the seminal residue (τὸ σπερμα-τικὸν περίττωμα) more stable';[181] this in turn helps to prevent excessive sexual excitation and, apparently, premature ejaculation.

While there were other models of spermatogenesis in antiquity, these three – the encephalogenetic, pangenetic, and haematogenous models – were probably best known in Herophilus' time. Here again, as so often, we find Herophilus siding with Aristotle against the Hippocratic Corpus: he rejects the encephalogenetic and pangenetic theories and instead accepts Aristotle's theory that seed has its origin in blood.

Herophilus does not accept all the details and presuppositions of the Aristotelian view (see below), in part perhaps because of his

[180] On the testicles as loom weights see Aristotle, *Generation of Animals* 1.4.717a34–36; cf. 5.7.787b24–6.
[181] *Ibid.*, 717a29–31.

superior anatomical knowledge of the reproductive organs, but he
does embrace the central thesis of Aristotle's theory – i.e. that human
seed is a product of blood – and he even defends it on anatomical
grounds, a step of considerable significance since he was arguably the
most renowned anatomist of pre-Galenic antiquity. According to a
famous fragment, De semine, in a Latin codex now in Brussels (a
fragment thought by most scholars to be the work of St Augustine's
friend Vindician), Herophilus said[182] that dissection proves the
haematogenous theory of seed to be correct, because the bloodvessels
leading into the genitalia contain more blood when they are at a
greater distance from the genitalia, but less blood – and more of a
seed-coloured substance – the closer they get to the genitalia. The
author of the fragment presents this argument as the first of five proofs
of the haematogenous origin of human seed, and there can be no
doubt that this one is attributed to Herophilus himself: 'primo igitur
ut Herofilus ait, abruptio [apertio Jaeger] corporum testatur . . . ' If
the rest of this argument is also attributable to Herophilus, as Werner
Jaeger maintained,[183] Herophilus accepted as a subsidiary argument
a further element of Aristotle's theory of blood residues, namely that
mother's milk, like seed, is a residue or surplus product of blood:[184]
when blood is no longer needed to nourish the foetus in the uterus
because the woman has already given birth, 'the blood flows to the
breasts by a natural course, and through the power of the breasts,
grows white and takes on the quality of milk.'[185]

It is possible that the remaining four 'proofs' advanced in defence of
the haematogeneous theory of seed in this part of Vindician's
fragment were also by Herophilus. But Jaeger's analysis does not
prove their Herophilean authorship quite as conclusively as he
claims: 'Es ist also keine Ausflucht möglich vor der Folgerung', says
Jaeger 'dass das Herofilus ait [sc. preceding the first proof] alle fünf
folgenden Beweise umfasst'; and the five proofs '[werden] ausdrücklich
dem Herophilos zugeschrieben.'[186] While no one is eager to be guilty
of resorting to an impossible Ausflucht, it should be noted that the
formulations in the fragment are in fact less explicit and conclusive

[182] T191.   [183] Jaeger, 1938a: 198–201.
[184] On lactation see Aristotle, Generation of Animals 4.8.776a15–777a27.Cf. Galen, De
         placitis Hp. et Plat. 7.3.29.
[185] T191, lines 13–16. Cf. Isidorus, Etymologiae XI.1.77.
[186] Jaeger, 1938a: 200.

than Jaeger would have us believe. Having enumerated five adherents of the haematogenous theory at the outset – Diogenes of Apollonia, Erasistratus, Herophilus, Herophilus' follower Alexander Philalethes (see Chapter XXII *infra*), and the Stoics – the author of the fragment adds 'and *different authors* explain it by providing different proofs which, as it were, are brought together [seized upon; grasped] for one and the same purpose. First, then, as Herophilus says, . . . dissection is a witness to this . . . ' Even if one reads 'different Stoics' for 'different authors' – a reading the Latin text permits[187] – the entire collection of five proofs does not seem to be introduced as the sole responsibility of Herophilus. Furthermore, only the first proof is explicitly attributed to Herophilus – and probably because it resorts to a branch of medicine associated more firmly and consistently with Herophilus than with any other ancient physician except Galen: anatomy.

In none of the other proofs is Herophilus mentioned again. The second proof simply states that excessive intercourse results in an emission of blood instead of seed (since excessive seminal depletion causes blood which has not yet been converted into seed to enter the spermatic duct system). The third proof, a syllogism, again is not attributed to any specific author: what is most important (*summum*) can only arise from what is more important, but seed is the most important of all the moistures in us, and so is blood, therefore seed is generated out of blood. According to the fourth proof, the symptoms following bloodletting (paleness, loss of weight, weakness) are the same as the ones attending exhaustion from sexual intercourse, therefore seed is formed in the blood. And in the fifth proof it is argued that, since blood congeals when removed from its own vessels (i.e. from veins and arteries), and since seed does so too – dissections, the author says, show that seed congeals when it has been deposited in the uterus – the essence of seed must come from blood. While Herophilus' name is not prefixed to any of these last four 'proofs', it is striking that the series ends with a further appeal to observations made in dissection, and this points to considerations not raised by Jaeger.

Jaeger attributed these five proofs to Herophilus mainly on stylistic

[187] T191, lines 4–6: 'hoc idem Stoici philosophi de materiali semine senserunt. et demonstrationes alii alias deferentes . . . enarrant.' Especially if one punctuates differently (e.g. a comma after 'senserunt'), it is possible to read 'alii' as referring to various Stoics.

grounds – i.e. on the basis of the sequence 'primo igitur, ut Herophilus ait, . . . secundo . . . tertio . . . quartum . . . quintum' (but ignor-
ing the introductory statement) – yet at least as strong an argument
for Herophilean authorship can be made on the basis of the contents
and focus of these proofs. The arguments advanced in these proofs are
more consistent with the theory and practice of Herophilus than with
that of any other author mentioned in Vindician's introductory
enumeration of defenders of the hematogenous theory. Thus the first
proof not only mentions Herophilus by name but also refers to two of
his areas of expertise: (a) dissection and (b) the male reproductive
organs. (Among the haematogenous theorists introduced in this
fragment Erasistratus of course also was a pioneer of dissection – none
of the others practised systematic dissection, as far as we know – but
he cannot be shown to have been particularly renowned for his
anatomy of the male genitalia.) The second proof again alludes to a
problem of particular interest to Herophilus – i.e. the contributions
made to seed production by various parts of its 'transportation
system'[188] – but, as far as we know, not discussed by Diogenes,
Erasistratus, Alexander Philalethes,[189] and the Stoics (although it
must be stressed in this case that the scant nature of the extant
evidence deprives this judgment of much value). The third argument,
about blood and seed as *summa*, could presumably have been
advanced by any of the adherents of the haematogenous view, but the
fourth, with its reference to bloodletting, is striking. If it is simply a
statement based on observing the practice of others, it too could have
been made by any of the philosophers or physicians on Vindician's
list, but if it is based on personal clinical or experimental observation – as the first and fifth proofs seem to be – then the range of
possible authors can be narrowed down radically. The Stoics and the
Presocratic Diogenes of Apollonia are philosophers who were almost
certainly not among the ancient 'phlebotomers', and none of the

[188] Cf. T 192. It is striking that a variation of this second argument (i.e. that excessive
    intercourse results in the ejaculation of blood or 'unconcocted seed', but not of
    seed) was also used by Aristotle to prove that seed derives from blood: *Generation
    of Animals* 1.19.726b7–10. Much of this account is ultimately indebted to
    Aristotle (see also n. 190 *infra*), but in this form the arguments undoubtedly post-
    date Aristotle.
[189] Cf. Diogenes of Apollonia, 64A24-27DK, 64B6DK. About Erasistratus' views on
    reproduction we know next to nothing. For Alexander Philalethes see *infra*
    Chapter XXII, especially *AP*. 9–11.

ancient testimonia concerning Alexander Philalethes (see *infra*, Chapter xxii) refers to his use of bloodletting. Erasistratus, as we know from Galen's extensive polemics,[190] rejected bloodletting as a therapeutic device. This leaves Herophilus, for whom indeed the use – though not the indiscriminate use – of bloodletting as a therapeutic measure is attested, as I shall argue below (Chapter VIII.A). Finally, the fifth proof recorded in the Brussels fragment again introduces not only dissection but also a subject on which Herophilus, more than any other author on Vindician's list, was an authority: the female reproductive system.[191] From the point of view of internal consistency and historical probability, it therefore seems possible and even likely that all or most of these five proofs of the haematogenous origin of seed were advanced by Herophilus. They are 'refuted' one by one in a subsequent part of Vindician's fragment, and hence appear to have been regarded as influential – and about Herophilus' stature and impact there cannot be much doubt. But this tentative conclusion about the authorship of the proofs cannot make the confident claim to certainty with which Werner Jaeger tried to invest it, especially since it relies on several arguments *e silentio*.

Aristotle's central thesis concerning the origin of seed was, then, accepted and defended by Herophilus. But Herophilus also staked out his independence from Aristotle. While Aristotle thought the production of seed was completed in the blood vessels and therefore granted no role in seed production to the testes or to the spermatic duct, Herophilus maintains that both play a role in the generation of seed.[192] It is true that Galen criticises Herophilus for not attributing a greater role in seed production to the testicles than to the 'seminal vessel' or ductus deferens, but Galen is quick to add that Herophilus at least 'was not quite as mistaken as Aristotle, who compared the testicles to loom weights'.[193]

In Herophilus' theory male seed is apparently thought of as being

---

[190] See especially Galen, *De venae sectione adversus Erasistratum* (xi, pp. 147–86k). As in the case of the second 'proof', it is striking that an inchoate version of this fourth proof was first introduced by Aristotle. In *Generation of Animals* (1.19.726b12–13) he says the discharge of seed from the system causes exhaustion (it is ἐκλυτικόν), just like the 'excretion' (ἀποχώρησις) of pure, healthy blood. But Aristotle seems to be referring to loss of blood generally, not to bloodletting; moreover, the description of the symptoms in 'Vindician' is more specific. See above, n. 188.
[191] Cf. Chapter VI, T105–T114 and T61; *infra*, T193–T204; Chapter VIII. T247.
[192] Cf. T189.   [193] *Ibid.* (See also above, n. 180).

only imperfectly formed when it arrives from the blood vessels in the testicles. In a continuing process of further refinement it passes from the testes to the epididymis, and from there the seed is apparently thought of as being drawn up into the ductus deferens and the seminal vessels. Herophilus does not, however, seem to have given a clear or satisfactory account of the mechanism or 'faculty' by which the seed gets from the testicles to the penis, and Rufus of Ephesus concludes that 'this provided Herophilus, too, with an insoluble difficulty'.[194] Both the vasa deferentia and the seminal vesicles are called 'assistants' (παραστάται),[195] and they presumably 'assisted' not only in the production but also in the transportation of male seed. But whereas Herophilus accounted for most other forms of bodily movement – respiration, pulsation, tremor, spasm, palpitation, and voluntary muscle movements – by resorting to concepts such as 'natural faculty', 'natural tendency', and 'voluntary motor nerves', we are not much better informed than Rufus appears to have been concerning Herophilus' view of the principles of movement within the male genitalia.

6 Herophilus' 'Midwifery'; gynaecology

When we turn from Herophilus' discussion of the functions of the male reproductive organs to the female, it is striking that an interest in pathology, which is largely absent from the testimonia concerning the male organs, looms large in his discussion of the female. This is undoubtedly due in part to the nature of the treatise to which the testimonia concerning women seem to belong – Herophilus' *Midwifery* or *On Delivery* – but it also reveals an acute general interest in gynaecology which some might consider unusual in a physician with a 'Coan', rather than a 'Cnidian' background (if, in fact, this distinction has any merit).[196]

Yet Herophilus' *Midwifery*, the first such treatise from antiquity

---

[194] T192.
[195] Cf. Chapter VI. A.5, and T101–T105. On the 'assistants' (*parastatai*) see also *Comments*, T189, T101–3, and T61 ('varix-like assistants').
[196] W. D. Smith (1973), Lonie (1978), and Thivel (1981) have challenged the traditional distinction between 'Coan' and 'Cnidian'. But the views of J. Ilberg, Lonie (1965b) and others who have tried to preserve and clarify this distinction are still being defended with various modifications, especially by J. Jouanna and H. Grensemann. For the relevant literature see *infra*, Chapter XIV (Bacchius), n. 15.

(although a rich gynaecological tradition is preserved in some of the so-called Cnidian treatises of the Hippocratic Corpus), was not exclusively concerned with pathological conditions. It also contained some of his physiological views, for example that the uterus is constituted of the same material elements as the rest of the body and is regulated by the same faculties. (Some of the anatomical details concerning the uterus, the ovaries, and parts of the Fallopian tubes that were discussed above (Chapter VI.A.5; Fr61, T105–T114) might also have been presented in Herophilus' *Midwifery* rather than in his *Anatomy*.)

The primary aim even of the physiological observations in *Midwifery* seems to be, however, to provide a basis for a pathology which would demystify the female organs by depicting them as subject to the same faculties, and hence to the same disorders, as the rest of the human body, whether male or female. 'There is no disease peculiar to women', is Herophilus' reassurance, 'because the uterus becomes diseased through the agency of the same things' as any other part of the male or female body, for example by quantitative excesses (of humours?), by 'thickness' or growth, and by disharmony.[197]

Despite these reassurances Herophilus had to concede, however, that certain 'affections' are peculiar to women: menstruation, conception, childbirth, breast-feeding, concocting or 'ripening' of the mother's milk, and 'the opposites of these' (i.e. presumably infertility, miscarriage, lack of lactation).[198] It is to these exceptions, and in particular to obstetrical problems, that most of the extant testimonia concerning his *Midwifery* belong. The degree to which 'the mouth of the uterus' is dilated at childbirth and during various stages of pregnancy (as opposed to during menstruation), the clinical problem of inserting a probe into both the healthy uterus and the prolapsed cervix – these are the kinds of questions Herophilus also dealt with in what seems to have been a wide-ranging work.[199]

While several ancient texts refer to or are based on Herophilus' *Midwifery*, the only fragment (or literal quotation) from *Midwifery* is a

---

[197] T193–T194. A useful general survey of Greek views on whether (and how) the female differs from the male is provided by Diepgen, 1937: 123–30. Cf. also Lesky, 1950; Manuli, 1980; Rouselle, 1980; Lloyd, 1983: 58–111.

[198] T193.

[199] Cf. T200 on the question of the dilation of the cervix (see also *Comments*, T200). On the prolapsus of the cervix cf. T201 (and see *Comments ad loc.*)

lengthy passage concerning the reasons for difficult childbirth.[200]
Among the 'internal conditions' that cause difficult childbirth,
Herophilus lists an oblique position of the foetus, inadequate dilation
of the neck of the uterus, failure of the amniotic sac to break before
birth, 'atonic' uterus, multiple births (ranging from triplets to
quintuplets). Herophilus became famous throughout antiquity for
mentioning a case of quintuplets,[201] and this seems to indicate that
such cases were much more rare in the ancient world than they have
become today, in part undoubtedly because the Greeks did not
possess the fertility drugs which are in use at present.

Among the 'external conditions' – i.e. conditions external to the
uterus – which can cause difficult childbirth, Herophilus mentions[202]
diet, the nature of one's activities, discharge of too much 'blood-like
moisture', excessive cold or heat, a tumour or abscess in the intestines,
a 'concavity' of the loin or spine, and excessive fat in the hips or in the
upper abdominal cavity. His choice of some of these 'external causes'
is not particularly felicitous, but in his observations on the 'internal
causes' of difficult childbirth Herophilus cannot be accused of having
been entirely imperceptive.

Embryological questions also seem to have been dealt with in
Herophilus' *Midwifery*. We saw earlier that he dealt with the question
whether a foetus is a living being, and that he apparently gave the
qualified answer that it possesses involuntary motions, such as
pulsation, but not voluntary motions that are subject to the nervous
system[203] – an interesting shift from Aristotle's emphasis on the
sentient soul contributed to the embryo by the male seed and the
nutritive soul contributed by menstrual blood.[204]

The duration of pregnancy is a related question which intrigued
Greek physicians from 'Hippocrates' onward, and according to the
Neoplatonist Proclus' commentary on Plato's *Republic*, Herophilus,
with his new knowledge of female anatomy, expressed his opposition
to one of the traditional, erroneous answers, namely that pregnancy
normally lasts seven months.[205] Proclus' explanation of the roots of

[200] T196 (see also *Comments*, T196).
[201] T196, T197a, T197b. Cf. Heiberg, 1912: 194, lines 3–4.
[202] T196, lines 12ff.
[203] T202a and 202b; cf. T199.
[204] Cf. Aristotle, *Generation of Animals* 1.19–22, and especially 2.3.736a24–737a7.
[205] T198. Cf. Hp., *On the Eight-Month Child* (vii, pp. 436–52L). Cf. also Herodotus
       6.69, and Aristotle, *Historia animalium* 7.4.584a35–b25 (conception can last

this common error, namely that many women become aware of their pregnancy only two months after conception, may be on target. If Proclus' report may be trusted – and this is not certain by any means, because the textual basis for attributing this view to Herophilus is flimsy[206] – it would provide another striking example of the explicit criticism of a traditional error in the 'new', scientific medicine of Alexandria.

7 Herophilus' 'Against Common Opinions'

With this work Herophilus initiated an Alexandrian doxographic tradition which endured within his own school until the last visible generation of Herophileans (see Chapter x.a). It is a tradition to which we undoubtedly owe the survival of much of the evidence concerning Herophilus and his followers.[207] The doxographic polemics of later Herophileans often focused on subtle, esoteric controversies that pitted Herophilean against Herophilean. Herophilus' treatise, by contrast, appears to reflect the position of the bold, confident founder of a 'new' medicine: he goes on the offensive not against esoteric theories and definitions developed within his own circle of followers, but against 'common opinions'.

Only one ancient text can be assigned unequivocally to this work. It suggests that *Against Common Opinions* not only attempted to refute mistaken conceptions which had become prevalent by Herophilus' time, but also contained his own positive doctrines. Soranus of Ephesus, a distinguished physician who lived at the time of the Emperors Trajan and Hadrian (A.D. 98–138), reports[208] that Herophilus in this treatise attacked the notion that menstruation is advantageous not only for one's general health but also for childbearing. Instead, Herophilus adopted the discriminating view that menstruation is helpful to some women but harmful to others,

---

seven, eight, or nine months, but usually lasts ten months, sometimes also eleven); Aëtius, *Placita* 5.18 (*DG*, pp. 427–9); ps.-Galen, *Definitiones medicae* 450 (xix, p. 454K); ps.-Galen, *De historia philosopha* 122 (*DG*, p. 644) [= Chapter 34, xix, pp. 331–4K].

[206] See critical apparatus, T198.

[207] Cf. Chapter x.a; Chapter xxv; Chapter iii.a.1.

[208] T203. On Greek theories concerning menstruation and other forms of vaginal discharge cf. Diepgen, 1937: 190–9. See also below, Chapter xvi, *DA*.17, for a later Herophilean's classification of vaginal discharges. Cf. also T204.

depending on their individual circumstances. While Soranus mentions that Herophilus tried to verify this hypothesis by means of clinical examples, more evidence about the reasons he advanced for these variations has not been transmitted. (Soranus himself, it should be noted, firmly rejects Herophilus' view, claiming that menstruation is invariably harmful but that its effects are noticeable to varying degrees; despite the disagreement, he gives a place of unusual prominence to Herophilus throughout his *Gynaecology*, also providing the extensive quotation from Herophilus' *Midwifery*.[209])

The fact that the only testimonium attributable to *Against Common Opinions* is of a gynaecological nature confirms what his *Midwifery* already established: that Herophilus was particularly interested in obstetrics and gynaecology. But it cannot be interpreted as evidence that *Against Common Opinions* was confined to gynaecological questions. The title suggests a far-ranging work that might have dealt with popular or commonly held pathophysiological and therapeutic views as well. Whether it extended beyond medical questions to include other 'opinions' – as did the treatise *On False Beliefs* by Herophilus' pupil Andreas (see *infra*, Chapter XI, *An.* 45). – is unclear, but what we know about Herophilus' interests makes this unlikely.

The doxographic genre was growing in popularity in the early Hellenistic period, inspired in part by the example of Aristotle, who often collected, classified, and criticized popular as well as more technical opinions on scientific and philosophical questions. Two of Aristotle's pupils, Theophrastus and Meno, were the authors of influential doxographic works on philosophy and medicine respectively, and a third, Demetrius of Phaleron, may have had a considerable impact on Alexandrian approaches to the systematization of knowledge. Although strictly speaking Herophilus' work does not seem to have been a specialized 'doxography' in the Peripatetic tradition, his work perhaps belongs in this general context of collecting and criticizing the views of others. It is the first such work

---

[209] Among the testimonia drawn from Soranus' *Gynaecia* are T193–T196, T201, T203–T204, T106, T113. Two of Herophilus' followers, Demetrius of Apamea and Alexander Philalethes, are also cited more than once in Soranus' *Gynaecia* (cf. *infra*, Chapter XVI, *DA.*3, *DA.*17–21, *DA.*25, and Chapter XXII, *AP.* 10–11), and several others are mentioned at least once (Andreas, Apollonius Mys, Mantias, and possibly Bacchius). See Chapter XI, *An.* 9; Chapter XVIII, *Ma.* 11–12; Chapter XXIII, *AM.* 7; Chapter XIV, *Ba.* 79. Caelius Aurelianus also supplies rich but non-gynaecological 'Soranian' evidence about Herophileaus.

from the new centre of science, Alexandria. Like Aristotle, Theophrastus and Meno, Herophilus did not, however, use collections of opinions only to schematize, summarize, and attack the views of predecessors; he also tried to use it as a means of establishing himself as a new scientist who no longer was enslaved to the errors of the past.

8 General pathological evidence; semiotics

In the discussion of the humours (*supra*), it was pointed out that Herophilus made the humours a basis not only of his physiology but also of his pathology. More specifically, an 'affection' is defined by Herophilus and the Herophileans as something 'which is difficult to resolve and to alleviate [or: to change] and which has its cause in the humours [or: moistures] of the body'.[210] The question of humours vs. moistures was dealt with earlier; here the question of what Herophilus means by 'affection' deserves brief consideration.

A second definition of 'affection' attributed to 'the Herophileans' in the pseudo-Galenic *Medical Definitions* (*c.* A.D. 100?) is: 'An affection is that which is not throughout dissolved [resolved] in the same time but sometimes in less time, sometimes in more.'[211] Since 'Herophileans' here is not used in opposition to 'Herophilus' – as in some texts included below (see especially Chapter x) – it seems reasonable to include Herophilus among those who adhered to this definition. If so, it would indicate that the pathological perspectives which Herophilus insisted on include not only the degree of curability – as in the first definiton – but also the durational variability of diseases.

The notion of variability seems to have been put to even broader use by Herophilus. According to Caelius Aurelianus, a fifth-century A.D. physician who depended heavily on Soranus, Herophilus also extended the notion of variability to the question of health. Whereas Herophilus' contemporary Erasistratus denied that there are degrees of health, insisting that there are no peaks or valleys in health, Herophilus anticipated the Methodists' theory that health is a variable 'since it increases and decreases'.[212] From a theoretical point of view the insistence on varying degrees of health and illness might have produced problems in antiquity, because it virtually invites the kind of sorites that was gaining popularity with Herophilus' contemporaries. The Megarian logician Diodorus Cronus, who once sought

[210] T205.   [211] T206.   [212] T207.

Herophilus' help with a dislocated shoulder,[213] would probably have been tempted to ask the physician: 'If there are varying degrees of health and illness, exactly where does poor health cease and disease begin? Exactly at what point does good health cross the border into excellent health?' But from a practical point of view it was undoubtedly a useful approach to problems confronting the physician.

Beyond developing these general pathological perspectives, Herophilus attempted to determine the specific cause of individual disorders. There is tempting though not conclusive evidence that he used the heuristic tool which made him famous, dissection, not only for anatomical exploration but also for pathological examination. Vindician reports that Herophilus was one of the physicians practising in Alexandria who 'found it proper to examine the bodies of the dead *in order to know for what reason and in what manner they died'*.[214] Although the value of this text is compromised by considerations raised above,[215] historical probability is strongly in favour of accepting this part of Vindician's statement as accurate.

For all Herophilus' emphasis on the provisionality and hypothetical nature of causal explanation,[216] the evidence presented in this chapter (especially T205–T225) leaves no doubt that Vindician is right, at least to the extent that Herophilus engaged in causal explanation not only for physiological but also for pathological purposes. While Herophilus' cautious, sceptical strain breaks through in his statement that 'people sometimes suffer from fever although there is no antecedent [i.e. proximate] cause',[217] Pliny confirms that 'Herophilus established examining the causes of diseases' (causas morborum scrutari . . Herophilus instituerat).[218] And other ancient sources ascribe not only the development of a general humoral theory of causation but also the description of the proximate causes of a variety of diseases to Herophilus: cardiac disorders can be due to poor diet or spoiled food and indigestion,[219] the extraction of a tooth can

---

[213] See Chapter II, T15.   [214] T208.   [215] See Chapter II, *Comments* on T5.
[216] Cf. Chapter V.A.   [217] T217.   [218] T209.
[219] T214. The vague phrase 'tamquam sectator Herophili' leaves unsettled whether Herophilus himself also held this view. Caelius Aurelianus seems to be translating οἱ περὶ τὸν Ἡρόφιλον or οἱ Ἡροφίλειοι – from his Greek source (Soranus' lost work *On Acute and Chronic Diseases*) – fairly consistently as *sectator(es) Herophili*, but these Greek phrases are notoriously ambiguous, as pointed out above.

cause death,[220] 'paralysis' of the heart causes a sudden death,[221] pneumonia is caused by an inflammation of the entire lung,[222] and so on.

In addition to examining the causes of diseases, Herophilus paid considerable attention to their symptoms: phrenitis, which he defined as a violent attack of madness (*deliratio*), is said to have as its symptoms fever and loss of reason (*alienatio*);[223] pleurisy is an affection of the lung – in this he disagreed with Diocles and Erasistratus, but agreed with his teacher Praxagoras – accompanied by fever, a slight cough, and a swelling of the lung, but not by redness, protrusions, swelling, and pain in the sides;[224] slight fever is a sign that tetanic recurvation is about to be alleviated.[225] In addition, Caelius Aurelianus reports more ambiguously that 'the followers of Herophilus' (*sectatores Herophili*) mention the symptoms which are attendant upon those who are affected by paralysis'[226] – but unfortunately the author does not specify what these symptoms are. Galen and Caelius Aurelianus also confirm that Herophilus wrote on various kinds of intestinal disorders – obstruction, lientery, dysentery, constipation – but frustratingly little is known about his views concerning these diseases (except that they are at odds with Erasistratus').[227]

Finally, in a passage which is introduced in hypothetical terms and hence might be of questionable value,[228] Sextus Empiricus says Herophilus might regard the following symptoms in feverish patients

---

[220] T218.
[221] T212. It seems significant that Herophilus does not say sudden death occurs 'for no cause' – the cause is, after all, 'paralysis of the heart' – but 'for no apparent cause', 'nulla ex manifesta causa'. This seems to vindicate the characterization of his theory of method and causation provided above (Chapter v): one can and must start with the phenomena only, but there might be more to reality.
[222] T215.   [223] T211.
[224] T216. (This entire extract is included, because Herophilus seems to belong to the *primi* of line 6.)
[225] T222.   [226] T213.
[227] T219–T221. T221 is, however, of questionable value; the 'Galenic' commentary in which it occurs is a forgery compiled in the Renaissance from various Galenic texts. Cf. Wenkebach, 1917. For Galen's genuine commentary on *Epidemics* II see *CMG* v.10.1, ed. Pfaff (Leipzig/Berlin, 1934).
[228] T225. An abbreviated version of a similar sceptic argument is presented in T224; as in T225, Sextus' trio of 'dogmatists' who typically give the same signs contradictory interpretations consists of Herophilus, Erasistratus, and Asclepiades.

as 'signs of good blood': flushing, a prominence of the bloodvessels,
moist skin, high temperature, vehemence of the pulse. But Sextus, a
sceptic, is constructing an argument of a type frequently used by the
Greek sceptics. It is based on either real or hypothetical διαφωνία,
disagreement, between 'dogmatists' or 'rationalists': faced with the
same question or with the same set of signs, the 'dogmatists' would
offer conflicting answers and interpretations; and, he adds, it is
impossible to ascribe intrinsic superiority to any of these interpretations – hence one can only suspend judgment. For example, the very
symptoms which Herophilus might interpret as 'signs of good blood',
says Sextus, Erasistratus would interpret as 'signs of the transference
from the veins into the arteries', while Asclepiades would interpret
them as signs of 'the impaction of intelligible molecules in intelligible
interstices'. Sextus appears to be having fun at the expense, first, of
Erasistratus' theory of *synanastomoses* between veins and arteries and
Erasistratus' general pathological principle of plethora (i.e. the
notion that morbid conditions are generally attributable to hyperaemia, which causes the blood to spill over from the veins into the
arteries which in a healthy condition contain only pneuma).[229]
Secondly, Sextus' example alludes mockingly to Asclepiades' atomistic theory of subsensory – and hence only intelligible – molecules
(ὄγκοι) and interstices or passages (πόροι).[230] Since the success of
Sextus' allusions to the theories of Erasistratus and Asclepiades
clearly depends on the fact that these physicians actually held views
somehow identifiable with Sextus' characterizations, the same would
seem to hold true for the allusion to Herophilus' 'good blood' theory.
But just what Herophilus' theory was, and what symptoms actually
were associated with it, leaves us with yet another tantalizing mystery
to which his views on the humours might have held the key.

  In all likelihood Herophilus was, however, not content only to

---

[229] Cf., for example, *De usu partium* 6.17 (I, pp. 358–9 Helmreich); *id., De venae sectione
adversus Erasistratum* 3 (XI, pp. 153–6K); *id., An in arteriis natura sanguis contineatur*
2–4 and *passim* (IV, especially pp. 706–17K); Anonymus Londinensis 26.39–
28.12. The relation of Erasistratus' theory to the so-called *horror vacui* principle
developed by Strato of Lampsacus (cf. Hero of Alexandria, *Pneumatica*, pp. 4–10,
16–20, 24–8 Schmidt; Strato, fr. 54–67 Wehrli) is not as clearly derivative as
Diels suggested (1893a) – but an analysis of this question belongs elsewhere. Cf.
Furley/Wilkie, 1984: 31–7.

[230] CF. S.E., *M* 9.363 (= *Adv. Phys.* 1.363) and the passages cited below in Chapter
XXII, n. 11. (See also Chapter XXII.A and n. 5, on Asclepiades.) Cf. Galen, *De
elementis ex Hippocrate* 2.3 (I, p. 499K).

observe and record countless symptoms. The strong systematizing thrust of much of his pathophysiology – most manifest in his taxonomy of the pulse – probably also informed his approach to symptomatology. But the only evidence that supports this view[231] is compromised by an ambiguous phrase which has dogged our steps throughout this volume: οἱ περὶ τὸν Ἡρόφιλον, literally 'those around Herophilus', which, as I pointed out earlier, could mean (i) 'Herophilus and his followers' or (ii) 'the followers of Herophilus' or (iii) simply 'Herophilus' (LSJ, s.v. περί, c.I.2). Referring to the Alexandrian Empiricists' τρίχρονος σημείωσις or 'triple-timed inference from signs', Galen in his *On Repletion* adds that 'those around Herophilus introduced it in a manner similar to the Empiricists' (T223a, lines 3–4). If the Empiricist theory of the interpretation of signs does date back to Herophilus himself – as several aspects of Empiricist doctrine do (and perhaps not surprisingly so, since the founder of the Empiricist school had been a student of Herophilus)[232] – then the scheme adopted by Herophilus would be the following. The interpretation of signs has to be threefold: from present signs or symptoms the physician makes pathological inferences about the current condition of the patient; from past signs he infers the history of the patient's illness and its proximate causes, while 'future signs' refer to the inferences made from what happened to other patients (who had been in this condition but were cured), i.e. 'future signs' indicate how a similar cure might be effected by similar measures in the patient currently under treatment. But whereas the Empiricists' emphasis seems to have been primarily on symptomatology as an exercise which directly provides therapeutic criteria[233] – after all, they rejected aetiology – Herophilus' emphasis was probably at least as much on the aetiological potential of a 'triple-timed' interpretation of signs. The attribution of this temporal classification of symptoms to Herophilus himself must, however, remain as tentative as the frustrating phase οἱ περὶ τὸν Ἡρόφιλον is ambiguous.

---

[231] T223a, lines 2–4. Cf. Deichgräber, 1965: fr. 122 and p. 310.

[232] Philinus of Cos; see Deichgräber, 1965: fr. 6 and pp. 163–4, 254–5. Cf. above, Chapter II, T1. See also Kollesch, 1968.

[233] Cf. Deichgräber, 1965: 308–13. Deichgräber's observation, 'der Empiriker sieht in dem Symptom die direkten Kriterien der geforderten Therapie' (p. 308), is substantiated by the evidence: fr. 78–93. Cf. Galen, *CMG* v.9.2, p. 202.25.

9 Dream theory

'I am far from seeking to maintain that I am the first writer to
have had the idea of deriving dreams from wishes . . . Those
who attach any importance to anticipations of this kind may
go back to classical antiquity and quote Herophilus . . . '

SIGMUND FREUD, *The Interpretation of Dreams*

Herophilus' discussion of a mental disorder, phrenitis,[234] indicates
that his interest in the interpretation and classification of symptoms
also extended to mental or psychic conditions. One of the psychic
conditions or activities upon which he brought his taxonomic passion
to bear is dreams, which he divided into three general types.

A first type of dream – dreams sent by a god – is described in less
detail than the other two. God-inspired dreams simply are said to
occur 'inevitably' or 'by necessity'.[235] Herophilus thus rejects
Aristotle's argument (*On Divination in Sleep* 462b12–464b18) that
dreams, though perhaps 'demonic', never are god-sent but are
attributable only to natural causes. The Alexandrian instead reverts
to a traditional belief, of a kind richly reflected in Greek literature,
that the gods are responsible for at least some of our dreams.

Second, 'natural dreams' are described as arising 'when the soul
forms for itself an image of what is to its advantage and of what will
happen next'. This category, *pace* Kessels (1969), does not seem to be
the same as the 'predictive' class of dreams associated, for example,
with the Homeric Gates of Horn (*Odyssey* 19.560–7). Herophilus'
'natural dreams' are not occasioned by any external agent, such as a
god or a demon or even a recent percept. Rather, they are, as
Schrijvers (1977) observed, 'endogenous', and in them the psyche
images not only the future but specifically its own interest.

Finally, 'mixed' or 'compound' dreams are described, in an
interesting anticipation of the sexual emphasis of some modern dream
theories, as 'arising spontaneously (or: 'accidentally') according to
the impact of the images, whenever we see what we wish to see, as
happens in the case of men who in their dreams make love to (or: 'see')
the women they love'.[236] The phrase 'the impact of the images'

---

[234] T211.
[235] T226a–c: κατ' ἀνάγκην. Cf. 'divine dreams' in Hp., *Regimen* 4.87.
[236] T226a–c. For parallels see Plato, *Republic* 9.571c–d4; *id.*, *Timaeus* 45d3–46a2;
Aristotle, *De Insomniis* 3.461a15, 462a11–19. See also Schrijvers, 1977: 15ff.

(*eidōla*) might conjure up an atomistic model of a stream of *eidōla* or atomic film-like images impacting on a person continuously,[237] but if this is what Herophilus meant, he would be providing an uncharacteristic physiological foundation for his 'mixed' or 'compound' dreams. In all probability this cryptic phrase represents a different use of *eidōlon*, especially since the soul, in the case of 'natural dreams', is said to be capable of producing its own *eidōla*. Be this as it may, in both these classes of dreams there is no reference to dreams as anything but mental or psychic activities.

The 'compound' or 'mixed' dreams appear to derive their name from having elements in common with both 'god-sent' and 'natural' dreams. With the former they share an external agency ('god' or 'the impact of images'), and with the latter an internal stimulus ('autonomous psychic imaging' or 'what we wish'). Impressive attempts have been made to argue for more complicated solutions – most recently, for example, Schrijver's (1977) suggestion that the Platonic and Aristotelian division of the origins of 'things that come into being' (*gignomena*) into *technē*, *physis*, and *tychē* (or *automaton*; see Plato, *Laws* 10.888E4–6 and *Metaphysics* Z.7.1032a12–13) served as the model for Herophilus' tripartition, with *technē* said to correspond to Herophilus' god-sent dreams – but such interpretations appear to put the Herophilean texts under unacceptable strain.

As Sigmund Freud acknowledged, Herophilus' emphasis on the fulfilment of sexual and other wishes or desires in both the 'natural' and 'compound' dream categories is striking from a modern perspective. It should be noted, however, that, as far as we know, Herophilus did not attach pathological and therapeutic significance to these observations. Rather, he seems to have been interested in developing a taxonomy of dreams by origin, and while his classification therefore has an aetiological orientation, there is no evidence that he put it to therapeutic use.

With his tripartite classification of dreams Herophilus seems to have launched a remarkably rich Hellenistic and patristic tradition of

---

[237] Cf. Lucretius, *De rerum natura* 4.757–815 (less relevant in this context is the more famous passage on dreams, 4.962–1036). Cf. also Epicurus' use of προσπίπτω in fr. 24 [45].20–1 Arrighetti (= Pap. Herc. 993.3.VII). A very different use of *eidōlon* – but in an erotic context remarkably similar to that of T226a and T226b – occurs in Plato's *Phaedrus* 255D8-E1. Cf. also Aristotle's discussion of the function of 'images' (*phantasmata*) in dreams: *De insomniis* (*passim*), *De somno et vigilia* 2.456a24–6.

dream theory. In Greek literature antedating Herophilus, there admittedly are many examples of dreams which, in some respect or other, resemble Herophilus' dream types. Dreams in Homer, Herodotus, the Greek tragedians, and Plato (for example, *Crito* 44A5–B4; *Republic* IX. 571C–572B) could be introduced with some legitimacy as precursors of one or another of Herophilus' dream types. Efforts had also been made – notably by Aristotle in his treatises *On Dreams* and *On Divination in Sleep* – to give an account of the psycho-physiological causes of dreams. But Herophilus' attempt to provide a systematic classification of dreams by origin seems to represent something novel and unusually influential.

Although the Herophilean model is explicitly attributed to Herophilus by only three ancient sources,[238] a modified version of his threefold classification was developed by the Stoics and attained a popularity commensurate with that of Stoicism generally. The Stoic division of dreams is perhaps best known in a form popularized by Posidonius (*c*. 135–50 B.C.): (1) in some dreams the soul foresees things by itself; (2) in other dreams 'immortal souls stamped with the truth' fill the air and cause us to dream; (3) and, finally, there are dreams in which the gods themselves converse with sleeping humans.[239] Posidonius' third class of dreams is virtually identical with Herophilus' class of 'dreams sent by god' (although it must be emphasized that Posidonius characterizes all three kinds of dreams as ultimately caused by divine impulse, and that he discusses them in the context of divination). The Stoic's first class likewise reveals a strong affinity with Herophilus' characterization of 'natural dreams' as the autonomous imaging activity of the soul. The second type of dreams mentioned by Posidonius, the ones caused by *immortales animi* filling the air, therefore is the only one which, prima facie at least, does not correspond closely to one of Herophilus' three dream types. The remaining class in Herophilus' classification is, of course, 'mixed' or 'compound' dreams, and Herophilus attributes these dreams not to a divine agency but to the impaction of images, while Posidonius'

---

[238] Aëtius and the pseudo-Galenic *De historia philosopha* are the main sources. The latter is, however, heavily dependent on Aëtius (or on Aëtius' source); it therefore does not represent independent evidence. Ps.-Plutarch (T226b) is identical with Aëtius.

[239] Posidonius, F108 Edelstein/Kidd (= Cicero, *De divinatione* 1.64). Cf. Reinhardt, 1921: 457–60; Blankert, 1940: 204–6; Behr, 1968: 175–6; Theiler, 1982: vol. II, p. 296.

attribution of these dreams to 'immortal souls' seems to be a clear allusion to the *daimones* that are prominent in the Stoic theory of divination.[240] Yet even here there is some affinity, because both in Posidonius' revision and in the Herophilean original this class of dreams fulfils the same function: it covers all dreams which are neither sent by gods nor attributable to autonomous, self-initiated psychic activity.

The Herophilean-Posidonian classification of dreams was adopted with some modification by numerous authors. Thus Philo of Alexandria distinguishes between (1) dreams in which the 'divine' (τὸ θεῖον) sends us our dream images (*phantasiai*); (2) dreams in which our mind (νοῦς), moving in unison with the mind of the whole, seems to be possessed or inspired and can prognosticate; (3) dreams in which the soul is moved by itself, agitating itself, and predicting the future.[241] Again, Philo's first dream type is similar to Herophilus' 'dreams sent by a god', while his third type shows strong affinities with Herophilus' 'natural dreams'. Philo's second class of dreams might appear to fall outside the basic scheme, but it partially resembles Posidonius' 'immortal soul' class, inasmuch as the 'mind of the whole' is itself 'full of immortal souls'.[242]

Similar classifications of dreams became entrenched in early Christian literature, too, but with two differences: first, the 'immortal souls' of Posidonius (or the 'compound dreams' of Herophilus) are replaced by the devil or by evil demons, and secondly, dream taxonomy is gradually divested of the emphasis on predictive dreams which started with Posidonius, and in this respect again reverts to Herophilus' more comprehensive approach. Tertullian, for example, distinguishes between (1) edifying, revelatory dreams sent by God, (2) fallacious, confused dreams sent by demons, and (3) dreams in which the soul more or less autonomously contemplates things. These Tertullian, like Herophilus, calls 'natural'.[243] Similarly, Prudentius

---

[240] Cf. *SVF* III, 605 (= Stobaeus, *Eclogae* II, p. 114 Wachsmuth): dreams come from gods or demons. See also *SVF* II, 1198 (= Calcidius, *Commentary on Plato's Timaeus*, Chapter 251, pp. 260–1 Waszink), and Switalski, 1902: p. 37 n. 1.

[241] Philo, *De somniis* 1.1–2; 2.1–4; cf. Waszink, 1941: 77–8, and see n. 247 *infra*.

[242] On the relation of Philo's second dream type to Posidonius' 'immortal soul' class, see Waszink, 1941: 77–8; Reinhardt, 1921: 458; Blum, 1936: 66; Volker, 1938: 289 n. 4; Theiler, 1930: 136. Cf. n. 247 infra.

[243] Tertullian, *De anima* 47. Waszink, 1947, provides a useful analysis and source history of this passage in his commentary *ad loc.*, pp. 500–6.

divides dreams into those sent by Christ, those sent by the devil, and dreams initiated by the soul itself.[244] A similar distinction is made by Cassianus,[245] and St Augustine likewise differentiates between dreams sent directly by God, dreams originating with angels or demons, and dreams initiated by the soul itself.[246]

Throughout this long history of tripartite dream classifications, two of the three dream types introduced by Herophilus therefore remained remarkably intact: dreams sent directly by god, and dreams arising through autonomous psychic activity (i.e. what Herophilus called 'natural dreams', φυσικοὶ ὄνειροι). But Herophilus' third type, 'combined dreams', which 'arise spontaneously according to the impact of images', in later literature is replaced by 'dreams sent by demons or the devil'. Herophilus had illustrated this third kind of dream in non-pathological, apparently value-free terms with the example of sexual wish fulfilment in one's dreams; the Christians illustrate it with examples of deceptive, confused, demonic dreams. Yet even here some continuity might lurk in Herophilus' use of 'compound' or 'mixed' (συγκραματικοὶ ὄνειροι): cognates of this word are often used to refer to 'confusion', and later Latin writers may have invested Herophilus' term with this meaning.[247]

From Herophilus' innovative taxonomy of dreams by origin to its Christian expropriation there is therefore much continuity, but it is also emblematic of the fate of Herophilus' theory that the Alexandrian's sexual dream is usurped by the Christians' demonic dream.

[244] Prudentius, *Cathemerinon liber* 6.37–40, 73–6, 137–40.
[245] Johannes Cassianus, *Collationes Patrum* 1.19: 'tria cogitationum principia'.
[246] St Augustine, *Epistulae* 162.5, 9.3 (cf. also *De trinitate* 11.7; *De civitate Dei* 18.18.2).
[247] Cf., for example, Aeschylus, *Choephoroi* 744. The affinities pointed out above seem to constitute a reasonable case for the Herophilean–Stoic–Christian genealogy suggested here. For different views of the historical place of Herophilus' dream theory, cf. Gelzer, 1907: 40–51; Wellmann, 1924–5: 70–2; Blum, 1936: 69–70; Waszink, 1947: 502; Dodds, 1951: 124 n. 28; Edelstein, 1967: 205–46; Behr, 1968: 174–8; Kessels, 1969: especially 414–24; Schrijvers, 1977: 13–27.

B · TEXTS

1 *Humours,* * *Faculties*

130 Ps.-Galenus, *Introductio sive medicus* 9 (xiv, pp. 698–9K)

(περὶ στοιχείων ἐξ ὧν ὁ ἄνθρωπος συνέστηκεν·) . . . οἱ μὲν μόνοις τοῖς χυμοῖς τῶν τε κατὰ φύσιν τὴν σύστασιν καὶ τῶν παρὰ φύσιν τὴν αἰτίαν ἀνέθεσαν, ὡς Πραξαγόρας καὶ Ἡρόφιλος.

130 [Concerning the elements out of which humans are constituted:] . . .
Some people attributed both the constitution of things that are in accordance with nature and the cause of things that are contrary to nature to the humours alone, as did Praxagoras and Herophilus.

131 Galenus, *De pulsuum dignotione* 2.3 (viii, p. 870K)

. . . οὐ πολὺ μέντοι βέλτιον ἦν μὴ περὶ τοῦ τέτταρας ὑφ' Ἡροφίλου λέγεσθαι τὰς διοικούσας τὰ ζῷα δυνάμεις ζητεῖν . . . ; *(Vid. Herophili T184 infra.)*

131 . . . Wouldn't it be much better not to inquire about the fact that four faculties were said by Herophilus to govern living beings . . . ? *(See T184 infra.)*

132 Galenus, *De placitis Hippocratis et Platonis* 8.5.24 (*CMG* v.4.1.2, p. 510 De Lacy)

οὐ μόνος δὲ Πλάτων, ἀλλὰ καὶ Ἀριστοτέλης καὶ Θεόφραστος οἵ τε ἄλλοι μαθηταὶ Πλάτωνός τε καὶ Ἀριστοτέλους [οἳ] τὸν περὶ τῶν χυμῶν λόγον ἐζήλωσαν Ἱπποκράτους, ὥσπερ γε καὶ τῶν παλαιῶν ἰατρῶν οἱ δοκιμώτατοι, Διοκλῆς, Πλειστόνικος,
5 Μνησίθεος, Πραξαγόρας, Φιλότιμος, Ἡρόφιλος.

2 οἳ *del. Cornarius*   5 φιλότιμος *H: corr. DeLacy*

* On the 'humours' or 'moistures' cf. also T205a–b below.

132 Not only Plato but also Aristotle, Theophrastus, and the other pupils of Plato and Aristotle tried to emulate Hippocrates' account of the humours, as did also the most reputable of the ancient physicians: Diocles, Plistonicus, Mnesitheus, Praxagoras, Phylotimus, and Herophilus.

133 A. Cornelius Celsus, *Medicina* 1 (*Artes* 6), *prohoem.* 14–15 (*CML* 1, p. 19 Marx)

> neque enim credunt (sc. qui rationalem medicam profitentur) posse eum scire, quomodo morbos curare conveniat, qui unde sint ignoret; neque esse dubium quin alia curatione opus sit, si ex quattuor principiis vel superans aliquod vel deficiens adversam
> 5 valetudinem creat, ut quidam ex sapientiae professoribus dixerunt; alia, si in umidis omne vitium est, ut Herophilo visum est; alia, si in spiritu, ut Hippocrati . . .

> 2–3 qui unde sint ignoret *FV*: quod unde hi ignorat sint *J*   4 aliquid *J*
> 6 ut Herophilo visum est *om. F, add. m¹ in marg.*

133 For they [sc. those who profess 'rationalist' medicine] believe that a person who does not know where diseases come from cannot know how to treat them properly. And, they say, there is no doubt that a different treatment is required if either some excess or some deficiency among the four principle elements produces an adverse state of health, as some of the teachers of wisdom have said; and a different treatment again, if every defect lies in the moistures [of the body], as Herophilus thought; and yet a different treatment, if it lies in the pneuma, as Hippocrates thought . . .

134 Ps.-Galenus, *In 'Hippocratis' De alimento Comment.* 3.21 (xv, p. 346K)

> περὶ δὲ μελαίνης χολῆς λέγει μὲν (sc. Πλάτων) ἐκεῖνα, ἅπερ ἡμεῖς ἤδη γεγράφαμεν, ταὐτὰ δὲ λέγουσι καὶ ᾿Αριστοτέλης καὶ Θεόφραστος καὶ τῶν ἰατρῶν οἱ δοκιμώτατοι, Διοκλῆς, Πλειστόνικος, Φυλότιμος, ῾Ηρόφιλος καὶ ἄλλοι πολλοί.

134 As far as black bile is concerned, he [Plato] says exactly what we

have already written, and the same things are also said by Aristotle, Theophrastus, and the most reputable of physicians: Diocles, Plistonicus, Phylotimus, Herophilus, and many others. *(This 'Galenic' commentary is a Renaissance compilation of very limited value.)*

135 Galenus, *Adversus Iulianum* 5.11 (*CMG* v.10.3, p. 51 Wenkebach)

οὔτε γὰρ Ἱπποκράτης οὔτε Διοκλῆς οὔτε Πλειστόνικος οὔτε Πραξαγόρας οὔτε Φυλότιμος οὔτε Μνησίθεος οὔτε Ἐρασίστρατος οὔτε Ἡρόφιλος οὔτε ἄλλος τις ἰατρὸς οὔτε λογικὸς οὔτε ἐμπειρικὸς ἠρέσθη ταῖς Θεσσαλοῦ κοινότησι.

135 For, neither Hippocrates nor Diocles nor Plistonicus nor Praxagoras nor Phylotimus nor Mnesitheus nor Erasistratus nor Herophilus nor any other physician – neither rationalist nor Empiricist – was satisfied with the 'common qualities' of Thessalus.

2 Control Centre, Nerves*

136 Galenus, *De usu partium* 1.8 (I, p. 15 Helmreich)

ὁ μὲν γὰρ τὴν καρδίαν, ὁ δὲ τὰς μήνιγγας, ὁ δὲ τὸν ἐγκέφαλον ἐν ἑαυτῷ φησιν ἔχειν τὸ τῆς ψυχῆς ἡγεμονοῦν, ὥστε καὶ τῶν ἐν αὐτοῖς μορίων τὴν ὠφέλειαν ἄλλος ἄλλην ἐρεῖ ... οὐδὲ γὰρ νῦν αὐτῶν (sc. τῶν ἀρεσκόντων) ἐμνημονεύσαμεν ἄλλου τινὸς ἕνεκεν
5 ἢ τοῦ μηνῦσαι τὰς αἰτίας, δι' ἃς περὶ χρείας μορίων ἐνεχειρήσαμεν γράφειν, οὕτω μὲν Ἀριστοτέλει πολλῶν καὶ καλῶς εἰρημένων, οὕτω δ' οὐκ ὀλίγοις ἄλλοις ἰατροῖς τε καὶ φιλοσόφοις, ἧττον μὲν ἴσως Ἀριστοτέλους, καλῶς δ' οὖν καὶ αὐτοῖς, ὥσπερ ἀμέλει καὶ Ἡροφίλῳ τῷ Καλχηδονίῳ. ἀλλ' οὐδὲ τὰ Ἱπποκρά-
10 τους ἦν ἱκανά ...

2–3 τῶν ἐν αὐτοῖς μορίων τὴν *CD*: τὴν ἐν τοῖς μορίοις αὐτῶν *U*
8 ἀριστοτέλους *U*: ἀριστοτέλει *CD*   9 Καλχηδονίῳ *scripsi*: καρχηδονίῳ *CD*: Χαλκηδονίῳ *Marx, Helmreich (sed cf. Herophili T2 supra et comment. ad T2)*

* *On the nerves cf. also Chapter* VI *supra,* T80–T89.

136 The one says that the heart contains in itself the command centre of the soul, another says the meninges do, still another the brain, so that one will claim one use for the parts in them, another will claim another use . . . I have not mentioned these [differing opinions] now for any other purpose than to disclose the reasons for which I undertook to write about the usefulness of parts, although Aristotle has written much, and well, about it, and although not a few other physicians and philosophers have done so too, perhaps less fully than Aristotle, but also well – just as, of course, Herophilus of Chalcedon. But not even the writings of Hippocrates are adequate . . .

137a Aëtius Doxographus, *Placita* 4.5.1–6 (*DG*, p. 391)

137b Ps.-Plutarchus, *Placita* 4.5 (*Moralia* 899A, vol. v.2.1 (Teubner), p. 117 Mau)

137c Eusebius, *Praeparatio evangelica* 15.61.1–6 (*GCS*, Eus. 8.2), p. 421 Mras

137d Galenus, *De historia philosopha* 28 (xix, p. 315K)

τί τὸ τῆς ψυχῆς ἡγεμονικὸν καὶ ἐν τίνι ἐστίν· Πλάτων, Δημόκριτος ἐν ὅλῃ τῇ κεφαλῇ. Στράτων ἐν μεσοφρύῳ. Ἐρασίσ-τρατος περὶ τὴν μήνιγγα τοῦ ἐγκεφάλου, ἣν ἐπικρανίδα λέγει. Ἡρόφιλος ἐν τῇ τοῦ ἐγκεφάλου κοιλίᾳ, ἥτις ἐστὶ καὶ βάσις.
5 Παρμενίδης ἐν ὅλῳ τῷ θώρακι καὶ Ἐπίκουρος. οἱ Στωικοὶ πάντες ἐν ὅλῃ τῇ καρδίᾳ ἢ τῷ περὶ τὴν καρδίαν πνεύματι . . .

1–6 *hunc locum Charterius (*II [1679], p. 49D–E) *et Kühn (*xix *p. 315) in editionibus libri* De historia philosopha *(cap. 28) Galeno ascripti habent, sed Diels (*DG p. 639) om.*　　1 περὶ (τοῦ) ἡγεμονικοῦ *Eusebius*　　1–2 Δημόκριτος καὶ Πλάτων *Galenus (Kühn)*　　2 *post* κεφαλῇ *habet* καθίζουσι *Galenus*　　4 ἐν ταῖς τοῦ ἐγκ. κοιλίαις *Galenus*　　ἥτις–βάσις *om. Galenus (sic etiam* T137e)　　5 Παρμενίδης καὶ Ἐπίκουρος B (*Aët.), Galenus (*καὶ Ἐπίκ. *olim schol. in marg. fuisse susp. Diels, fort. recte)*　　6 ἐν *ante* τῷ *add. Galenus*　　τὴν *om.* BP (*Plut.)*　　ἢ –πνεύματι *om. Eusebius*

137a–d Concerning the command centre: Plato and Democritus [locate it] in the entire head; Strato in the space between the eyebrows; Erasistratus in the area of the meninx of the brain, which he calls 'on the skull' (*epikranis*); Herophilus in the ventricle of the brain which is also its 'base' (*basis*); Parmenides in the entire thorax, and so too Epicurus; and all the Stoics, in the entire heart or in the pneuma around the heart . . .

137e Theodoretus Cyrrhensis, *Graecarum affectionum curatio* 5.22 (*Sources Chrétiennes* 57, vol. 1, pp. 232–3 Canivet; p. 128 Raeder)

ὅσα δὲ καὶ περὶ τῆς τοῦ ἡγεμονικοῦ χώρας διηνέχθησαν (sc. οἱ Ἕλληνες) πρὸς ἀλλήλους, ῥᾴδιον διαγνῶναι. Ἱπποκράτης μὲν γὰρ καὶ Δημόκριτος καὶ Πλάτων ἐν ἐγκεφάλῳ τοῦτο ἱδρῦσθαι εἰρήκασιν· ὁ δὲ Στράτων ἐν μεσοφρύῳ· Ἐρασίστρατος δὲ ὁ
5 ἰατρὸς περὶ τὴν τοῦ ἐγκεφάλου μήνιγγα, ἣν ἐπικρανίδα λέγει· Ἡρόφιλος δὲ ἐν τῇ τοῦ ἐγκεφάλου κοιλίᾳ· Παρμενίδης δὲ καὶ Ἐπίκουρος ἐν ὅλῳ τῷ θώρακι· Ἐμπεδοκλῆς δὲ καὶ Ἀριστοτέλης καὶ τῶν Στωικῶν ἡ ξυμμορία τὴν καρδίαν ἀπεκλήρωσαν τούτῳ . . .

7 ἀριστοτέλης *KMSCV*: ἀριστοκλῆς *BLV*: Ἀριστοτέλης Διοκλῆς *Diels* (*DG*, p. 204 n. 1)

137e It is easy to discern all the disagreements they [the pagan Greeks] had with each other concerning the location of the command centre. For, while Hippocrates, Democritus and Plato said that it has its seat in the brain, Strato [said] in the space between the eyebrows. But Erasistratus, the physician, [said it is] in the area of the meninx of the brain, which he calls 'on the skull' (*epikranis*); Herophilus, in the ventricle of the brain; Parmenides and Epicurus in the entire thorax; Empedocles, Aristotle, and the Stoic school assigned the heart to it [sc. to the command centre] . . .

138 Galenus, *De usu partium* 8.11 (1, p. 484 Helmreich)

καὶ οἷς γε τετάρτη τις αὕτη κοιλία (sc. τὸ ὑπὲρ τὴν κοινὴν κοιλότητα μόριον ἐγκεφάλου ἢ καμάριον) νενόμισται, κυριωτάτην εἶναί φασιν αὐτὴν ἁπασῶν τῶν καθ᾽ ὅλον τὸν ἐγκέφαλον. Ἡρόφιλος μὴν οὐ ταύτην, ἀλλὰ τὴν ἐν τῇ παρεγκεφαλίδι
5 κυριωτέραν ἔοικεν ὑπολαμβάνειν.

4 μὴν *L²U*: μὲν *cett.*

138 Those who hold the view that this cavity [sc. the fornix] is a fourth ventricle, say that, of all the ventricles in the entire brain, it exercises most control. Herophilus, however, seems to assume that not this ventricle, but the one in the cerebellum (*parenkephalis*), exercises more control. (= *T78, p. 199.*)

139 Tertullianus, *De anima* 15.2–5 (pp. 19–20 Waszink)

(2) Messenius aliqui Dicaearchus, ex medicis autem Andreas et Asclepiades ita abstulerunt principale (sc. ab anima), dum in animo ipso volunt esse sensus quorum vindicatur princi-pale . . . (3) sed plures et philosophi adversus Dicaearchum,
5 Plato Strato Epicurus Democritus Empedocles Socrates Aristo-teles, et medici adversus Andrean et Asclepiaden, Herophilus Erasistratus Diocles Hippocrates et ipse Soranus, iamque omnibus plures Christiani, qui apud deum de utroque deduci-mur, et esse principale in anima et certo in corporis recessu
10 consecratum. (4) si enim 'scrutatorem et dispectorem cordis' deum legimus, si etiam prophetes eius occulta cordis traducendo probatur, si deus ipse recogitatus cordis in populo praevenit . . . simul utrumque dilucet, et esse principale in anima, quod intentio divina conveniat, id est vim sapientialem atque vita-
15 lem . . . , et in eo thesauro corporis haberi, ad quem deus respicit, (5) ut neque extrinsecus agitari putes principale istud secundum Heraclitum, neque per totum corpus ventilari secun-dum Moschionem, neque in capite concludi secundum Plato-nem, neque in vertice potius praesidere secundum Xenocratem,
20 neque in cerebro cubare secundum Hippocraten, sed nec circa cerebri fundamentum, ut Herophilus, nec in membranulis ut Strato et Erasistratus, nec in superciliorum meditullio, ut Strato Physicus, nec in tota lorica pectoris, ut Epicurus, sed quod et Aegyptii renuntiaverunt et qui divinarum commentatores
25 videbantur, ut et ille versus Orphei vel Empedoclis: 'namque homini sanguis circumcordialis est sensus'.

1 aliqui *A*: aliquis *B Gel*   2 abstulerint *A corr.*   4 adverdi ce arcum *A*
5 Socrates *codd.*: Xenocrates *Diels (DG, p. 204)*   8–9 ducimur *A*:
docemur *Mercerus*: deducimus *Iun*   10 despectorem *A*   12 deus]
dominus *A*   13 quod] quo *A*   15 ad quem] atque *A*
21 herophilo *A*   membranullis *A corr.*: membranula eius *Iun susp.*
22 Strato et *secl. Diels (l.c.)*   25 et (*sec*)] ei *B Gel*: ii *Urs*: ut *Hartel*

139 (2) A certain Dicaearchus, a Messenian, and among the physicians Andreas and Asclepiades, have thus removed the ruling power [from the soul], while wanting the senses to be in the mind and while claiming the ruling power for the senses . . . (3) But very many people are opposed to this view: the philosophers Plato, Strato, Epicurus, Democritus, Empedocles, Socrates, and Aristotle [are opposed] to Dicaearchus, and the physicians Herophilus, Erasistratus, Diocles, Hippocrates, and Soranus, himself, are opposed to Andreas and Asclepiades – and, in fact, more than all others, we Christians [are opposed], we who are led by God concerning both these questions, namely that there is a ruling power in the soul and that it is enshrined in a certain recess of the body. (4) For if we read of God as the 'investigator and examiner of the heart'[Wisdom of Solomon 1:6]; if, furthermore, his prophet is tested by revealing to him the hidden secrets of the heart; if God himself anticipates in the people the reflections of their heart . . . then both points become clear at once, namely that there is in the soul a ruling power with which the divine purpose is in agreement, i.e. a wisdom and life, and that it is contained in that treasurehouse of the body to which God looks. (5) Consequently you should not think, with Heraclitus, that this ruling power is stirred up from outside, nor, with Moschion, that it breezes through the whole body, nor, with Plato, that it is enclosed in the head, nor, with Xenocrates, that it rather sits in command in the crown of the head, nor, with Hippocrates, that it reclines in the brain, nor indeed around the base of the brain, as Herophilus [said], nor in its little membranes, as Strato and Erasistratus [said], nor in the middle, between the eyebrows, as Strato the physicist [said], nor in the entire enclosure of the chest, as Epicurus [said]; but rather, what the Egyptians have declared and the authors of divine scriptures also seemed [to say] – as does that famous verse of Orpheus or Empedocles too: 'For the blood around the heart is a human being's sense.'

140a Galenus, *De usu partium* 10.12 (II, p. 93 Helmreich)*

τῶν γὰρ ἐπὶ τοὺς ὀφθαλμοὺς ἀπ' ἐγκεφάλου κατιόντων

* See also Chapters VI (T84–T89) and VIII (T260) for opthalmological texts. Cf. Appendix, IV.

318   HEROPHILUS

νεύρων τῶν αἰσθητικῶν, ἃ δὴ καὶ πόρους ὠνόμαζεν
Ἡρόφιλος, ὅτι μόνοις αὐτοῖς αἰσθηταὶ καὶ σαφεῖς εἰσιν αἱ τοῦ
πνεύματος ὁδοί, ὥσπερ αὐτὸ τοῦτο [τὸ] παράδοξόν τε καὶ
5 ὑπὲρ τὰ λοιπὰ τῶν νεύρων ἐστίν, οὕτω καὶ τὸ φύεσθαι μὲν ἐκ
διαφερόντων τόπων, προιόντα δ' ἀλλήλοις ἑνοῦσθαι, κᾆπειτα
πάλιν ἀποχωρεῖν τε καὶ διασχίζεσθαι.

1 ἀπὸ τοῦ B   2 ἃ γὰρ δὴ AU   4 τὸ om. B: del. Helmreich

140a As regards the sensory nerves that descend to the eyes from the
brain, which Herophilus in fact also calls 'passages' (poroi) since they
alone have clear, perceptible paths for the pneuma – just as this itself
is contrary to expectation and 'beyond' the rest of the nerves, so too is
the fact that they grow out from different places but, as they proceed
forward, are united, and then again go away from each other and are
separated.

140b Galenus, *De symptomatum causis* 1.2 (VII, pp. 88–9K)

See Chapter VI, T85, supra.

140c Galenus, *De libris propriis* 3 (Scr. Min. II, p. 108 Mueller)

See Chapter VI, T84 (cf. also T86) supra.

141 Galenus, *De tremore, palpitatione, convulsione et rigore* 5 (VII,
pp. 605–6K)

πεπονθὼς δὲ τόπος εἷς οὐδείς ἐστιν ἐξ ἀνάγκης ἐν τρόμοις, καὶ
μέμφομαί γε ἐνταῦθα Πραξαγόρᾳ καὶ Ἡροφίλῳ, τῷ μὲν ἀρτηριῶν πάθος εἰπόντι τὸν τρόμον, Ἡροφίλῳ δὲ φιλοτιμουμένῳ
δεῖξαι περὶ τὸ νευρῶδες αὐτὸ γένος ἀεὶ συνιστάμενον. ὁ μὲν οὖν
5 Πραξαγόρας πόρρω τοῦ ἀληθοῦς ἥκει· ὁ δὲ Ἡρόφιλος ἠπατήθη
τὸ τῆς δυνάμεως πάθος ἀναφέρων τοῖς ὀργάνοις· ὅτι μὲν γὰρ
τὸ νευρῶδες γένος, οὐ τὸ ἀρτηριῶδες, ὑπηρετεῖ ταῖς κατὰ
προαίρεσιν κινήσεσιν, ὀρθῶς ἐγίνωσκεν· ὅτι δὲ οὐκ αὐτὸ τὸ
σῶμα τῶν νεύρων αἴτιον κινήσεως, ἀλλὰ τοῦτο μὲν ὄργανον, ἡ
10 κινοῦσα δ' αἰτία ἡ διήκουσα δύναμις διὰ τῶν νεύρων ἐστίν,

ἐνταῦθα μέμφομαι αὐτῷ μὴ διορίσαντι δύναμίν τε καὶ ὄργανον. εἰ γὰρ διώρισεν, εὐθὺς ἂν ἔγνω διότι βλαβήσεται τοὔργον οὐκ ὀργάνων μόνων, ἀλλὰ καὶ δυνάμεως πάθει. ἐπὶ μὲν οὖν τεθ-νεώτων οὐδὲν οὔτε τὰ νεῦρα πέπονθεν οὔθ' οἱ μύες ὅσα πάθη
15 πάσχειν αὐτὰ νομίζουσιν Ἡρόφιλός τε καὶ Πραξαγόρας. ἀπολέ-λοιπε δ' αὐτῶν πᾶσα κίνησις εὐθὺς ἅμα τῇ ψυχῇ, μύες δὲ καὶ νεῦρα ταύτης ὄργανα. (Vid. etiam T144sqq. infra.)

141 In cases of tremor there is necessarily not just one single place that is affected. And here, at least, I reproach Praxagoras and Herophilus, the former for having said that tremor is an affection of the arteries, but Herophilus for having the ambition to demonstrate that it always arises in association with the nerve-like class [of bodily parts]. Praxagoras, then, is further from the truth, but Herophilus was mistaken in attributing the affection of the [motive] faculty to its organs [instruments]. For, while Herophilus recognized correctly that the nerve-like, and not the arterial, class [of parts] serves the voluntary motions, [he did not recognize that] the body of the nerves is not itself the cause of motion but rather its instrument (*organon*), whereas its moving cause is the faculty (*dynamis*) which extends through the nerves. Here I reproach him for not having distinguished faculty from instrument. For, if he had made the distinction, he would have recognized immediately that the function will be impaired by an affection not of the organs alone, but also of the faculties. Thus, in the case of the dead neither the nerves nor the muscles are in the state of suffering all the affections which Herophilus and Praxagoras think they do: all motion has deserted them instantly with the soul, for muscles and nerves are just the instruments of the soul.
(*See also T144–T177 below, especially T152–T153.*)

142a Aëtius Doxographus, *Placita* 1.23.6 (*DG*, p. 320)

142b Ps.-Plutarchus, *Placita* 1.23 (*Moralia* 884C, vol. v.2.1 (Teubner), p. 74 Mau)

142c Iohannes Stobaeus, *Eclogae* 1.19.1 (i, p. 162 Wachsmuth)

Ἡρόφιλος κινήσεως τὴν μὲν λόγῳ θεωρητήν, τὴν δ' αἰσθητήν.

1 τὰς . . . αἰσθητάς M (*a.c.*): τὴν . . -ήν M (*p.c.*)EB

142a–c Herophilus [says] that one kind of motion is perceptible by reason, the other by the senses.

3 Respiration

143a Aëtius Doxographus, *Placita* 4.22.3 (*DG*, pp. 413–14)

143b Ps.-Plutarchus, *Placita* 4.22 (*Moralia* 903F-904B, vol. v.2.1 (Teubner), pp. 130–1 Mau)

Ἡρόφιλος δυνάμεις ἀπολείπει περὶ τὰ σώματα τὰς κινητικὰς ἐν νεύροις, ἐν ἀρτηρίαις, ἐν μυσί· τὸν οὖν πνεύμονα νομίζει μόνον ὀρέγεσθαι διαστολῆς τε καὶ συστολῆς φυσικῶς· [εἶτα δὲ καὶ τἆλλα.] ἐνέργειαν μὲν < οὖν > εἶναι τοῦ πνεύμονος τὴν ἔξωθεν

5 τοῦ πνεύματος ὁλκήν· ὑπὸ δὲ τῆς πληρώσεως τῆς θύραθεν γινομένης ἐφέλκεται· παρακειμένως δὲ διὰ τὴν δευτέραν ὄρεξιν ἐφ' αὐτὸν ὁ θώραξ τὸ πνεῦμα μετοχετεύει, πληρωθεὶς δὲ καὶ μηκέτι ἐφέλκεσθαι δυνάμενος πάλιν εἰς τὸν πνεύμονα τὸ περιττὸν ἀντιμεταρρεῖ, δι' οὗ πρὸς τὰ ἐκτὸς τὰ τῆς ἀποκρίσεως

10 γίνεται, τῶν σωματικῶν μερῶν ἀντιπασχόντων ἀλλήλοις. ὅτε μὲν γὰρ διαστολή, < ὅτε δὲ συστολή, > γίνεται πνεύμονος, ταῖς ἀλλήλων ἀντιμεταλήψεσι πληρώσεώς τε καὶ κενώσεως γινομένης, ὡς τέσσαρας μὲν γίνεσθαι κινήσεις περὶ τὸν πνεύμονα, τὴν μὲν πρώτην καθ' ἣν ἔξωθεν ἀέρα δέχεται, τὴν δὲ δευτέραν

15 καθ' ἣν τοῦθ' ὅπερ ἐδέξατο θύραθεν ἐντὸς αὐτοῦ πρὸς τὸν θώρακα μεταρρεῖ, τὴν δὲ τρίτην καθ' ἣν τὸ ἀπὸ τοῦ θώρακος συστελλόμενον αὖθις εἰς αὐτὸν ἐκδέχεται, τὴν δὲ τετάρτην καθ' ἣν τὸ ἐξ ὑποστροφῆς ἐν αὐτῷ γινόμενον θύραζε ἐξερᾷ. τούτων δὲ τῶν κινήσεων δύο μὲν εἶναι διαστολάς, τήν τ' ἔξωθεν τήν τ' ἀπὸ

20 τοῦ θώρακος· δύο δὲ συστολάς, τὴν μὲν ὅταν ὁ θώραξ ἐφ' αὐτὸν τὸ πνευματικὸν ἑλκύσῃ, τὴν δ' ὅταν αὐτὸς εἰς τὸν ἐκτὸς ἀέρα ἀποκρίνῃ· δύο γὰρ μόναι γίνονται περὶ τὸν θώρακα, διαστολὴ μὲν ὅταν ἀπὸ τοῦ πνεύμονος ἐφέλκηται, συστολὴ δ' ὅταν τούτῳ πάλιν ἀνταποδιδῷ.

2 μόνον *codd.*: πρῶτον *Diels*   3–4 εἶτα δὲ καὶ ἄλλα *E*: εἶτα δὴ τὰ ἄλλα *B*: *del. Diels*   δὲ ... πνεύμονος *om. M*   4 οὖν *suppl. Diels sec. Galen.*   6 ἐφέλκεται *codd.*: < ἐπειδὰν μηκέτι > ἐφέλκηται, *vel* παύεται *coni. Mau Galeno (T143c) collato, fort. recte*   6 παρακειμένως ... ὄρεξιν *del. Mau ut glossema*   6 περικείμενος *coni. Mau*   7 ἐπ' αὐτὸν *MΠ*

7 μετοχετεύων ΜΠ 9 ἀντεμετερᾷ coni. Bernardakis 11 ὅτε δὲ
συστολή add. Diels 11 πνεύματος B 13 μὲν del. Reiske
15 ἐντός] ἐκτὸς coni. Bernardakis 16 μεταρρεῖν M: μετερᾷ
Bernardakis 17 τὸν αὐτὸν B ἦν καὶ τὸ Π 18 γενόμενον
MB 20 ὁ om. M. ὑπ' αὐτὸν ΒΠ: ὑπ' αὐτὸ M: corr. Diels
21 ἐκτός] κόλπον Π 23 ταὐτὸ ΜΒα: αὐτὸ AE: corr. Diels

143a–b Herophilus admits motor capacities for bodies in the nerves,
arteries, and muscles. He thinks that the lung alone has a natural
tendency to dilate and contract. The drawing in of pneuma from
outside, he says, is accordingly the activity of the lung, and it draws it
in through the repletion which occurs without. Next, on account of a
second [natural] tendency, the thorax diverts the pneuma to itself,
and when it is filled and no longer capable of drawing it in, it lets the
excess flow back again into the lung, through which the exhalation of
what is excreted occurs. The parts of the body are thus affected in
turn. For now dilation, then contraction of the lung occurs, since
filling up and emptying occur through reciprocal exchange, so that
four motions in fact occur in the lung: the first is the one by which it
receives air from outside; the second by which the pneuma which it
has received from outside changes its flow internally toward the
thorax; the third by which it receives again into itself the contracted
pneuma from the thorax; the fourth by which it evacuates to the
outside that which is in it after rounding the turn. Of these motions of
the lung, he says, two are dilations – the one from outside and the one
from the thorax – while two are contractions, namely one when the
thorax draws the pneumatic substance to itself, the other when the
lung itself excretes pneuma into the external air. Only two motions,
you see, occur in the thorax: dilation when it draws pneuma from the
lung, contraction when it delivers it back again to the lung.

143c Ps.-Galenus, *De historia philosopha* 103 (*DG*, p. 639)

Ἡρόφιλος δὲ δύναμιν ἀπολείπει περὶ τὰ σώματα κινητικὴν ἐν
νεύροις καὶ ἐν ἀρτηρίαις καὶ μυσί· τὸν οὖν πνεύμονα νομίζει
προσορέγεσθαι διαστολῆς τε καὶ συστολῆς. φυσικὴν ἐνέργειαν
μὲν οὖν εἶναι τοῦ πνεύμονος τὴν ἔξωθεν τοῦ πνεύματος ὁλκήν,
5 ὑπὸ δὲ τῆς πληρώσεως τῆς ἔξωθεν γινομένης ἐφέλκεσθαι μὴ
δυνάμενον, εἰς τὸν θώρακα τὸ περιττὸν ἀναπέμπειν, τὸν δὲ εἰς
τὸν ἔξωθεν ἀέρα ἀπωθεῖν.

1 δύναμιν *om.* B   ἀπολείπειν A   2 γοῦν B   3 προσορέγεσθαι A:
προορέγεσθαι B   3 *in* φυσικὴν *latere* φυσικῶς *susp.* Diels   4 οὖν εἶναι
Diels: συνεῖναι AB   5 ἀπὸ B   γιγνόμενον AB   7 *post* ἀπωθεῖν
Kühn (XIX, *pp.* 318.12–319.7), *edd. vett. habent* ὡς τέσσαρας μὲν γίνεσθαι
κινήσεις *usque ad* ὅταν τούτῳ πάχιν ἀνταποδιδῷ (*T143a–b.13–24*)

143c Herophilus admits a motor capacity for bodies in the nerves,
arteries, and muscles. He accordingly thinks the lung has an
additional tendency to dilate and contract. The natural activity of
the lung, he says, is, then, the drawing in of pneuma from the outside;
but when a repletion from outside occurs and the lung is not able to
draw in [more pneuma], it sends on the excess into the thorax, and it
expels it into the external air.

4   *Vascular physiology; pulse-lore ('On Pulses')*

144   Galenus (ex Aristoxeno?), *De pulsuum differentiis* 4.6 (VIII,
p. 733K)

τοῖς δὲ περὶ τὸν Ἡρόφιλον ἀρέσκει τὰς ἀρτηρίας συνεχεῖς
οὔσας τῇ καρδίᾳ διὰ τῶν χιτώνων ἐπιρρέουσαν ἔχειν τὴν παρ'
αὐτοῖς δύναμιν, ᾗ χρώμεναι παραπλησίως αὐτῇ τῇ καρδίᾳ
διαστελλόμεναι μὲν ἕλκουσι πανταχόθεν, ὅθεν ἂν δύνωνται, τὸ
5 πληρῶσον αὐτῶν τὴν διαστολήν, συστελλόμεναι δὲ ἐκθλίβουσι,
καὶ διὰ τοῦτο φαίνεσθαι καθ' ἕνα χρόνον ἅμα πάσας αὐτὰς
διαστελλομένας τε καὶ συστελλομένας, τὴν αὐτὴν προθεσμίαν
τῇ καρδίᾳ τῶν κινήσεων ἀμφοτέρων φυλαττούσας.

144 Herophilus and his followers hold the opinion that the arteries
are continuous with the heart and that they have a faculty that flows
to them through their coats. Using this faculty they dilate in a manner
similar to the heart itself and draw, from everywhere they can, that
which will fill their dilation; but when they contract, they expel it. For
this reason all of the arteries are observed to dilate at one and the same
time and to contract [simultaneously], preserving for the heart the
same fixed time for both motions.

145a   Galenus, *An in arteriis natura sanguis contineatur* 8 (pp. 18–19
Albrecht; 176–8 Furley/Wilkie)

ὥσθ' ὅταν ἀπορῶσι (sc. οἱ περὶ τὸν Ἐρασίστρατον) πῶς εἰς ὅλον τὸ σῶμα παρὰ τῆς καρδίας κομισθήσεται τὸ πνεῦμα πεπληρωμένων αἵματος τῶν ἀρτηριῶν, οὐ χαλεπὸν ἐπιλύσασθαι τὴν ἀπορίαν αὐτῶν, μὴ πέμπεσθαι φάντας, ἀλλ' ἕλκεσθαι,
5 μήτ' ἐκ καρδίας μόνης, ἀλλὰ πανταχόθεν, ὡς Ἡροφίλῳ τε καὶ πρὸ τούτου Πραξαγόρᾳ καὶ Φυλοτίμῳ καὶ Διοκλεῖ καὶ Πλειστονίκῳ καὶ Ἱπποκράτει καὶ μυρίοις ἑτέροις ἀρέσκει. ὅτι μέντοι τῆς διαστελλούσης τὰς ἀρτηρίας δυνάμεως οἷον πηγή τίς ἐστιν ἡ καρδία, καὶ τοῦθ' ἑτέρωθί τε πρὸς ἡμῶν ἐπιδέδεικται καὶ τοῖς
10 προειρημένοις ἅπασιν ἀνδράσιν ὡμολόγηται.

6 φιλοτίμῳ LV Aldus: Φιλοτίμῳ Kühn, Furley/Wilkie: corr. Wellmann post quem Albrecht (cf. Diller, 1941: 1030)   9 τε om. V Aldus

145a Consequently, whenever [Erasistratus and his followers] are at a loss to explain how – if the arteries are filled with blood – pneuma will be carried from the heart to the entire body, it is not difficult to solve their problem by saying that the pneuma is not 'sent' but 'drawn', and not from the heart alone but from everywhere, as Herophilus thought, and before him Praxagoras, Phylotimus, Diocles, Plistonicus, Hippocrates, and countless others. All the aforementioned men agree, however – and it has been demonstrated elsewhere by me – that the heart is something like a source of the faculty which dilates the arteries.

145b Galenus, De sententiis, ed. V. Nutton (CMG, in preparation)

Et sicut non refert apud medicum in medicando egritudines utrum anima sit mortalis aut immortalis, ita etiam non refert utrum anima sit incorporea prout vult aut sit corporea prout vult, cum iudicavit quod substantia anime sit spiritus; et non
5 manifestavit, prout manifestavit Erasistratus, utrum spiritus anime contineatur in corporibus animalium in concavitatibus vel expandatur per omnia membra radicalia vel dividatur in minutas partes prout voluit Herophilus, dicens quod sit in unaquaque parte partium membri radicalis, ita quod nulla pars
10 partium sit quod non sit in ipsa.

8 Herophilus coni. Nutton: Elemirephilis et similia codd.

145b And just as it is not important for the physician, in healing illnesses, whether the soul is mortal or immortal, so too it is not important whether the soul is incorporeal, if he wishes, or corporeal, if he wishes, since he has decided that the substance of the soul is pneuma. And he has not shown clearly, as Erasistratus did, whether the pneuma of the soul is contained in the bodies of living creatures in the ventricles or is spread out through all the ducts [?'root-like parts'] or is divided into small parts as Herophilus wanted, saying that it is in every single part of the parts of the root member, such that there is no part of [these] parts in which it is not.

146 *P. Londinensis* 137 (Anonymus Londinensis, *Iatrica Menonia*), 28.46–29.23 (*Supplementum Aristotelicum* iii.1, pp. 53–4 Diels)

ὁ μέντοι γε Ἡρόφιλος ἐναντίως διείληφεν· οἴεται γὰρ πλείονα μ(ὲν) γί(νεσθαι) ἀνάδοσιν ἐν ταῖς ἀρτηρίαις, ἧσσ[ον]α δὲ ἐν ταῖς φλεψὶ διὰ δύο ταῦτ[α]· ἃ μ(έν), ἐπειδήπερ ἀμφότεραι μ(ὲν) ὀρεκτικ[ῶ]ς ἔχουσι τῆς τροφῆς, ἥ τε φλὲψ κ[α]ὶ ἡ ἀρτηρία, ἐπεὶ
5 δὲ κατ' ἴσον ὀρέγονται τῆς τροφῆς, κατ' ἴσον καὶ ἡ ἀνάδοσις ε[ἰς] αὐτ[ὰς] γενήσεται. δεύτερον δὲ αἱ μ(ὲν) ἀρτηρίαι, φ(ησίν), συστέλ < λ > ονταί τε καὶ διαστέλλονται τόν τε σφυγμὸν ἀποδι-δόασιν, αἱ δὲ φλέβες οὔτε συστέλ[λ]ονται οὔτε διαστέλλονται οὐδὲ σφυγμωδῶς κεινοῦνται . ἐπεὶ τοιγ(άρ)τοι αἱ μὲν ἀρτηρί(αι)
10 σφυγμωδῶς κεινοῦνται, αἱ δὲ φλέβες οὐ κεινοῦνται [σ]φυγμωδῶς, ταύτῃ ἐπὶ τ(ῶν) ἀρτηριῶν [διὰ [τ]ὴν ὥσ[ιν ἐ]κ[εί]ν[η]ν] εὔ[λο]γον πλείονα γί(νεσθαι) τὴν ἀνάδοσιν ἤπερ ἐπὶ τ(ῶν) φλεβῶν διὰ τὴν εἰρημένην α(ἰτίαν). οὐκ ὀρθ[ῶ]ς δὲ ὁ προκείμενος ἀνὴρ ἐποίησεν. οὐ γ(ὰρ) ἐνόησεν, ὡς εὐρυκοιλιώ-
15 τεραί (εἰσιν) αἱ φλέβες παρὰ τὰς ἀρτηρίας, εὐρυκοιλιώτεραι δὲ οὖσαι πλείονα δεόντως ἕξουσι καὶ τὴν ἐν αὐταῖ[ς] γινομένην ἀνάδοσιν. καὶ π(ρὸς) μ(ὲν) τὸ ἃ τούτου κεφάλαιον τοῦτο καθήξει λέγειν, πρὸς δὲ τὸ δεύτερον ἐροῦμ(εν), διότι [[ὡσπέρ]] αἱ ἀρτηρίαι σφυγμωδῶς κεινοῦνται συστε[λ] < λ > όμεναι καὶ
20 διαστελλόμεναι, ο(ὕτως) δὲ κεινούμεναι ἐκθλείψουσιν εἰς τὸ ἐκτὸς τὴν τρο[φήν].

6 εἰς αὐτὰς *corr. ipse* P *ex* ἐξ αὐτῶν   16 ἐν *ex* εἰς P

146 Herophilus, however, has taken the opposite view. For he thinks greater distribution [sc. of nourishment] occurs through the arteries

and less through the veins for the following two reasons. First, since both of them have a desire for nourishment – I mean vein and artery – and since they derive nourishment equally, distribution into them will also occur equally. Secondly, the arteries, he says, dilate and contract, and produce a pulse, whereas the veins neither contract nor dilate, and do not move in a pulsating manner. Since, then, the arteries move in a pulsating manner whereas the veins do not, it is probably because of this pushing action that, for the reason given, greater distribution takes place [through the arteries] than in the case of the veins. But the author under consideration here [sc. Herophilus] did not do this correctly. For he did not grasp that the veins have a wider cavity than the arteries and, because they have a wider cavity, will necessarily also have a greater absorption occurring in them. And against his first main point it will be appropriate to make the preceding reply; but against his second point we will say that because the arteries move in a pulsating manner, dilating and contracting, they will expel the nourishment to the outside, moving in this manner . . .

147 Galenus, *De experientia medica* 13.6 (translated into English from the Arabic translation of the lost original by Richard Walzer, pp. 109–110)

Herophilus . . . is a man who is known by everybody to have surpassed the great majority of the ancients, not only in width of knowledge but in intellect, and to have advanced the art of medicine in many ways; as, for instance, by his logos of the pulsation of 'veins',* which one needs more now and finds more useful than any other logos, for deriving benefit therefrom, while those before overlooked it and neglected to investigate it. We find, however, that this Herophilus concedes no small importance to experience . . .

148 Galenus, *De pulsuum differentiis* 4.2 (VIII, pp. 716–17K)

ὅταν δ' αὖ πάλιν ἀναγνῶμεν Αἰγιμίου τὸ περὶ παλμῶν βιβλίον,

* The original must have read ἀρτηριῶν, 'arteries', since Herophilus attributed pulsation only to the arteries, not to the veins. Cf. T144–T146, T148ff.

εὑρίσκομεν, ὃ νῦν ἡμεῖς καλοῦμεν σφυγμόν, ὑπ' ἐκείνου παλμὸν
ὀνομαζόμενον. ἐναντίως δ' αὐτῷ τὸν Ἡρόφιλον εὕροις ἂν εὐθὺς
ἐν ἀρχῇ τῆς περὶ σφυγμῶν πραγματείας διορίζοντα σφυγμὸν
5 παλμοῦ. φαίνεται γὰρ ὁ ἀνὴρ οὗτος ἅπασαν ἀρτηριῶν κίνησιν,
ἣν ὁρῶμεν ἐξ ἀρχῆς ἡμῖν ἕως τέλους ὑπάρχουσαν, ὀνομάζων
σφυγμόν, ἐξ οὗ καὶ τὰς διαγνώσεις τῶν παρόντων καὶ τὰς
προγνώσεις τῶν ἐσομένων ποιούμεθα, μηδὲν τοῦ κατὰ τὴν
καρδίαν, ἢ τὸν ἐγκέφαλον, ἢ τὰς μήνιγγας δεόμενοι σφυγμοῦ.

148 Whenever, once again, I read Aegimius' book *On Palpitations*, I
find that what we now call 'pulse' was called 'palpitation' by him. But
you would find Herophilus, right at the beginning of his treatise *On
Pulses*, taking a view opposed to Aegimius', inasmuch as he distinguishes 'pulse' from 'palpitation'. For this author [sc. Herophilus]
seems to call all the motion of the arteries that we see existing in us,
from beginning to end, 'pulse', and on the basis of this [arterial]
pulsation we also make diagnoses of what is present and prognoses of
what is to be, without requiring any pulsation of the heart, the brain
or the meninges at all.

149 Rufus Ephesius (?), *Synopsis de pulsibus* 2 (pp. 220–1
Daremberg/Ruelle)

Πραξαγόρας μὲν οὖν ὑπέλαβε ταῦτα (sc. τὸν σφυγμόν, τὸν
παλμόν, τὸν σπασμόν, τὸν τρόμον) ἀλλήλων διαφέρειν
ποσότητι, οὐκέτι δὲ καὶ ποιότητι . . . καὶ ταῦτα μὲν ὁ Πραξαγόρας, ἀνὴρ οὐχ ὁ τυχὼν οὔτε ἐν τοῖς κατὰ τὴν ἰατρικὴν
5 θεωρήμασιν, οὔτε ἐν τῷ ἄλλῳ βίῳ· ὁ δὲ Ἡρόφιλος ἀκριβέστερον
ἐπιστήσας τῷ τόπῳ ἐν ποιότητι μᾶλλον αὐτῶν τὰς διαφορὰς
εὗρεν· γίγνεσθαι γὰρ τὸν σφυγμὸν περὶ μόνας ἀρτηρίας καὶ
καρδίαν, τὸν δὲ παλμὸν καὶ τὸν σπασμὸν καὶ τὸν τρόμον περὶ
μύας τε καὶ νεῦρα· καὶ τὸν μὲν σφυγμὸν συγγεννᾶσθαι τῷ ζῴῳ
10 καὶ συναποθνήσκειν, ταῦτα δὲ οὔ· καὶ τὸν μὲν σφυγμὸν πληρου-
μένων τε καὶ κενουμένων τῶν ἀρτηρίων, ταῦτα δὲ οὔ. καὶ τὸν μὲν
σφυγμὸν ἀπροαιρέτως ἡμῖν πάντοτε παρακολουθεῖν, ἐπεὶ καὶ
φυσικῶς ὑπάρχει, ταῦτα δὲ εἶναι καὶ ἐν τῇ ἡμετέρᾳ προαιρέσει,
ἀποπιεσθέντων πολλάκις καὶ βαρυνθέντων τῶν μερῶν.

7 γίνεσθαι *P*   8 καὶ τὸν τρόμον *om. FG*   11–14 ταῦτα δὲ . . . μερῶν
om. G   12 ἡμῖν *om. P*

149 Praxagoras, then, assumed that these things [sc. pulse, palpitation, spasm, tremor] differ from each other in quantity but not in quality as well . . . And this is what Praxagoras said, who was not an inconsequential figure either in his medical theories or in the other aspects of life. But Herophilus, who had a more accurate knowledge of this topic, found the differences of these affections to lie in quality instead. For, he says, pulse occurs only in the arteries and the heart, whereas palpitation and spasm and tremor occur in muscles as well as nerves. And the pulse, he says, is born with a living being and dies with it, whereas these other motions do not. Also, the pulse, he says, occurs both when the arteries are filled and when they are emptied, whereas these others do not; and the pulse at all times attends us involuntarily and exists naturally, whereas the others are within our power to choose, namely by pressing out and depressing the parts [sc. muscles and nerves?] frequently.

150 Galenus (ex Aristoxeno?), *De pulsuum differentiis* 4.3 (VIII, pp. 723–4K)

οὐ σμικρὰ δ' ἀντιλογία περὶ τῶν παθῶν τούτων (sc. σπασμῶν, τρόμων, παλμῶν) γέγονεν Ἡροφίλῳ πρὸς τὸν διδάσκαλον Πραξαγόραν, οὐκ ὀρθῶς ἀποφηνάμενον ἀρτηριῶν πάθος εἶναι καὶ παλμὸν καὶ τρόμον καὶ σπασμόν, οὐ γένει διαφέροντα τῆς
5 σφυγμώδους ἐν αὐταῖς κινήσεως, ἀλλὰ μεγέθει. κατὰ φύσιν μὲν γὰρ ἐχόντων ἄνευ πάσης περιστάσεως γίνεσθαι τοὺς σφυγμούς, αὐξηθείσης δὲ τῆς κινήσεως αὐτῶν εἰς τὸ παρὰ φύσιν πρῶτον μὲν σπασμὸν ἀποτελεῖσθαι, δεύτερον δ' ἐπ' αὐτῷ τρόμον, καὶ τρίτον τὸν παλμόν, ἀλλήλων διαφέροντα μεγέθει
10 πάντα ταῦτα τὰ πάθη.
διὰ τοῦτ' οὖν Ἡρόφιλος εὐθέως ἐν ἀρχῇ τῆς περὶ σφυγμῶν πραγματείας ἀνατρέπειν πειρᾶται τὴν τοῦ διδασκάλου δόξαν, ἀλλ' ὡς ἔθος Ἡροφίλῳ, δι' ἑρμηνείας ἀσαφοῦς, ἣν ἐπὶ τὸ σαφὲς οἱ ἀπ' αὐτοῦ μεταλαμβάνοντες ἔγραψαν ἐν αἷς ἐπ<οι>ήσαντο
15 πραγματείαις περὶ τῆς Ἡροφίλου αἱρέσεως. ὥστε εἰ μνημονεύω νῦν αὐτῆς Ἡροφίλου ῥήσεως, ἣν ἐν ἀρχῇ τοῦ πρώτου περὶ σφυγμῶν ἔγραψεν, ἢ τῶν εἰρημένων τοῖς ἀπ' αὐτοῦ, μέγεθος ἑνὸς βιβλίου γενήσεται . . . (*Cf. Herophili T22 supra.*)

5 αὐταῖς *coni. Steckerl*: αὐτοῖς *vulg.*: earum *Chartier*

150 There was no paltry dispute between Herophilus and his teacher Praxagoras concerning these affections [sc. spasm, tremor, palpitation], since Praxagoras had stated incorrectly that palpitation, tremor, and spasm are an affection of the arteries, differing not in kind but in size from the pulsating motion in them. For the pulse, Praxagoras said, occurs when the arteries are in a natural condition, in the absence of every difficult circumstance. But when their motion is increased to an unnatural extent, first spasm is caused; secondly, following upon it, tremor; third, palpitation. All these affections differ from each other in size.

For this reason, then, Herophilus right at the beginning of his treatise *On Pulses* tries to overturn his teacher's opinion. But, as is Herophilus' custom, he does so in an unclear form of expression which his followers clarified and recorded in the treatises they composed about Herophilus' school. Consequently, if I now were to recall the statement Herophilus recorded at the beginning of Book 1 of his *On Pulses*, or the things said by his successors, it would be the size of one [whole] book . . . (*Cf. Chapter* III, *T22 supra.*)

151 Galenus, *De pulsuum differentiis* 1.2 (VIII, p. 498K)

καὶ πολὺ παρὰ τὸ τῶν ἄλλων οὐκ ἰατρῶν μόνον, ἀλλὰ καὶ ἰδιωτῶν ἔθος ἅπασαν ἀρτηριῶν κίνησιν παλμὸν ὀνομάζει (sc. ὁ Αἰγίμιος). ἡ δὲ Πραξαγόρου τε καὶ Ἡροφίλου χρῆσις ἔτι καὶ εἰς τάδε κρατεῖ. σφυγμὸν γὰρ οὗτοι πᾶσαν ἀρτηριῶν κίνησιν τὴν
5 αἰσθητὴν καλοῦσιν.

151 And very much contrary to the custom of others – not only of physicians, but also of laymen – [Aegimius] gives the name 'palpitation' to all motion of the arteries. But the usage of Praxagoras and of Herophilus still prevails, even to the present: for they call all *perceptible* motion of the arteries 'pulse'.

152 Galenus, *De tremore, palpitatione, convulsione et rigore* 5 (VII, p. 594K)

ἀλλ' εἴτε μυῶν ἐστι πάθος μόνον ὁ παλμός, ὡς Ἡρόφιλος ἐνόμιζεν, ἢ καὶ τοῦ δέρματος, ἢ ἀρτηριῶν, ὡς ὑπελάμβανε Πραξαγόρας, αὖθις τοῦτο σκεψόμεθα. (*Vid. etiam T141 supra.*)

152 But whether palpitation is an affection of the muscles only, as Herophilus thought, or also of the skin, or of the arteries, as Praxagoras supposed – this we shall examine again. (*See also T141 supra.*)

153 Galenus, *De placitis Hippocratis et Platonis* 6.1 (*CMG* v.4.1.2, p. 362 De Lacy)

ἡ τῆς καρδίας κίνησις ἡ μὲν κατὰ τοὺς σφυγμοὺς ἐνέργειά ἐστιν, ἡ δὲ κατὰ τοὺς παλμοὺς πάθος. ἐξ ἑαυτῆς μὲν γάρ ἐστι καὶ ἡ κατὰ τοὺς παλμούς, ἀλλ᾽ οὐ κατὰ φύσιν, ἐξ ἑαυτῆς δὲ καὶ ἡ τῶν σφυγμῶν, ἀλλὰ κατὰ φύσιν. δεῖ δὲ τοῦ σφυγμὸς ὀνόματος
5 ἀκούειν οὕτως νῦν ὡς Πραξαγόρας καὶ Ἡρόφιλος ἅπαντές τε σχεδὸν οἱ μετ᾽ αὐτοὺς ἐχρήσαντο μέχρι καὶ ἡμῶν, ὡς ἥ γε παλαιοτέρα χρῆσις, ἣ κἂν τοῖς Ἐρασιστράτου τε καὶ Ἱπποκράτους εὑρίσκεται γράμμασιν, ἑτέρα τίς ἐστι καὶ λεχθήσεται περὶ αὐτῆς ἐν τοῖς μετὰ ταῦτα. τὴν μέντοι τῆς καρδίας ἰδίαν κίνησιν
10 ὀνομαζόντων ἡμῶν σφυγμὸν ὁ παλμὸς μὲν πάθος εἶναι λεχθήσεται κατά γε τὸ δεύτερον τῆς πάθος φωνῆς σημαινόμενον (sc. ἡ παρὰ φύσιν κίνησις), ὁ σφυγμὸς δ᾽ οὐ πᾶς ἐνέργεια.

1 ἡ τῆς] ἥτις *L*   2 ἐστι καί] ἐστιν *L*   3 τῶν σφυγμῶν *ex* κατὰ τὸν σφυγμὸν *corr. H*   4 σφυγμός] σφυγμοῦ *HL corr. Kühn*   5 ἀκούειν ὀνόματος *L*   7 ἢ (*ante* κἂν) *ex* ἢ *corr. H*   10 ὑμῶν *L*   12 ὁ] οὐ *L*

153 The motion of the heart is an activity (*energeia*) in the case of pulsation, but in the case of palpitation it is an affection (*pathos*). For, the palpitating motion too arises within the heart itself, but not according to nature, whereas the pulsating motion, while also arising within the heart, is in accordance with nature. But here you must understand the noun 'pulsation' (*sphygmos*) in the way that Praxagoras and Herophilus and almost all those after them, up to us too, have used it. For, the more ancient usage, which is also found in the writings of Erasistratus and Hippocrates, is a different one, and there will be a discussion about it in a subsequent section. Since we give the name 'pulsation' to the motion proper to the heart, however, palpitation must be called an affection (*pathos*) in the second meaning of the word *pathos* [sc. motion contrary to nature]; but not all 'pulsation' is [cardiac] activity (*energeia*).

154 Galenus, *De pulsuum usu* 4 (v, pp. 163-4K; pp. 208–10 Furley/Wilkie)

ταύτης δὲ τῆς διπλῆς καὶ συνθέτου τῶν ἀρτηριῶν κινήσεως, ἣν δὴ καὶ σφυγμὸν ὀνομάζομεν, ἐξηγεῖται μὲν ἡ καρδία, καθάπερ καὶ ἡμῖν ἐν ἑτέροις καὶ μυρίοις ἄλλοις πρὸ ἡμῶν ἀποδέδεικται, οὐ μὴν καθ' ὃν Ἐρασίστρατος ὑπελάμβανεν τρόπον, ἀλλ' ὡς
5 Ἡρόφιλός τε καὶ Ἱπποκράτης καὶ σχεδὸν οἱ δοκιμώτατοι πάντες τῶν παλαιῶν ἰατρῶν τε καὶ φιλοσόφων.

3 πρὸ ἡμῖν S: πρὸς ἡμῖν *Ald*: *corr. Kühn* (ante nos *Linacri interpretatio*)

154 This double, compound motion of the arteries, to which, of course, we also give the name 'pulse' (*sphygmos*), is governed by the heart, as has been demonstrated both by me in my other works and by countless others before me – I do not mean the way in which Erasistratus assumed that it happens, but the way Herophilus as well as Hippocrates and almost all very reputable ancient physicians and philosophers assumed it happens [sc. the *dynamis* in the body of the heart, by which it expands and contracts, flows out through the arterial coats to all the arteries, expanding and contracting them].

155 Galenus (ex Aristoxeno?), *De pulsuum differentiis* 4.2 (viii, pp. 702–3K)

ἔτι δὲ μείζων ἄλλη διαφορὰ τοῖς ἰατροῖς ἐκ παλαιοῦ περὶ τῶν ἀρτηριῶν ἐγένετο, τινῶν μὲν ἡγουμένων αὐτὰς ἐξ ἑαυτῶν σφύζειν, σύμφυτον ἐχούσας ὁμοίως τῇ καρδίᾳ τὴν τοιαύτην δύναμιν, ὧν ἐστι καὶ ὁ Πραξαγόρας, ἐνίων δὲ σφύζειν μὲν αὐτοῦ
5 τοῦ χιτῶνος αὐτῶν διαστελλομένου τε καὶ συστελλομένου, καθάπερ ἡ καρδία, τὴν δύναμιν δὲ οὐκ ἐχουσῶν σύμφυτον ᾗ τοῦτο δρῶσιν, ἀλλὰ παρὰ καρδίας λαμβανουσῶν. ἧς γνώμης ἔχεται καὶ Ἡρόφιλος. Ἐρασιστράτῳ δὲ οὐδέτερον ἀρέσκει . . .

5 *post* αὐτοῦ *interpunxit Kühn*   7 καρδίας *ABL*: καρδίαν *vulg.*

155 A still bigger difference arose among physicians of ancient times concerning the arteries. Some, among them also Praxagoras, thought that the arteries pulsate by themselves, possessing – like the heart – an innate faculty of such a kind. Others, by contrast, thought that while they pulsate because the arterial coat itself dilates as well as contracts,

just like the heart, it is not because they possess an innate faculty by means of which they do this, but rather because they receive [this faculty] from the heart. To this judgment Herophilus, too, adhered. But Erasistratus held neither of these views . . .

156 Galenus (ex Aristoxeno?), *De pulsuum differentiis* 4.10 (VIII, p. 744K)

τῷ δ' ὑπὸ ʒωτικῆς καὶ ψυχικῆς δυνάμεως γίνεσθαι τὸν σφυγμὸν ὑπὸ Χρυσέρμου λελεγμένῳ προσέθηκεν ὁ Ἡρακλείδης τὸ πλεισ-τοδυναμούσης, ἐπειδὴ καὶ ἄλλα τινὰ συντελεῖν εἰς τὴν τῶν σφυγμῶν γένεσιν ὁ Ἡρόφιλος αὐτός φησι καὶ πάντες οἱ ἀπ'
5 αὐτοῦ κληθέντες Ἡροφίλειοι. (*Vid. infra HE.2a; Cr. 1-2; Caput* x.a.)

156 To what was said by Chrysermus, namely that the pulse arises through the agency of a vital and psychic faculty, Heraclides added 'which is dominant', since Herophilus and all those who are called 'Herophileans' after him say that other things, too, contribute to the generation of the pulses. (*See Chapters* x.a, xx.a, xxiv.a *infra.*)

157 Galenus (ex Aristoxeno?), *De pulsuum differentiis* 4.10 (VIII, pp. 747-8K)

ἀλλὰ τὰ μὲν τοιαῦτα πρὸς τοὺς ἀφ' ἑτέρων αἱρέσεων ἀμφισβη-τεῖται καὶ τούτῳ καὶ τοῖς ἄλλοις Ἡροφιλείοις, αὐτῷ δὲ τῷ Ἡροφίλῳ φαίνοιτ' ἂν διαφερόμενος ἐν τῷ τὸν σφυγμὸν ἐνέργειαν μὲν εἶναι νομίζειν ἀρτηριῶν καὶ καρδίας, μέρη δ' αὐτῷ τίθεσθαι
5 τὴν διαστολήν τε καὶ συστολὴν καί ποτε καὶ τὰς ἠρεμίας. ἐὰν γὰρ ἀκριβῶς ἕπηται τοῖς Ἡροφίλου δόγμασιν, ἡ συστολὴ μὲν ἐνέργεια τῶν ἀρτηριῶν ἐστιν, ἡ διαστολὴ δὲ εἰς τὴν οἰκείαν τε καὶ φυσικὴν κατάστασιν τοῦ σώματος αὐτῶν ἐπάνοδος. βούλεται γάρ, ὥσπερ ἐπὶ τῶν τεθνεώτων ὁρᾶται διεστὼς ὁ χιτὼν τῆς
10 ἀρτηρίας, οὕτω κἀπὶ τῶν ʒώντων ὅσον ἐφ' ἑαυτῷ διεστάναι, τοὐναντίον Ἀσκληπιάδου δοξάζοντος.

157 Both he [Aristoxenus; *Chapter* xxv] and the other Herophileans argue about such points [pulse definitions] against adherents of other

'schools', yet Aristoxenus would seem to differ with Herophilus himself, on the one hand in so far as he considers the pulse an activity of the arteries *and* of the heart, on the other hand in so far as he attributes 'dilation', 'contraction', *and* sometimes also the 'pauses' [intervals of rest] to the pulse as its parts. For, if one follows Herophilus' teachings very closely, contraction (*systolē*) is an activity (*energeia*) of the arteries, while dilation (*diastolē*) is a return (*epanodos*) to the proper and natural condition of their body. The intention of his view is in fact that just as the coat of the artery is seen to be distended in the case of those who are dead, so too in those who are alive it is distended as much as is in its power – although Asclepiades holds the opposite opinion.

158 Galenus, *De pulsuum differentiis* 4.12 (VIII, p. 754K)

ἐκ διαστολῆς τε καὶ συστολῆς ὡς μερῶν συγκεῖσθαι νομίζουσι τὸν σφυγμὸν οἱ πνευματικοὶ πάντες, ἐνεργείας ἡγούμενοι τὰς κινήσεις ἀμφοτέρας εἶναι, τῶν περὶ τὸν Ἡρόφιλόν τε καὶ Ἀσκληπιάδην οὐχ ὁμοίως δοκούντων φέρεσθαι. τὸν μὲν οὖν
5 Ἡρόφιλον περὶ διαστολῆς τε καὶ συστολῆς ἀρτηριῶν ζήτησιν ἰδίαν ἔχειν μακροτέραν· ἐνίοτε μὲν γάρ σοι δόξει καὶ τὴν διαστολὴν καὶ τὴν συστολὴν ἐνέργειαν νομίζειν, ὡς τὸ πολὺ δὲ μόνην τὴν συστολήν.

158 All the Pneumatics think that the pulse is composed of contraction and dilation, as though composed of parts, and they regard both motions as activities (*energeiai*); but the followers of Herophilus and Asclepiades do not seem to have had a similar opinion. Herophilus, it seems, conducted his own rather long investigation into the dilation and contraction of arteries. Sometimes, it will seem to you, he considered both the dilation (*diastolē*) and contraction (*systolē*) an activity (*energeia*), but for the most part only the contraction.

159 Galenus, *De pulsuum dignotione* 1.1 (VIII, p. 771K)

πολλοῖς μὲν γὰρ ἔτεσιν οὐδ' εἰ σαφῶς ἐστι τῇ ἁφῇ διαγνῶναι τὴν συστολὴν τῆς ἀρτηρίας ἠπιστάμην, ἀλλ' ἦν ἄπορόν μοι

πότερον οἱ περὶ τὸν ᾽Αρχιγένην καὶ ῾Ηρόφιλον ἢ οἱ περὶ τὸν
᾽Αγαθῖνον καὶ σχεδὸν ἅπαντας τοὺς ἐμπειρικοὺς ἀληθεύουσι,
5 τοσοῦτον ἀπελειπόμην τοῦ πότερον ὅλης αὐτῆς αἰσθάνεσθαι
δυνατόν ἐστιν ἢ μορίου τινὸς καὶ πόσον τούτου σαφές τι
γινώσκειν.

159 For many years I did not know whether it is even possible to
discern the contraction of the artery clearly with one's touch. In fact,
I was at a loss as to whether the followers of Archigenes and
Herophilus, or the followers of Agathinus and of virtually all the
Empiricists, speak the truth – so far was I from recognizing clearly
whether it is possible to perceive the contraction in its entirety, or only
some part of it, and how much of this.

160 Galenus, *De pulsuum dignotione* 1.3 (VIII, pp. 786–8K)

᾽Αγαθίνου τοίνυν λέγοντος ἀναίσθητον εἶναι τὴν συστολὴν τῆς
ἀρτηρίας, ῾Ηροφίλου δὲ διὰ παντὸς ὡς ὑπὲρ αἰσθητῆς διαλεγο-
μένου, χαλεπὸν ὄντως ἦν καὶ ἄπορον ἑτέρῳ πρὸ θατέρου
πιστεῦσαι, τοσαύτην μὲν ἀμφοτέρων σπουδὴν εἰσενηνεγμένων
5 εἴς τε τἄλλα τῆς ἰατρικῆς καὶ τὴν περὶ τοὺς σφυγμοὺς τέχνην
αὐξῆσαι, μακρῷ τε χρόνῳ τόν τε λογισμὸν καὶ τὴν αἴσθησιν
ἱκανῶς γεγυμνασμένων. ἐδόκει δή μοι δίκαιον εἶναι πρῶτον μὲν
ἀσκῆσαι τὴν ἀφήν τῆς παρὰ μικρὸν αἰσθάνεσθαι διαφορᾶς, ἵν'
εἴπερ ἡμῖν αὐτοῖς ποτε καταφανὴς ἐναργῶς γένοιτο ἡ συστολή,
10 μηκέτ' ἄλλου δεοίμεθα μάρτυρος· δεύτερον δὲ καὶ τὴν τῶν
πρεσβυτέρων ἱστορίαν ἀναλέξασθαι ... εὑρίσκοντες οὖν τοὺς
μὲν ῾Ηροφιλείους σχεδὸν ἅπαντας αἰσθητὴν εἶναι λέγοντας, τοῦ
δὲ περὶ τὸν ᾽Ερασίστρατον χοροῦ τοὺς μὲν ὁμολογοῦντας, τοὺς
δ' ἀρνουμένους, καὶ τρίτους τοὺς ἀπ' ᾽Αθηναίου τοῦ ᾽Αττα-
15 λέως, ὧν εἷς ἦν καὶ ᾽Αγαθῖνος, ὡσαύτως πρὸς ἀλλήλους
διαφερομένους, ὅσον μὲν ἐπὶ τῇ τῶν πρεσβυτέρων ἱστορίᾳ πλέον
οὐδὲν ἡμῖν ἔγνωμεν ἐσόμενον ...

160 Now, since Agathinus says the contraction of the artery is
imperceptible, whereas Herophilus discourses throughout as though
about a perceptible contraction, it was really difficult, in fact
impossible, to believe the one in preference to the other. For, both

have contributed so great a zeal toward the growth of the other branches of medicine and especially to the growth of the art concerning the pulse, and both have trained their reasoning capacity as well as their sense-perception sufficiently over a long period of time. It did seem right to me first to practise one's touch to perceive a small difference, so that, if ever the contraction were to become clearly manifest to us ourselves, we would no longer require another witness; second, also to read through the inquiries of older authors . . . I accordingly found that almost all the Herophileans say it [sc. the contraction] is perceptible, whereas some members of the chorus around Erasistratus agree and others deny it; and a third group, descendants of Athenaeus of Attalia, one of whom is Agathinus, likewise disagree among themselves. I recognized that, as far as the reports of the older authors are concerned, they will be of no profit to us . . .

161　Galenus, *De pulsuum dignotione* 4.2 (VIII, p. 941 K)

ἀλλ' εἰ τοῦτο λέγουσιν, ὡς ἔστιν ἐκ τῶν κατὰ τὴν ἀφὴν παθῶν
συλλογίσασθαί τι περὶ τῶν κατὰ τὰς ἀρτηρίας διαθέσεων, οὐκ
ἀντιλέγω. καὶ γὰρ Πραξαγόρας αὐτὸ ποιεῖ καὶ Ἡρόφιλος καὶ
πάντες ὀλίγου δεῖν, οἱ μὲν μᾶλλον, οἱ δὲ ἧττον, καὶ οἱ μὲν
5　χεῖρον, οἱ δὲ βέλτιον.

161　But if this is what they say, namely that it is possible to make an inference concerning the states of the arteries on the basis of the experiences of the sense of touch, I do not contradict them. For, Praxagoras also does this, and so does Herophilus and almost all [physicians], some more so, some less, and some worse, some better.

162　Galenus, *De pulsuum dignotione* 4.3 (VIII, pp. 954–61 K)

καίτοι πῶς ἄν τις πιστεύσειε τοῖς δι' ἑνὸς χιτῶνος τοῦ κατὰ τὸν
ἀσκὸν μὴ δυναμένοις διαγνῶναι τοῦ περιεχομένου τὴν ποιότητα
δυνατοῖς εἶναι διά τε δέρματος οὐχ ἧττον ἢ κατ' ἀσκὸν παχέος
καὶ ὑμένων τοὐλάχιστον δυοῖν καὶ χιτώνων ἐξ ἀνάγκης δυοῖν
5　τὴν ἐντὸς τῆς ἀρτηρίας διαγνῶναι ποιότητα; ταῦτ' οὖν αὐτοὶ
μὲν λεγέτωσαν, Ἡροφίλου δὲ μὴ καταψευδέσθωσαν, μηδὲ δυσω-

πείτωσαν ὀνόματι σεμνῷ τοὺς ἀμαθεῖς τῶν Ἡροφίλου γραμμάτων, μηδ᾽ ἐκ τούτου τὴν πίστιν τῷ λόγῳ πορίζέσθωσαν
(Τ39). αἰσχρὸν γὰρ ἐπὶ μαρτύρων ἀγωνίζεσθαι, καθάπερ ἐν
10 δικαστηρίῳ. εἰ λέγειν ἔχεις εἰς ἀπόδειξιν, ἡδέως ἀκουσόμεθά
σου. τὸ δ᾽ Ἡρόφιλόν τε καὶ Ἡροφιλείους καλεῖν μάρτυρας,
ἀποδιδράσκοντός ἐστι τὸν ἐξ εὐθείας ἀγῶνα, καὶ λόγον καὶ
διαδύσεις τε καὶ μηχανὰς ἐξευρίσκοντος ἐλέγχου φόβῳ. δῆλον,
ὡς ἕνεκα τοῦ μὴ περὶ πράγματος ἔτι ζητεῖν, ἀλλ᾽ ἱστορίας οἱ
15 κατεψευσμένοι μάρτυρες ἐπεισάγονται. "λέγει τοῦθ᾽ Ἡρόφιλος;" "οὐ μὲν οὖν." "ἀλλὰ οὐδὲ ψεύσῃ;" "δεῖξον πῶς ψεύδομαι,
δεῖξον πῶς λέγει." κἄπειτα λέξις, εἰ οὕτως ἔτυχεν, ἀμφίβολος
προβάλλεται καὶ πόλεμος ἄμφ᾽ αὐτῇ συνίσταται· "τί ποθ᾽ ἡ
λέξις λέγει;" καὶ "τί ποτε βούλεται . . ."
20   τί γὰρ οὐκ εἴρηται τοῖς νεωτέροις ἰατροῖς εἰς τὸ πρόβλημα,
τοῖς μὲν κατασκευάζουσιν ἐπίστασθαι τὸν Ἡρόφιλον καὶ ταύτην
τοῦ σφυγμοῦ τὴν διαφοράν, τοῖς δ᾽ ὡς οὐκ οἶδεν ἐγχειροῦσι
δεικνύειν; ταλαίπωροι μὲν οὖν ἑκάτεροι καὶ ἐλεεῖσθαι δίκαιοι, τῆς
μὲν ἀμαθείας οἱ πρότεροι, τῆς φιλονεικίας δ᾽ οἱ δεύτεροι.
25 ταλαίπωροι δὲ καὶ ἡμεῖς, οἷς γε οὐκ ἀρκεῖ τὴν ἰδίαν ἀσκεῖν
θεωρίαν τῆς τέχνης, ἀλλὰ τί μὲν Ἡρόφιλος εἶπεν, τί δ᾽
Ἡρακλείδης τε καὶ Χρύσερμος καὶ Ἡγήτωρ οὐκ ὀρθῶς ἐξηγήσαντο, τί δ᾽ ἀντεῖπον Ἀπολλώνιός τε καὶ Βακχεῖος καὶ Ἀριστό-
ξενος εἰδέναι βουλόμεθα. καὶ εἰ μὴ βουλόμεθα δέ, πάντως
30 ἀναγκαζόμεθα καὶ διττῶν ἀπολαύομεν κακῶν, ὅτι τε φλυαροῦμεν
οὐδὲν δέον ὅτι τε μὴ βουλόμενοι τοῦτο δρῶμεν, ὥσπερ ἐκεῖνοι·
νῦν γοῦν ἐμὲ δεῖ δυοῖν θάτερον, ἢ δοκεῖν Ἀρχιγένει τε καὶ
Ἡροφίλῳ καὶ μυρίοις ἄλλοις τἀναντία λέγειν, ἢ δεικνύειν ὅτι
καθ᾽ Ἡρόφιλον οὐδείς ἐστι πλήρης σφυγμός . . .
35   . . . ὅσοι δὲ καὶ ἱστορίαν ἐκμανθάνειν παλαιὰν ἐθέλουσι, καὶ
χρόνον εἰς τοῦτ᾽ ἔχουσιν, ἅπαντα προσθήσω, δεικνὺς ὅτι
μηδαμοῦ χρῆται πρὸς μηδὲν Ἡρόφιλος τῷ πλήρει σφυγμῷ.
   πρῶτον δ᾽ ἀπ᾽ αὐτῆς ἄρξομαι τῆς λέξεως, ἧς ἐκεῖνοι
προβάλλουσιν, ἐν τῷ πρώτῳ [περὶ] τῶν Ἡροφίλου περὶ
40 σφυγμῶν γεγραμμένης, ἣν καὶ μόνην ἀνεγνωκέναι μοι δοκοῦσιν
(Τ23). ἔχει δὲ οὕτως· "καθόλου μὲν οὖν δοκεῖ διαφέρειν σφυγμὸς
σφυγμοῦ πλήθει, μεγέθει, τάχει, σφοδρότητι, ῥυθμῷ."
   ταύτην γὰρ προβάλλοντες ἐρωτῶσι τί ποτ᾽ ἐστὶ τὸ πλῆθος,
ὥσπερ εἰ μὴ γιγνώσκοιμεν ὁποῖόν τι δηλοῖ τῷ πλήθει τῆς
45 πληρότητος ἐξ ἀνάγκης ὑπ᾽ αὐτοῦ δηλουμένης. ἐγὼ τοίνυν, ὡς

νομίζω, χαριέντως ἀποκρίνομαι. τὸ γὰρ πλήθει πυκνότητά φημι
δηλοῦν. αὖθις δ᾽ ἂν ἑτέροις ἀποκριναίμην, τὸ πλήθει σφοδρότητα δηλοῦν, καὶ πάντα μᾶλλον ἢ πληρότητα φήσαιμ᾽ ἄν, ἵνα
γνῶσιν ὅση τοῖς φλυαρεῖν βουλομένοις ἐστὶν ἐξουσία. διὰ τί γὰρ
50 πληρότητι μᾶλλον, οὐ πυκνότητι δηλώσει τὸ πλῆθος; ἢ ὅτι τὴν
πρώτην συλλαβὴν ἔν τε τῇ πληρότητι καὶ πλήθει διὰ τῶν αὐτῶν
στοιχείων λέγομεν;
    ... ἀλλ᾽ εὔλογον, φασίν, ἔστι καὶ τὴν κατὰ πληρότητα
διαφορὰν ὑπάρχουσαν ἐν τοῖς σφυγμοῖς εἰρῆσθαι νῦν καὶ
55 γινώσκεσθαι πρὸς Ἡροφίλου. τί δ᾽ οὐκ εὔλογον καὶ τὴν
⟨πυκνότητα καὶ τὴν⟩ σκληρότητα γινώσκεσθαι καὶ λέγεσθαι;
καὶ γὰρ καὶ αὗται διαφοραί τέ εἰσι σφυγμῶν καὶ πάντως αὐτὰς
ἐγίνωσκεν Ἡρόφιλος.
    πόθεν οὖν τὴν κατὰ πληρότητα λέγει, κάλλιον ἦν, οἶμαι,
60 μακρῷ πρότερον ἀναγνῶναι πάντ᾽ αὐτοῦ τὰ περὶ σφυγμῶν
συγγράμματα. καὶ γάρ μοι καὶ νόμος οὗτος ἐξηγήσεως,
ἕκαστον τῶν ἀνδρῶν ἐξ ἑαυτοῦ σαφηνίζεσθαι καὶ μὴ κεναῖς
ὑπονοίαις καὶ φάσεσιν ἀναποδείκτοις ἀπολήρειν ὅ τι τις
βούλεται. ποῦ τοίνυν εὗρες ἀλλαχόθι τό τοῦ πλήρους ὄνομα
65 παρ᾽ Ἡροφίλῳ; τὸ μὲν γὰρ τοῦ πυκνοῦ μυριάκις. ὅταν οὖν ἡ μὲν
κατὰ πληρότητα διαφορὰ μήτ᾽ εἰς διάγνωσιν ἥκει, καθότι
δέδεικται, μήθ᾽ Ἡρόφιλος αὐτῆς ἑτέρωθι μνημονεύει, ἡ δὲ κατὰ
πυκνότητα καὶ πρὸς ἁπάντων ὡμολόγηται, καὶ μυριάκις αὐτὴν
Ἡρόφιλος εὑρίσκεται γράφων, εὐλογώτερον ἂν εἴη, πυκνότητα
70 νομίζειν εἰρῆσθαι μᾶλλον ἢ πληρότητα, καὶ οὐ τοῦτό φημι νῦν,
ὡς τὸ πλήθει γέγραφεν Ἡρόφιλος ἀντὶ τοῦ πυκνότητι, γελοῖος
γὰρ ἂν εἴην ὁμοίως ἐκείνοις ἐξηγητής, εἰ τοῦτο λέγοιμι, ἀλλὰ ὅτι
ῥᾷον ἔστι καὶ πυκνότητα καὶ σκληρότητα καὶ πάντα μᾶλλον ἢ
τὴν πληρότητα δεῖξαι δηλούμενα.
75   ἐγὼ δὲ τί μὲν δηλοῖ τὸ πλήθει παρ᾽ Ἡροφίλῳ δι᾽ ἑτέρων οἶμαι
σαφῶς ἐξηγήσασθαι, νῦν δὲ ὅτι οὐ δηλοῖ πληρότητα, πῶς οὖν
ἀποδείκνυμεν αὐτό; πρῶτον μὲν ἐπιφέρων εὐθύς φησιν ὡδί –
γράψω γὰρ τὴν ῥῆσιν ὅλην, ἵνα μᾶλλον θαυμάσῃς τὴν ἄνοιαν
τῶν ἀνθρώπων πληρότητα τῷ πλήθει νομιζόντων λέγεσθαι·
80   ''καθ᾽ ὅλου μὲν οὖν δοκεῖ διαφέρειν σφυγμὸς σφυγμοῦ πλήθει,
μεγέθει, τάχει, σφοδρότητι, ῥυθμῷ. ἐκ τοῦ κατὰ ταῦτα διαφέρειν
φανερὸς γίνεται ἐνίοτε ὅ τε οἰκεῖος καὶ οὐκ οἰκεῖος. φαίνεται δὲ
διαφέρειν καὶ ἐπιγινώσκεσθαι καθόλου μὲν ἕτερος ἑτέρου σφυγμός, ὡς εἴρηται, ῥυθμῷ, μεγέθει, τάχει, σφοδρότητι. εἰ δὲ ἐν τῷ

85 αὐτῷ ῥυθμῷ φαίνεται διαφέρειν ἕτερος ἑτέρου σφυγμὸς σφυγμοῦ, τάχει, μεγέθει, σφοδρότητι."

τίνα βούλει πιστότερον Ἡροφίλου λαβεῖν μάρτυρα τῆς
Ἡροφίλου γνώμης; "φαίνεται", φησίν, "ἕτερος ἑτέρου διαφέρειν
σφυγμός, ὥσπερ εἴρηται, ῥυθμῷ, μεγέθει, τάχει, σφοδρότητι".

90 πῶς οὖν εἴπερ ὅλως διαφοράν τινα σφυγμῶν τὸ πλήθει δηλοῖ,
παρέλιπεν αὐτὴν νῦν, ἐπαναλαμβάνων τὸν λόγον, οὐχ ἁπλῶς,
οὐδ᾽ ἀργῶς, ἀλλὰ μετὰ τοῦ προσθεῖναι "ὡς εἴρηται"; πῶς δὲ
τοὺς ἐν ταὐτῷ ῥυθμῷ σφυγμούς φησι τάχει καὶ μεγέθει καὶ
σφοδρότητι διαφέρειν;

95 πῶς δ᾽ ἐφεξῆς τὰς καθ᾽ ἡλικίαν διαφορὰς ἐκτιθέμενος, ταῖς
μὲν ἄλλαις διορίζει τοὺς σφυγμούς, παρέλιπε δὲ τὴν
πληρότητα; καὶ κατὰ τὰ πάθη δὲ καὶ τὰς ὥρας καὶ τὰ
ἐπιτηδεύματα καὶ τἆλλα πάντα διορίζων τοὺς σφυγμοὺς τῶν
μὲν ἄλλων πασῶν ἀεὶ μνημονεύει διαφορῶν, τῆς πληρότητος δ᾽

100 οὐδαμοῦ. καὶ τὸ μεῖζον, αὐτὴν ταύτην τὴν λέξιν σχεδὸν καθ᾽
ἕκαστον αὐτῶν προσγράφων οὐδαμοῦ τὸ πλήθει προσέθηκεν,
ἀλλ᾽ ἐν τῷ α᾽ βιβλίῳ μόνον, οὐκ ἐν τοῖς ἅπασι λόγοις, οὐκ ἂν
παραλιπών, εἴπερ ὄνομα διαφορᾶς ἦν σφυγμῶν. ταῦθ᾽ ὥσπερ
ἐπιτομὴ τῶν εἰρημένων ἡμῖν ἐν τοῖς περὶ τῆς καθ᾽ Ἡρόφιλον ἐν

105 τοῖς σφυγμοῖς διαφορᾶς ἔστω λελεγμένα. δι᾽ ἐκείνων γὰρ ἐπὶ
πλέον ἐξηγησάμεθα τὴν Ἡροφίλου τῶν κατὰ σφυγμοὺς ὀνομάτων συνήθειαν.

(*Vid. etiam T163a–b; T276; T164sqq infra.*)

23–25 ταλαίπωροι *Schöne*: ἀταλαίπωροι *vulg.*   26 ἂν εἴπεν *vulg.: corr.*
Schöne   39 περὶ *delevi* (cf. T162.65–74)   56 πυκνότητα καὶ τὴν *add. De*
Lacy (*cf.* T162.73)   79 πληρότητι τὸ *vulg.: corr. De Lacy*   86–87
σφοδρότητι, τίνα *vulg.: correxi*

162 Yet how could one believe that people who cannot discern the
quality of the contents through a single coat in the case of a wineskin,
can discern the quality inside the artery through a skin which is not
less thick than that of a wineskin, and through at least two
membranes, and through what must be two [arterial] coats? Let
them then maintain this themselves, but let them not falsify
Herophilus, and let them not embarrass – with a revered name –
those who are ignorant of Herophilus' writings, and let them not
procure belief in their argument on this basis [*Chapter* III, T39]. For, it
is shameful to contend with witnesses as in a court. If you can say

something with a view to providing proof, I will gladly listen to you. But calling on Herophilus and Herophileans as one's witnesses is characteristic of someone who runs away from the direct contest and, for fear of cross-examination, discovers a pretext and evasions and contrivances. It is clear that falsified witnesses are introduced not for the sake of inquiring further into the matter but for historical sanction. 'Does Herophilus say this?' 'Of course not.' 'But then surely you must be lying,' 'Show how I am lying; show how he argues!' And then, it may be, an ambiguous text is put forward and a battle is joined concerning it: what could the text possibly mean? and what is its intention? . . .[*See Chapter* x, *T276 infra.*]

What then has not been said by the more recent physicians regarding this problem, some establishing that Herophilus knew this difference between pulses [sc. their degree of 'fullness'], too, others trying to show that he did not know it? Both sides are pathetic and worthy of our pity, the first for their ignorance, the second for their competitiveness. We, too, are in fact pitiful – at least in so far as it is not enough for us to cultivate our own theory of the art [of sphygmology], but we want to know what Herophilus said; what Heraclides, Chrysermus, and Hegetor did not explain correctly; what Apollonius, Bacchius, and Aristoxenus said in opposition. Even if we do not want to know, we are simply compelled to and [thus] have the benefit of two evils: that we speak rubbish although it is not necessary, and that, although we do not want to, we do this just as they do. I must, therefore, now do one of two things: either appear to say the opposite of Archigenes and Herophilus and a host of others, or demonstrate that there is no 'full pulse' (*plērēs sphygmos*) according to Herophilus.

. . . But for all those who want to learn ancient history, and who have the time for it, I shall add everything, showing that Herophilus did not use the 'full pulse' at all for any purpose.

First, I shall start from the passage they put forward, which is recorded in Book ɪ of Herophilus' *On Pulses*. This is also the only passage they seem to have read [*Chapter* ɪɪɪ, *T23*]. It runs as follows: 'In general, then, pulse is thought to differ from pulse in mass (*plēthos*), in size, in speed, in vehemence, and in rhythm.'

This passage they put forward, asking what 'mass' (*plēthos*) is, just as if we would not recognize what kind of thing he signifies with 'mass' and as if 'fullness' (*plērotēs*) were necessarily what it means. I then answer – cleverly, I think: for I say the expression 'in mass' (*plēthos*) signifies 'frequency' (*pyknotēs*). Then again, I would answer others: 'in mass' signifies 'vehemence' (*sphodrotēs*), and I would say everything rather than 'fullness', so that they may recognize how great a scope there is for those who wish to speak nonsense. You see, for what reason would he rather signify 'mass' by 'fullness' (*plērotēs*), and not by 'frequency' (*pyknotēs*)? Or is it because we pronounce the first syllable in both 'fullness' (*plē-rotēs*) and 'mass' (*plē-thos*) with the same letters?

. . . But it is probable, they say, that the difference in 'fullness' (*plērotēs*) that occurs in pulses was mentioned at this time [sc. in this passage] and was recognized by Herophilus. Why, then, is it not probable that [frequency and] hardness (*sklērotēs*) were mentioned and recognized? For these, too, are differences between pulses and Herophilus certainly recognized them.

On whatever ground one therefore mentions the distinction by 'fullness', it would be far better, I think, first to have read all his writings on the pulse. And this is also my law of interpretation, to explain clearly each author out of himself and not to spout forth empty conjectures and unproven assertions [about] what any [author] intends to say. Where else, then, in Herophilus did you find the word 'full' (*plērēs*)? 'Frequent' (*pyknon*), by contrast, yes, ten thousand times. So, since the difference in 'fullness' neither reached the point of being discerned, as was shown, nor is mentioned elsewhere by Herophilus, whereas the difference in frequency (*pyknotēs*) is conceded by all, and Herophilus is found to record it ten thousands of times, it would be more reasonable to think that 'frequency' was meant rather than 'fullness'. And with this I am not saying that Herophilus wrote 'in mass' (*plēthei*) for 'in frequency' (*pyknotēti*), for, if I were to say it, as an interpreter I would be subject to the same kind of ridicule as they. Rather. I am saying that it is easier to demonstrate that frequency, hardness, and all the other [pulse qualities] are signified than that 'fullness' is.

In other books, I think, I have explained clearly what 'in mass' signifies in Herophilus; but now, how do I demonstrate that it does not signify 'fullness'? First, right at the outset, when he introduces the subject, Herophilus says this – I am actually recording the passage in its entirety, so that you may be more amazed at the foolishness of those people who think that 'fullness' is meant by 'mass':

'In general, then, pulse seems to differ from pulse in mass, in size, in speed, in vehemence, and in rhythm. From the fact that they differ in these respects, the pulse clearly at times becomes proper (*oikeios*), at times not proper. One pulse appears to differ from another, and in general to be recognized [as different], in rhythm, size, speed, and vehemence, as was said. But if, in the same rhythm, one pulse appears to differ from another, then in speed, size, and vehemence.'

What more reliable witness to Herophilus' view do you wish to get than Herophilus? 'One pulse appears', he says, 'to differ from another in rhythm, size, speed, and vehemence, as was said.' If indeed the expression 'in mass' actually signifies some difference between pulses, why, then, did he omit it here [in the second enumeration] when he resumed his argument, not simply or lazily, but with the addition 'as was said'? And why does he say that pulses *in the same rhythm* differ in speed, size, and vehemence?

And, subsequently, when he sets forth the pulse differences according to stages of life, why does he define pulses by other differences but omit 'fullness'? He distinguishes the pulses according to afflictions, seasons, living habits, and all the rest, and always mentions all the other differences; but 'fullness'? Nowhere. And what's more, while he appended these very words in just about every case, he nowhere added 'in mass'. Rather, only in Book I, not in all his works [did he add it], although he would not have omitted it if indeed it were a name of a difference between pulses. Let this stand as a summary of what I said in my books *On the difference in pulses according to Herophilus*. For in them I gave a more elaborate exposition of Herophilus' customary use of names involving the pulse. (*See also T163a–T163b; T276; and T164ff infra.*)

163a Archigenes apud Galenum, *De pulsuum differentiis* 2.6 (VIII, pp. 592–3K)

... ἐν τῷ περὶ τάξεως καὶ ἀταξίας ὁμαλότητός τε καὶ ἀνωμαλίας λόγῳ τὰ γένη τούτων τῶν διαφορῶν (sc. τῶν σφυγμῶν) ἀκατονόμαστα λέγων εἶναι, τόνδε τὸν τρόπον ἄρχεται (sc. ὁ Ἀρχιγένης). "ὁ δὲ Ἡρόφιλος κατὰ γένος τὰς ἄλλας διαφορὰς 5 τῶν σφυγμῶν ἐκθέμενος οὕτως, 'μέγεθος, τάχος, σφοδρότης,

ῥυθμός', ἀσυζύγως κατ' εἶδος τάξεως ἐμνήσθη καὶ ἀταξίας
ὁμαλότητός τε καὶ ἀνωμαλίας. ἐγκαλεῖται τοίνυν ὑπὸ τῶν
μικραιτίων ὡς γένεσιν εἴδη ἀντιδιαστειλάμενος." ταῦτα μὲν
κατὰ τὴν ἀρχὴν τοῦ λόγου· κατωτέρω δὲ οὐκέτι τὸ Ἡροφίλῳ
10 δοκοῦν ἐξηγούμενος, ἀλλὰ τὴν ἑαυτοῦ γνώμην γράφων (sc. ὁ
Ἀρχιγένης) ἐν τῷ περὶ τάξεως καὶ ἀταξίας λόγῳ, τί φησι; . . .

163a In his discussion of the regularity and irregularity [of pulses],
and of their evenness and unevenness, [Archigenes] says that the
genera of these [pulse] differences are nameless, and this is the way he
starts: 'Although Herophilus expounded the other differences
between pulses by genus as follows, namely by "size, speed,
vehemence, and rhythm", he also mentioned regularity (*taxis*) and
irregularity (*ataxia*) and evenness (*homalotēs*) and unevenness (*anōmalia*) by species without combining them [sc. into genera]. He is,
therefore, charged by petty accusers with having contrasted species
with genera.' This is at the beginning of his discussion. Later,
however, when Archigenes is no longer expounding Herophilus' view
but recording his own opinion in his discussion of regularity and
irregularity, what does he say? . . .

163b Archigenes apud Galenum, *De pulsuum differentiis* 2.10 (VIII,
p. 625K)

τοῦ μὲν δὴ μὴ καινοτομεῖν πρῶτος Ἀρχιγένης μάρτυς, ὡδί πως
γράφων κατὰ τὴν ἀρχὴν τοῦ περὶ τάξεώς τε καὶ ἀταξίας
ὁμαλότητός τε καὶ ἀνωμαλίας λόγου· "Ἡρόφιλος κατὰ γένος
τὰς ἄλλας διαφορὰς τῶν σφυγμῶν ἐκθέμενος οὕτως· 'μέγεθος,
5 τάχος, σφοδρότης, ῥυθμός', ἀσυζύγως κατ' εἶδος τάξεως
ἐμνήσθη καὶ ἀταξίας ὁμαλότητός τε καὶ ἀνωμαλίας." ἐν ταύτη
τῇ λέξει σαφῶς ὁ Ἀρχιγένης οὐ μόνον ὅτι διαφοραὶ περὶ τοὺς
σφυγμούς εἰσιν, ἀλλὰ καὶ ὡς αἱ μέν τινες αὐτῶν κατὰ γένος, αἱ
δὲ κατ' εἶδος ἐμνημόνευσεν.

3 λόγου *ABHLV*: γένους *Kühn (sed* tractatus *in versione latina)*

163b Archigenes is my first witness that I am not instituting
innovations, since he writes as follows at the beginning of his
discussion of regularity and irregularity and of evenness and

unevenness: 'Although Herophilus expounded the other pulse differences by genus as follows, namely by "size, speed, vehemence, and rhythm", he also mentioned regularity (*taxis*) and irregularity (*ataxia*), and evenness (*homalotēs*) and unevenness (*anōmalia*), by species without combining them [sc. into genera].' In this statement Archigenes clearly not only mentions that there are differences in pulses, but also that some differences are generic, others specific.

164 Galenus, *De pulsuum differentiis* 3.2 (VIII, p. 645K)

Ἡρόφιλος μὲν γάρ φησι ῥώμην τῆς κατὰ τὰς ἀρτηρίας ζωτικῆς δυνάμεως αἰτίαν εἶναι σφοδροῦ σφυγμοῦ.

1 τὰς *coni. De Lacy:* τῆς *Kühn,* edd. vett.

164 For Herophilus says that the strength of the vital faculty in the arteries is the cause of a vehement (*sphodros*) pulse.

165 Galenus, *De pulsuum differentiis* 2.10 (VIII, p. 632K)

ὅσα μὲν οὖν Χρύσιππος εἰς τὴν τῶν Ἀθηναίων ἐξυβρίζει διάλεκτον, τάχ' ἄν ποτε καὶ αὖθις ἡμῖν διελθεῖν γένοιτο· τὰ δ' Ἀρχιγένους ταυτὶ τὰ νῦν ἡμῖν προκείμενα θαυμαστῶς ὁρᾷς ὁμόλογα, φοβηθέντος μὲν εἰπεῖν πρῶτα γένη καὶ πρώτας
5 διαφορὰς καὶ γενικὰς διαφορὰς καὶ γένη διαφορῶν, καίτοι τούτων ἁπάντων συνήθων μὲν τοῖς Ἕλλησιν ὄντων, ὑπὸ Ἡροφίλου δὲ καὶ τῶν Ἡροφιλείων σχεδὸν ἁπάντων μυριάκις εἰρημένων, ἐξευρόντος δὲ τὸ τῆς ποιότητος ὄνομα κατὰ πάντων κοινόν.

165 All of Chrysippus' outrages against the dialect of the Athenians I could perhaps expound upon again at some point, but you see these amazingly similar outrages by Archigenes that now lie before us. He feared, on the one hand, to mention primary genera and primary differences, also generic differences and genera of differences, although all these things were not only customary among the Greeks, but were also mentioned countless times by Herophilus and almost all the Herophileans. Yet, on the other hand, he 'discovered' the word 'quality', which is common to all of them.

166 Galenus, *De pulsuum differentiis* 2.7 (VIII, p. 602K)

'Αρχιγένης δὲ – τούτου γὰρ πρώτου δίκαιον μνημονεύειν μετά
γε τὸν Ἡρόφιλον ἐπιφωνήσαντας τὸν Ὅμηρον· 'οἷος πέπνυται,
τοὶ δὲ σκιαὶ ἀίσσουσιν' – οὐ μόνον ἐν τοῖς ὀνόμασιν ἔοικεν, ἀλλὰ
καὶ πολὺ πρότερον ἐν τοῖς πράγμασιν αὐτοῖς τεταράχθαι.

166 Archigenes, however – for it is right to mention him first, at least
after Herophilus, having invoked Homer: 'He alone understands,
and the shades flit around' – seems to be in a state of confusion not
only with reference to names but even much more so with reference to
the facts themselves.

167 Galenus, *De pulsuum differentiis* 3.1 (VIII, p. 643K)

ἄλλο δέ τι μεῖζον ἁμάρτημα (sc. τοῦ 'Αρχιγένους) τῆς ἐν τοῖς
ὀνόμασι μικρολογίας ἁμαρτάνουσι σχεδὸν ἅπαντες οἱ μεθ'
Ἡρόφιλον περὶ τῶν σφυγμῶν γεγραφότες.

167 Almost all people who wrote about the pulse after Herophilus
made some other mistake, bigger than [Archigenes'] hair-splitting in
matters of nomenclature.

168 Marcellinus, *De pulsibus* 27 (p. 467 Schöne)

τῶν δὴ σφυγμῶν ἀναγκαῖον καὶ τὰ ὀνόματα ἐκθέσθαι. οὕτω γὰρ
ἂν εὐσημότερον διδαχθείημεν τὰς προσηγορίας κατατάξαντες
αὐτῶν. κεῖται δὲ καὶ παρ' Ἡροφιλείοις καὶ παρὰ 'Αρχιγενείοις
τούτων κατάλογος. καλεῖται γὰρ ὁ μέν τις ἐκλείπων σφυγμός, ὁ
5 δὲ διαλείπων, ὁ δὲ παλινδρομῶν καὶ δορκαδίζων καὶ τρομώδης
καὶ μύουρος.

1 τῶν . . . γὰρ *om. PV*   δὴ *AM*: δὲ *BFH*   ἀναγκαῖόν ἐστιν ἐκθέσθαι
καὶ τὰ ὀνόματα *FH*: ἀναγκαῖον κατονομασθέντα *B*   2 διδαχθείημεν
ABFH: διδαχθεῖναι *M*: *fort.* διαλεχθείημεν *Schöne*   κατατάξαντες *ABM*:
κατάρξαντες *FH*   3 αὐτῶν *AFH*: αὐτῆς *B*: αὐτοῖς *M*   κεῖται δὲ *om.*
M in lac.: κεῖται δ *F*   παρ' *ABM*: παρὰ *FH*   παρὰ *om. H*
'Αρχιγενείοις *BFH*: 'Αρχιγενίοις *M*: 'Αρχιγένει οἷς *A*   6 μείουρος *F*

168 It is a matter of necessity also to set forth the nomenclature of the pulses, for in this way, having set down their appellations in order, we would be more distinctly instructed. A list of these is also found in the works of the followers of Herophilus and Archigenes. One is called a 'fading' pulse, another 'discontinuous', and others 'recurrent', 'gazelle-like' [*caprizans*: capering], 'quivering' ['trembling'], and 'tapering off' ['mouse-tailed'].

169 Galenus, *De pulsuum differentiis* 1.28 (VIII, p. 556K)

καὶ ὁ δορκαδίζων δὲ κληθεὶς ὑπὸ Ἡροφίλου σφυγμός ἐστι μὲν ἐκ τῶν κατὰ μίαν διαστολὴν ἀνωμάλων, σύνθετος δὲ καὶ αὐτός ἐστιν, οὐδετέρας ἐφαπτόμενος τῶν προσιουσῶν τοῖς πρώτοις πέντε γένεσιν ἀνωμαλιῶν, ἀλλ' ὅταν καθ' ἓν μόριον ὁτιοῦν
5 διακόπτηται τὴν κίνησιν ἡ ἀρτηρία, τηνικαῦτα μάλιστα γενόμενος, οὐχ ἁπλῶς. οὐ γὰρ ὅλον τοῦτο τὸ γένος δορκαδίζων ἐστὶ σφυγμός, ἀλλ' ὅταν ἡ μετὰ τὴν ἡσυχίαν δευτέρα κίνησις ὠκυτέρα τε καὶ σφοδροτέρα τῆς προτέρας ᾖ.

169 And the pulse called 'gazelle-like' (*dorkadizōn* (*caprizans*: capering)) by Herophilus consists of uneven beats in one dilation, but is itself also a compound pulse, attaining neither of the unevennesses that attach to the five primary kinds; but, whenever the artery in any given single part interrupts its motion, then especially, but not absolutely, it occurs. For, this kind of pulse is not 'gazelle-like' in its entirety, but only when the second motion after the pause is both faster and more vehement than the first.

170 Marcellinus, *De pulsibus* 31 (pp. 468–9 Schöne)

Ἡρόφιλος μὲν ὁ πρῶτος ὀνομάσας δορκαδίζοντα σφυγμόν φησιν ἅπαξ ἑωρακέναι, ἐπί τινος εὐνούχου, ἡμῖν δὲ συνεχῶν ἐπὶ τῶν ἔργων ἐπέπεσεν ἔν τε φρενητικαῖς καὶ καρδιακαῖς διαθέσεσι.

1–3 *om.* BH   1 καὶ *post* ὁ *add.* F   σφυγμὸν *om.* P   2 φασιν *AM*
3 ἐνέπεσεν *F*   φρενιτικαῖς *FM*   διάθεσιν *V*

170 Herophilus, who was actually the first to give the 'gazelle-like' (*dorkadizōn* (*caprizans*)) pulse its name, says that he saw it once in the

case of a certain eunuch, but it has fallen under our observation continually in actual practice in conditions of delirium and heart disease.

171 Marcellinus, *De pulsibus* 35 (pp. 470–1 Schöne)

τίς ὁ τρομώδης σφυγμός . . . τῶν δὲ διαστολῶν καὶ τῶν συστολῶν ὑπὲρ εὐσήμου διδασκαλίας ἐροῦμεν καὶ παράδειγμά τι παρὰ τοῖς Ἡροφιλείοις τιθέμενον τοιοῦτον. ὥσπερ γάρ, φασί, τρυπήμασιν αὐλῶν περιτεθέντων λεπτοτάτων ἀραχναίων,
5 ἔπειτα ἐμπνευσθέντων ὑπὸ τοῦ μουσουργοῦ τῶν αὐλῶν πρὸς τὴν διαδρομήν τε καὶ τὴν ἔμπτωσιν τρομώδης αὐτῶν ὁρᾶται κίνησις ἐπὶ τοῖς τρυπήμασιν, οὐκ ἴσης οὐδὲ ὁμαλῆς γινομένης αὐτῶν τῆς διασαλεύσεως ὅλων, ἀλλὰ μετεωριζομένων κατ' ἄλλα μὲν μέρη μᾶλλον, κατ' ἄλλα δ' ἧττον, καὶ καθ' ἃ μὲν
10 εὐτονώτερον ἐπανισταμένων, καθ' ἃ δὲ ἀσθενέστερον, οὕτω δὴ καὶ τὴν ἀρτηρίαν κινεῖσθαι λέγουσιν ἀνωμάλως κατὰ μέν τι διαστελλομένην μέρος ἐπὶ πλέον, κατὰ δέ τι ἔλαττον καὶ πῆ μὲν βιαιότερον, πῆ δὲ ἀσθενέστερον.

1–13 *om.* FH   1 τίς ὁ τρομώδης σφυγμός *om.* M   1–13 τῶν (*pr.*) . . . ἀσθενέστερον *om.* B   2 ὑπὲρ εὐσήμου *AMP*: ὑπερευσημένου V   παραδείγματι *codd.*: *corr. Schöne*   3 Ἡροφιλίοις *APV*: ἡροφίλοις M   4 τυπήμασιν M   λεπτοτάτων . . . ἐμπνευσθέντων *om.* M.   5 μυσουργοῦ *APV*   6 τε *coni. Schöne*: δὲ *codd.*   αὐτῶν *om.* M   ὁρᾶται *AM* (*P corr. ex* ὁρᾶσθαι *u.v.*): ἐβαφαιται V   7 τοῖς *AM*: τῆς PV   οὐκ ἴσης *APV*: οὐ κίνησις M   8 διὰ ἐλεύσεως ὅλον M   μετεωριζόμενον M   9 δ' *om.* PV: δὲ M   ἧττον *Schöne*   13 πῆ *corr.* e τη V

171 What the quivering (*tromōdēs*) pulse is: . . . For the sake of clear instruction we shall also cite the following example – established among the Herophileans – of its dilations and contractions. For, they say, the artery moves unevenly, dilating more in one part, less in another, also more forcefully here, more weakly there, just as when very thin web-like [covers] have been placed around the holes in flutes and a musician then breathes into the flutes: at the holes a motion is observed that quivers in relation both to the passage of the breath and to its pressure. The vibration which arises is, however, neither equal nor even in the web-like covers as a whole, but they are raised more in some parts, less in others, rising more tautly in some, more weakly in others – so the artery, too, moves unevenly.

172 Ps.-Soranus, *Quaestiones medicinales* 172 (*Anecdota Graeca et Graecolatina*, vol. II, p. 265 Rose)

quid est rhythmos pulsus? Herophilus: 'rhythmos est motio in temporibus ordinationem habens definitam'. *(Cf. Ba. 3 infra).*

172 What is the rhythm of a pulse? Herophilus: 'Rhythm is a motion which has a defined regulation in time.' *(Cf. Chapter XIV, Ba. 3 infra.)*

173 Galenus, *De pulsuum dignotione* 3.3 (VIII, pp. 911–13K)

κατὰ ταῦτ' οὖν ἅπαντα τὰς ἐν ταῖς αἱρέσεσι πολλὰς ἀπορίας ἀνάγκη συμπίπτειν ἐν ταῖς τῶν ῥυθμῶν διαγνώσεσι, καὶ διὰ τοῦτ' οἶμαι μηδ' ἐπιχειρῆσαί τι γράψαι τοὺς μεθ' Ἡρόφιλον εἰς τὴν ἀπ' αὐτῶν πρόγνωσιν. αὐτὸς δὲ ὁ Ἡρόφιλος πολλαχόθι μὲν
5 ῥυθμῶν εἰς τὰς προγνώσεις μνημονεύει, χαλεπὸν μὴν ἐξευρεῖν τί ποτε καὶ λέγει τὸν ῥυθμόν, ἆρά γε τὸν λόγον τοῦ τῆς διαστολῆς μόνον χρόνου πρὸς τὸν τῆς συστολῆς μόνης, ἢ καὶ αὖ τὸν τῆς ἑπομένης ἑκατέρᾳ τῶν κινήσεων ἠρεμίας προσνέμει. καὶ διὰ τοῦτο οὐδὲ τοῖς ἀπ' αὐτοῦ κληθεῖσιν Ἡροφιλείοις ὁμολογεῖται,
10 τί ποθ' ὑπὲρ αὐτῶν φρονεῖ γε ὄντως. οὔτε γὰρ ἡ λέξις αὐτοῦ θάτερον ἐνδείκνυται σαφῶς οὔθ' ἡ τῶν πραγμάτων φύσις ἱκανὴ πιστώσασθαι ...
κείσθω τοίνυν διὰ τὴν χρείαν ἐν τῷ λόγῳ τοῦ χρόνου τῶν κινήσεων τὸν ῥυθμὸν συνίστασθαι, ζητησόντων ἡμῶν ἰδίᾳ ποτὲ
15 τὸ δοκοῦν Ἡροφίλῳ.

7 αὖ τὸν (*vel* [αὐ]τὸν) *coni.* De Lacy: αὐτὸν *vulg.*   9 ἀπ' *conieci:* ὑπ' *vulg.*   10 γε ὄντως *BLV:* δεόντως *vulg.*

173 In all these things many insoluble difficulties necessarily occur in the [medical] factions in differentiation of rhythms, and I think it is for this reason that physicians after Herophilus did not even attempt to write anything on prognosis based on rhythms. And while Herophilus himself in many places mentions rhythms with a view to prognoses, it is very difficult to discover just what he means by

'rhythm' (*rhythmos*): is it the ratio (*logos*)of the time of dilation (*diastolē*) to the time of contraction (*systolē*) only, or does he also attribute to 'rhythm' the time of the pause (*ēremia*) which follows upon each of the two motions? This is why there is no agreement, not even among those who are named 'Herophileans' after him, concerning just what Herophilus really thought about rhythms. For his words do not indicate one of the two alternatives clearly, nor is the nature of these things capable of providing confirmation . . .

Let it then be established, for practical purposes, that rhythm consists in the ratio of the time of the motions, since we will at some point make a separate inquiry about Herophilus' view.

174 Galenus, *De pulsuum dignotione* 3.3 (VIII, pp. 913–14K)

πῶς οὖν Ἡρόφιλος πρῶτός τινα πρὸς αἴσθησιν (sc. τῶν τοῦ
σφυγμοῦ ῥυθμῶν) ὑποτίθεται χρόνον, ᾧ τοὺς ἄλλους μετρῶν ἢ
δυοῖν, ἢ καὶ τριῶν ἢ καὶ πλειόνων εἶναι φάσκει, ἤτοι τελέων τε καὶ
ὡς αὐτοὶ καλοῦσιν ἀπαραύξων, ἢ καὶ ἀπηυξημένων ἐπ᾽ ὀλίγον,
5 ἢ ἐπὶ πλεῖον, ἢ ἐπὶ πλεῖστον; ὡς γὰρ ἐπὶ πάντων ἀκριβῶς τῶν
σφυγμῶν διαγινώσκων τοὺς χρόνους εἴτε τῶν κινήσεων μόνων
εἴτε καὶ τῶν μετ᾽ αὐτοὺς ἡσυχιῶν, οὐδὲν γὰρ διαφέρει πρός γε
τὴν παροῦσαν ἀπορίαν, ἔοικε ταῦτα γράφειν, εἰ μή τι οὐκ ἐπὶ
πάντων, ἀλλ᾽ ἐφ᾽ ὧν δυνατόν, ἐπὶ τούτων μόνον ἡγητέον αὐτὸν
10 τὰ τοιαῦτα γράφειν. τοῦτο μὲν οὖν τάχ᾽ ἂν ἰδίᾳ ποθ᾽ ὕστερον
ἐπισκεψόμεθα. νυνὶ δ᾽ οὐ γὰρ πρόκειται τὸ δοκοῦν Ἡροφίλῳ
ζητεῖν, ἀλλὰ τἀληθές τε ἅμα καὶ χρήσιμον ἐξευρεῖν, τοῦτο
πειρατέον ἐνδείξασθαι σαφῶς ὡς ἐπ᾽ αὐτῶν τῶν ἔργων ἡμῖν
πειρωμένοις εὑρέθη.

4 ἀπαραύξων dub. l.

174 Why then is Herophilus the first to establish a time-unit in relation to sense-perception [sc. for the rhythms of the pulse], a unit with which he measures other units, saying that they consist of two or also of three or even more [of the units], whether of complete units and, as they themselves call it 'units not subject to increase', or also of ones which have been diminished by a small amount or a greater or the greatest amount [i.e., fractions]? He seems to write these things as though, in *all* pulses, he were accurately discerning the time-units

either of their motions only or also of the pauses that follow the time-units of motion. (As regards the present difficulty, this actually makes no difference.) Or, if not in *all* pulses, but [only] in pulses where it is possible [to discern the time-units], we must then suppose that Herophilus made such statements with reference only to these. This I shall perhaps examine separately at some later time. But now, since the task which lies before us is not to inquire into what Herophilus thought, but to discover what is at once both true and useful, we must try to show this clearly as it is found by us when we experience it in actual practice.

175 Galenus, *Synopsis librorum suorum de pulsibus* 14 (IX, pp. 470–1K)

ἐν δὲ τῷ παραβάλλειν τὸν χρόνον τῆς διαστολῆς (sc. τοῦ σφυγμοῦ) τῷ χρόνῳ τῆς συστολῆς, ὡς Ἡρόφιλος ἠξίου, τὸ μὲν ὅτι παρὰ φύσιν ὁ κάμνων ἔχει δυνατόν ἐστι γνωσθῆναι, καὶ πρὸς τούτῳ γε ὅτι μεγάλως παρὰ φύσιν ἢ μικρῶς. αἱ μὲν γὰρ μεγάλαι
5 τῶν κατὰ φύσιν ῥυθμῶν εἰς τὸ παρὰ φύσιν ἐκτροπαὶ μεγάλην σημαίνουσι τὴν βλάβην, αἱ δ' ἥττους μικροτέραν. βραχεῖαν μὲν οὖν ἐκτροπὴν οἱ παράρυθμοι δηλοῦσι σφυγμοί, μείζονα δὲ οἱ ἑτερόρρυθμοι, μεγίστην δὲ οἱ ἔκρυθμοι.

175 In comparing the time of the dilation [of the pulse] to the time of the contraction, as Herophilus thought one should, it can be recognized that the ill person has [a pulse] contrary to nature, and in addition that it is greatly or negligibly contrary to nature. For, great deviations from the natural rhythms into that which is contrary to nature signify great harm, whereas lesser deviations signify smaller harm. For the pararhythmic pulses display the smallest deviation, hetero-rhythmic pulses a greater deviation, and ecrhythmic pulses the greatest.

176 Galenus, *De praesagitione ex pulsibus* 2.3 (IX, pp. 278–9K)

ἑξῆς δ' ἐστὶν ἐπί γε τῇ τάξει τοῦ λόγου περὶ ῥυθμῶν (sc. τῶν σφυγμῶν) διελθεῖν, ὑπὲρ ὧν Ἡροφίλῳ μὲν ἐπὶ πλέον εἴρηται τήρησίν τινα καὶ ἐμπειρίαν ἱστοροῦντι μᾶλλον ἢ λογικὴν μέθοδον

ἐκδιδάσκοντι. τοὺς γὰρ καθ' ἑκάστην ἡλικίαν ὡς τὸ πολὺ
5 φαινομένους ῥυθμοὺς τῶν σφυγμῶν ἔγραψε, πρῶτον μὲν οὐδ'
ἐφ' ὧν τινων φύσεων ἐτήρησεν αὐτοὺς οὐδὲν ἡμῖν εἰπών· εἶτ' ἐξ
αὐτῶν ὧν διδάσκει δῆλον ὅτι συγκέχυταί τε καὶ ἀδιάρθρωτός
ἐστι περὶ τὴν τῆς συστολῆς τε καὶ τῶν ἠρεμιῶν διάγνωσιν. εἴπερ
γὰρ ἡγεῖταί ποτε δύνασθαι γενέσθαι συστολὴν ἐπὶ τῶν γεγη-
10 ρακότων ἄχρι δὴ τῶν δέκα πρώτων χρόνων ἐκτεταμένην,
εὔδηλός ἐστι τῆς ὄντως συστολῆς ἀναισθήτως ἔχων. αὕτη γὰρ
ἐνίοτε μὲν ὀλιγοχρονιωτέρα τῆς διαστολῆς ἐστιν, ἐνίοτε δ'
ἰσόχρονός ἐστιν, ὁτὲ δέ, ὡς ἐκεῖνος γράφει, πολυχρονιωτέρα
μέν, οὐ μήν, ὡς οἴεται, πενταπλασίων, ἀλλὰ βραχεῖ τινι μείζων.
15 ὅσα δ' ἄλλα μοχθηρὰ καὶ ἀδιάρθρωτα καὶ ἀδύνατα πρὸς τὰς
προγνώσεις ἔχει τὰ περὶ ῥυθμῶν ὑφ' Ἡροφίλου λεγόμενα, τὰ μὲν
ἐκ τοῦ τρίτου περὶ τῆς διαγνώσεως τῶν σφυγμῶν ἔνεστι μαθεῖν,
τὰ δ' ἐξ ὧν ἰδίᾳ γράψομεν ὑπὲρ τῆς Ἡροφίλου περὶ τοὺς
σφυγμοὺς τέχνης.

176 Next in the sequence of my account I can expound upon
rhythms [of the pulse], concerning which quite a lot was said by
Herophilus, who gave an account of observation and experience,
rather than teaching a 'rational' (logikē) method. For, he described
the rhythms which appear predominantly in each stage of life. At first
he did not even tell us at all in which natures he observed them, but
then it became clear, on the basis of the things he did teach, that he is
confused and does not clearly articulate the distinction between
contraction and rest [pause]. For, if he actually thinks that a
contraction which is extended for as long as ten primary time-units
can arise in old people, he very clearly is not perceptive about what a
contraction really is. You see, sometimes it is of shorter duration than
the dilation, sometimes of equal duration, and at other times, as he
writes, of longer duration – but not, as he thinks, five times as long;
rather, only a little more. As regards all the other erroneous and
indistinctly articulated things, and also things impossible to use for
prognosis, that are contained in what Herophilus said about rhythms:
some of these can be learnt from Book III of my *On Differentiating
Between Pulses* [cf. T173, T174], others from what I shall write
separately about Herophilus' art concerning the pulse.

177 Rufus Ephesius (?), *Synopsis de pulsibus* 4 (pp. 223–5
Daremberg/Ruelle)

τούτων δὲ οὕτως ἐχόντων, ἐροῦμεν πρῶτον τὰς διαφορὰς τῶν
φυσικῶς ἑκάστῃ ἡλικίᾳ παρεπομένων σφυγμῶν, ἔπειτα τὰς
γινομένας ἐπὶ τῶν πυρεσσόντων, καὶ μετὰ ταῦτα τοὺς εὑρισκο-
μένους κατὰ τὰ πάθη, τελευταῖον δὲ τοὺς παρὰ τοῖς ἀρχαίοις
5 κατονομασθέντας. τῶν μὲν οὖν ἀρτιγενῶν παίδων ὁ σφυγμὸς
ὑπάρχει βραχὺς παντελῶς καὶ οὐ διωρισμένος ἔν τε τῇ συστολῇ
καὶ τῇ διαστολῇ. τοῦτον τὸν σφυγμὸν Ἡρόφιλος ἄλογον
συνεστάναι φησίν· ἄλογον δὲ καλεῖ σφυγμὸν τὸν μὴ ἔχοντα πρός
τινα ἀναλογίαν· οὔτε γὰρ τὸν διπλάσιον, οὔτε τὸν ἡμιόλιον,
10 οὔτε ἕτερόν τινα λόγον ἔχει οὗτος, ἀλλά ἐστι βραχὺς παντελῶς
καὶ τῷ μεγέθει βελόνης κεντήματι ὁμοίως ἡμῖν ὑποπίπτει· διὸ
καὶ πρῶτον αὐτὸν Ἡρόφιλος ἄλογον δεόντως εἶπεν. προβαι-
νούσης δὲ τῆς ἡλικίας καὶ τοῦ σώματος εἰς αὔξησιν ἐρχομένου,
καὶ ὁ σφυγμὸς πρὸς λόγον μεγεθύνεται, πρὸς λόγον τὴν
15 διαστολὴν τῆς συστολῆς λαμβάνων πλατυτέραν· ὅ τε λοιπὸν
ἔστιν αὐτοῖς καὶ ἐφαρμόσαι πρὸς ἀπόδειξιν ἐκ τοῦ ποδισμοῦ τῆς
γραμματικῆς· ὁ μὲν γὰρ πρῶτος ἐπὶ τῶν ἀρτιγενῶν παίδων
εὑρισκόμενος σφυγμὸς ῥυθμὸν λήψεται τὸν τοῦ βραχυσυλλά-
βου· καὶ γὰρ ἐν τῇ διαστολῇ καὶ τῇ συστολῇ βραχὺς ὑπάρχει,
20 καὶ διὰ τοῦτο δίχρονος νοεῖται· ὁ δὲ τῶν πρὸς αὔξησιν ὄντων
ἀναλογεῖ τῷ τε παρὰ ἐκείνοις ποδὶ τροχαίῳ. ἔστι δὲ οὗτος
τρίχρονος, τὴν μὲν διαστολὴν ἐπὶ δύο χρόνους λαμβάνων, ἐπὶ
ἕνα δὲ τὴν συστολήν. ὁ δὲ τῶν ἀκμαζόντων ταῖς ἡλικίαις ἐν
ἀμφοτέροις ἴσος ὑπάρχει, ἔν τε τῇ διαστολῇ καὶ τῇ συστολῇ,
25 συγκρινόμενος τῷ καλουμένῳ σπονδείῳ, ὃς τῶν δισυλλάβων
ποδῶν μακρότατός ἐστιν· ἔστιν οὖν συγκείμενος ἐκ χρόνων
τεσσάρων. τοῦτον τὸν σφυγμὸν Ἡρόφιλος διὰ ἴσου καλεῖ. ὁ δὲ
τῶν παρακμαζόντων καὶ σχεδὸν ἤδη γερόντων καὶ αὐτὸς ἐκ
τριῶν σύγκειται χρόνων, τὴν συστολὴν τῆς διαστολῆς διπλῆν
30 παραλαμβάνων καὶ χρονιωτέραν.

6 καὶ δεδιορισμένος F   11 κεντήματος ἡμῖν F   16–17 ἀπόδειξιν τοῦ
ἐκ τῆς γραμματικῆς ποδισμοῦ F   18 τὸν *om.* P   19 τῇ *(sec.) om.*
F   25 συγκρινόμενος . . . σπονδείῳ *om.* P   26 κείμενος *codd.: corr.*
Daremberg/Ruelle   29–30 τὴν διαστολὴν τῆς συστολῆς FG

177 These things being the case, I shall first treat the differences

between the pulses which naturally attend each stage of life, then those that occur in people having a fever, after that the pulses found in diseases [in different parts of the body], and finally the pulses to which the ancients gave particular names. The pulse of newborn children, then, is completely short and not distinct in its contraction and dilation. Herophilus says this pulse is constituted 'without definable ratios' (*a-logos*; 'irrational'). He calls the pulse which is without a relation to some ratio (*ana-logia*) a pulse 'without definable ratios', for it has neither a double ratio, nor a ratio of one and a half to one, nor any other proportion (*logos*), but rather is completely short, and we observe it to be similar in size to the prick of a needle. For this reason Herophilus first called it 'without definable ratios', as one should. But when one's age progresses and one's body comes into its full growth, the pulse, too, increases with reference to ratio, getting a dilation which is proportionately more extended than the contraction. For the rest, one can also adapt their [proportions] to a demonstration based on the scansion that belongs to the art of philology. You see, the first pulse found in newborn children will have the rhythm of a short-syllabled metrical foot, since it is short in both dilation and contraction, and it therefore is conceived of as consisting of two [short] time-units, whereas the pulse of children who are growing is analogous to the metrical foot [known] among them as trochee. This pulse consists of three time-units, holding its dilation for two time-units, but its contraction for one. And the pulse of those in the prime stage of their lives is equal in both, that is, in dilation and contraction, and it is compared to the foot called spondee, which is the longest of the disyllabic feet. It is actually composed of four [short] time-units. This pulse Herophilus calls 'in equal quantity' (*dia isou*). The pulse of those who are beyond their prime, and almost old, is itself also composed of three time-units, holding its contraction for twice as long as its dilation and longer [i.e., an iambic pulse].

178 Galenus, *Synopsis librorum suorum de pulsibus* 21 (IX, p. 499K)

οὐ γὰρ μόνον φλεβοπαλία παιδικὴ γέροντι κακόν, ἀλλὰ γερον-
τικὴ παιδί. δέκα γοῦν χρόνων τῶν πρώτων, ὡς Ἡρόφιλος
ἐμέτρει τοὺς σφυγμούς, εἰ παιδίῳ γεννηθείη ποτὲ τὸ μεταξὺ δύο
πληγῶν διάστημα, ψύξεως ἐσχάτης καὶ διὰ τοῦτο καὶ νεκρώ-

5 σεώς ἐστι σημεῖον· ὡσπερεὶ γέροντι πάλιν παιδίων σφυγμός, ἐν
ᾧ τῆς διαστολῆς ὁ χρόνος ἴσος ἐστὶ τῷ τῆς συστολῆς,
ἐκπεπυρῶσθαι σημαίνει τὴν φύσιν.

3 γενηθείη coni. De Lacy

178 Not only is the pulse-beat of children bad in an old man, but also
that of old men in a child. Accordingly, if ever in a child the interval
between the two pulse-beats increases to ten 'primary time-units', as
Herophilus used to measure pulses, it is a sign of extreme chilling and
therefore also of mortification. Just as, conversely, in an old man the
children's pulse, in which the time of the dilation is equal to that of the
contraction, signifies that his nature (*physis*) has become excessively
heated.

179 Galenus, *Synopsis librorum suorum de pulsibus* 21 (ix, p. 493K)

... κἀπὶ τῶν παίδων ἔνιοι τὸν σφυγμὸν εἶναι μικρὸν λέγουσιν,
οὐ τῇ κατὰ τὴν ἀρτηρίαν εὐρυχωρίᾳ παραβάλλοντες τὴν
διαστολήν, ἀλλὰ τῇ τῶν ἀκμαζόντων. ὡς ἐάν γε λογίσηταί τις,
ὁπηλίκη κατὰ κύκλον οὖσα τῶν παίδων ἡ ἀρτηρία τὸν σφυγμὸν
5 πηλίκον ἐργάζεται, γνώσεται ὅτι καλῶς ὁ Ἡρόφιλος ἔφη τὸν
σφυγμὸν αὐτῶν ἱκανὸν εἶναι τῷ μεγέθει.

179 .... Also in the case of children some people say that the pulse is
small, but they compare its dilation not to the capaciousness of the
artery, but to the [pulse dilation] of people in their prime. So, if
someone would calculate how large a pulse the artery of children
produces, being of how large a circumference, he will recognize that
Herophilus said correctly that their pulse is adequate in size.

180 Galenus, *Synopsis librorum suorum de pulsibus* 8 (ix, p. 453K)

τὸν γοῦν τοῦ παιδὸς σφυγμὸν ὁ μὲν Ἡρόφιλος ἱκανὸν τῷ μεγέθει
φησὶν ὑπάρχειν, ὁ δ' Ἀρχιγένης μικρόν. οὕτω δὴ καὶ τὸν
μυρμηκίζοντα ταχὺν εἶναι φησὶν ὁ Ἀρχιγένης, Ἡρόφιλος δὲ οὐ
ταχύν.

180 Herophilus therefore says the pulse of a child is adequate in size,

whereas Archigenes says it is small. Archigenes likewise says the 'ant-like' pulse (*myrmēkizōn* (*formicans*)) is fast, whereas Herophilus says it is not fast.

181 Galenus, *De pulsuum dignotione* 2.2 (VIII, p. 853K)

... ἀναγκαῖον ἐπίστασθαι τὸν σύμμετρον (sc. σφυγμόν). ἴσως γὰρ καὶ ὁ τοῦ παιδὸς ὑπὲρ τὸν σύμμετρόν ἐστιν. Ἡρόφιλος γοῦν ποτὲ μὲν εὐμεγέθη τὸν σφυγμὸν τοῦτον ὀνομάζει.

181 It is necessary to know the moderate [pulse]. For it is possible that the pulse of a child can also be beyond the moderate. Herophilus accordingly at times also called this pulse [sc. a child's] 'of a good size'.

182 Marcellinus, *De pulsibus* 11 (p. 463 Schöne)

τίς ἡ Ἡροφίλου στάσις περὶ τοῦ σφυγμοῦ τῶν πυρεσσόντων· ὁ δὲ Ἡρόφιλος πυρέσσειν ἀπεφήνατο τὸν ἄνθρωπον, ὁπόταν πυκνότερος καὶ μείζων καὶ σφοδρότερος ὁ σφυγμὸς γένηται μετὰ πολλῆς θερμασίας ἔνδον. εἰ μὲν οὖν προαπαλλάξειε τὴν
5 σφοδρότητα καὶ τὸ μέγεθος, ἔνδοσιν τοῦ πυρετοῦ λαμβάνοντος· τὴν δὲ πυκνότητα τῶν σφυγμῶν ἀρχομένων τε τῶν πυρετῶν πρώτην συνίστασθαι καὶ συμπαραμένειν μέχρι τῆς τελείας αὐτῶν λύσεως λέγει. οὕτω δὲ τῇ πυκνοσφυξίᾳ τὸν Ἡρόφιλον θαρρεῖν λόγος ὡς βεβαίῳ σημείῳ χρώμενον, ὥστε κλεψύδραν
10 κατασκευάσαι χωρητικὴν ἀριθμοῦ ῥητοῦ τῶν κατὰ φύσιν σφυγμῶν ἑκάστης ἡλικίας εἰσιόντα τε πρὸς τὸν ἄρρωστον καὶ τιθέντα τὴν κλεψύδραν ἅπτεσθαι τοῦ πυρέσσοντος· ὅσῳ δ' ἂν πλείονες παρέλθοιεν κινήσεις τῶν σφυγμῶν παρὰ τὸ κατὰ φύσιν εἰς τὴν ἐκπλήρωσιν τῆς κλεψύδρας, τοσούτῳ καὶ τὸν σφυγμὸν
15 πυκνότερον ἀποφαίνειν, τουτέστι πυρέσσειν ἢ μᾶλλον· ἢ ἧττον.

1 τίς ... πυρεσσόντων *om. M* ἡ *om. B* στάσις *ABF*: σύστασις *H*: τάσις *PV* τοῦ σφυγμοῦ *om. FH* 2 ὁ πόταν *ABMFH* (ὁπότ' ἂν *FH*): ὁπότε *P*: ὅπερ *V* 4 προαπαλλάξειε *AP*: προαπαλάξειεν *B*: πρὸ ἀπαλάξει ἐν *V*: ἀπαλλάξειε *FH*: ἀπαλάξειε *M* 5 ἔνδοσιν *AMPV*: ἔνδοσι *B*: ἔνωσιν *F*: ἄνεσιν *H* 6 δὲ *om. FHM* τε *om. FHMPV* 7 μέχρι τῆς] μετὰ *P* 8-15 λέγει ... ἧττον *om. B.* 8-9 οὕτω ... λόγος *om.*

F 8 οὔπω *HM* τὴν πυκνοσφυξίαν *HM* 9 βεβαίως *V*
χρώμενος *F* 10 τῶν *AFHM*: τῆς *PV* 11 τε *om.* *F* 12 ὅσαι
FHM 13 κινήσεις *om.* *FHM* τῶν σφυγμῶν *FHM*: τῷ σφυγμῷ
APV τὸ *APV*: τῶν *FHM* 14 ἐκλήρωσιν *APV*: πλήρωσιν *FHM*:
fort. ἐκκένωσιν *Schmidt*: ἐκπλήρωσιν τοῦ χρόνου *Diels* τοσούτῳ *corr.*
Schöne e τοσοῦτο *A*: τοσούτων *P*: τοσοῦτον *rell.* 15 ἢ βραδύτερον *post*
πυκνότερον *add.* *Diels*

182 What Herophilus' position concerning the pulse of those
suffering from fever is: Herophilus gave the opinion that a person has
a fever whenever his pulse becomes more frequent, bigger, and
stronger, [and is] accompanied by a high internal temperature. So, if
the pulse loses its strength and magnitude, [it is] because the fever is
getting [some] relief. The frequency of the pulse-beats, on the other
hand, not only first arises when the fevers begin, but then also
continues to linger up to the complete remission of the fever – thus
Herophilus. There is a story that Herophilus had such confidence in
the frequency of the pulse, using it as a reliable diagnostic sign, that he
constructed a water-clock capable of containing a specified amount
for the natural pulses of each age. And, upon entering to visit a
patient, he would set up his water-clock and feel the pulse of the
person suffering from a fever. By as much as the movements of the
pulse exceeded the number that is natural for filling up the water-
clock, by that much he declared the [patient's] pulse too frequent –
that is, that [the patient] had either more or less of a fever.

183 Galenus, *Synopsis librorum suorum de pulsibus* 12 (IX,
pp. 463–5K)

γέγραπται μὲν οὖν καὶ Ἡροφίλῳ τὰ κατὰ τοὺς χρόνους μετὰ
τῆς διαστολῆς τε καὶ συστολῆς (sc. τῶν σφυγμῶν), ἕνεκα τῶν
ἡλικιῶν εἰς ῥυθμοὺς ἀνάγοντι τὸν λόγον. ὥσπερ γὰρ ἐκείνους οἱ
μουσικοὶ κατά τινας ὡρισμένας χρόνων τάξεις συνιστῶσι
5 παραβάλλοντες ἀλλήλαις ἄρσιν καὶ θέσιν, οὕτως καὶ Ἡρόφιλος
ἀνάλογον μὲν ἄρσει τὴν διαστολὴν ὑποθέμενος, ἀνάλογον δὲ
θέσει τὴν συστολὴν τῆς ἀρτηρίας, ἀρξάμενος ἀπὸ τοῦ νεογε-
νοῦς παιδίου τὴν τήρησιν ἐποιήσατο, πρῶτον χρόνον αἰσθητὸν
ὑποθέμενος ἐν ᾧ διαστελλομένην εὕρισκε τὴν ἀρτηρίαν, ἴσον δ'
10 αὐτῇ καὶ τὸν τῆς συστολῆς εἶναι φησίν, οὐ πάνυ τι διοριζόμενος
ὑπὲρ ἑκατέρας τῶν ἡσυχιῶν.

οἷς γὰρ ἀναίσθητός ἐστιν ἡ τῆς ἀρτηρίας συστολή, τούτοις
εἰς δύο χρόνους τοὺς πάντας ὁ ῥυθμὸς τοῦ σφυγμοῦ μερίζεται,
τόν τε τῆς αἰσθητῆς κινήσεως, ἡνίκα πλήττει τὴν ἀφὴν ἡμῶν ἡ
15 ἀρτηρία διαστελλομένη, καὶ τὸ λοιπὸν ἅπαντα συγκείμενον ἔκ τε
τῆς ἐκτὸς ἠρεμίας καὶ τῆς μετ' αὐτὴν συστολῆς, καὶ τῆς ἐπ'
ἐκείνῃ πάλιν ἠρεμίας καὶ τῶν πρώτων τῆς διαστολῆς, ἅπερ
ἐστὶν ἀναίσθητα καὶ αὐτά. καὶ διὰ τοῦτο εἰς πληγὴν καὶ
διάλειμμα μερίζουσι τὸν σφυγμόν, ἐν τῷ τοῦ διαλείμματος πόσῳ
20 πυκνότητα καὶ ἀραιότητα τιθέμενοι, καθάπερ ἐν τῷ τῆς πληγῆς
τάχος καὶ βραδυτῆτα.

καθ' ὅσον μὲν οὖν δι' ἴσου (sc. χρόνου) τὸν τοῦ σφυγμοῦ
ῥυθμὸν εἶναί φησιν ἐπὶ τῶν ἀρτιγενῶν ὁ Ἡρόφιλος, κατὰ
τοσοῦτο διαγινώσκειν ἔδοξέ μοι τὴν ἀρχὴν τῆς συστολῆς· καθ'
25 ὅσον δὲ πάλιν ἄχρι δέκα χρόνων τῶν πρώτων ἐκτείνει τὴν
συστολὴν τῆς τῶν γερόντων ἀρτηρίας, κατὰ τοσοῦτο μηκέτι
διαγινώσκειν, ἀλλὰ τὴν διαστολὴν ταῖς αἰσθηταῖς κινήσεσι
γνωρίζειν, ἃς ἐκ τοῦ πλήττεσθαι τοὺς δακτύλους ἡμῶν δια-
γινώσκομεν, τὴν συστολὴν δὲ πᾶν τὸ λοιπὸν τίθεσθαι καθ' ὃ
30 κινήσεως οὐκ ἠσθάνετο. ἀλλὰ περὶ μὲν τῆς Ἡροφίλου περὶ τοὺς
σφυγμοὺς τέχνης ἐατέον.

22–3 τὸν τοῦ σφυγμοῦ ῥυθμὸν *coni. DeLacy*: τὸν τοῦ ῥυθμοῦ σφυγμὸν *vulg.*

183 The time-units in the dilation and contraction [of pulses]
actually are also recorded by Herophilus, who refers his argument to
the rhythms for the sake of [accounting for] the stages of life. For, just
as musicians establish rhythms according to certain defined sequences
of time-units, comparing up-beat (*arsis*) and down-beat (*thesis*) with
each other, so too Herophilus supposes that the dilation of the artery
is analogous to the up-beat, while the contraction is analogous to the
down-beat. He made his observation having started from the
newborn child, and, on the supposition that a primary perceptible
time-unit is that in which he usually found the artery [of a newborn
child] dilating, he says that the time-unit of the contraction is also
equal to it, not making any distinctions at all concerning either of the
moments of rest [between contractions and dilations].

For those to whom the contraction of the artery is imperceptible,
the rhythm of the pulse is divided into two time-units in all: (i) a unit
of perceptible motion, when the dilating artery beats against our
touch; and, (ii) for the rest, the entire time-unit composed of the

'external' pause and of the contraction after this pause, and then again, of the pause following upon this contraction, and of the first parts of the dilation – which themselves, too, are imperceptible. And for this reason they divide the pulse into 'beat' (*plēgē*) and 'interval' (*dialeimma*), locating frequency and infrequency in the amount [of time] of the interval, just as they locate speed and slowness in that of the beat.

In so far as Herophilus, therefore, says the pulse in the newborn occurs with a rhythm of equal time-units [sc. in diastole and systole], to that extent it seemed to me that he is distinguishing the *beginning* of the contraction; but in so far as he then extends the contraction of the artery in old people up to ten primary time units, to that extent he no longer seemed to be making this distinction, but to be determining the dilation by the perceptible motions which we distinguish on the basis of their beating against our fingers, and to be making the contraction the entire remaining part in which he was not perceiving motion. But we must leave aside Herophilus' art concerning the pulses.

184 Galenus, *De pulsuum dignotione* 2.3 (VIII, pp. 869–72K)

δι' οὐδὲν ἄλλο ἢ ὅτι πεφυρημένον τε καὶ ἀδιάρθρωτον ὑπὲρ
αὐτῶν (sc. σφυγμῶν) ἔχοντες τὸν νοῦν, ἑνί γε τῷ πρώτῳ
σφαλέντι πάντες ἠκολούθησαν, εἶτα περὶ τῶν ἀξιόλογον οὐδε-
μίαν εἰς αὐτὰ τὰ τῆς τέχνης ἔργα βλάβην ἢ ὠφέλειαν εἰσφερο-
5 μένων πικρῶς ἐρίζουσιν οὐκ ἀλλήλοις μόνον, ἀλλὰ καὶ Ἡροφίλῳ
. . . ἀλλὰ μικρὸν μὲν τὸν τοῦ παιδὸς εἰρήκασι σφυγμόν,
ὡσαύτως δὲ καὶ τὸν τοῦ γέροντος μικρόν, ὁπότερος δ' αὐτῶν
μικρότερος, οὐκέτι γράφουσι, καίτοι σαφῶς Ἡροφίλου τοῖς γε
μὴ παρέργως ἐντυγχάνουσιν αὐτοῦ τοῖς βιβλίοις ὑπὲρ ἀμφο-
10 τέρων γεγραφότος (Τ38) . . . μικρόν γ' οὖν λέγουσι τὸν τοῦ
παιδὸς σφυγμόν, Ἡροφίλου μηδεπώποτε μικρὸν εἰρηκότος,
ἀλλὰ ποτὲ μὲν ἱκανὸν τῷ μεγέθει, ποτὲ δὲ ἀξιόλογον, ἤ πως
οὕτως ὀνομάζοντος.

εἶτα τίς μὲν ἡ κινοῦσα τὰς ἀρτηρίας αἰτία ζητοῦσι καὶ τῶν εἰς
15 τοῦθ' Ἡροφίλῳ γεγραμμένων οὐδὲν παραλείπουσι, τῶν δ' εἰς τὰ
ἔργα τῆς τέχνης διαφερόντων θεωρημάτων, οὔτ' εἰ καλῶς οὔτ'
εἰ μὴ καλῶς ἔγραψεν Ἡρόφιλος, οὐδενὸς ἔτι μέμνηνται· ὦ πρὸς
τῶν θεῶν, οὐ πολὺ μέντοι βέλτιον ἦν μὴ περὶ τοῦ τέτταρας ὑφ'

'Ηροφίλου λέγεσθαι τὰς διοικούσας τὰ ӡῷα δυνάμεις ӡητεῖν
20 (Τ131), μηδὲ πικρῶς ἐρίӡειν τε καὶ ἀντιλέγειν αὐτῷ περί γε
τούτων, ἀλλ' εἴπερ ἐβούλοντο καταβάλλειν τε καὶ διεξελέγξαι
αὐτὸν εἰκῆ ληροῦντα, τῶν τοιούτων αὐτοῦ μνημονεύειν, ἃ
φανερῶς τοῖς ἐναργέσι μάχεται, καὶ ταῦτα μαρτύρων ἀριθμὸν
οὐκ ὀλίγον ἀθροῖσαι κατ' αὐτοῦ δυνάμενοι; τούς τε γὰρ μεθ'
25 'Ηρόφιλον τὰ περὶ σφυγμῶν πραγματευσαμένους καὶ σχεδὸν
τοὺς νῦν ἅπαντας ἕξουσι μαρτυροῦντας, ὡς ὁ τῶν παίδων
σφυγμὸς μικρότερός ἐστι τοῦ τῶν γερόντων, καὶ πολλῷ γέ
τι⟨νι⟩ σμικρότερος . . .
    τοιούτους οὖν μυρίους ἔχοντες μάρτυρας καὶ τἄλλα φιλονεικ-
30 οῦντες ἀεὶ πρὸς 'Ηρόφιλον, οὐκ οἶδ' ὅπως τὰ τοιαῦτα παραλε-
λοίπασι τὴν ἀρχήν, οὐδ' εἰ γέγραφεν αὐτὰ γιγνώσκουσιν
. . . ταῦτ' οὖν ἐκλέγουσι μόνον τῶν 'Ηροφίλου βιβλίων τὰ
κεφάλαια, τὰ δὲ ἄλλα παντάπασιν ὑπερβαίνουσι, καὶ διὰ τοῦτ'
οὐδ' ὅλως ἴσασι τί γέγραφεν 'Ηρόφιλος εἰς μὲν τὰ τῆς τέχνης
35 ἔργα μεγάλως διαφέρον, ἐναντίον δ' οἷς οὗτοι λέγουσι . . .
    ἀλλ' 'Ηρόφιλός γε τὴν ἐναντίαν ὁδὸν ἰὼν αὐτοῖς παραλείπει
μὲν ἃ παρὰ τοῖς μουσικοῖς ἐχρῆν μεμαθηκέναι τὸν ἀξίως τῆς
τέχνης πεπαιδευμένον, ὡς ἐπισταμένοις δ' αὐτοῖς διαλέγεται,
τὸ χρήσιμον εἰς τὴν ἰατρικὴν ἐξ αὐτῶν λαμβάνων. οἱ δ' ὅταν τὴν
40 θαυμαστὴν ταύτην, ὡς αὐτοὶ καλοῦσι, τεχνολογίαν τὴν περὶ
τῶν ῥυθμῶν διεξέλθωσιν, οὐκέτ' αὐτοῖς μέλει δεῖξαι, πῶς ἄν τις
ἱκανὸς προγνῶναί τι δι' αὐτῶν ἢ σημειώσασθαι γένοιτο. ταῦτ'
ἄρα καὶ τὸν παίδων σφυγμὸν μικρὸν λέγουσιν, 'Ηροφίλου
τἀναντία γράφοντος, οὐδὲ μέχρι τοσούτου διασκέψασθαι σπου-
45 δάӡοντες, ὡς ἐννοῆσαι δυνηθῆναι, ποία τις παρὰ τοῖς ἀνθρώποις μεγάλη καὶ μικρὰ διαστολὴ λέγεται.

3 ἀξιόλογον De Lacy: ἀξιολόγων vulg.   5 ἐρίӡουσιν BLV: ἐριӡόντων
vulg.   8 γε ABL: τε vulg   28 τι⟨νι⟩ σμικρότερος coni. De Lacy: τις
μικρότερος vulg.

184 For no other reason than that they have a confused and
disjointed mind concerning them [sc. pulses], they all followed the
one person who first stumbled, and then they argued bitterly, not
only with each other, but also with Herophilus, about matters which
contribute no appreciable harm or benefit to the actual tasks of our
art . . . Now, they say the pulse of a child is small, just as the pulse of
an old man is small, too; but which of them is smaller, they do not

record at all, although Herophilus wrote clearly about both, at least
for those who do not have just a casual encounter with his books
[T38] . . . They say, then, that the pulse of a child is small, although
Herophilus never said it is small, but sometimes named it 'adequate in
size', sometimes 'remarkable', or something like this.

Then they inquire which cause moves the arteries, and they omit
nothing Herophilus wrote on this; but when his theories are in
disagreement with the facts of our art, they no longer mention at all
whether what Herophilus wrote is correct or incorrect. For God's
sake, wouldn't it be much better not to inquire about the fact that
four faculties were said by Herophilus to govern living beings (T131),
or to argue bitterly and to speak against him, at least concerning these
things? But rather, if they did wish to revile and refute him for talking
idle nonsense, to mention such of his views as clearly are in conflict
with what is evident, and all the more since they can collect no small
number of witnesses against him? They will have as their witnesses
those who dealt with pulses after Herophilus, and almost all those
who do so now – witnesses to the fact that the pulse of children is
smaller than that of old men, and that it is, in fact, smaller by some
considerable amount . . .

Although they therefore have countless such witnesses and always
enter into contentious rivalry with Herophilus on other matters, they
somehow from the outset have omitted such matters, and they do not
even know whether he has actually written these things . . . In fact,
they excerpt only these chapters from Herophilus' books, but the
others they pass over completely, and for this reason they do not even
know at all what Herophilus has written that is not only greatly at
odds with the facts of the art, but also the opposite of what these
people say . . .

Herophilus, however, goes the opposite way and omits what
someone who is educated in a manner worthy of the art should have
learnt from the musicians, and he discourses with them as though they
understand this, taking from them [sc. the musicians] what is useful
for the art of medicine. But whenever they give an exposition of this
'amazing scientific system' (*technologia*) – as they call it – concerning
the rhythms, they are no longer interested in demonstrating how a
person could become competent at prognosticating or interpreting
something through them. That, then, is why they also call the pulse of
children small, although Herophilus wrote the opposite, because they

are not even serious about examining [it] far enough to be able to conceive what kind of dilation is called 'large' and 'small' in human beings.

185 C. Plinius Secundus, *Naturalis historia* 29.4.5–29.5.6

alia factio, ab experimentis se cognominans empiricen, coepit in Sicilia, Acrone Agragantino Empedoclis physici auctoritate commendato, dissederuntque hae scholae et omnes eas damnavit Herophilus, in musicos pedes venarum pulsu discripto per
5 aetatum gradus. deserta deinde et haec secta est, quoniam necesse erat in ea litteras scire.

> 1 se *V²E*: *om.* *VRdT*   cognominans *VREr²*: -nant *dTr*   2 physici
> *d vett.*: pysci *V¹*: chysippi *E*: chry. *r in ras.* crisippi *V²*   3 hae scholae
> *Detlefsen*: hae disolae *Vd* (-le): eae scholae *vett.*: hae diu scholae
> *Hardouin*   4 discripto *V*: de- *Rd*: discerpto *E*

185 Another school [of medicine], which gave itself the name 'Empiricist' [since it was] based on experience, started in Sicily with Acron of Agrigentum, who was commended by the authority of the natural philosopher Empedocles. And these schools were in disagreement and were all condemned by Herophilus, who divided the pulse of the bloodvessels into musical feet according to the different stages of life. Then this school [sc. Herophilus'?], too, was abandoned since its members had to have a literary learning.

186 C. Plinius Secundus, *Naturalis historia* 11.89.219

inter hos (sc. nervos) latent arteriae, id est spiritus semitae; his innatant venae, id est sanguinis rivi. arteriarum pulsus in cacumine maxime membrorum evidens, index fere morborum, in modulos certos legesque metricas per aetates, stabilis aut
5 citatus aut tardus, discriptus ab Herophilo medicinae vate miranda arte nimiam propter suptilitatem desertus, observatione tamen crebri aut languidi ictus gubernacula vitae temperat.

> 2 innatant *DF*: natant *REa*   3 morborum *R vett.*: membrorum
> *MEa*   4–5 stabilis aut citatus aut tardus, discriptus *MF²R*: *om. rell.*

4 stabilis F^2R: tantis M 5 discriptus MR: de- F^2: descriptas
vett.   7–8 temperat MDF:temperant RF^2: temperet E

186 Between the nerves lie hidden the arteries, i.e., the ducts for
pneuma. The veins, i.e., the channels for blood, float among them.
The pulsation of the arteries is most apparent in the extremity of the
limbs. In general, it is an indicator of diseases, and it was divided by
Herophilus, an oracle of medicine, into definite measures and
metrical laws according to age: regular, or in rapid motion, or slow.
But this [nowadays] is abandoned on account of its excessive subtlety;
nevertheless, through our observation of the frequent or feeble beat it
[still] regulates the steering of one's life.

187 Censorinus, *De die natali* 12.4-5 (p. 22 Sallmann)

> . . . Pythagoras, ut animum sua semper divinitate imbueret,
> prius quam se somno daret et cum esset expergitus, cithara ut
> ferunt cantare consueverat, et Asclepiades medicus phreneti-
> corum mentes morbo turbatas saepe per symphonian suae
> 5 naturae reddidit. Herophilus autem, artis eiusdem professor,
> venarum pulsus rhythmis musicis ait moveri. itaque si et in
> corporis et in animi motu est harmonia, procul dubio a
> natalibus nostris musica non est aliena.

2 cythara V: sythara CP 5 ierophilus CPV: Herophilus *pr. vulgo*
artis] mortis CP: *corr. V*

187 . . . Before he went to sleep and when he was awakened,
Pythagoras used to sing to the lyre, they say, in order always to fill his
soul with divinity. And the physician Asclepiades restored the minds
of people suffering from phrenitis [delirium] – minds agitated by
disease – to their own nature through musical harmony. But Herophilus, a practitioner of the same art, says the pulsations of the
bloodvessels move in musical rhythms. If, therefore, there is harmony
in the movement of both the body and the soul, then doubtless music
is not alien to the days of our birth.

188a Martianus Capella, *De nuptiis Philologiae et Mercurii* 9.926
(p. 356 Willis)

Herophilus aegrorum venas rhythmorum collatione pensabat.

1 erofilius *B*¹*D*¹*P*: ergo filius *AR*¹

188a Herophilus used to examine the bloodvessels of the ill through a
comparison of their rhythms.

188b Remigius Autissiodorensis, *Commentum in Martianum Capellam*
9.493.7 (II, p. 327 Lutz)

Erofilus interpretatur fortis amor; *ero* fortis, *filos* amor; *aegrorum
venas* id est pulsus venarum; *rithmorum* id est numerorum;
collatione pensabat computabat, considerabat. nam si pulsus
venarum fuerit secundum pedes naturales, id est convenientes,
5 sanus erit homo.

1 amor *L*: amator *PΠGC*   3 considerabat *om. ΠGC*

188b 'Erofilus' is translated 'Strong Love': 'ero' is strong, 'filos' is
love. 'Bloodvessels of the ill': that is, pulse of the bloodvessels. 'Their
rhythms': that is, their measures. 'He used to examine through a
comparison': he used to calculate, he used to look at attentively. For if
the pulse of the bloodvessels were in accordance with natural – i.e.,
appropriate – metrical feet, the person would be healthy.

5 *Male reproductive physiology; spermatogenesis**

189 Galenus, *De semine* 1.16 (IV, pp. 582-3K)

καὶ τὸ κατὰ τὴν ἐπιδιδυμίδα περιεχόμενον (sc. ὑγρὸν) ἐκ τούτου
(sc. τοῦ ὄρχεως) μετείληπται πρὸς αὐτήν, ὥσπερ ἐκ ταύτης εἰς
τὸ σπερματικὸν ἀγγεῖον, οὗ παραστάτην κιρσοειδῆ τὸ πρὸς τῷ
καυλῷ μέρος Ἡρόφιλος ὠνόμασεν, ἁμαρτάνων μὲν καὶ αὐτός,
5 ὅτι τῷ σπερματικῷ πλέον ἢ τοῖς ὄρχεσιν ἀναφέρει τῆς τοῦ
σπέρματος γενέσεως, οὐ μὴν ἴσα Ἀριστοτέλει σφαλλόμενος
εἰκάζοντι λείαις τοὺς ὄρχεις.

* Cf. also the sections on the anatomy of male organs, Chapter VI.A.5; T101–T105.

1 ἐπιδιδυμίδα *P Ald*: διδυμίδα *M*　　3 κιρσοειδῆ *MP Ald*: corr.
Kühn　　3–4 τὸ πρὸς τ.κ. μέρος *P Ald*: τῷ πρός τ.κ. μέρει *M*　　5 τῷ
σπερματικῷ *Ald*: τὸ σπερματικὸν *MP*　　6 σφαλόμενος *MP*?　　7 λείας
P: fort. λαίαις *coni.*

189 And the seminal fluid contained in the epididymis is transferred
from the testicle to the epididymis, just as it is from there into the
seminal vessel. To the part of the seminal vessel bordering on the shaft
[penis] Herophilus gave the name 'varicose assistant' (*parastatēs
kirsoeidēs*). Even Herophilus is mistaken inasmuch as he attributes a
greater role in the generation of seed to the seminal vessel than to the
testicles, but he was not quite as mistaken as Aristotle, who compared
the testicles to loom weights.

190　Galenus, *De semine* 1.15 (IV, pp. 565–6K)

καὶ μὲν δὴ καὶ ὁ πόρος ὁ σπερματικός, ὃν ὀνομάζουσιν ἔνιοι
κιρσοειδῆ παραστάτην, ἐντεῦθεν (sc. ἀπὸ τῆς ἐπιδιδυμίδος)ἀρ-
υόμενος τὴν γονήν, ἐπὶ τὴν ἔκφυσιν ἀναφέρει τοῦ αἰδοίου. καὶ διὰ
τοῦτο οἶμαι καὶ τὸν Ἡρόφιλον οἰηθῆναι μηδέν τι μέγα συνεργά-
5　ζεσθαι τῇ γενέσει τοῦ σπέρματος. μέχρι μὲν γὰρ ἐντὸς τῶν
λαγόνων ἐστὶν ἡ ἀρτηρία καὶ ἡ φλέψ, ἅμα τοῖς ἄλλοις ἅπασι
σπλάγχνοις καὶ τῷ κοινῷ πάντων καλύπτεται σκεπάσματι, τῷ
περιτοναίῳ καλουμένῳ.

2–3 ἀρυόμενος] ἀρχόμενος Oribasii cod. F (*lib. inc. 9; vol.* IV, p. 91
Raeder　　4 τὸν *M*: om. *P Ald*　　ἡρόφιλος *P*　　λέγων post οἰηθῆναι
add. *P*　　5–6 ἐντὸς τῶν λαγόνων *M Ald* Oribasius (*loc. cit.*): τῶν
λαγόνων ἐντὸς *P*　　6 τοῖς] τοῖς γε Oribasius　　7 σπλάγχνοις καὶ
(*ante* τῷ) *MP*: σπλάγχνοις *Ald*: τοῖς τῇδε Oribasius　　τῷ κοινῷ
Oribasius: τῶ κοινῶν *P*

190 And indeed the seminal duct, to which some people give the
name 'varicose assistant' (*kirsoeidēs parastatēs*), draws seed from there
[sc. from the epididymis] and carries it up to the projection of the
pudendum. For this reason too I think even Herophilus thought that
they [the testicles] do not contribute very much to the generation of
seed. For, as long as the artery and the vein are on the inside of the
flanks, they too, along with all the rest of the internal organs, are
hidden by the covering that is common to all of them, the one called
the 'stretched over membrane' (*peritonaion* (peritoneum)).

191 Vindicianus (?), *Fragmentum Bruxellense de semine* 1, e codice Bruxellensi 1348–59, fol. 48r (Wellmann, 1901: 208; Werner Jaeger, *Diokles von Karystos* (Berlin, 1938; ²1963), pp. 191–2)

Alexander amator veri appellatus, discipulus Asclepiadis, libro primo de semine spumam sanguinis eius essentiam dixit Diogenis placitis consentiens. item Erasistratus et Herofilus essentiam seminis dicunt sanguinem. hoc idem Stoici philosophi de
5 materiali semine senserunt, et demonstrationes alii alias deferentes quasi in unum comprehensas enarrant.

primo igitur, ut Herofilus ait, abruptio corporum hoc testatur quam Graeci ἀνατομήν vocant. etenim seminalium vasculorum interiora atque secretius remota sanguinulenta videntur,
10 sequentia vero sive secunda plurimum a praescriptis demutata sunt, inferiora ac proxima seminis colorem habent. quo probatur in seminales vias sanguinem venire, sed earum virtute albescere atque mutatum in seminis transire qualitatem. sicut etiam in feminis post partum, si quid sanguinis nondum fuerit
15 uteri nutrimento consumptum, naturali meatu fluit in mammas et earum virtute albescens lactis accipit qualitatem. secundo: [cum] illi, qui frequentius usu venerio depurgantur, sanguinis sustinent per seminales vias emissionem, siquidem celeritatis causa essentia sanguinis in seminales venire non sinitur vias.
20 tertio: summum quicquam ex summo fieri necesse est. summum est autem semen ex omnibus in nobis liquoribus, summus est sanguis. semen igitur ex sanguine generatur. quartum: quicumque flebotomantur, sustinent post sanguinis detractionem pallorem, tenuitatem, debilitatem. haec etiam peracta venere
25 corpora comitantur, siquidem semen ex sanguine fieri videtur. quintum: semen matrici appositum congelatur ut declarant corporis abruptiones, quod est signum seminis [atque] essentiae de sanguine venientis et ad suam originem redeuntis, quippe praeter sua vascula constituti.

3,7 erofilus B *(utroque loco)* 7 abruptio B *Neu Wellmann:* apertio *coni.*
Jaeger fort. recte 11 habentia B *Neu: corr. Wellmann* 12 virtutem B
Neu: corr. Wellmann 13 mutatam B *Neu: corr. Wellmann* se
ministrans ire *Neu: corr. Rose (Aristot. fragm. p. 220)* 14 feminis *Neu:*
seminis B 15 fluit *Neu:* suo B 17 cum *del. Wellmann*
23 flebotomati B 26 *fort.* impositum 27 apertiones *coni. Jaeger*
atque *del. Wellmann*

191   Alexander, called 'Philalethes' ['truth-lover'], a pupil of Asclepiades, says in Book I of his *On Seed* that the essence of seed is the froth
of the blood, and therein he agrees with the opinion of Diogenes
[*Chapter* XXII, *AP.9*]. Erasistratus and Herophilus likewise say that the
essence of seed is blood. The Stoic philosophers felt the same way
about material seed, and different authors explain it by providing
different proofs which, as it were, are seized upon for one and the
same purpose.

First, then, as Herophilus says, tearing open bodies, which the
Greeks called 'dissection' (*anatomē*), is a witness to this. For the
internal parts of the seminal vessels which are also at a more remote
distance [sc. from the genitalia] appear full of blood, whereas the ones
that follow next are changed very much compared to the aforementioned ones, and the lower, more accessible ones have the colour of
seed. This proves that blood enters into the seminal ducts but then
through the power of these ducts becomes white and, having
changed, is transformed into the quality of seed. Similarly in females,
too, if after child-birth no blood is any longer used up as nourishment
for the uterus, the blood flows to the breasts by a natural course and,
through the power of the breasts, grows white and takes on the quality
of milk.

Second, men who deplete themselves too frequently through sexual
intercourse suffer an emission of blood through their seminal ducts,
since the essence of the blood is in fact not allowed to enter into the
seminal ducts on account of the speed [sc. of seminal depletion].

Third, anything that is most important must arise from something
that is most important. But of all the moistures in us seed is the most
important. Blood, too, is most important. Seed therefore is generated
out of blood.

Fourth, whoever is subjected to bloodletting suffers from paleness,
loss of weight, and weakness, after the blood has been drawn. These
things also attend bodies that have been exhausted in sexual
intercourse, since seed in fact seems to be formed from blood.

Fifth, when seed is placed in the uterus, it congeals, as dissections of
the body make clear. This is a sign of the fact that its essence comes
from the blood and that it returns to its own origin because it has been
placed outside its own vessels.

192 Rufus Ephesius, *De satyriasmo et gonorrhoea* 7–8 (p. 67 Daremberg/Ruelle)

τὸ δὲ σπέρμα τῶν σατυριώντων καὶ γονορροούντων δαψιλὲς εὑρίσκεται. πῶς οὖν ἀπὸ τῶν διδύ⟨μων εἰς τὸ αἰδοῖον τὸ σπέρμα ἔρ⟩χεται; τοῦτο γὰρ δοκεῖ μοὶ καὶ τῷ Ἡροφίλῳ ⟨ἀπορίαν παρα⟩σχεῖν.

2–3 -μων ... ἔρ- *add. Daremberg*   3 ἀπορίαν παρα- *add. Daremberg*

192 The seed of people suffering from satyriasis and spermatorrhoea [*gonorrhoia*] is found to be excessive. How then does the seed get from the testicles to the penis? For this seems to me to have provided Herophilus, too, with an insoluble difficulty.

6 *Herophilus' 'Midwifery'; gynaecology**

193 Soranus, *Gynaecia* 3, prooem. 3.4 (*CMG* IV, p. 95 Ilberg)

καὶ Ἡρόφιλος ἐν τῷ Μαιωτικῷ φησι τὴν ὑστέραν ἐκ τῶν αὐτῶν τοῖς ἄλλοις μέρεσι πεπλέχθαι καὶ ὑπὸ τῶν αὐτῶν δυνάμεων διοικεῖσθαι καὶ τὰς αὐτὰς παρακειμένας ἔχειν ὕλας καὶ ὑπὸ τῶν αὐτῶν αἰτιῶν νοσοποιεῖσθαι, καθάπερ πλήθους, πάχους, δια-
5 φορᾶς τῶν ὁμοίων· οὐδὲν οὖν ἴδιον πάθος γυναικῶν πλὴν τοῦ κυῆσαι καὶ τοῦ τὸ κυηθὲν ἐκθρέψαι καὶ ἀποτεκεῖν καὶ τὸ γάλα πεπᾶναι καὶ τὰ ἐναντία τούτοις.

3 παρεγκειμένας *Ermerins*

193 And in his *Midwifery* Herophilus says that the uterus is woven from the same things as the other parts, is regulated by the same faculties, has the same material substances at hand, and is caused to be diseased by the same things, such as excessive quantity, thickness, and disharmony in similars. Accordingly, says Herophilus, there is no affection peculiar to women, except conceiving, nourishing what has been conceived, giving birth, 'ripening' the milk, and the opposites of these.

* Cf. the section on female reproductive anatomy, Chapter VI (T105–T114), and Chapter VIII (T247) on abortion; some of those testimonia might belong to Herophilus' treatise *Midwifery*. See also below, T203–T204, for gynaecological views, and above, Chapter VI, Fr 61.

366   HEROPHILUS

194 Soranus, *Gynaecia* 3, proem. 2 (*CMG* IV, pp. 94–5 Ilberg)

ἡ δὲ ζήτησις εὔχρηστος ἕνεκα τοῦ μαθεῖν, εἰ καὶ ἰδίας τινὸς
θεραπείας χρῄζουσιν αἱ γυναῖκες. καὶ γεγένηται δὲ διαφωνία·
τινὲς μὲν γὰρ ὑπολαμβάνουσιν ἴδια πάθη γίγνεσθαι γυναικῶν,
καθάπερ οἱ ἀπὸ τῆς ἐμπειρίας καὶ Διοκλῆς ἐν τῷ πρώτῳ τῶν
5 Γυναικείων καὶ τῶν Ἐρασιστρατείων Ἀθηνίων ... τινὲς δὲ μὴ
γίνεσθαι, καθάπερ κατὰ τοὺς πλείστους Ἐρασίστρατος καὶ
Ἡρόφιλος, ὡς παρασεσημείωται ...

5 ἀθηνιω[ν *f*: Ἀθηναίων *p*: Ἀθηναῖος Rose (*cf. Wellmann, 1985a: 9 n. 8*)

194 The inquiry is very useful for the sake of learning whether
women also need some treatment that is peculiar to them. But a
disagreement has arisen. For, some assume that diseases arise which
are peculiar to women, as do the Empiricists, Diocles in Book I of his
Gynaecology, and among the Erasistrateans Athenion ... Others,
however, assume that no diseases peculiar to women arise, for
example, in the opinion of most people, Erasistratus and Herophilus,
as has been implied ... (*Cf. Chapters* XVI (*DA. 18*), XXII (*AP. 11*), *and*
XXIII (*AM. 7*) *infra.*)

195 Soranus, *Gynaecia* 3, prooem. 4.2-3 (*CMG* IV, p. 96 Ilberg)

κἂν μὴ διαφέρῃ (sc. μέρος τι ἐπὶ θηλειῶν) τῶν ἄλλων, ἐνδέχεται
πάσχειν αὐτὸ διαφόρως, ὅτι καὶ τὸ αὐτὸ μέρος ποτὲ μὲν
στεγνοπαθεῖ, ποτὲ δὲ ῥευματίζεται. τὰ δὲ ὅμοια καὶ πρὸς
Ἡρόφιλον λεκτέον καὶ πρὸς Ἀσκληπιάδην, καταψευδόμενον μὲν
5 τῶν στοιχείων, καταψευδόμενον δὲ καὶ τῆς αἰτίας.

2 αὐτῶ (*prim.*) P: *corr. Rose*   3 στεγνοπαθεῖν P: *corr. Dietz*   4 *post*
λεκτέον *lacunam statuit Rose*

195 Even if some part in women does not differ from the others, it
can be affected differently, since the same part sometimes is affected
by constriction, but sometimes suffers from flux. Similar things must
also be said against Herophilus and Asclepiades: against the former
for being mistaken about the elements, against the latter for being
mistaken about the cause.

196 Soranus, *Gynaecia* 4.1 [53]. 4–5 (*CMG* IV, pp. 130–1 Ilberg)

Ἡρόφιλος δὲ ἐν τῷ Μαιωτικῷ λέγει· "δυστοκεῖται γοῦν ὡς παρὰ Σίμωνος τοῦ Μάγνητος ὡράθη, ὅτι πολλά τις, ⟨οἷον⟩ τρεῖς ἀνὰ πέντε, ἐκύησεν ἐργωδῶς. γίνεται δὲ δυστοκία πλαγίου γεννωμένου τοῦ ἐμβρύου ἢ τοῦ αὐχένος τῆς μήτρας ἢ καὶ τοῦ
5 στόματος οὐχ ἱκανῶς διεστῶτος ἢ τοῦ ὑμένος τοῦ περιέχοντος τὸ ἔμβρυον, ὅπου τὸ ὕδωρ συλλέγεται, παχυτέρου ὄντος καὶ μὴ δυναμένου πρὸ τοῦ τόκου ῥαγῆναι." ἑωρᾶσθαι δέ φησιν ἔμβρυα προπεπτωκότα ἄνευ τοῦ τὸν ὑμένα ῥαγῆναι, τὰ δὲ τοιαῦτα ἔτι ἐργωδῶς τίκτεσθαι.
10 ⟨γίνεσθαι⟩ δὲ δυστοκίαν καὶ παρὰ τὸ ἀτονεῖν τὴν μήτραν ἢ τὸ στόμα. ἀπορία δέ ἐστιν τὸ ἀτονεῖν τὴν μήτραν ἐν τῷ σώματι.
"καὶ παρὰ τὰ ἔξωθεν δὲ προσπίπτοντα καὶ προσφερόμενα καὶ ποιούμενα καὶ τὰ ἐκ τοῦ σώματος ἐκκρινόμενα αἱματώδη πλείονα ὑγρὰ δυστοκία γίνεται. καὶ παρὰ τὸ διαταθῆναι ὑπὸ
15 τοῦ ἐμβρύου τὴν μήτραν ὠδῖσι τοῦ τίκτειν γίνεται δυσέργεια παρά τε ψῦχος ἢ καῦμα ἢ φῦμα ἢ ἀπόστημα ἐν τοῖς ἐντέροις, ἐν ἐπιγαστρίῳ. καὶ τὸ ἐν ὀσφύι δὲ καὶ ῥάχει γινόμενον κοίλωμα αἴτιον δυστοκίας γίνεται, καὶ διὰ πιμελῶδες ἐν ἐπιγαστρίῳ καὶ ἐν ἰσχίῳ δυστοκία γίνεται ὡς ἂν ἀποπιεζομένης τῆς μήτρας,
20 καὶ διὰ τὸ τεθνηκέναι τὰ ἔμβρυα."
καὶ τοσαῦτα μὲν Ἡρόφιλος.

1 δυστοκεῖται γοῦν ὡς παρὰ *conieci:* δυστοκεῖσθαι γοῦν ὡς γὰρ *P:*
δυστοκεῖσθαι (*fort.* δυστοκεῖται) γοῦν ⟨παρὰ τὸ πλῆθος⟩ †ὡς γὰρ *Ilberg:*
δυστοκεῖσθαι γοῦν < καὶ διὰ τὰ πολλὰ κυίσκεσθαι. οὔτ > ὡς γὰρ ⟨ἡ⟩
Rose 2 πολλά τις *scripsi (et tr.):* πολλάκις *P ante* Μάγνητος: παλλακὶς
Rose οἷον *addidi* ἑωράθη *Dietz, Rose* τρεῖς *P:* τρὶς *Rose,*
Ilberg 3 ἐκύησαν *Dietz* 7 πρὸς *P: corr. Dietz* 10 γίνεσθαι *add.*
Ermerins 11 στόμα *P:* σῶμα *Reinhold* ἀπορία ... σώματι *secl.*
Reinhold ἀπορία *P (scil.* τῆς ἀποτέξεως *Ilberg):* ἀφορία *Rose* τὸ
Rose: τοῦ *P* 14 διατεθῆναι *P: corr. Ermerins* 15 ὠδῖσι *Ilberg (cf.*
Sorani p. 134.17): ἢ διὰ *P:* ἰδίᾳ *Rose* 15 τοῦ *Ermerins:* τὸ *P* 16 παρὰ
τε *Ilberg:* παρὰ τὸ *P:* καὶ παρὰ τὸ *Ermerins:* ἢ παρά τι *Rose* 16–17 ἢ ἐν
ὑπογαστρίῳ *Ermerins* 17 γενόμενον *Rose* 18 τὸ *ante* πιμελῶδες *add.*
Rose

196 In his treatise *Midwifery* Herophilus says:
'Difficult labour accordingly occurs because a woman has had a troublesome pregnancy with many foetuses, for example with three to five, as was observed by Simon the Magnesian. Difficult labour

also occurs when the foetus is born in an oblique position or when the neck [*isthmus*] of the uterus or also its orifice is not distended sufficiently, or when the membrane containing the foetus, in which the water collects, is too thick and not capable of being broken before the birth.'

He says that foetuses have been seen to issue forth without the membrane being broken, but such foetuses are also born with difficulty.

Difficult labour, he says, also occurs because the uterus or its orifice is slack [atonic]. And that the uterus is slack, is a problem with the body.

'But also because of external things – things that happen to one, things consumed, things done – and because too much blood-like moisture is excreted from the body, difficult labour occurs. Difficulty also arises because the uterus is distended by the foetus through pains during birth, and because of cold or heat or a tumour or an abscess in the intestines, in the upper abdominal cavity.

'When a concavity arises in the loin and spine, it, too, becomes a cause of difficult labour. On account of fat in the upper abdominal cavity and in the hips, difficult labour also occurs as if the uterus is squeezed, and because the foetuses are dead.'

And this much Herophilus says.

197a Paulus Aegineta, 3.76.1 (*CMG* ix.1, pp. 294–5 Heiberg)

ἡ δυστοκία γίνεται ἢ παρὰ τὴν τίκτουσαν ἢ παρὰ τὸ τικτόμενον
ἢ παρὰ τὸ χόριον ἢ παρὰ τὰ ἔξωθεν ... παρὰ δὲ τὸ κυόμενον ἢ
ὑπερμέγεθες ὂν ἢ μικρὸν καὶ ὀλιγοβαρὲς ἢ ἁδροκέφαλον ἢ
τεράστιον οἷον δικέφαλον ἢ τεθνηκὸς ἢ ζῶν μέν, ἀσθενὲς δὲ καὶ μὴ
5 δυνάμενον προιέναι πρὸς τοὔκτός, ἢ διὰ τὸ πλείονα τυγχάνειν
ἔμβρυα (πέντε γὰρ ἱστόρησεν Ἡρόφιλος) ἢ διὰ τὸ παρὰ φύσιν
ἔχειν τὸ σχῆμα.

2 κυούμενον *EFG*   3 ὑπὲρ μέγεθος *D*

197a Difficult labour in childbirth arises either because of the woman who is giving birth, or because of what is born, or because of the

chorion, or because of the external parts . . . But if it is because of the
foetus, then because it is over-sized or small and of a light weight or
large-headed or monstrously malformed – for example, two-
headed – or dead or, though alive, weak and incapable of proceeding
to the outside, or on account of the fact that there happen to be several
foetuses – for Herophilus recorded five – or because it has an unnatural shape.

197b Nicolaus Rocheus, *De morbis mulierum curandis* 27
(*Gynaeciorum libri*, ed. Casparus Vuolphius Tigurinus
(Basileae, 1566), p. 524)

> de difficultatis partus causis: . . . culpa vero foetus vel quum
> supra modum ingens est, aut nimium pusillus et nec magnopere
> ponderosus, aut amplissimi capitis, aut monstrum: verbi causa
> biceps, aut mortuus, aut vivens quidem sed inbecillis neque
> 5 potens in lucem progredi: aut quod complures partus sortita sit:
> quinque nanque simul a quadam in lucem editos asserit
> Herophilus: aut quod non naturaliter dispositus sit foetus, neque
> ad exitum quadrans corporis figura.

197b On the causes of difficult labour: . . . the foetus is responsible
either when it is immoderately large or excessively small and not very
heavy, or has a very large head, or is a monster (for example, two-
headed), or dead, or, though alive, weak and unable to proceed to the
light, or again, because it was the woman's lot to get several foetuses –
for Herophilus claims that five were brought forth into the light at the
same time by a certain woman – or because the foetus is not arranged
naturally and the shape of its body is not at the right angle to the exit.

198 Proclus (Diadochus), *In Platonis Rem Publicam comment.* 13: *De
vaticinio Musarum* 32 (II, p. 33 Kroll)

> ὅτι Ἡρόφιλος ὁ ἰατρὸς καὶ ἄλλοι πολλοὶ τῶν ἐλλογίμων ἕνα
> χρόνον φασὶν εἶναι γενέσεως ⟨ὡς⟩ καὶ τοῖς ἄλλοις ζῴοις· τὸν δὲ
> ἑπτάμηνον ἠπατημένων ὑποληφθῆναι τῶν γυναικῶν, διὰ τὸ καὶ

μετὰ σύλληψιν καὶ ἐπὶ δύο μῆνας καθαίρεσθαί τινας καὶ οἴεσθαι
5 διὰ τὴν κάθαρσιν μὴ γεγονέναι σύλληψιν.

1 ὅτι Ἡρόφιλος ὁ Ἰατρὸς *m*³ *in marg.*: φιλόστρατος *m*¹ *sed exp.*   2 ὡς
suppl. Kroll: τοῖς ἀνθρώποις ὡς *Reitzenstein*

198 The physician Herophilus and many others of those held in high
repute say that there is a single duration for generation [i.e.,
pregnancy], as in other animals, too. They say that a seven-month
duration was assumed because women were mistaken about it on
account of the fact that some women menstruate for as long as two
months even after conception and, on account of their menstruation,
think that conception has not taken place.

199 Vindicianus, *Gynaecia*, praef. 1 (p. 464 Rose)

quomodo in utero materno contenemur vel portemur cum sit
artis medicinae grecis auctoribus placuit ⟨exponere⟩ . . . inter-
pretationem nobis hanc prioribus in virtute domini agentibus
medicinam⟨m⟩ Lupo et Pelope Erofilo et Erasistrato Yppo⟨c-
5 rate⟩ et Apolon⟨io⟩ et ceteris anatomicis licuit discutere.

1–5 *e cod.* E   1 contenimus vel portemus E   2 exponere *supplevi*
3 prioribus *correxi ex* in peioribus E   4 medicina E: *correxi*   Lupi
E   Pilupio E   4–5 Yppo E   5 Apolon. E   ceteris anatomicis
GC: ceteri anatomici E

199 Greek authors decided to expound how we are contained or
borne in the maternal uterus, since this belongs to the art of
medicine . . . We can discuss this explanation, since, by the grace of
God, earlier people practised medicine, namely Lycus, Pelops,
Herophilus, Erasistratus, Hippocrates, Apollonius, and the rest of the
anatomists. (*Cf. Chapter* VI, *T64a–b supra.*)

200 Galenus, *De naturalibus facultatibus* 3.3 (*Scr. Min.* III, pp. 209–
10 Helmreich)

Ἡρόφιλος μέν γε καὶ ὡς οὐδὲ πυρῆνα μήλης ἂν δέχοιτο τῶν
μητρῶν τὸ στόμα, πρὶν ἀποκυεῖν τὴν γυναῖκα, καὶ ὡς οὐδὲ
τοὐλάχιστον ἔτι διέστηκεν, ἢν ὑπάρξηται κυεῖν, καὶ ὡς ἐπὶ πλέον

ἀναστομοῦνται κατὰ τὰς τῶν ἐπιμηνίων φοράς, οὐκ ὤκνησε
5 γράφειν· συνομολογοῦσι δ' αὐτῷ καὶ οἱ ἄλλοι πάντες οἱ περὶ
τούτων πραγματευσάμενοι καὶ πρῶτός γ' ἁπάντων ἰατρῶν τε
καὶ φιλοσόφων Ἱπποκράτης ἀπεφήνατο μύειν τὸ στόμα τῶν
ὑστέρων ἔν τε ταῖς κυήσεσι καὶ ταῖς φλεγμοναῖς . . .

1 μέν γε καὶ LM: γε μὴν O   ἂν δέχοιτο Helmreich: δ' ἔχοιτ' ἂν M: οὐκ
ἂν δέχοιτο O   2 ἀποκύειν P: ἀκούειν M: κύειν LO   3 ἦν LO: πρὶν
M   6 πρῶτος] πρὸ L

200 Herophilus, at least, did not hesitate to write that until a woman
gives birth the mouth of the uterus [sc. in any pregnant woman] could
not even admit the head of a probe, and, once she has started being
pregnant, it no longer stands ajar even to the slightest degree; also,
that they open up increasingly at the time of the menstrual flow. All
others who treated of these matters are in full agreement with him,
especially Hippocrates, who was the first of all physicians and
philosophers to state that the mouth of the uterus closes both in
pregnancies and in inflammations.

201 Soranus, *Gynaecia* 4.36 [85].1–2 (*CMG* IV, p. 148 Ilberg)

ἔνιοι μὲν οὖν ὅλην λέγουσιν προπίπτειν (sc. τὴν μήτραν) τῶν
ἀντεχόντων αὐτὴν ὑμένων καὶ μυῶν ῥαγέντων ἐκ πληγῆς ἤ
τινος τῶν ἐμφερῶν ⟨ἢ⟩ χαλασθέντων καὶ ὅμοιόν τι παραλύσει
ἐργασθέντων. οἱ δὲ περὶ τὸν Ἱπποκράτην καὶ Ἡρόφιλον μόνον
5 τὸ στόμιον· γνωρίζεται δέ ἐκ τοῦ τρυφεροῦ προπῖπτον τὸ
σύγκριμα ὅμοιον κεφαλῇ πολύποδος, ὡς Ἡρόφιλος ἔλεγεν,
πόρον ἔχον ὡς παραδέξασθαι διπύρηνον.

3 ἢ add. Ermerins: aut relaxatis membranis Muscio   τι Ermerins: τῇ
P   5 προπίπτειν P: corr. Rose   6 κεφαλὴν P: corr. Dietz   7 πόνον
P: corr. Kind

201 Some, then, say that the whole uterus prolapses if the membranes and muscles which hold it in place have been ruptured by a
blow or by something similar, or if they have become relaxed and
have produced something resembling paralysis. But the followers of
Hippocrates and Herophilus say that only the orifice prolapses; the
prolapsing structure is recognized by its softness, being similar to the

head of an octopus, as Herophilus said, with a duct so as to admit a two-knobbed probe. (*Cf. Chapter* vi, *T111a–b supra.*)

202a Aëtius Doxographus, *Placita* 5.15.5 (*DG*, p. 426)

202b Ps.-Plutarchus, *Placita* 5.15 (*Moralia* 907c-d, vol. v.2.1 (Teubner), pp. 141–2 Mau)

εἰ τὸ ἔμβρυον ζῷον·
... Ἡρόφιλος κίνησιν ἀπολείπει φυσικὴν τοῖς ἐμβρύοις, οὐ πνευματικήν· τῆς δὲ κινήσεως αἴτια νεῦρα· τότε δὲ ζῷα γίνεσθαι, ὅταν προχυθέντα προσλάβῃ τι τοῦ ἀέρος.

2 ἀπολείπειν (*lig.*) B

202a–b Whether a foetus is a living being:
... Herophilus grants foetuses natural motion but not pneumatic motion. And the nerves are responsible for the motion. They [sc. the foetuses] become living beings whenever they are poured forth and take in some air.

202c Ps.-Galenus, *De historia philosopha* 119 (*DG*, p. 643)

εἰ τὸ ἔμβρυον ζῷον·
... Ἡρόφιλος· κίνησις ἀπολείπεται φυσικὴ ἐν τοῖς ἐμβρύοις, οὐ δὲ πνευματική· τῆς δὲ κινήσεως αἴτια τὰ νεῦρα. τότε ζῷα γίνεσθαι, ὅταν προχυθέντα προσλάβῃ τοῦ ἀέρος.

2 Ἡρ. κίνησιν ἀπολείπει φυσικὴν (ἐν *om.*) *Kühn* (xix p. 330)   2–3 οὐ δὲ *scripsi*: οὐ *Kühn*: τοῦ *codd. Diels*   3 πνευματική *scripsi*: πνευματικήν *Kühn*: πνευματικοῦ *codd. Diels*   αἰτιᾶται τὰ *AB*: αἴτια (τὰ *om.*) *Kühn*   τότε δὲ *Kühn*: του *codd.*   ζῷα *Kühn*: ζῴου *codd.*   4 προσλάβῃ *Kühn, Diels*: προσβῇ *AB*

202c Whether a foetus is a living being:
... Herophilus: Natural motion in foetuses is granted, but not pneumatic motion. And the nerves are the causes of the motion. They [sc. foetuses] become living beings whenever they are poured forth and take in air.

7 Herophilus' 'Against Common Opinions'

203 Soranus, *Gynaecia* 1.27.2 (*CMG* IV, p. 17 Ilberg)

ἔνιοι μὲν οὖν τῶν ἔμπροσθεν, ὡς καὶ Ἡρόφιλος ἐν τῷ πρὸς τὰς
κοινὰς δόξας ἐμνημόνευσεν, ἐπὶ συμφέροντι λέγουσιν γεγονέναι
τὴν κάθαρσιν καὶ πρὸς ὑγείαν καὶ πρὸς παιδοποιίαν, Θεμίσων
δὲ καὶ οἱ πλεῖστοι τῶν ἡμετέρων πρὸς μόνην παιδογονίαν, τινὲς
5 δὲ τῶν ἐπισημοτέρων οὔτε πρὸς ὑγείαν οὔτε πρὸς παιδοποιίαν.
Ἡρόφιλος δὲ καὶ Μνασέας κατὰ διαφόρους ἐπιβολὰς τισι μὲν
τῶν γυναικῶν πρὸς ὑγείαν ὠφέλιμον λέγουσιν εἶναι τὴν κάθαρσιν, τισὶ δὲ βλαβεράν.

2 λέγομεν P: corr. Dietz   5 ἐπισημοτέρων Ilberg: εὐσημοτέρων P
6 ἐπιβουλὰς P: corr. Dietz

203 Now, some previous physicians, as Herophilus also mentioned
in his *Against Common Opinions*, say that menstruation is advantageous
both for one's health and for childbearing. Themison, however, and
most of our people say [it is advantageous] for childbearing alone,
while some of the more distinguished physicians say [it benefits]
neither health nor childbearing. But Herophilus and Mnaseas, with
different approaches, say that menstruation is helpful to the health of
some women, but harmful to others.

204 Soranus, *Gynaecia* 1.29.1 et 4 (*CMG* IV, p. 19 Ilberg)

(1) Ἡρόφιλος δὲ ποτὲ μὲν καί τισιν τῶν γυναικῶν βλαβερὰν
φησιν εἶναι τὴν κάθαρσιν, καὶ γὰρ ἀνεμποδίστως τινὰς ὑγιαίνειν
μὴ καθαιρομένας καὶ πολλάκις τοὐναντίον καθαιρομένας ὠχρο-
τέρας γίνεσθαι καὶ ἰσχνοτέρας καὶ παθῶν λαμβάνειν ἀφορμάς,
5 ποτὲ δὲ καὶ ἐπί τινων ὠφέλιμον, ὥστε πρότερον ἀχροούσας καὶ
ἀτροφούσας ὕστερον καὶ μετὰ τὴν κάθαρσιν εὐχροῆσαί τε καὶ
εὐτροφῆσαι . . .
(4) κοινῇ δὲ πρὸς τοῦτον (sc. Μνασέαν) καὶ πρὸς Ἡρόφιλον
λεκτέον, ὅτι βλάπτει μὲν ἡ κάθαρσις πρὸς τὸ ὑγιαίνειν ἁπάσας,
10 ἤδη δὲ τῶν μὲν εὐπαθεστέρων καθάπτεται μᾶλλον, διαλανθάνει
δὲ τὸ βλαβερὸν αὐτῆς ἐφ' ὧν δυσπαθῆ τὰ σώματα κέκτηνται.

9 ἅπασα P: corr. Gomperz   11 κέχρηται P: corr. Ermerins

204 (1) Herophilus, however, says that at certain times, and for
certain women, menstruation is harmful. Some women, he says, are
actually in a state of unimpeded health when they are not menstruating, whereas the opposite often happens while they are menstruating:
they become paler and thinner and contract the beginnings of
diseases. At other times, however, and in certain cases, menstruation
is beneficial, so that women who previously were wan and emaciated,
later, after menstruation, have good colour and are well nourished . . .

(4) Against him [sc. Mnaseas] and Herophilus one must raise an
objection in common, namely that with regard to health, menstruation is harmful to all women, although it affects those who are rather
prone to illness more, while its harmfulness goes entirely unnoticed in
the case of those who possess bodies that are not easily affected.

8 General pathological evidence; semiotics*

205a Ps.-Galenus, *Definitiones medicae* 149 (XIX, p. 391 K)

νόσημα ἔμμονόν ἐστιν ἔμμονος κατασκευὴ παρὰ φύσιν περὶ τὰ
μετέχοντα τοῦ ζῆν σώματα· οἱ Ἡροφίλειοι πάθος λέγουσιν εἶναι
τὸ δύσλυτον καὶ ἀκίνητον οὗ τὴν αἰτίαν ἐν ὑγροῖς εἶναι.

205a A chronic disease is a chronic constitution contrary to nature in
bodies that partake of living. The Herophileans say it is an affection
(*pathos*) which is hard to resolve and to change, the cause of which lies
in moistures [of the body].

205b Ps.-Soranus, *Quaestiones medicinales* 103 (*Anecdota Graeca et
Graecolatina*, vol. II, p. 259 Rose)

quid est pathos? Herophilus dixit esse passionem quae ⟨non⟩
bene solvitur et bene mollitur. huius enim dixit esse causam in
humoribus constitutam.

1 non *addidi (cf. T205a supra)*

* On the 'moistures' or 'humours' see also T130–T134 above.

205b What is an affection (*pathos*)? Herophilus said it is an affliction which is not easily resolved and alleviated. For its cause, he said, is constituted in the humours.

206 Ps.-Galenus, *Definitiones medicae* 134 (XIX, pp. 386–7K)

πάθος ἐστὶ παραποδισμὸς τῆς κατὰ φύσιν ἐνεργείας νοσώδης ἤ τινος ἤ τινων ἤ μιᾶς ἤ πάντων τῶν τῆς φύσεως ἐνεργημάτων. τινὲς δὲ οὕτως ὡς Ἡροφίλειοι· "πάθος ἐστὶ τὸ μὴ διὰ παντὸς ἐν τῷ αὐτῷ χρόνῳ λυόμενον, καὶ ἐλάττονι δέ ποτε καὶ ἐν πλείονι."

4 ἐν *fort. ante* ἐλάττονι *addendum est*

206 An affection (*pathos*) is an unwholesome impeding of the natural activity either of a certain, or of some, or of a single, or of all the operations of nature. Some people [define it] this way, as do the Herophileans: 'An affection (*pathos*) is that which is not throughout resolved in the same time, but sometimes in less, sometimes in more.'

207 Caelius Aurelianus, *Medicinales responsiones: De salutaribus praeceptibus* 10 (*Anecdota Graeca et Graecolatina*, ed. V. Rose, vol. II (1870), p. 197)

uniformis est sanitas, an varia cum extenditur et minuitur? secundum Asclepiadem et Erasistratum uniformis: nolunt enim summum sanitatis et quantitudinem esse. secundum Herophilum et methodicos varia, cum extenditur et minuitur.

207 Is health uniform or is it variable, since it increases and diminishes? According to Asclepiades and Erasistratus it is uniform, for they deny that there is a 'peak' and a 'quantitative degree' of health. According to Herophilus and the Methodist physicians, health is variable since it increases and diminishes.

208 Vindicianus, *Gynaecia*, praef. (vel 2), cod. L (K. Sudhoff, *AGM* 8 (1915), pp. 417–18)

(See Chapter VI, *T64a supra.)*

209 C. Plinius Secundus, *Naturalis historia* 26.8.14

trahebat (sc. Asclepiades) praeterea mentes (sc. aegrorum) artificio amabili, iam vinum promittendo aegris dandoque tempestive, iam frigidam aquam et, quoniam causas morborum scrutari prius Herophilus instituerat, vini rationem inlustra-
5 verat Cleophantus apud priscos, ipse cognominari se frigida danda praeferens, ut auctor est M. Varro.

1 mentes *RdE*: mentis *V*   2 amabili iam *coni. Ernout*: animalia *VRd*: mirabili *d(?) Ha*: mirabili iam *Sillig*: inani alias *Ma*: animos iam *Ianus Detlefsen*   vinum *Rd*: vina *V*: vino *E*   3 iam *VRdTF*: tam *Er*: tum *vett.*   5 cognominaris se *dR vett.*: cognominaveris e *VRF*: cognomen ab aegris *Gronovius Sillig*: cognomen a vinis et *Urlich*

209 Asclepiades, moreover, influenced the minds [of his patients] with a likeable device, namely at one time promising the ill wine and giving it to them opportunely, at another cold water. And, since Herophilus had previously established examining the causes of diseases, while Cleophantus elucidated the regulation of wine-drinking among the ancients, Asclepiades preferred that he himself be surnamed 'Cold-Water Giver', as Marcus Varro reports.

210 A. Cornelius Celsus, *Medicina* 1 (*Artes* 6), prohoem. 28 (*CML* 1, p. 22 Marx)

non posse vero conprehendi (sc. naturam) patere (sc. Empirici contendunt) ex eorum, qui de his disputarunt, discordia, cum de ista re neque inter sapientiae professores, neque inter ipsos medicos conveniat. cur enim potius aliquis Hippocrati credat
5 quam Herophilo? cur huic potius quam Asclepiadi?

2 qui de his *FJ*: quid eis *V*: quid de eis *V²*

210 That [nature] cannot be comprehended is in fact patently clear, [the Empiricists claim,] from the disagreement among those who argue about these things: for, on this question there is not agreement either among teachers of philosophy or among the physicians themselves. Why, then, should anyone believe Hippocrates rather than Herophilus? Why Herophilus rather than Asclepiades?

211 Caelius Aurelianus, *Celeres vel acutae passiones* 1, praef. 4–5

nam Demetrius (*DA.4, infra*) Erophilum sequens libro sexto quem de passionibus scripsit hanc (sc. phrenitem) diffiniens delirationem dixit vehementem cum alienatione atque ⟨frequentius cum⟩ febre, et in interfectionem celerem, aliquando et
5 in sanitatem. sed neque a deliratione vehementi alienationem differre quisquam existimet . . .

3 frequentius *add. Bendz (Lunds Univ. Arssk. N.F. avd. 1, vol. 38.4 (1943), p. 77)*   4 cum *add. Drabkin*   4 aliquando *transposuit post* atque *P. Schmid (Contributions Cael. Aur., p. 75)*

211 For, in Book VI of his book *On Affections*, Demetrius, following Herophilus, defined phrenitis, saying that it is a violent attack of madness (*deliratio*) accompanied by loss of reason (*alienatio*) and quite frequently by fever, quickly leading to death but at times also back to health. But no one could think that 'loss of reason' (*alienatio*) is different from 'violent madness' (*deliratio*) . . . (*Cf. Chapter* XVI, *DA.4 infra.*)

212 Caelius Aurelianus, *Tardae passiones* 2.1.15

Herophilus denique repentinam mortem, nulla ex manifesta causa venientem, fieri inquit paralysi cordis.

212 In fact, Herophilus says that a sudden death, coming on without any apparent cause, occurs because of a paralysis of the heart.

213 Caelius Aurelianus, *Tardae passiones* 2.1.49

veterum autem medicorum Hippocratis atque Herophili sectatores memorant ea quae in passione constitutos sequuntur, curationem (sc. paralyseos) vero nullam tradiderunt.

213 Among the ancient physicians, however, the followers of Hippocrates and Herophilus mention the symptoms which are attendant upon those who are affected by this disease [sc. paralysis], but they handed down no treatment for it.

214 Caelius Aurelianus, *Celeres vel acutae passiones* 2.39.225

> hic (sc. Asclepiades) quoque secundo libro celerum vel acu-
> tarum passionum providens ne qua sit in corpore cruditas,
> clysteres adhibet operantissimos ob transversionem faciendam,
> primo nescius quae sit operans in cardiacis causa, et tamquam
> 5 Herophili sector indigestionem atque corruptionem intuen-
> dam existimans.

Herophilus *G: corr. R in marg.*

214 In Book II of his treatise *On Swift or Acute Diseases* Asclepiades,
too, tries to prevent the presence of undigested food in the body by
prescribing very 'effective' clysters to accomplish the transfer. In the
first place, he does not know what the efficient cause is in cases of
cardiac disorders, and, just like a follower of Herophilus, thinks that
indigestion and spoiled food are what must be examined.

215 Caelius Aurelianus, *Celeres vel acutae passiones* 2.28.147

> pati in peripneumonicis Diocles venas pulmonis inquit, Erasis-
> tratus vero arterias, Praxagoras eas inquit partes pulmonis pati
> quae sunt spinae coniunctae. etenim omnem inquit pulmonem
> pati Herophilus; si febrem, inquit, fuerint passi, pleuriticam
> 5 facit.

215 In the case of people suffering from pneumonia, Diocles says the
veins of the lung are affected, while Erasistratus says the arteries are
affected, and Praxagoras the parts of the lung which are joined to the
spine. But Herophilus says the whole lung is affected. If the patients
[also] suffer from fever, he says, it causes pleurisy.

216 Caelius Aurelianus, *Celeres vel acutae passiones* 2.16.96–7

> quaesitum etiam est a veteribus quis in pleuriticis locus patiatur,
> et quidam pulmonem pati dixerunt, ut Euryphon, Euenor,
> Praxagoras, Herophilus, Phylotimus. item quidam hypezocota
> membranam quae latera ex interiore cingit, ut Diocles, Erasis-
> 5 tratus, Asclepiades, et eorum plurimi sectatores.

horum primi aiunt non esse in lateribus tumorem, cum neque
extantia ulla earum partium inspectione sentiatur, neque rubor,
nec motu nec tactu dolor acutus vel fortis, tamquam manifestis
tumoribus. accedit etiam quod facile supra id latus quod patitur
10 iacere possint aegrotantes, supra aliud vero quod passione
liberum videtur si se iactaverint, difficultas spirationis accedat,
siquidem nunc sustentatae pulmonis partes iaceant, nunc veluti
pendere sentiantur. dehinc etiam tussicula signum est ex
accedentibus consequens fibrarum pulmonis esudati corporis
15 liquoris sive cannae gutturis. singula etiam et tussita de pulmone
venire manifestum est, qui neque venis neque arteriis neque
fibris contiguus vel admixtus esse lateri videatur, ut per ipsum
latere accepta excludi posse credamus.

　　　unde igitur dolores? numquidne pulmonis sensibiles partes in
20 passione constitutae causa sunt? an vero eius tumore latera
vicinantia comprimuntur et propterea dextrarum fibrarum
tumor dextri lateris dolorem facit, sinistrarum sinistri? sed in
peripneumonicis totus tumet pulmo nec ullus tamen sequitur
dolor.

25　　sed huic quidem sententiae contrarii aiunt propterea neque
ruborem neque extantiam vel dolorem aegrotantes consequi,
siquidem in alto tumor esse videatur . . .

2 Euriphon *edd.*　　　4 ex *Drabkin*: et *GRA*　　　14 accedentibus *GRA*:
accidentibus *coni. Drabkin*: antecedentibus *Bendz (p. 92)*　　　morbum *add.*
post consequens *R*　　　15 cannae *R*: canna *G*　　　et tussita *L*: extussita *R*
in marg.　　　18 latera *G: corr. R*

216 The ancients also asked what place is affected in cases of
pleurisy. Some said the lung is affected, and among them are
Euryphon, Euenor, Praxagoras, Herophilus, and Phylotimus; others
again, like Diocles, Erasistratus, Asclepiades, and most of their
followers, [said] that it is the pleural [*lit.*, 'undergirding'] membrane
which girds the sides internally [that is affected in pleurisy].

　　Those in the former group say there is no swelling in the sides, since
no protrusion of these parts is perceived upon inspection, or any
redness, and no sharp or severe pain when they are moved or touched,
as when swellings are clearly apparent. There is the further fact that
the patients could lie comfortably on the side which is affected, but if
they toss themselves onto the side which seems to be free from the

affection, difficulty in breathing sets in. This is so because in the first case the parts of the lung lie in a supported position, but in the second they feel as if they are hanging down. Then again, a slight cough is a sign (following from its attributes) that liquid of the body has been excreted from the interior parts of the lung or from the windpipe. Also, it is clear that what is coughed up each time comes from the lung – which does not seem to be bordering on, or to be connected with, the side through veins or arteries or filaments [in such a way] that we could believe that what is coughed up is received from the side and then excreted through the lung itself.

Where, then, do the pains [sc. in the sides] come from? Surely the sensitive parts of the lung that are in a diseased condition are not the cause? Or are the sides adjacent to the swelling of the lung compressed, and does the swelling of the right sections [right lobes of the lung?] therefore cause pain in the right side, and swelling of the left [lobes] pain in the left side? But in patients with pneumonia the entire lung is swollen, and yet no pain accompanies it.

But those [sc. of the latter group, not including Herophilus], who are opposed to this view – that the lung is affected in pleurisy – say that neither redness nor protrusion nor pain is attendant upon patients ill with pleurisy, for the reason that the swelling seems to be deep inside . . .

217a Ps.-Galenus, *De historia philosopha* 131 (*DG*, p. 647; cf. *DG* p. 441, ps.-Plutarchus, *Placita* 5.29.3)

Ἡρόφιλός φησιν ἐνίοτε μηδεμιᾶς αἰτίας προηγησαμένης πυρέττειν τινάς.

1–2 om. Mau (Plut. Mor. vol. v. 2.1: Placita 5.29)   1 Ἡρόφιλος corr. codd. ex. Ἡρόδοτος (cf. DG, p. 39)   ἐνίοτε om. B

217a Herophilus says people sometimes suffer from fever although there is no antecedent [proximate?] cause.

217b Aëtius Doxographus, *Placita* 5.29.3 (*Aetius Arabus*, p. 517 Daiber)

Herophilus refuted this [sc. Diocles' view that the visible

symptoms of fever are sores, boils, and swollen glands] and believed that the hot swelling does not precede fever but that fever precedes it. Fever for the most part arises in this way. Frequently fever occurs without a cause being apparent in it. Its cause provokes a movement of the chronic(?) diseases and the growth of hot sores.

218 Caelius Aurelianus, *Tardae passiones* 2.4.84

Herophilus denique et Heraclides Tarentinus mori quosdam detractione dentis memoraverunt.

218 Herophilus and Heraclides of Tarentum mentioned that some people die on account of the pulling of a tooth.

219 Caelius Aurelianus, *Celeres vel acutae passiones* 3.17.167

(de acuto tormento quod Graeci ileon appellant:) . . . Herophilus de his nihil locutus est.

219 [Concerning acute intestinal obstruction, which the Greeks call *(e)ileos:*] . . . Herophilus said nothing about these cases.

220 Galenus, *In Hippocratis Aphorismos comment.* 6.1 (ad Hp. iv, p. 562 L) (xviiiA, pp. 6–7K)

"εἰ δ ἄπεπτα εἴεν τὰ διαχωρούμενα, μεμιγμένα δὲ τοῖς αἱματώ-δεσί τε καὶ μυξώδεσι, λειεντερίαν (sc. τὸ πάθος ἐκάλουν οἱ πρότερον ἰατροί) . . ." ταυτὶ μὲν οὖν ὁ Ἐρασίστρατος εἶπεν, οὐκ οἶδα τί δόξαν αὐτῷ προσθεὶς τοῖς ἀπέπτοις διαχωρήμασιν
5 αἱματώδη τε καὶ μυξώδη. τοῦτο γὰρ οὐδεὶς προσέθηκεν οὔτε τῶν κατὰ τὸν αὐτὸν αὐτῷ γεγονότων χρόνον ἐπιφανεστάτων, οἷον Φυλότιμος, Ἡρόφιλος, Εὔδημος, οὔτε τῶν μετ' αὐτὸν γενομένων τις ἄχρι τῶν νεωτέρων τούτων τῶν περὶ τὸν Ἀρχιγένην.

6 χρόνων *Kühn: correxi*

220 'If the excreted things were undigested but mixed with blood-like and mucous matter, [then the earlier physicians used to call the affection] "lienteric diarrhoea" . . . ' This, then, is what Erasistratus said, and I do not know what he thought when he added 'blood-like and mucous matter' to the undigested excretions. For this is something no one had added: neither any of the most illustrious [doctors] who lived at the same time as he, for example Phylotimus, Herophilus, and Eudemus, nor any of those who lived after him, until these more recent followers of Archigenes.

221 Ps.-Galenus, *In Hippocratis Epidemiarum 2.2.21 comment.* 3.23 (ad Hp. v, p. 92L) (xviiA, p. 364 K)

αὕτη ἡ ῥῆσις μικρόν τε ἄλλως γεγραμμένη ἐν τοῖς ἀφορισμοῖς εὑρίσκεται, καὶ ἡμεῖς ἤδη αὐτὴν ἐξηγησάμεθα καὶ τὰς τοῦ Ἐρασιστράτου περὶ λειεντερίας τε καὶ δυσεντερίας καὶ τεινεσμοῦ ῥήσεις προσεθήκαμεν, καὶ ἐδείχθη ὅτι ἀλλότρια γράφει τῆς γνώμης τῶν ἐπιφανεστάτων ἰατρῶν, οἷον Φυλοτίμου, Ἡροφίλου, Εὐδήμου, Ἀρχιγένου, Διοκλέους, Πραξαγόρου καὶ τῶν ἄλλων παλαιῶν.

221 This passage [sc. Hp., *Epidemics* 2.2.21], though written a little differently, is also found in the *Aphorisms* [*Aph.* 6.1]. I have already explicated it and, in addition, have given the passages from Erasistratus concerning lientery as well as dysentery and constipation. It was also shown that he writes things that are very different from the judgment of the most illustrious physicians, such as Phylotimus, Herophilus, Eudemus, Archigenes, Diocles, Praxagoras, and the other ancients. (*This text is from a Renaissance compilation; cf. Wenkebach, 1917.*)

222 Caelius Aurelianus, *Celeres vel acutae passiones* 3.8.83

veterum medicorum Erasistratus tetanicam passionem non memoravit; Herophilus vero nihil plus inquit, nisi quod vehemens opisthotonia rectiora faciat ea quae nodorum spinae evulsione arcuata videntur, et quod febricula irruens passionem
5　solvat. item Serapion primo libro curationum sic inquit curandos tetanicos quemadmodum phreniticos . . .

222 Among ancient physicians, Erasistratus does not mention the disease of tetanus, while Herophilus says no more than that a violent attack of tetanic recurvation (*opisthotonia*) causes those things to be straighter which [normally] appear curved by the turning of the vertebrae of the spine, and that the onset of a slight fever breaks up the disease. Serapion, in Book I of his *Treatments*, says that cases of tetanus must be treated just like cases of phrenitis . . .

223a Galenus, *De plenitudine* 8 (VII, pp. 554–5K)

ὀλίγου τοίνυν ἐδέησεν αὐτῷ (sc. Ἐρασιστράτῳ) πᾶσαν ἡμῖν
γράψαι τὴν τῶν ἐμπειρικῶν συνδρομήν· ἀμέλει καὶ μέρος τι τῆς
τριχρόνου λεγομένης σημειώσεως ἣν οἱ περὶ τὸν Ἡρόφιλον
εἰσήγαγον ὁμοίως τοῖς ἐμπειρικοῖς, ἔγραψεν ἐν τῷ οὕτω φάναι·
5 "τῆς γὰρ ἀναδιδομένης τροφῆς μήτε καταπεττομένης μήτε
ἐκπονουμένης κατὰ τὸ εἰθισμένον ἑκάστῳ, μήτε ἄλλως πως
ἐκκρινομένης". οὐδὲν γὰρ διήνεγκεν ἢ ταῦτα εἰπεῖν ἢ, ὡς ἐκεῖνοι
λέγουσιν, ἀργὸν βίον, ἐπίσχεσίν τε συνήθων ἐκκρίσεων. ἀργὸν
μὲν γὰρ τὸν ἔμπροσθεν βίον ἐνεδείξατο, "μήτε ἐκπονουμένης"
10 φήσας "κατὰ τὸ εἰθισμένον ἑκάστῳ", τὴν δὲ τῶν ἐκκρίσεων
ἐπίσχεσιν ἐν τῷ προσγράψαι, "μήτε ἄλλως ἐκκρινομένης".
ἡ ⟨δὲ⟩ διὰ χρόνον σημείωσις τοῦ πλήθους· ἐκ μὲν τοῦ
προγεγονότος χρόνου λαμβάνων τὸν ἀργὸν βίον ἅμα τῇ τῶν
ἐκκρίσεων ἐπισχέσει· ἐκ δὲ τοῦ νῦν ἐνεστῶτος τό τε παρεμπίμ-
15 πλασθαι καὶ τὴν ἑλκώδη διάθεσιν, ὄκνον τε πρὸς τὰς κινήσεις,
καὶ βάρος ὅλου τοῦ σώματος, ὅσα τε ἄλλα τοιαῦτα προστιθέα-
σιν· ἐκ δὲ τοῦ μέλλοντος, ὅτι [περ] κενωθέντες οἱ οὕτως ἔχοντες
καλῶς ὤνηνται, ὅπερ Ἐρασιστράτῳ παραλέλειπται.

4 ἐν τῷ *Kühn: om. codd. (vid. Deichgräber, 1965: 156)*   12 δὲ *addidi*
διὰ χρόνον *vulg.*: τρίχρονος *conieci*   17 περ *seclusi (dittogr. u.v.)*

223a Erasistratus recorded almost the whole of the Empiricists' 'concurrence of symptoms' (*syndromē*) for us. Of course, he also recorded a part of their so-called 'triple-timed inference from signs' (*trichronos sēmeiōsis*) –which the followers of Herophilus introduced in a manner similar to the Empiricists – by speaking as follows: 'You see, when the food which is being distributed [in the body] is neither being digested nor being refined according to the habit of each, nor somehow being excreted in another way . . .'. For, it made no difference whether one said it was these things or, as the former [sc. the Empiricists?] say, an idle way of life and the stoppage of customary excretions. For he [sc. Erasistratus?] indicated that one's earlier way of life was idle, when he said 'nor is it refined to the habit of each', while he indicated the stoppage of the excretions by adding 'nor being excreted in another way'.

And for repletion the 'diachronic* inference from signs' (*dia chronon sēmeiōsis*) is this: from past time he grasps the idle mode of life at the same time as the stoppage of the excretions; from the present time, the fact of being replete, the ulcerous condition, the hesitation with regard to movements, the heaviness of the whole body, and all other such things which they attribute to it; from the future, that those who were in this condition enjoyed good health once they had been subjected to evacuations – which is exactly what is omitted by Erasistratus.

223b Galenus, *In Hippocratis Aphorismos comment.* 2.17 (ad Hp. IV, p. 474 L) (XVIIB, p. 480K)

ἡ δ' ἐπὶ τέλει τοῦ ἀφορισμοῦ προσγεγραμμένη λέξις, ἔνθα φησί, "δηλοῖ δὲ ἴησις," ἄμεινον ἂν εἶχε μετὰ τοῦ καὶ συνδέσμου γεγραμμένη κατὰ τόνδε τὸν τρόπον· "δηλοῖ δὲ καὶ ἡ ἴησις" . . . τίς οὖν ἐστιν αὕτη κατὰ τὸν προκείμενον λόγον; ἡ ἐπὶ ταῖς
5 κενώσεσιν ἴασις τῶν λυπούντων χυμῶν, ἥντινα καὶ Ἡρόφιλος ἐν τῇ τριχρόνῳ καλουμένῃ σημειώσει παρέλαβεν.

223b The phrase added at the end of the *Aphorism* [2.17], where he says, 'The treatment makes this clear', would have been better if it had been written in the following way, namely with the conjunction 'and': '*and* the treatment makes this clear' . . . What then is this [treatment] in the passage under discussion here? The treatment accompanying evacuations of those humours that cause pain, which Herophilus in fact also adopts in his so-called 'triple-timed inference from signs'.

---

* The text should perhaps be emended to read *trichronos* ('triple-timed'), to resume the thought of line 3, instead of *dia chronon* ('through time').

224 Sextus Empiricus, *Adversus logicos* 2.188 (= *Adversus Mathematicos* 8.188)

τὰ γὰρ αὐτὰ φαινόμενα λόγου χάριν ἐν ἰατρικῇ ἄλλου μέν ἐστι σημεῖα τῷδε, καθάπερ Ἐρασιστράτῳ, ἄλλου δὲ τῷδε, καθάπερ Ἡροφίλῳ, ἄλλου δὲ τῷδε, καθάπερ Ἀσκληπιάδῃ. οὐ τοίνυν λεκτέον αἰσθητὸν εἶναι τὸ σημεῖον. εἰ γὰρ τὸ μὲν αἰσθητὸν
5 πάντας ὁμοίως κινεῖ, τὸ δὲ σημεῖον οὐ πάντας ὁμοίως κινεῖ, οὐκ ἂν εἴη αἰσθητὸν τὸ σημεῖον.

2 καθάπερ (*sec.*) ς: οἷον *NLE*

224 Thus the same appearances, for instance in medicine, are signs of one thing to this person, like Erasistratus, but of another thing to that one, like Herophilus, and of yet another to this one, like Asclepiades. One must, therefore, not say that the sign is a sensible. For, if the sensible affects all people similarly, while the sign does not affect all similarly, the sign could not be a sensible.

225 Sextus Empiricus, *Adversus logicos* 2.219-20 (= *Adversus mathematicos* 8.219-20)

τὸ γοῦν ἐπὶ τῶν πυρεσσόντων ἔρευθος καὶ ἡ τῶν ἀγγείων προπάλεια καὶ ὁ ἔνικμος χρὼς καὶ ἡ πλείων θερμασία καὶ ἡ σφοδρότης τῶν σφυγμῶν καὶ τὰ λοιπὰ σημεῖα τοῖς ὁμοίως κατά τε τὰς αἰσθήσεις καὶ τὴν ἄλλην σύγκρισιν διακειμένοις οὐ
5 τοῦ αὐτοῦ προσπίπτει σημεῖα, οὐδ' ὡσαύτως πᾶσι φαίνεται, ἀλλ' Ἡροφίλῳ μὲν λόγου χάριν ὡς ἄντικρυς χρηστοῦ αἵματος σημεῖα, Ἐρασιστράτῳ δὲ ὡς μεταπτώσεως τῆς ἐκ φλεβῶν εἰς ἀρτηρίας, Ἀσκληπιάδῃ δὲ ὡς ἐνστάσεως νοητῶν ὄγκων ἐν νοητοῖς ἀραιώμασιν.

1 ἀγγείων Kalbfleisch (*cf.* ibid. 204 et [Galeni] 'Introductio sive Medicus' 14 p. 729K): αἰτίων LE ς   5 προσπίπτει Bekker: προπίπτει G
7 ἐρεσιστράτῳ ς   8 ἐντάσεως N

225 In the case of patients with fever, therefore, flushing, a prominence of the blood-vessels, a moist skin, higher temperature, vehemence of the pulses, and the rest of the signs do not strike those who are in a similar state with respect to their senses and the rest of their constitution, as signs of the same thing. And these signs do not

even appear in like manner to all, but to Herophilus, for the sake of argument, clearly as signs of good blood, while they appear to Erasistratus as signs of the transference from the veins into the arteries, and to Asclepiades as the impaction of intelligible corpuscles [onkoi] in intelligible interstices.

9 Dream theory

226a Aëtius Doxographus, *Placita* 5.2.3 (*DG*, 416)

226b Ps.-Plutarchus, *Placita* 5.2 (*Moralia* 904F, vol. v.2.1 (Teubner), p. 134 Mau)

Ἡρόφιλος τῶν ὀνείρων τοὺς μὲν θεοπνεύστους κατ' ἀνάγκην γίνεσθαι, τοὺς δὲ φυσικοὺς ἀνειδωλοποιουμένης τῆς ψυχῆς τὸ συμφέρον αὐτῇ καὶ τὸ πρὸς τούτοις ἐσόμενον, τοὺς δὲ συγκρα-ματικοὺς ἐκ τοῦ αὐτομάτου κατ' εἰδώλων πρόσπτωσιν, ὅταν ἃ 5 βουλόμεθα βλέπωμεν, ὡς ἐπὶ τῶν τὰς ἐρωμένας ἐχόντων ἐν ὕπνῳ γίνεται.

1 τοὺς ὀνείρους τοὺς θεοπνεύστους Π   θεοπνεύστους] θεοπέμπτους Diels e ps.-Galeno (*T226c*)   2 τῆς om. Diels   3 αὐτῇ Diels   πρὸς τούτοις] πάντως Diels sec. ps.-Gal.: πρὸς τούτους Kessels (*1969: 416 adn. 3*)   3-4 συγκραματικοὺς codd.: συγκριματικοὺς ps.-Galenus: συγκρουματικοὺς coni. Reiske: συγκυρματικοὺς coni. Wyttenbach: πνευματικοὺς coni. Diels ex Aëtii sive 'Plutarchi' Placitis 5.15.5 (*T202a supra*)   4 ἐκ τοῦ αὐτομάτου del. Diels   κατ'] καὶ κατ' susp. Bernardakis   πρόπτωσιν M   5 ἐχόντων codd.: ἐρώντων ps.-Galenus, *T226c*: ἔχειν δοκούντων coni. Mau, fort. recte: ὁρώντων Diels: βλεπόντων Reiske

226a–b Herophilus says that some dreams are inspired by a god and arise by necessity, while others are natural ones and arise when the soul forms for itself an image (*eidōlon*) of what is to its own advantage and of what will happen next; and still others are mixed and arise spontaneously [or: 'accidentally'] according to the impact of the images, whenever we see what we wish, as happens in the case of those who in their sleep make love to* the women they love.

* The MSS read 'have' or 'hold' for 'make love to', but the MSS of the pseudo-Galenic *De historia philosopha* (see T226c) unanimously read 'love' or 'make love to'; Jürgen Mau has emended the text to read 'who in their sleep seem to hold' – not an implausible suggestion. 'Seem to hold' sometimes has sexual connotations, also in dream literature; cf. Artemidorus 4.4 (p. 248. 9-11 Pack). See also Schrijvers, 1977: 14 n. 3.

226c Ps.-Galenus, *De historia philosopha* 106 (*DG*, p. 640)

Ἡρόφιλος τῶν ὀνείρων τοὺς μὲν θεοπέμπτους κατ' ἀνάγκην
γίγνεσθαι, τοὺς δὲ φυσικοὺς εἰδωλοποιουμένης τῆς ψυχῆς τὸ
συμφέρον αὐτῇ καὶ τὸ πάντως ἐσόμενον· τοὺς δὲ συγκριματικοὺς αὐτομάτως κατ' εἰδώλων πρόσπτωσιν, ὅταν ἃ βουλόμεθα
5 βλέπωμεν, ⟨ὡς ἐπὶ τῶν⟩ φιλούντων γίγνεται τὰς ἐρωμένας
ἐρώντων ἐν ὕπνοις.

1-2 γίγνεσθαι κατ' ἀνάγκην *B*   3-4 καὶ . . . αὐτομάτως *om. A*
4 αὐτὸν ὅτι κατ' εἰδώλων ἐστὶ *B*   4-5 ὅταν ἀπολλύμεθα βλέπομεν
AB   5 ὡς ἐπὶ τῶν *suppl. Diels*   5 γίγνεσθαι *B*   6 εἰς ὕπνους *A*

226c Herophilus says that some dreams are sent by a god and arise by
necessity, while others are natural and arise when the soul makes for
itself an image (*eidōlon*) of what is to its advantage and of what will
undoubtedly happen; but the 'compound' dreams [arise] spontaneously, according to the impact of the images whenever we see what
we wish, as happens in the case of men who harbour affection, when
in their dreams they make love to the women they love.

226d Ioannes Laurentius Lydus, *Liber de mensibus* 4.135 (pp. 161–
2 Wünsch)

Καλένδαις Ὀκτωβρίαις οἱ ἱερεῖς ἐθέσπιζον τῷ δήμῳ μὴ χρῆναι
προσέχειν τοῖς ὀνείροις διὰ τὰς ἐκ τῆς ὑγρᾶς ὀγκώσεως τῶν
τοῦ φθινοπώρου καρπῶν φαντασίας, ἀπὸ δὲ τῶν Αὐξιφωτίων
ἤγουν τοῦ Ἰανουαρίου ὡς μάλιστα προσέχειν κατὰ τὸ δοκοῦν
5 Ἡροφίλῳ, ὃς καὶ θεοπέμπτους ἐνέκρινε τοὺς ὀνείρους, ὁ δὲ
Δημόκριτος κατὰ τὰς παραστάσεις τῶν εἰδώλων.

226d On the calends of October the priests decree to the people that
they should not pay attention to their dreams because of the [idle]
images (*phantasiai*) caused by the wet swelling of the fruits of autumn.
But from the time of the increase of light, or January, they should pay
as much attention as possible, in accordance with the opinion of
Herophilus, who judged that dreams are god-sent, whereas Democritus said that they occur in accordance with the representation of the
[atomistic] images (*eidōla*).

C · COMMENTS

T132 Although Galen's attribution of a humoral pathology to all these authors is correct in some general sense, it must be read with more than a pinch of salt, as the example of Plato reveals. While the humours are mentioned in Plato's pathological theory (*Timaeus* 81e–86a), they play a secondary role. Plato seems to follow a Sicilian model, perhaps inspired by Philistion (Wellmann, 1901: Philistion fr. 4, p. 110), in which the four elements of Philistion–Empedocles and the four humours espoused by the author of the Hippocratic treatise *On the Nature of Humans* provide the first foundation of pathology. Plato's first class of diseases results from excess, deficiency or misplacement of one of the primary elements. The second class, affecting tissues, does involve the generation of two – not four – noxious humours, but it is primarily depicted as a reversal of the normal course of nutrition and growth: bile and phlegm are the morbid products of the decomposition of flesh. A third class of diseases is due to the blocking of respiration (or the morbid formation of air inside the body) and to the two noxious humours. In his fever theory, too, Plato uses the four elements rather than the four humours (*Timaeus* 86a). It is, moreover, striking that blood – one of the four 'Hippocratic' humours – is never ranked among the humours by Plato. For a fuller discussion of the motley masks of humoral theory in Greek antiquity see Schöner, 1964. Cf. also Kollesch, 1976.

Aristotle: The only passages in the Aristotelian corpus which refer explicitly to the applicability of a humoral theory to human beings or animals occur in the pseudo-Aristotelian *Problemata Physica*. Cf., for example, *Probl.* 5.27.883b29; 10.22.893a35; 18.1.916b6; 30.1. Cf. *Eth. Nic.* 7.8.1150b25, 7.11.1152a27–9; *Hist. An.* 3.2.511b9–10, 1.1.487a1–6. But even these references are only allusive and do not reveal clearly an acceptance of a fullfledged humoral pathology.

Diocles: cf. fr. 7–9 and pp. 74ff. Wellmann. Cf. Galen, *De naturalibus facultatibus* 2.8 (*Scr. Min.* III, pp. 181–6 Helmreich); *Methodus medendi* 1.2 (x, pp. 14–18K); *In Hp. De natura hominis comm.* 2.6 (*CMG* v.9.1, p. 70 Mewaldt). Cf. also Diocles, fr. 42–3 Wellmann.

On Praxagoras and his pupils Plistonicus and Phylotimus, see Steckerl, 1958: fr. 16–18 and pp. 108–26; also Bardong, 1951, and *id.*, 1954; *supra*, T10, T14, and Chapter II nn. 20 and 34.

Mnesitheus: a physician of the mid-fourth century B.C.; see Bertier, fr. 12–15 (= fr. 6–9 Hohenstein), and Deichgräber, 1932.

Cf. Galen, *De naturalibus facultatibus*, *loc. cit.*, for comparable enumerations in the context of praising his 'ancient' (*palaioi*) precursors' views on the humours. (Exempted from his praise is, however, once again Erasistratus.)

See also Galen's list of his 'ancient' (*archaioi*) predecessors in *In Hp. De natura hominis comm.*, *loc. cit.* (cf. Chapter VI, T69 *supra*).

T137–T139 Among the indirect testimonia might be the following:
    (a) Dionysius Aegaeus, *Dictyaca* 40 (in Photius, *Bibliothecae*, cod. 211, vol. III, p. 118 Henry): ὅτι διὰ τῶν νεύρων ἡ αἴσθησις καὶ ἡ κίνησις τοῦ ζῴου, καὶ ὅτι οὐχ οὕτως, 'That the sensation *and* movement of a living being [occur] through the nerves, and that this is not the case.' Dionysius is presenting topics for dialectical argument (pro and con), and the first view to which he alludes might be Herophilus', although other Greeks also held this view (cf. Dulière, 1965: 510).
    (b) Caelius Aurelianus, *Celeres vel acutae passiones* 1.8.53: quaesitum etiam quis locus in phreniticis patitur . . . aliqui igitur cerebrum pati dixerunt (sc. Hippocrates?), alii eius fundum sive basin (sc. Herophilus?), quam nos sessionem dicere poterimus, alii membranas (sc. Erasistratus?), alii et cerebrum et eius membranas (sc. Posidonius medicus?), alii cor (Praxagoras?), alii cordis summitatem . . . 'It is also asked which place is affected in people suffering from phrenitis [delirium]. Now some [sc. the Hippocratics?] say the brain is affected, others [sc. Herophilus?] its fundus or base, which we may translate 'seat' (*sessio*), others again [sc. Erasistratus?] its membranes, others the brain and its membranes [sc. Posidonius the physician?], others the heart [sc. Praxagoras?], others the apex of the heart . . . '
    Praxagoras:fr. 62, p. 76 Steckerl. Posidonius medicus: Aëtius, *Libri medicinales* 6.2 (*CMG* VIII. 2, p. 125 Olivieri); Wellmann, 1901: 14–20; Fuchs, 1894b: esp. pp. 540–1. Cf. also Galen, *Sympt. caus.* 2.7 (VII, p. 202K); ps.-Galen, *Introductio* 13 (XIV, p. 733K).
    Cf. also Dionysius Aegaeus, *Dictyaca* 50 (in Photius, *Bibliothecae*, cod. 211; vol. III, p. 118 Henry): ὅτι τὸ διανοητικόν ἐστι περὶ τὴν μέσην τοῦ ἐγκεφάλου κοιλίαν, καὶ ὅτι οὐχ οὕτως, 'That the capacity to think is [located] in the area of the central ventricle of the brain, and that this is not the case'. Deichgräber (1965: 340) apparently thinks that the first of these two views is attributable to Herophilus, but the location of the *dianoētikon* in the central ventricle might well be a post-Galenic development; see Nemesius, *On the Nature of Man* 12 (p. 201 Matthaei), and Posidonius medicus, in Aëtius, *loc. cit.* (p. 125, l.17): τῆς δὲ μέσης κοιλίας τοῦ ἐγκεφάλου βλαβείσης παρατροπὴ γίγνεται τοῦ λογιστικοῦ. Cf. Edelstein & Kidd, 1972: T114, under 'Dubia'; Flashar, 1966: 121; Sudhoff, 1913. *Dictyaca* 42 (Photius, *op cit.* 'That the liver is the source of the veins . . .') might be further evidence that Dionysius post-dates Galen, as Phillip De Lacy kindly pointed out to me.

T137a–e Aëtius' *Placita* is the primary source; all the others (137b–e) seem to depend on Aëtius, if not on his main source, the *Vetusta Placita*. Plato: cf. *Timaeus* 44D5–6; Democritus: 68A105DK; Strato: fr. 119–21 Wehrli;

Erasistratus: cf. Galen, *De Plac. Hp. et Plat.* 7.3; Parmenides: 28A45DK; Epicurus: cf. fr. 312 Usener and fr. 160 Arrighetti (and Arrighetti's comments, pp. 515f.); Stoics: *SVF* II, 838 (cf. II, 839).

T138 Cf. Chapter XI below, *An.* 6.

T142–143 On Aëtius' primacy as a source cf. above, *Comments*, T137a–e.

T149 Praxagoras: fr. 27, p. 62 Steckerl.

T150 Praxagoras: fr. 27, pp. 61–2 Steckerl.

T151 Praxagoras: fr. 26, p. 61 Steckerl.

T152 Praxagoras: fr. 27, p. 63 Steckerl.

T153 Praxagoras: fr. 26, p. 61 Steckerl.

Palpitation. Galen provides a fuller explanation of palpitation (παλμός) in *De tremore, palpitatione, convulsione et rigore* 5 (VII pp. 593–9K). For a discussion of Herophilus' use of 'pulsation' and 'palpitation,' see Introd. to this section (VII. A. 4). Cf. also Harris, 1973: 182–4. Galen's distinction (pulse-activity vs. palpitation-affection) is taken over by Nemesius of Emesa, *De natura hominis* 16 (p. 217 Matthaei).

Erasistratus. The 'more ancient usage' attributed to Erasistratus and Hippocrates is probably the use of *sphygmos* in the restricted sense of the perceptible throbbing especially in the cases of inflammation. Thus, in *De differentiis pulsuum* 4.17 (VIII, p. 761K), Galen says, on the basis of the first book of Erasistratus' *On Fevers*: 'Erasistratus indeed seems to give the name 'pulsation' (*sphygmos*) not to the natural motion in the arteries but only to the motion in inflammation (ἐπὶ φλεγμονῇ)'. Elsewhere, however, Galen clearly implies that Erasistratus also used 'pulsation' of the movement of the arteries in a mechanical process of diastole and systole: in its systole, the heart mechanically propels pneuma into the arteries, and the resulting expansion of the arteries is the systole of the pulse; the contraction is equally mechanical (*De diff. puls.* 4.2 (VIII, p. 714K); *Synopsis librorum de pulsibus* 22 (IX, pp. 507–8K); *De usu pulsuum* 5 (V, p. 167–8K). In *De diff. puls.* 1.2 (VIII, p. 497K), on the other hand, Galen again, as in this testimonium from *De placitis*, puts Hippocrates and Erasistratus in the same camp of sphygmological primitives. Galen's negative attitude to Erasistratus, which also emerges in his famous experiment on the arterial pulse (see von Staden, 1975: 182–3), was, in the case of pulse theory at least, probably fed by the mechanistic implications of Erasistratus' model.

Subsequent section: Galen, *De placitis Hp. et Plat.* 6.8 (*CMG* v. 4.1.2, p. 416, ll. 27–32 De Lacy).

T155 Praxagoras: fr. 28, p. 64 Steckerl.

T161 Praxagoras: fr. 84, pp. 84–5 Steckerl.

T162 Cf. Chapter xiv, *Ba* 4; Chapter xvii, *Hg*. 2; Chapter xx, *Cr*. 3; Chapter xxiii, *AM*. 3; Chapter xxiv, *HE*. 12; Chapter xxv, *Ar. 4*

T166 Cf. *Odyssey* 10.495. A popular Homeric verse throughout antiquity: Plato, *Meno* 100A5, *Republic* 3.386D7; Diogenes Laertius 7.183 (applied to Chrysippus the Stoic). Cato the Elder used the same verse of Scipio (concerning Carthage): Plutarch, *Cato Maior* 27.6 (I. 1, p. 324 Ziegler), *Moralia* 200A and 804F–805A; Diodorus of Sicily 32.9.a.2; Polybius 36.8.7; Suda s.vv. *aissousin* (α.691), *Katōn* (κ.1113).

T169 It is important to note that only the coinage 'gazelle-like pulse' – not the description or explanation offered in T169 – is attributed to Herophilus.

T175 It is far from certain (*pace* Pigeaud, 1978: 260, and Longrigg, 1981: 174) that Galen wishes to attribute the threefold pathological classification—'pararhythmic', 'hetero-rhythmic', 'ecrhythmic'—to Herophilus. Here all Galen says explicitly about Herophilus is that the Alexandrian proposed comparing the time of dilation to the time of contraction, and neither Galen nor any other ancient author ever unequivocally attributes the three terms to Herophilus. In the next sentence after T175 Galen refers his reader to an earlier work, *De pulsuum differentiis* 1.8 (viii, pp. 514–17K), for an explanation of these three kinds of abnormal pulse—a passage in which, once again, Herophilus is not depicted as the author of these distinctions. Similarly, in ps.-Galen, *Definitiones medicae* 220 (xix, pp. 408–9K)—a passage invoked by Pigeaud, Longrigg, and others in this context–the attributions of rhythm definitions are to the Herophileans Zeno (ch. xv, *Zn*.2), Bacchius (ch. xiv, *Ba*.3), and Hegetor (ch. xvii, *Hg*. 4; see Kollesch, 1973: 137 n.183). On the independence of later Herophileans from Herophilus, also in pulse theory, see below, ch. x. A, and von Staden, 1982: 85–93. Moreover, in *Definitiones medicae* 221–2 (xix, pp. 409–10) the definitions of eurhythmic, arhythmic, caco-rhythmic, pararhythmic, hetero-rhythmic and ecrhythmic are presented as the author's own definitions, not as those of any Herophilean, although the emphasis on stages of life both here and in *De puls. diff*. 1.8 suggests at least the oblique influence of Herophilus (see T176–T186). See also n. 162.

T176 In T177 there is no reference to any normal systole or contraction of the pulse that lasts more than two 'primary time-units'. The references to contractions that last five or ten primary time-units in T176 therefore seem to be allusions to pathological phenomena of the kind described in T178.

HEROPHILUS

T177 Herophilus apparently distinguished four stages of life, but it is striking that Marcellinus, who in his *On Pulses* often mentions Herophilus, refers to those who recognized four stages only as τινες, 'some people' (Chapter 25; Marcellinus himself, *ibid.*, reverts to a traditional sevenfold division of the stages of life, famous versions of which are Hp., *Hebd.* 5 (IX, p. 436; VIII, p. 636L); Philo, *De opificio mundi* 103–6 (35–6 Cohn/Wendland)). Fourfold divisions of the ages of man also occur prior to Herophilus. Cf., for example, Xenophon, *Symposium* 4.17; Aristotle, *On Generation of Animals* 5.3.784a17–20 (vs. three stages in Aristotle's *Rhetoric* 2.12–14); Hp., *On Regimen* 1.33 (*CMG* 1.2.4, p. 150 Joly/Byl); and D.L. 8.10, where it is said to be a Pythagorean division. Although one cannot be absolutely certain that this entire testimonium should be assigned to Herophilus, the fact that Rufus (?) here mentions Herophilus as the author of the characterizations both of the first and of the last of the four pulse types under discussion strongly suggests that the entire passage is based on Herophilus' theory. Cf. Ch. IX, T267–8 on *nēpion*.

alogos: A concept perhaps inspired by the extensive treatment of *alogoi* feet in the *Rhythmica* of Aristoxenus of Tarentum; cf. Westphal, 1883–93: vol. I, pp. 151–7; *Rhythmica* 2.20–1 and 25 (vol. II, pp. 82–3 Westphal). *Alogos* continued to be used widely by subsequent musical and metrical theorists, e.g. Aristides Quintilianus, *De musica* 1.14, 17, 19 (pp. 33–4, 37, 40 Winnington-Ingram); Bacchius Geron, *Isagoge* 95 (*Musici scriptores Graeci* p. 313 Jan); Cleonides, *Isagoge harmonica* 5, 8, 10 (pp. 187–9, 193, 199 Jan); *Anonyma de musica Bellermanniana* 58 (p. 16 Najock). In sphygmology it became a less central term.

T182 See also above *Comments*, T177, and n. 150.

Hermann Diels' conjecture ἢ βραδύτερον in line 14 (1920: 27 n. 4, adopted by Fraser, 1972: vol. II, p. 518 n. 113) is superfluous and, in fact, misleading. (i) The patient has a fever, hence his pulse rate will necessarily be πυκνότερος (i.e., more frequent than normal or '*too* frequent') in Herophilus' view: ὁ δὲ Ἡρόφιλος πυρέσσειν ἀπεφήνατο τὸν ἄνθρωπον, ὁπόταν πυκνότερος ... ὁ σφυγμὸς γένηται μετὰ πολλῆς θερμασίας ἔνδον (T182.1–4 *supra*). What the physician tries to determine with the help of his *clepsydra* is simply *by how much* the pulse is πυκνότερος; this will in turn reveal whether the patient has a high or slight fever. (ii) In ancient sphygmological theory the antonym of πυκνός tends to be *not* βραδύς but ἀραιός. βραδύς would be the antonym of ταχύς, which is distinct from πυκνός. Marcellinus devotes an entire chapter of his treatise to this very distinction: τίνι διαφέρει ταχύτης πυκνότητος (ch. 6, Schöne). See n. 156 (p. 284 *supra*).

T183 arsis and **thesis**: This too might be an echo of the *Rhythmica* (e.g. 2.20) of the Peripatetic philosopher Aristoxenus of Tarentum (although he seems to have preferred *arsis* and *basis*: Westphal, 1883–93: vol. II, p. 82). For the musical tradition concerning *arsis*   and *thesis* see, e.g., Aristides Quintilianus, *De musica* 1.13 (p. 31 Winnington-Ingram). (For a non-musical use see ps.-Aristotle, *Problemata* 5.41.885b6.)

primary time-unit: Herophilus' use of *chronos prōtos* might have been inspired by Aristoxenus' use of *prōtos chronos* in his *Rhythmica* (e.g., 2.10–12; cf. Westphal, 1883–93: vol. I, pp. 13–16, 485–6;vol. II, pp. CLII, 78–9, 94–5). See also Georgiades, 1949: 40–1. Aristoxenus defines his 'primary time unit' as the smallest unit of time which cannot be further divided by any of the three *rhythmizomena* (*lexis, melos,* somatic *kinēsis*). All other time-units are defined as multiples of the primary time-unit (*chronos disēmos, trisēmos, tetrasēmos,* etc.). Cf. by contrast *SVF* II, 509ff.: there are no indivisible units of time.

T187 Pythagoras: cf. Cicero, *Tusculan Disputations* 4.3; Seneca, *De ira* 3.9.2; Quintilian, *Institutiones orat.* 9.4.12; Iamblichus, *Vita Pythagorae* 25; Plutarch, *Moralia* 384A.

Asclepiades: cf. Martianus Capella 9.926 (p. 355 Willis).

harmony: This part of the testimonium is not attributed to Herophilus. Is is worth noting, however, that the Peripatetic Aristoxenus of Tarentum, whose *Rhythmica* apparently had at least some influence on Herophilus' pulse theories, also suggested an analogy between musical harmony, harmony in the body, and the soul as harmony (fr. 120a–d Wehrli; cf. also Dicaearchus, fr. 5–12 Wehrli). It is not impossible that Aristoxenus' version of this popular analogy, which might have originated with the Pythagoreans, played a role in Herophilus' assimilation of prosody to sphygmology. Cf. Pigeaud, 1978: 264; n. 136 *supra*; Huchzermeyer, 1974; Kümmel, 1977: 23ff.

T189 Varicose assistant (παραστάτης κιρσοειδής): Although *parastatēs* was used of genital parts as early as the fifth century B.C. (see Chapter VI, *Comments*, T101–3), this particular usage originated with Herophilus, and it seems to refer specifically to the ampullae of the vasa deferentia, as Galen apparently suggests here. At the end of the long fragment from his *Anatomy* (Fr61), Herophilus indicates that it is a designation normally limited to a part of the *male* reproductive system. The 'assistance' rendered by the 'varicose *parastatēs*' not only assumes the form of help in the transportation of seed from its source – the blood, according to Herophilus – to the penis, but apparently also 'assistance' in the final stage of seed formation prior to seminal discharge, as this testimonium and the next (T190) make clear. On the name see also T101–T103, T105, T190. (παραστάτης was, however, also used for a variety of other anatomical structures: testes, epididymis, etc. Cf. LSJ.) On the 'glandular assistants' see T101, T102, T105, and Galen, *On Seed* 2.6 (IV, pp. 642–651K). Cf. Ch. VI, *Comments*, T61.

καυλός means 'penis' as early as Hp., *On Internal Affections* 14 (VII, p. 202L).

Cf. also Galen, *Use of Parts* 14.12 (II, p. 324 Helmreich), *On Seed* 2.5 (IV, p. 636K); Rufus, *Onom.* 101 (p. 146 Daremberg/Ruelle).

One of Galen's major criticisms of Herophilus' reproductive theory is that Herophilus failed to attribute enough significance to the role of the testes in the generation of sperm. In the section immediately preceding T189, Galen discusses castration and raises the question 'why the whole [male] body is made feminine by the excision of the testicles'. The implication seems to be that Herophilus' theory could not account adequately for such phenomena. As I suggested above (VII.A.5), however, Herophilus perhaps does not take quite as dim a view of the contribution of the testes to seed formation as Galen and some of his readers have assumed.

Loom weights: Aristotle uses this image of the function of the testicles in *On the Generation of Animals* 1.4.717a35 and 5.7.787b26.

T192 satyriasis: A description of this affection of the penis – a sustained erection from which no relief can be obtained, not even by masturbation – is provided by Herophilus' follower Demetrius of Apamea; see *infra*, Chapter XVI, *DA.2*. On a closely related affection, priapism, see *ibid.*, *DA.1*.

T196 Herophilus seems to have classified cases of difficult childbirth by internal and external cause, and this provides another striking example of the strong aetiological orientation that characterizes his pathophysiology, despite the sceptical strain which is represented in his theory of scientific method (cf. Chapter V *supra*). For a further example of his aetiological approach to taxonomy cf. T226. One of Herophilus's pupils, Demetrius of Apamea, introduced a new aetiological classification of *dystokiai*, namely by causes which can be traced (a) to the foetus, (b) to the parturient's general constitution, and (c) to the female reproductive tract (see below Chapter XVI, *DA.* 21). This tripartite division apparently became the standard one; cf. Soranus, *Gynaecia* 4.2[54]–4.5[57] (*CMG* IV, pp. 131–5 Ilberg). The conditions Herophilus discusses all appear to be chronic in nature; see Most, 1981: 194–5 nn. 16–17. For further examples of the Greek tradition of discussing or classifying cases of difficult childbirth, see Diepgen, 1937: 207–12; Buess, 1968.

Most (1981) argues brilliantly that Callimachus' *Hymn to Delos* 206–11 displays the poet's 'unmistakeable wit' in applying 'the recent medical discoveries of Herophilus to the transmitted myth of the birth of Apollo' (i.e. Homeric *Hymn to Apollo* 117–18). Especially in view of Oppermann's (1925) demonstration of Herophilus' influence in a Callimachean allusion (see *Comments*, T87–T89), Most's argument is seductive. One should keep in mind, however, (a) that Herophilus is not known to have advocated the sitting position assumed by Callimachus' Leto; (b) Leto's position in Callimachus' *Hymn* (but not in the Homeric Hymn) is the normal position of

Greek women in childbirth. Leto's Callimachean position therefore requires neither Herophilean invention nor Callimachean allusion to Alexandrian medical discoveries for its pointed subversion and inversion of the Homeric Hymn.

T200 Herophilus' view that the mouth of the uterus closes so tightly immediately upon conception that not even the tip or head of a probe could be inserted into it was adopted by later Greek authors. The closing of the mouth of the uterus was regarded as one of the most prominent early indications of pregnancy. Some Greek authors used this symptom to argue that the 'closed uterus' prevents the volatile pneuma in the seed from escaping. Cf. Soranus, *Gynaecia* 1.44 (*CMG* IV, p. 31 Ilberg); Galen, *De usu partium* 14.3 (II, p. 288 Helmreich). See also *ibid.*, 15.7 (II, pp. 363–4 Helmreich): 'There is no one who does not know that the orifice of the uterus is tightly constricted and closed during pregnancy while it is open as wide as possible at the time of birth.' Cf. also Diepgen, 1937: 144–5. **Hippocrates:** *Aphor.* 5.51 and 5.54 (IV, pp. 550–2L).

T201 Herophilus' observation that only the orifice of the uterus (i.e. cervix?) and not the entire uterus prolapses comes close to the modern understanding of prolapsus. Cases of prolapsus apparently were fairly common; it is discussed or alluded to from the Hippocratic Corpus onward. Cf., for example, Hp., *On the Nature of Woman* 4–5, 81 (VII, pp. 316–18, 406L); *Diseases of Women* 2.143–5, 147, 153, 204 (VIII, pp. 316–20, 322ff., 328, 392L); *On Barren Women* (*Steril.*) 213(1), 247(35)–248(36) (VIII, pp. 414, 460L); *On Places in Man* 47 (VI, p. 344L). See also Soranus, *Gynaecia* 4.35–40 (*CMG* IV, pp. 147–52). For a more detailed discussion cf. Diepgen, 1937: 228–32. (See also Diepgen, 1937: 244–5, on the use of probes in antiquity as a gynaecological diagnostic device.)

T203 The title of Herophilus' work, *Against Common Opinions*, has Aristotelian overtones (cf., for example, Ar., *Physics* 4.6.213a21-2: one should examine the 'pro' views regarding the existence of void, the 'con' views, 'and, in the third place, the commonly held opinions, *koinai doxai*, concerning these issues'). It is possible that Herophilus' treatise dealt with 'commonly held opinions' in this Aristotelian sense and hence was not doxographic in an orthodox sense. Be this as it may, the title suggests that Herophilus at least had an interest in *doxai* other than those reported in the Hippocratic Corpus. For further details on Herophilean doxography see Chapters X–XI, XIV, XXII–XXV; Schöne, 1893.

T218 In his catalogue of mediaeval Latin medical manuscripts in France, Ernest Wickersheimer (1966: 159–71, no. CIX) describes an eleventh-century manuscript from Rouen – cod. 1407 (O.55), from the Abbey of Saint-

Ouen – which contains *inter alia* a medley of excerpts and summaries of various diseases and their cures (fol. 202–214v). One of the excerpts reports that *Yrofilus auctor quoque Irralicles* wrote about toothaches. Wickersheimer, 1966: 171, observes that some of the excerpts appear to be passages, or echoes of passages, from Book III of Galen's *Ad Glauconem methodus medendi*, while others recur in Gariopontus' *Passionarius* (a derivative eleventh-century Salernitan compilation, sometimes also attributed to Galen). The excerpt concerning Herophilus appears to be neither derived from Galen's *Ad Glauconem* nor independent evidence. Rather, it depends on T218 (and ultimately on Caelius Aurelianus' source, Soranus): Aurelianus' *Herophilus denique Heraclides Tarentinus* has been transformed into *Yrofilus auctor quoque Irralicles* by the time of the medieval compilation. On the manuscript see also Beccaria, 1956: 183–5.

T220   The aphorism concerned is Hp., *Aphorism* 6.1 (IV, p. 562L): 'In cases of chronic lientery, it is a good sign if acid eructation [or: heartburn], not having occurred previously, supervenes.'

VIII · REGIMEN
AND THERAPEUTICS

'Let us . . . take our Phlebothomer with us to let hym bloud.'

WILLIAM BULLEIN, *Bulwarke of defence against*
all sicknesse, soarenesse and woundes (1562)

A · INTRODUCTION

It has been said that the history of therapeutics is a history of errors, and those who glance back more than two thousand years, from the contemporary perspectives of psychopharmacology, chemotherapy, hormone treatment, antibiotics, and cardiac surgery, might be inclined to agree. Many therapeutic measures employed by the Greeks seem to have been not only inefficacious but also harmful, and much seems to have been outrageous and amusing quackery.[1] Herophilus' use of crocodile dung and hyena bile to cure day-blindness[2] might confirm the worst suspicions of some modern critics, and it might deal a blow to those neo-Romantics who, like Mr Crotchet of *Crotchet Castle*, think that 'where [the Greeks] had anything that exalts, delights, or adorns humanity, we have nothing but cant, cant, cant . . .'.[3]

Yet not all was foul in the land of the Ptolemies. The comprehensive nature of the Alexandrians' approach to the problem of health strongly echoes positions being advocated today. Herophilus, for example, stressed that therapeutics should encompass not only the symptomatic treatment of disorders by means of drugs and dietary regulation, but also causal treatment – despite his insistence on the provisional nature of all causal explanation[4] – and, at least equally significantly, he insisted that health care included preventive care through athletic and other forms of exercise and through a sound diet.

[1] For general accounts see Ackerknecht, 1973; Ebstein, 1911; Neuburger, 1926: 5–21; Petersen, 1877; Schelenz, 1904; Majno, 1975: 141–206.
[2] Fr260 (below).   [3] Peacock, 1831: 136.   [4] See Chapter v.

In the absence of health, Herophilus said in his treatise *Regimen*,[5] one's wisdom cannot be demonstrated, one's scientific skill or craft remains invisible, one's strength cannot be exerted in contest, one's wealth is useless, and one's power of speech powerless. Wisdom, scientific skill, strength in contest, wealth, power of speaking: a vivid, revealing enumeration of Alexandrian values – and all these cherished values can, in Herophilus' view, be undermined radically just by the absence of health. That this view is presented in a work apparently devoted largely to regimen in the service of preventive care[6] seems to illustrate the importance attached by Herophilus to a comprehensive approach to health care. Already in antiquity Herophilus was given credit for this comprehensive emphasis. In a polemical discussion of whether 'the part of the art concerning health' (*to hygieinon*) belongs to 'the art of medicine' (*iatrikē*) or to 'the art of athletic exercises' (*gymnastikē*), Galen twice refers approvingly to Herophilus as a person knowledgeable 'about the *whole* art concerning the body',[7] i.e. both about 'the art of healing' or therapeutics proper and about 'the art of health' (*hygieinē*). The latter, Galen explains, also includes 'the art of athletic exercise'; and so firmly did this part of the 'art of health' become associated with Herophilus that a ball used in athletic exercises 'along with some other gymnastic instruments' were included in a sculpture of Herophilus mentioned by a twelfth-century Byzantine monk, Eustathius, in his commentary on the Homeric *Odyssey*.[8]

To general therapeutics Herophilus contributed a treatise entitled *Ways of Healing* or *Therapeutics* in at least two books.[9] Although much of the ancient information concerning it is in the form of negative

[5] T230. Cf. Hp., *Regimen* 3.69.

[6] Although regimen was often used for therapeutic purposes by ancient physicians (including Herophilus; cf. T256), the main emphasis of a treatise simply called 'regimen' would probably have been on preserving health. Cf. Edelstein, 1967: 307: 'Medicine in Hellenistic times, like earlier medicine, is concerned with the dietetics of the *healthy*' (italics mine). On the preventive and therapeutic functions of regimen in ancient medicine cf. also Temkin, 1962a; Petersen, 1903; Dustmann, 1938; Edelstein, 1967: 303–16. See also above, ch. IV.A.1.

[7] T227–T228. Schneider, 1967–9: vol. II, p. 412, claims that Herophilus recommended 'breathing lots of fresh air'. Presumably on a *Spaziergang*? There is no evidence for this assertion. Cf. Plato, *Gorgias* 464B vs. *Republic* 3.410B–D.

[8] T229.

[9] Caelius Aurelianus refers to Herophilus' *primo libro Curationum* (T231), and the conclusion that the work consisted of more than one book therefore seems reasonable.

data – for example, that Herophilus recorded no treatments for phrenitis, cholera, pleurisy, pneumonia, inflammation of the throat, and lethargic fever[10] – four general therapeutic ideas seem to emerge from the positive evidence.

First, for therapeutic purposes at least, Herophilus apparently abandoned the potential of the Aristotelian distinction between 'uniform' or 'homoeomerous' parts of the body (e.g. blood, marrow, bile, veins, sinew, seed) and 'instrumental' parts (e.g. eye, finger, arm, leg, liver, heart).[11] Instead, Herophilus limited his treatment to remedies indicated by the 'instrumental' parts of the body, i.e. by the position, colouration, sensation, and so on of individual 'instrumental' parts.[12] Galen argues that this, along with the abandonment of any therapeutic analysis in terms of the elements and their qualities – the hot and cold, the dry and wet – seriously restricts the number of remedial options within the physician's purview, and condemns Herophilus as a mere 'half-dogmatic'.[13] The inchoate histological possibilities lurking in the Aristotelian investigation of 'uniform' parts were indeed not exploited for their therapeutic potential, and Galen's strictures are perhaps not misdirected.

The usual lag between scientific and clinical medicine, between theory and therapy, seems to be illustrated by Herophilus' adherence to a relatively one-sided range of remedial indicators: while 'instrumental' parts alone serve to indicate remedies, Herophilus in his physiological theory by contrast deals extensively with the origins and functions of what Aristotle had called 'uniform' parts (especially with blood, bloodvessels, and seed), producing striking theoretical advances over some of his predecessors.

A second general therapeutic principle adopted by Herophilus seems to have been treatment by contrary remedies.[14] This allopathic principle did not originate with Herophilus;[15] it represents a further

[10] See T239–T244.
[11] T232–T233. Cf. Aristotle's discussion of this distinction in *On Parts of Animals* 1.1 640b17ff.; 2.1 646a20–4, 647a1–24; 2.2 647b10ff., etc. Not all later Herophileans seem to have abandoned this distinction.
[12] Cf. T232. See Harig, 1974: 58.
[13] T233: ἐξ ἡμισείας . . . ὄντες δογματικοί.   [14] T234.
[15] Already by the time of Aristotle the allopathic principle had become a commonplace; cf. *Nicomachean Ethics* 2.3.1104b18: 'medicines work *naturally* by means of opposites'. Examples from the Hippocratic Corpus include *Aphorisms* 2.22 and 5.19, *On Breaths* 1.

example of how the 'new' Alexandrian medicine tended to intertwine strands of conservatism with innovative strands.

A third, and related, theapeutic policy endorsed by Herophilus is the liberal use of drugs. 'Medicaments', Herophilus says, 'are the hands of the gods.'[16] Although it is not the hands of human beings that are extended beyond their normal reach through drugs, but those of the gods, the divine 'hands' require a human agent in order to be efficacious. Drugs are nothing *per se*, Herophilus also seems to have said, if they are not employed correctly by humans.[17]

Celsus' claim that Herophilus and his followers used drugs not only liberally but licentiously – 'they did not treat *any* kind of disease without drugs'[18] – is an exaggeration, as demonstrated, for example, by Herophilus' treatment of consumption by means of dietary regulation only (salted pickled fish with bread and water).[19] But Herophilus without question made very active use of drugs derived both from plants and from animals. Pliny and Galen refer to him primarily as an expert on simple drugs,[20] but four of his compound prescriptions – one for the expectoration of blood, one for an anal affection, one for day-blindness, and one (his 'green plaster') for a skin condition similar to lichen – are also recorded by ancient sources, and Galen refers to him reverentially in the context of the history of compound drugs.[21] Although Herophilus never receives the praise

[16] T248–T249. The value of the passage from Plutarch (T248c) depends, however, on an emendation suggested by Wellmann and accepted by Deichgräber; see critical apparatus *ad loc*. On the drug 'hand of Asclepius' see Aëtius of Amida 12.53 (p. 90 Costomiris).

[17] In T249 Galen seems to be saying that '*each of two things*' (ἑκάτερον) said by Herophilus is true: (a) 'that drugs alone *per se* are nothing, . . . for they are nothing if they do not have a person who employs them correctly'; and (b) that 'drugs are just like the hands of the gods'.

[18] T251.   [19] T256.

[20] T253 (Galen): Herophilus is a witness for simple drugs; T254 (Pliny): Herophilus thought 'that there is nothing which cannot be accomplished by *plants*, but that the powers of most plants are unknown'; T255: Herophilus used to compare *hellebore* to a very courageous general: 'when it has aroused all inside, it marches out in the vanguard' (and hence can be taken in large doses). On hellebore see Majno, 1979: 181, 496 n. 212.

[21] T258 (a prescription for expectoration of blood); T259 (a prescription for anal affections); Fr260 (an ointment for day-blindness, from Herophilus' *On Eyes*); T257 (his 'green plaster' apparently for 'mentagra', or a lichen-like condition). Michler's description (1968: 35) of T257 as a prescription for use 'bei Wunden und Geschwüren' is probably too general; the context in which Galen enumerates prescriptions in this chapter, starting as early as XII, p. 830K and continuing up to

bestowed upon a later Herophilean, Mantias,[22] as the father of the elaborate 'compound drug' tradition of antiquity, it is clear that 'the hands of the gods', in Herophilus' view, did not consist only of simple drugs such as hellebore, and that Herophilus might in fact have provided much of the impetus for the active development of the complex pharmacological tradition.

A fourth therapeutic principle adopted by Herophilus – and again one which did not originate with him – is phlebotomy, i.e. opening a vein to draw blood from a patient.[23] The belief that bloodletting had decisive therapeutic value in a wide range of diseases had become widespread no later than the fourth century B.C. – among others Hippocratics, Diocles, Mnesitheus, and Herophilus' teacher, Praxagoras, practised venesection[24] – and Herophilus, unlike his contemporary Erasistratus (who strongly opposed the indiscriminate use of bleeding[25]), here is uncritically accepting a reasonably entrenched

p. 844K, is specifically the treatment of lichen-like eruptions on the skin and related problems (cf. XII, pp. 830–1: πρὸς τοὺς . . . λειχῆνας; p. 832: τροχίσκος λειχηνικός; p. 834: πρὸς λειχῆνας χρονίους; p. 835: λειχηνική; p. 837: ἔμπλαστρα λειχηνικά; p. 841: πρὸς τὰς μεντάγρας; p. 842: χλωρὰ λειχηνικά and χλωρὸν . . . ἐπὶ τῆς μεντάγρας; p. 844: μετὰ τὴν τῶν λειχήνων ἐκδοράν, etc.). For Galen's general admiration for Herophilus as a pharmacologist cf. T252, T250; similarly, Celsus in T251.

[22] See Chapter XVIII below.

[23] T237–T238. Michler (1968: 13, 15) comes to exactly the opposite conclusion, viz. that Herophilus rejected phlebotomy: 'Die grundsätzliche Ablehnung der venae sectio durch Erasistratos *und schon durch Herophilos* und auch Xenophon musste aber in Alexandrien *mit einem Schlage* den unseligen Bann brechen' (p. 13; italics added); also, of physicians like Herophilus, Erasistratus, and Xenophon, Michler (p. 15) says that they 'mit ihren *blutsparenden Massnahmen* zum ersten Mal grösseren chirurgischen Eingriffen die Aussicht auf Erfolg öffneten'. While this might be true of Erasistratus, T237–T238 suggest the contrary: that the 'unselige' spell of phlebotomy was not broken 'with a single stroke' by Herophilus, but that the spell continued to bewitch even this remarkable physician. That Herophilus used bandaging and ligations in cases of *involuntary* bleeding – T231 – is a different matter and does not refute Galen's unequivocal reports that Herophilus subscribed to the use of phlebotomy.

[24] Cf. T237–T238; Diocles, fr. 89 Wellmann; Dieuches, fr. 3 Bertier; Mnesitheus, fr. 5 Bertier (= fr. 18 Hohenstein); Praxagoras, fr. 98 Steckerl. For the use of phlebotomy as a method of evacuation in the Hippocratic Corpus, cf. *Regimen in Acute Diseases (Spur.)* 3–6 [= 2–4L] (I, pp. 147–9Kw); *Prognostic* 15 (I, p. 93Kw); *Aphorisms* 5.31 and 6.47 (IV, pp. 542, 574L); *Coan Predictions* 288 (V, p. 648L); *De nat. hom.* 11 (*CMG* I.I.3, pp. 194–6 Jouanna).

[25] Cf., for example, Galen, *De venae sectione adversus Erasistratum, passim*, especially Chapters 1 (XI, pp. 148ff. K) and 7 (XI, pp. 175ff. K). See also *id., Methodus medendi*

tradition. Although Herophilus has been granted heroic status in modern scholarship for breaking the spell of phlebotomy,[26] there is no ancient evidence to support such a view. But before passing judgment too hastily on Herophilus' apparently uncritical acceptance of the putative value of phlebotomy, one should consider this practice in historical perspective. Bloodletting was not only accepted in pre-Alexandrian medicine but was actively advocated also by Galen,[27] and it remained in general use until the nineteenth century. In the Renaissance the view to which Herophilus and most ancient physicians had adhered remained the norm: 'We may not, in Phlebotomizatione, bee too timorouse and fearfull.'[28] Even the metaphorical potential of the practice was often exploited: 'Body politiques, . . . as well as the frayle bodies of men . . . must have an evacuation for their corrupt humours, they must be phlebotomiz'd.'[29] Well into the nineteenth century this view endured as the prevailing attitude to bloodletting – an attitude also summarized in an infelicitous couplet from an English *Faust*:

> For spirits sinking, spirits rising
> The one cure is phlebotomising.[30]

When the famous Parisian clinician Magendie (1783–1855) finally challenged tradition by ordering his interns not to practise bloodletting, 'his colleagues reacted in gay laughter . . . [and] his interns were so firmly convinced of the lifesaving function of bleeding that they did not dare, in the interest of their patients, to obey the orders of their chief, and bled secretly. This shows that at that time bloodletting must have held in France, and not only in France, a truly divine position.'[31]

Herophilus' faith in bloodletting therefore puts him in the mainstream of Western medicine rather than rendering him a

5.15 (x, p. 377K); *id.*, *De venae sectione adversus Erasistrateos Romae degentes* 7 (xi, pp. 230f. K).

[26] See n. 23.

[27] See, for example, Galen, *De venae sectione adversus Erasistratum* (xi, pp. 147–86K), *De venae sectione adversus Erasistrateos Romae degentes* (xi, pp. 187–249K), *De curandi ratione per venae sectionem* (xi, pp. 250–316K). Cf. also Bauer, 1870.

[28] *Guillemeau's French chirurgerye or the manualle operations of chirurgerye*, transl. A. M. (1597), 49/2.

[29] Howell, 1644: 160.

[30] *Faust*, tr. Anster (London, 1887), 292.   [31] Ackerknecht, 1973: 111–12.

regressive deviant. Galen clearly regarded Herophilus, along with 'Hippocrates' and most significant medical scientists of the fourth century B.C., as a patriarch of this tenacious bloodletting tradition. Furthermore, Galen's admiration for Herophilus as phlebotomist is due to more than Herophilus' general acceptance of this practice: '*To know when* one should cut the vein in the forehead, and *when* the veins next to the corners of the eyes or the ones under the tongue or the so-called "shoulder vein" [humero-cephalic vein] or the vein that goes through the armpits or the veins behind the thigh and the knee or along the ankle'[32] – this is the kind of precise knowledge, says Galen, that Herophilus displayed when he drew blood for therapeutic purposes.

The range represented by these four therapeutic principles seems to indicate that Herophilus was an aggressive, if not particularly innovative, therapist. Perhaps his most striking clinical innovation was the portable water-clock he used on his medical rounds to measure his patients' pulses (T182). From the point of view of *therapeutic* (rather than diagnostic) principles and measures it might not be particularly informative, but it again confirms his interest in clinical matters.

One area in which ancient sources meet us largely with silence is Herophilus' use of surgery.[33] The testimonia offer a relatively inconsequential reference to the extraction of a tooth,[34] and we also have Herophilus' general obstetrical observations on problems arising during or after delivery,[35] but the only reasonably firm knowledge we have of actual surgical intervention by Herophilus is the following: Herophilus, according to an indignant Tertullian, possessed an 'infanticidal' surgical instrument called *embryosphaktēs* or 'foetus slayer', and he used it even though he recognized that a foetus possesses life.[36] (Under what circumstances Herophilus regarded

[32] T237. (But Galen grants several other precursors the same expert status.)
[33] A useful discussion of Herophilus' position in the history of ancient surgery is provided by Michler, 1968: 10–15 and 90–1 (but see above, n. 23).
[34] Cf. Chapter VII, T218. T15 (Ch. II) perhaps has only anecdotal value.
[35] Cf. Chapter VII, T196–T197, T200–T201, and see Pinoff, 1847; Buess, 1968.
[36] T247 ('... utique viventis infantis peremptorium'). It is possible that the *anuloculter* or ring-shaped surgical knife to which Tertullian refers as an instrument of abortion is likewise attributed to Herophilus, but the exact referent of 'hoc' in 'hoc ... habuit' is unclear, and it is probably safer to read it as referring only to the 'foetus slayer' itself. Tertullian's source was probably Soranus (cf. Waszink's

abortion as advisable is, however, unknown.) As Tertullian points out, 'Hippocrates' already possessed a similar – or the same – instrument for embryotomy.[37] Herophilus might therefore simply have continued to use surgical methods and instruments already employed by earlier clinicians.[38]

In the light of the prominence of orthopaedic surgery and orthopaedic instruments in the Hippocratic Corpus,[39] and in view of the famous attempts by Herophilus' student, Andreas, to apply principles of Alexandrian mechanics to the construction of an instrument for reducing dislocations, it is striking that the only significant surgical testimonium concerning Herophilus does not belong to this branch of medicine. Instead, it seems to belong to the obstetrical discussion in his treatise Midwifery, just like his observations on difficult labour, on inserting a probe into the uterus, and on prolapse of the uterus at birth[40] – i.e. it belongs to a gynaecological rather than to a purely surgical context. Furthermore, this testimonium too suggests that he was a clinical traditionalist.

Three further testimonia might pertain to surgery, but their value is compromised by inadequate knowledge of the original context to which they belong. First, in an account of the amazing recovery of a slave boy whose heart had been laid bare, Galen reports that Herophilus too knew that 'the pericardium does not bring any exceptional danger of its own'.[41] It is unclear whether Herophilus made this observation on the basis of surgical experience or of vivisection (if he did in fact conduct vivisectory experiments) or, as seems more likely, on the basis of observing the convalescence of a badly wounded patient. This text therefore cannot be claimed with certainty as a surgical testimonium.

The second text deals with the question why round wounds heal with greater difficulty than others.[42] Since it refers to the making of

commentary, 1947: 318ff.), although it is puzzling that the two instruments mentioned by Tertullian are not discussed in the relevant chapters of Soranus' Gynaecia, viz. 4.9 [61]–13 [65] (CMG IV, pp. 140–4 Ilberg). Cf. also Waszink, 1947: 326–9, for a detailed commentary on this testimonium.
[37] Cf. Hp., On cutting out the foetus 1 (VIII, pp. 512ff. L).
[38] For a discussion of the history of the instruments used cf. Waszink, 1947: 327–8.
[39] E.g. Hp., On Joints, On Fractures, Instruments of Reduction (II, pp. 46–274Kw).
[40] Cf. Chapter VII, T196–T197, T200–T201.
[41] T235.   [42] T236. Cf. Majno, 1975: 155.

cross-incisions, apparently to aid the healing of wounds that are circular in shape, it might be regarded as evidence of a surgical procedure. But the formulation of the procedure is hypothetical, and the argument primarily concerns the above-mentioned question (i.e. why round wounds do not heal easily), not the surgical procedure itself; this passage hence has more of the overtones of a theoretical debate than of a clinical account or a surgical recommendation.

A final text concerns Herophilus' extensive use of ligations of the head, the arms, and the thighs to combat haemorrhage.[43] But this text again is of a general nature, and does not refer specifically to situations associated with surgical intervention.[44]

In general, then, it seems reasonable to conclude that Herophilus' extraordinary anatomical discoveries provided a necessary basis for the subsequent development of surgery.[45] But to what extent he himself succeeded in bridging the gap between (a) the observations or theories derived from minute dissection and (b) the clinical use of this anatomical knowledge in surgery remains unclear.

Herophilus' apparently limited contribution to surgery, and the inhibiting traditionalism which characterizes much of his therapeutics, should not, however, be allowed to obscure the fact that he was both an aggressive therapist and a thoughtful physician, and that he approached the problem of health care not only on an *ad hoc*, case by case basis, but from a comprehensive perspective which actively accommodated the idea of preventive care. For all the ridicule and abuse adherents of the ancient Empiricist school heaped upon Herophilus as a 'theoretical' physician who pursued ethereal matters of no clinical relevance and who would be helpless when actually confronted with a patient, the texts examined in this chapter establish beyond doubt that Herophilus did not only try to unveil what nature had concealed but also contributed actively to clinical medicine.

[43] T231, from Book I of Herophilus' treatise *Therapeutics*.
[44] The active use of ligations to check bleeding does not, however, allow the conclusion (recently advocated) that Herophilus opposed bloodletting as a therapeutic measure; cf. n. 23 above.
[45] A point developed especially well by Michler, 1968: 7–16. Gossen, 1956, sees T245 as evidence of Herophilus' surgical activity – a questionable inference; cf. Rawson, 1982: 367.

B · TEXTS

1 *Gymnastics*

227 Galenus, *Thrasybulus* (= *Utrum medicinae sit an gymnasticae hygieine*) 47 (*Scr. min.* III, p. 99 Helmreich)

οἱ νῦν ἅπαντες ἰατροὶ ... ἴσασι ... μόρια τῆς τέχνης αὐτῆς δύο τὰ μέγιστα, θεραπευτικόν τε καὶ ὑγιεινόν. αὐτοῦ δ' αὖ πάλιν τοῦ ὑγιεινοῦ μέρους ἴσασι τὸ γυμναστικόν, ὡς καὶ πρόσθεν ἐπιδέδεικται. καθάπερ οὖν Ἱπποκράτης καὶ Διοκλῆς καὶ Πραξα-
5 γόρας καὶ Φυλότιμος καὶ Ἡρόφιλος ὅλης τῆς περὶ τὸ σῶμα τέχνης ἐπιστήμονες ἦσαν, ὡς δηλοῖ τὰ συγγράμματα αὐτῶν, οὕτως αὖ πάλιν οἱ περὶ Θέωνα καὶ Τρύφωνα τὴν περὶ τοὺς ἀθλητὰς κακοτεχνίαν μετεχειρίσαντο ...

5 Φιλότιμος *codd.*: *corr. Wellmann*   6 συγγράμματα *L*: γράμματα *PAld*
(*cf. p. 99.21 Helmreich*)   8 μετεχειρίσαντο *Helmreich*: μεταχειρίσαντες *codd.*

227 All contemporary physicians ... know ... the two parts of the art itself that are the most important: therapeutics and hygiene. They also know gymnastics, which in turn belongs to this hygienic part of medicine, as has been demonstrated previously as well. So, just as Hippocrates, Diocles, Praxagoras, Phylotimus, and Herophilus were knowledgeable about the whole art concerning the body, as their writings make clear, so again the followers of Theon and Tryphon have pursued the base art concerned with athletic contestants ...

228 Galenus, *Thrasybulus* (= *Utrum medicinae sit an gymnasticae hygieine*) 38 (*Scr. min.* III, p. 85 Helmreich)

τούτους οὖν ἀποπέμψαντες (sc. οἱ τοὺς ἀθλητὰς γυμνά-ζουσι), ... τοὺς τῆς ὄντως γυμναστικῆς ἐπιστήμονας ἤδη καλῶμεν, Ἱπποκράτην τε καὶ Διοκλέα καὶ Πραξαγόραν καὶ Φυλότιμον, Ἐρασίστρατόν τε καὶ Ἡρόφιλον ὅσοι τ' ἄλλοι τὴν
5 ὅλην περὶ τὸ σῶμα τέχνην ἐξέμαθον.

2 ὄντας *PAld*: *corr.* P²

228 So, having dismissed these [sc. trainers of athletic contestants]

... let us now call on those who are knowledgeable about the true art of gymnastics: Hippocrates, Diocles, Praxagoras, Phylotimus, Erasistratus, Herophilus, and all the others who have learnt thoroughly the whole art concerning the body.

229 Eustathius, *Commentarii ad Homeri Odysseam* 1601.39-41 (ad *Odyss.* 8.372)

ὅτι δὲ τὸ σφαιρίζειν οὐκ ὀλίγη μοῖρα ἐνομίζετό φασι γυμναστικῆς, ἔστι συμβάλλειν καὶ ἐκ τῆς Ἡροφίλου τοῦ ἰατροῦ εἰκόνος. παράκειται γάρ φασιν αὐτῇ σὺν ἑτέροις τισὶ γυμναστικοῖς ὀργάνοις καὶ σφαῖρα.

229 That playing games with balls used to be considered no small part of the art of gymnastics can be inferred, they say, also from the statue of Herophilus the physician. For, they say, along with some other instruments of gymnastics, a ball too is present in the statue.

2   Herophilus' 'Regimen'

230 Sextus Empiricus, *Adversus mathematicos* 11 (= *Adv. ethicos*).50

Ἡρόφιλος δὲ ἐν τῷ διαιτητικῷ καὶ σοφίαν φησὶν ἀνεπίδεικτον καὶ τέχνην ἄδηλον καὶ ἰσχὺν ἀναγώνιστον καὶ πλοῦτον ἀχρεῖον καὶ λόγον ἀδύνατον ὑγείας ἀπούσης.

230 Herophilus says in his *Regimen* that, in the absence of health, wisdom cannot be displayed, science is non-evident, strength not exerted in contest, wealth useless, and rational speech powerless.

3   Herophilus' 'Therapeutics'; general evidence

231 Caelius Aurelianus, *Tardae passiones* 2.13.186

item de ligationibus pugnaverunt (sc. in curatione sanguinis fluoris), siquidem Xenophon et Dionysius et Herophilus primo libro Curationum et Erasistratus probent articulorum facien-

dam constrictionem: Herophilus vero capitis et brachiorum et
5 femorum, Erasistratus magis inguinum et alarum, etenim
laxatione sensus sanguinis approbat fieri retentionem; Asclepiades vero ad ipsum scribens libros Parasceuasticos ligationem
excludit . . .

6 laxationem *S: corr. R in marg.*

231 They also were in conflict about ligations [sc. in the treatment of
haemorrhages], since Xenophon, Dionysius, Herophilus in Book I of
his *Therapeutics*, and Erasistratus approve of bandaging limbs. But
Herophilus [approves of bandaging] the head, arms, and thighs,
whereas Erasistratus prefers [bandaging of] the groin and the
armpits; in fact, he holds the view that stoppage of the haemorrhage
takes place through a relaxation of the senses. Asclepiades, however,
when he writes against Erasistratus in his work *On Preparations*, shuts
the door on ligation . . .

232 Galenus, *Methodus medendi* 5.2 (x, pp. 309–10K)

αἱ δὲ τῶν βοηθημάτων ἐνδείξεις ἕτεραι μὲν ἀπὸ τῶν ὁμοιομερῶν
εἰσιν, ἕτεραι δὲ ἀπὸ τῶν ὀργανικῶν· ἀμφοτέρας μὲν οὖν οἱ τὴν
Ἱπποκράτους μέθοδον ἀσπαζόμενοι γινώσκουσι, διότι καὶ τὴν
ἑκατέρων τῶν μορίων φύσιν ἐπίστανται· τὴν δ' ἑτέραν ἐξ αὐτῶν
5 μόνην τὴν ἀπὸ τῶν ὀργανικῶν οἱ περὶ τὸν Ἐρασίστρατόν τε καὶ
Ἡρόφιλον· ὥστε κἂν τοῖς ἐφεξῆς λόγοις ὅσα μὲν ἀπὸ τοῦ θερμοῦ
καὶ ψυχροῦ καὶ ξηροῦ καὶ ὑγροῦ σώματος ἢ πάθους εἰς τὴν
ἔνδειξιν λαμβάνεται, τούτων οὐδενὸς ἕξουσι μέθοδον οἱ περὶ τὸν
Ἐρασίστρατόν τε καὶ Ἡρόφιλον· ὅσα δὲ ἀπὸ τῆς διαπλάσεως ἢ
10 θέσεως ἢ κυριότητος ἢ εὐαισθησίας ἢ τῶν ἐναντίων οὐκ
ἀγνοήσουσι.

232 And some indications for remedies are derived from homoeomerous parts [e.g. blood, humour, tissue, bone], others from
instrumental parts [e.g. lungs, liver, brain, heart, vessels]. Those who
hail Hippocrates' method therefore recognize both, because they
know the nature of each of these two kinds of parts, whereas
Erasistratus and Herophilus and their followers recognize only the
second of these kinds, viz. the one from instrumental parts. Conse-

quently, also in the discussions which follow, Erasistratus, Herophilus, and their followers will not possess a method for any of those things that are taken for the purpose of indication from the hot and cold body or disease and from the dry and wet body or disease. On the other hand, they will not be ignorant of all the things taken from conformation or position or dominance or keen sensation or their opposites.

233 Galenus, *Methodus medendi* 3.3 (x, pp. 184–5K)

ὁ δ᾽ ἐμπειρικὸς ὅτι μὲν οὐκ ἐσάρκωσε τόνδε τινὰ (sc. ἔχοντα ἕλκος κοῖλον) τὸ προσαχθὲν φάρμακον ὁρᾷ· μὴ γινώσκων μέντοι πότερον τῷ μᾶλλον ἢ τῷ ἧττον ξηρᾶναι, μεταβαίνειν ἐφ᾽ ἕτερον ἀδυνατεῖ. κατὰ δὲ τὸν αὐτὸν τρόπον καὶ οἱ περὶ τὸν Ἐρασίστρα-
5 τόν τε καὶ Ἡρόφιλον ἐξ ἡμισείας, ὥσπερ καὶ πρόσθεν ἐδείξαμεν, ὄντες δογματικοὶ κακῶς ἰατρεύουσιν ἕλκος. μόνα γὰρ ἐπιχειροῦσι λογικῶς θεραπεύειν ὅσα τῶν ὀργανικῶν ἐστι μορίων ἴδια νοσήματα· τὸ δ᾽ ἕλκος, ὥσπερ καὶ πρόσθεν εἴρηται, κοινόν ἐστιν ὁμοιομερῶν τε καὶ ὀργανικῶν, ὥστε καὶ τοῦτο κατὰ τοσοῦτον
10 ἐμπειρικῶς θεραπεύουσι, καθ᾽ ὅσον ἐν τοῖς ὁμοιομερέσι πέφυκε γίνεσθαι. καὶ μὲν δὴ κἂν τῷ τὰς ἀπολωλυίας τελέως οὐσίας ἢ κεκολοβωμένας ἐπιχειρεῖν θεραπεύειν, κἀνταῦθα ἀναγκαῖον αὐτοῖς ἐστιν ἀποπίπτειν πολλαχῇ τοῦ λογικῶς.

233 The Empiricist sees that the drug which was applied did not restore the flesh of some particular person [suffering from a 'hollow sore'] but since he does not know whether he could restore the flesh by drying it more or drying it less, he is incapable of making 'a transition to a different drug'. In the same way, Erasistratus and Herophilus and their followers, being only half-dogmatics, as I also showed previously, cure sores poorly; for they try to treat rationally only those diseases which are peculiar to the instrumental (*organika*) parts. But the sore, as was also said previously, is common to both homoeomerous and instrumental parts, so that they treat it empirically as well, to the extent that it naturally arises in the homoeomerous parts. And, in fact, even in the course of trying to treat substances that are completely destroyed or mutilated, here too they necessarily secede from the 'rationalist' [method of treatment] in many respects.

234 A. Cornelius Celsus, *Medicina* 3 (*Artes* 8).9.2 (*CML* 1, p. 116 Marx)

neque Hercules ista curatio nova est, qua nunc quidem traditos sibi aegros, qui sub cautioribus medicis trahebantur, interdum contrariis remediis sanant. siquidem apud antiquos quoque ante Herophilum et Erasistratum maximeque post Hippocra-
5 tem fuit ⟨celebris.⟩ (*Cf. T281 infra.*)

1 quidam *J* 4 herophllum *V* 5 celebris *suppl. Marx*

234 Nor, God knows, is that treatment new, with which nowadays from time to time they cure patients who have been handed over to them after receiving protracted treatment under more cautious physicians, namely treatment with contrary remedies [sc. here honeyed or diluted wine for fever-induced chills]. Even among the ancients, also before Herophilus and Erasistratus, but especially after Hippocrates, this treatment was frequently used. (*Cf. Chapter* x, *T281.*)

235 Galenus, *De placitis Hippocratis et Platonis* 1.5 (*CMG* v.4.1.2, pp. 74–6 DeLacy)

τὸ μὲν οὖν παιδάριον ἐσώθη σαρκωθέντων τε τῶν περὶ τὸ στέρνον καὶ συμφύντων ἀλλήλοις καὶ ⟨εἰς⟩ τοιοῦτον ἐπίθεμα γενομένων τῆς καρδίας οἷόν περ ἡ ἔμπροσθεν ἦν κορυφὴ τοῦ χιτῶνος. καὶ οὐ χρὴ θαυμάζειν, εἰ γυμνωθείσης τῆς καρδίας
5 ἐσώθη τὸ παιδάριον. οὐδὲν γὰρ περιττότερον ἡ διάθεσις εἶχε τῶν ὁσημέραι γινομένων εἰς τὸν θώρακα συντρήσεων. οὐ μὴν οὐδὲ ὁ περικάρδιος ἴδιον ἐξαίρετον ἐπιφέρει τινὰ κίνδυνον, ὥσπερ που καὶ Ἡρόφιλος εἴρηκε καὶ ἄλλοι πολλοὶ τῶν ἰατρῶν.

2 εἰς *add. DeLacy* 2 τοιοῦτον ἐπίθεμα *C²*: τοιοῦτ.....θεμα *C*:
τοιούτου ἐπιθέματος *Müller*: τοιούτων ἐπιθεμάτων *recens. anon.*
2 γενόμενον *C: corr. Caius* 3 ἔμπροσθεν] ἔμ.....*C, suppl. C²*

235 The little boy, then, was saved, since the parts around the sternum had taken on flesh and grew together, and formed a cover for the heart, of the kind that the apex of the tunic [of the heart] had previously been. And one should not be surprised that the boy was saved although his heart had been laid bare. For this condition is no more extraordinary than the perforations of the chest that take place every day. Nor does the pericardium bring any exceptional danger of its own, as indeed both Herophilus and many other physicians have said.

236   Cassius Iatrosphista, *Problemata* 1 (*Physici et medici Graeci minores*, vol. 1 (Berlin, 1841), p. 144 Ideler)

διὰ τί τὰ στρογγύλα ἕλκη δυσαλθέστερα καθέστηκε τῶν ἄλλων; οἱ μὲν οὖν Ἡροφίλειοι τὴν αἰτίαν ἀποδιδόασι γεωμετρικῇ χρώμενοι ἀποδείξει· φασὶ γὰρ ὅτι τὰ κυκλικὰ σχήματα τῶν ἑλκῶν μικρὰ μὲν φαίνεται τῇ περιοχῇ, οὐ τοιαῦτα δ᾽ ἐστίν, ἀλλ᾽
5   ἔχει τῇ δυνάμει μείζονα τὰ ἐμβαδὰ ἤπερ φαίνεται. τὸ μεῖζον δὲ πλείονος χρόνου δεῖται πρὸς τὴν ἐπούλωσιν· ὥστε εἰκότως τὰ τοιαῦτα ἕλκη φαίνεται δυσαλθῆ, εἴ γε καὶ μικρὰ φαίνεται· κατὰ δὲ τὸ ἀληθὲς οὐχ οὕτως ἔχει, ἀλλ᾽ ἐστὶ μείζονα. τοῦτο δὲ περικειμένως διεκρούσατο Ἀσκληπιάδης· εἴ τις στρογγύλου
10   ἕλκους ὑποκειμένου ἐπιδιέλῃ τὰ παρακείμενα σώματα, ὥστε ἐκ τῆς ἐπιδιαιρέσεως γενέσθαι ἐπιμηκέστερον τὸ σχῆμα τοῦ ἕλκους, θᾶττον ἂν γένοιτο ἡ ἐπούλωσις· τοῦτο δ᾽ ἐναντίον τῷ τοῦ Ἡροφίλου ἀρέσκοντι. εἰ γὰρ τὸ μέγεθος τοῦ ἕλκους, ὡς αὐτοί φασιν, αἴτιον γίνεται τῆς δυσθεραπευσίας, ἐχρῆν τοῦ
15   αὐτοῦ ὑποκειμένου μεγέθους καὶ ἑτέρου προσγινομένου ἐκ τῆς ἐπιδιαιρέσεως, μᾶλλον γίνεσθαι δυσιατότερα ταῦτα τὰ ἕλκη.

236   For what reason do round wounds heal with more difficulty than other wounds? The Herophileans actually account for its cause by using a geometric demonstration. For, they say, the circular shapes of wounds appear small in circumference, but are not such; rather they have surfaces larger in area than they appear. And that which is larger requires more time for scar tissue to form. It is consequently likely that such wounds appear to heal with difficulty, even if they also appear small. In truth, however, this is not so, but they are larger. Asclepiades, however, evaded this problem completely. If a round wound existed, and someone made a cross-incision in the body lying next to it, so that the shape of the wound became more elongated as a result of the cross-incision, scar tissue would form more quickly. This is the opposite of what Herophilus thinks. For, if the magnitude of the

wound is the cause of the difficulty in curing it, as they claim, then these wounds should rather have become more difficult to heal, when the same magnitude existed and, as a result of the cross-incision, another one arose in addition.

237 Galenus, *De venae sectione adversus Erasistratum* 6 (xi, pp. 169–70K)

τὸ γὰρ ἐπίστασθαι πηνίκα μὲν χρὴ τέμνειν τὴν ἐν τῷ μετώπῳ
φλέβα, πηνίκα δὲ τὰς παρὰ τοὺς κανθοὺς τῶν ὀφθαλμῶν ἢ τὰς
ὑπὸ τῇ γλώττῃ ἢ τὴν ὠμιαίαν ὀνομαζομένην ἢ τὴν διὰ
μασχαλῶν ἢ τὰς κατ' ἰγνύας ἢ παρὰ σφυρόν, ὑπὲρ ὧν ἁπασῶν
5 ἐδίδαξεν Ἱπποκράτης, τοῦτον ἐγὼ νομίζω τὸν λογισμὸν ἰατρῶν
εἶναι . . . ἄχρι μὲν γὰρ τοῦδε καὶ Διοκλῆς ἠπίστατο καὶ Πλειστόνικος, Ἡρόφιλός τε καὶ Πραξαγόρας καὶ Φυλότιμος ἄλλοι τε
πολλοὶ τῶν ἰατρῶν· οὐκ αὐτοὶ μὲν ἐξεῦρον, ἑπόμενοι δὲ Ἱπποκράτει, πηνίκα χρὴ τέμνειν ἑκάστην ὧν εἶπον φλέβα.

5 Ἱπποκράτη *U*

237 To know when one should cut the vein in the forehead, and when the veins next to the corners of the eyes or the ones under the tongue or the one called 'shoulder-vein' [humero-cephalic vein] or the vein that goes through the armpits or the veins behind the thigh and the knee, or along the ankle, about all of which Hippocrates taught [when they should be phlebotomized] – this I regard as the reasoning task of physicians . . . This much Diocles, too, had knowledge of, as did Plistonicus, Herophilus, Praxagoras, Phylotimus, and many others among the physicians; not that they discovered by themselves when one should cut each of the veins I mentioned, but rather by following Hippocrates.

238 Galenus, *De venae sectione adversus Erasistratum* 5 (xi, pp. 162–3K)

μεταβήσωμεν δὲ ἐπὶ τοὺς ἄλλους ἄνδρας ἑκατέρας αἱρέσεως
(sc. ἰατρικῆς), ἐμπειρικῆς τε καὶ λογικῆς. οὐδὲ γὰρ τούτων
οὐδένα εὑρίσκω τῆς φλεβοτομίας ἀποστάντα. δογματικῶν μὲν
γὰρ οἶδα καὶ Διοκλέα καὶ Πλειστόνικον καὶ Διευχῆ καὶ Μνησίθεον

5 Πραξαγόραν τε καὶ Φυλότιμον καὶ Ἡρόφιλον καὶ Ἀσκληπιάδην
φλεβοτομοῦντας.

1 μεταβήσομεν A: μεταβήσομαι U   3 δογματικῶν scripsi: δογματικὸν
UA Kühn   4 Δι' εὐχῆ A: δι' εὐχῆ U

238 Let me pass on to the rest of the authors of either school [of
medicine], viz. the empiricist and rationalist schools. I actually find
that not a single one of them has been adverse to the letting of blood
(*phlebotomia*). For, I know that among the Dogmatics Diocles as well
as Plistonicus, Dieuches, Mnesitheus, Praxagoras, Phylotimus, Herophilus, and Asclepiades practise bloodletting.

239 Caelius Aurelianus, *Celeres vel acutae passiones* 1.12.100

Hippocrates igitur solum nomen videtur tetigisse passionis (sc.
phreniticae) libro quem de ptisana scripsit, item libro praedic-
tivo quem prorrheticum appellavit; nam curationem nullam
tradidit. sed neque Praxagoras neque Herophilus.

239 Hippocrates therefore seems to have touched only on the name
of the disease [sc. phrenitis] in the book he wrote *On the Ptisan*, and
likewise in the prognostic book which he called *Prorrhetic*; for he
transmitted no treatment. But neither did Praxagoras or Herophilus.

240 Caelius Aurelianus, *Celeres vel acutae passiones* 3.21.215

at Herophilus cholericorum curationem secundum se aliis
nullam tradidit.

240 But Herophilus did not hand down to others any treatment of
his own for those who are ill with cholera.

241 Caelius Aurelianus, *Celeres vel acutae passiones* 2.18.112

antiquorum vero Erasistratus et Herophilus de pleuriticis nihil
dixerunt.

241 Of the ancients, however, Erasistratus and Herophilus said nothing about [the treatment of] patients with pleurisy.

242 Caelius Aurelianus, *Celeres vel acutae passiones* 2.29.153

Ex antiquis autem Erasistratus et Herophilus de ista passione (sc. de peripneumonia) nihil dixerunt.

242 Of the ancients, however, Erasistratus and Herophilus said nothing about this affection [sc. about pneumonia].

243 Caelius Aurelianus, *Celeres vel acutae passiones* 3.4.33

Herophilus de synanchicis nihil dixit.

243 Herophilus said nothing about [the treatment of] cases of inflammation of the throat (*synanche*).

244 Caelius Aurelianus, *Celeres vel acutae passiones* 2.6.32

antiquorum vero Hippocrates et Erasistratus et Herophilus ad eorum (sc. lethargicorum) curationem nihil posuerunt; sed Serapion Empiricus in primo libro quem ad sectas scribit obscura nimium atque pauca ordinavit, quorum nihil est
5 dignum enarrare.

3 quem *Wellmann*: quae *G*   3 *fort.* scripsit *Drabkin*

244 Of the ancients, however, Hippocrates, Erasistratus, and Herophilus proposed nothing with reference to treating those [sc. who suffer from lethargy]; Serapion the Empiricist admittedly gives a few very obscure rules in Book I of his *Against the Sects*, but nothing among these is worth expounding.

245 M. Terentius Varro, *Menippeae* 444 (*Quinquatrus* 5) (p. 75 Astbury) (apud Nonium Marcellum, *De conpendiosa doctrina* 2, p. 69M = I, p. 97 Lindsay (*aquilex*); 4, p. 371M = II, p. 591 Lindsay (*praestare, antecellere*))

an hoc praestat Herophilus Diogeni, quod ille e ventre aquam
mittit? et hoc te iactas? at hoc pacto utilior te Tuscus aquilex.

1 Herophilus *Iunius*: herofilius *codd.*   Diogeni *Turnebus*: diogenis *codd.*
(*Non. p. 69*): diogene *codd.* (Non. p. 371): Diogenem *Lindsay*   2 et
Bolisani: ad *codd.*: an *Bentinus*: del. *Riese*: at *Onions*   2 at ed. *Non. Venet.*
1471: ad *codd.*

245 Does Herophilus surpass Diogenes in this respect, namely that
he sends forth water from the stomach? Is this what you are boasting
about? But on these terms the Tuscan water-diviner is more useful
than you are.

246 Plutarchus, *De curiositate* 7 (= *Moralia* 518D)

οὕτω δ' ἑκάστῳ λυπηρόν ἐστιν ἡ τῶν περὶ αὐτὸν κακῶν
ἀνακάλυψις, ὥστε πολλοὺς ἀποθανεῖν ἂν πρότερον ἢ δεῖξαί τι
τῶν ἀπορρήτων νοσημάτων ἰατροῖς. φέρε γὰρ Ἡρόφιλον ἢ
Ἐρασίστρατον ἢ τὸν Ἀσκληπιὸν αὐτόν, ὅτ' ἦν ἄνθρωπος,
5 ἔχοντα τὰ φάρμακα καὶ τὰ ὄργανα, κατ' οἰκίαν παριστάμενον
ἀνακρίνειν, μή τις ἔχει σύριγγα περὶ δακτύλιον ἢ γυνὴ καρκίνον
ἐν ὑστέρᾳ, καίτοι σωτήριόν ἐστι τῆς τέχνης ταύτης τὸ
πολύπραγμον.

1 *fort.* αὐτὸν   2 ἂν add. *post vel ante* ἀποθανεῖν Λ   5 κατ'] παο' C
5 παριστάμενον M²ΠΔ: περιστ- M: προσιστ- JV, YNRh: προ . . ιστάμενον
G: προιστάμενον CWX Λ   6 παρὰ Π   7 ἐν om. D

246 So painful for each of us is the unveiling of our own troubles that
many people die rather than show any of their secret diseases to
doctors. For, imagine Herophilus or Erasistratus or Asclepius himself,
when he was a human being, going from house to house with his drugs
and instruments and inquiring whether someone has an abscess in his
anus or whether a woman has a cancer in her womb – although the
curiosity of this art is salutary.

247 Tertullian, *De anima* 25.5 (p. 36 Waszink)

itaque est inter arma medicorum et cum organo, ex quo prius
patescere secreta coguntur tortili temperamento, cum anulocultro, quo intus membra caeduntur anxio arbitrio, cum hebete

unco, quo totum facinus extrahitur violento puerperio. est etiam
5 aeneum spiculum, quo iugulatio ipsa dirigitur caeco latrocinio;
ἐμβρυοσφάκτην appellant de infanticidii officio, utique viventis
infantis peremptorium. hoc et Hippocrates habuit et Asclepiades et Erasistratus et maiorum quoque prosector Herophilus
et mitior ipse Soranus, certi animal esse conceptum atque ita
10 miserti infelicissimae huiusmodi infantiae, ut prius occidatur, ne
viva lanietur.

1 est *A*: et *B Gel*   et om. *A*   cum organia *A*: organa *B Gel*: organon
Urs   ex] est *Gel*: aes *Lindner*   2–3 anulocultro *Rig*: anulo cultro *A*:
anulo, cultro *B*: anulo cultrato *Gel*   4 facinus] pecus *Gel*: pignus *coni.*
Reifferscheid   attrahitur *B Gel*   6 ἐμβρυοσφάκτην *Urs*:
ΕΜΒΡΥΟΡΣΕΚΤΗΝ *A*: ἐμβρυοπάκτην *B* (ἐμβρυορσέκτην *in marg.*):
ἐμβρυορέκτην *Gel*: ἐμβρυονέκτην *Lat*: ἐμβρυορήκτην *Scal*   8 maiorum]
vivorum *Diels (DG p. 206 adn. 2)*   9 animal esse] animales se *A*
corr.   10 miserati *B Gel*   10–11 ne viva lanietur *Gel*: ne vivat lanietur
B: ne vivat *A*

247 Accordingly, among the physicians' tools there is also an
instrument [sc. a distender] with which things previously hidden are
forced to become exposed by means of a moderate rotating motion,
along with a ring-shaped surgical knife with which the members
within [the womb] are cut with anxious control, and along with a
blunted hook with which the entire victim of the crime is extracted
through a violent delivery. There is also a bronze, sharp-pointed
instrument with which the actual slaughter is managed in this furtive
robbery. From its function – infanticide – they call it 'foetus slayer'
(*embryo-sphaktēs*), and for the live infant it certainly is deadly. This
instrument Hippocrates possessed, and so did Asclepiades, Erasistratus, Herophilus – that dissector even of adults – and the milder
Soranus himself. They all were certain that a living being had been
conceived and thus felt pity for such most unfortunate infants, that
they had to be killed first, in order not to be butchered alive.*

4 *Materia medica*

248a Scribonius Largus, *Conpositiones*, praefatio (p. 875
Deichgräber; p. 1 Sconocchia)

* This testimonium might belong to Herophilus' *Midwifery*; cf. Chapter VII, T193ff.

248b Marcellus, *'Epistula Cornelii Celsi' De medicamentis* (*CML* v, 36 Niedermann/Liechtenhan)

inter maximos quondam habitus medicos Herophilus, Cai Iuli Calliste, fertur dixisse medicamenta divum manus esse, et id quidem non sine ratione, ut mea fert opinio: prorsus enim quod tactus divinus efficere potest, id praestant medicamenta usu
5 experientiaque probata.

1 Hierophilus *PLAT*   2 divum manus *Susemihl (1891–2: I, p. 796, adn. 104), Deichgräber:* divinum munus *Ru:* deorum immortalium manus *M:* deorum manus *vel* divinas manus *malunt Rhodius Helmreich*   2 et id quidem *om. M:* et *T*   4 usus experientia conprobata *M*

248a–b They say, Gaius Julius Callistus, that Herophilus, who was once held to be among the greatest physicians, said that medicaments are the hands of the gods, and indeed, not without reason, in my opinion. For certainly, what divine touch can effect, medicaments tested by use and experience also accomplish.

248c Plutarchus, *Quaestiones symposiacae* 4.1.3 (*Moralia* 663B–C)

... ὅταν μιγνύῃ (sc. Φίλων) τὰς βασιλικὰς καὶ ἀλεξιφαρμάκους ἐκείνας δυνάμεις, ἃς "θεῶν χεῖρας" ὠνόμαζεν ⟨'Ηρόφιλος⟩, 'Ερασίστρατος δ' ἐλέγχει τὴν ἀτοπίαν καὶ περιεργίαν, ὁμοῦ μεταλλικὰ καὶ βοτανικὰ καὶ θηριακὰ καὶ τὰ ἀπὸ γῆς καὶ
5 θαλάττης εἰς τὸ αὐτὸ συγκεραννύντος.

2 'Ηρόφιλος *add. Wellmann, Deichgräber* (ὁ 'Ηρ-)   3 δ' ἐλέγχει *codd.:* διέλεγχε *ab Leonico edd.*   5 συγκεραννύντας *T corr. Turnebus*

248c ... When [Philo] mixes those regal and potent substances – which Herophilus* used to call 'hands of gods' – mixing together into the same compound mineral, vegetable, and animal products from both land and sea, Erasistratus exposes his absurdity and excessive elaboration.

* The MSS read 'Erasistratus'; Max Wellmann, Karl Deichgräber, and others have suggested emending the text to read 'Herophilus ... [lacuna], Erasistratus'.

249 Galenus, *De compositione medicamentorum secundum locos* 6.8 (XII, pp. 965–6K)

ἀκαίρως γοῦν ἔνιοι χρησάμενοι φαρμάκοις οἷς εἶχον, εἶτ᾽ ἐκ τοῦ παροξῦναι τὸ πάθος ἐφ᾽ ἕτερα μεταβάντες ἄνευ μεθόδου. καὶ μηδὲν τούτοις ἀνύσαντες τὴν τρίτην ἐφεξῆς ἐφ᾽ ἕτερα μετάβασιν, ἔστι δ᾽ ὅτε καὶ τετάρτην ἀλόγως ποιήσαντες καὶ νομίσαντες τὸ
5 πάθος εἶναι κακόηθες, ἐκάλεσάν με συμβουλεῦσαί τι. κἀγὼ κελεύσας αὐτοὺς ἃ κέκτηνται φάρμακα δεῖξαί μοι τὸ συμφέρον τῇ παρούσῃ καταστάσει συνεβούλευον. καὶ φάντων αὐτῶν δι᾽ οὗ συνεβούλευσα φαρμάκου παροξυνθῆναι τὸν κάμνοντα καὶ διὰ τοῦτο χρῆσθαι δεδιότων, ἀλλὰ νῦν γε πεισθέντας ἐμοὶ χρήσασ-
10 θαι προτρέψας, ἐπέδειξα κἀκείνοις καὶ ὑμῖν ἑκάτερον ὧν ἔλεγεν Ἡρόφιλος ἀληθὲς ὑπάρχον. ἐάν τε γὰρ εἴπῃς οὐδὲν εἶναι τὰ φάρμακα μόνα καθ᾽ αὑτά, προσηκόντως ἐρεῖς, οὐδὲν γάρ ἐστιν, ἐὰν μὴ τὸν χρώμενον ὀρθῶς σχῇ, ἐάν τε πάλιν οἷόν περ θεῶν χεῖρας εἶναι τὰ φάρμακα, καὶ τοῦτο ὀρθῶς ἐρεῖς. ἀνύει γὰρ
15 μεγάλα τὸν χρώμενον αὐτοῖς ἔχοντα γεγυμνασμένον ἐν λογικῇ μεθόδῳ μετὰ τοῦ καὶ συνετὸν εἶναι φύσει.

249 It was, then, at the wrong time that some people used the drugs they had, and then, because this [inopportune use] exacerbated the disease, they made a transition to other drugs, without an inquiry, and when they accomplished nothing with these, they next went to a third transition to other drugs, and sometimes also to a fourth. And when they had done this irrationally, thinking the illness was malignant, they summoned me for a consultation. After telling them to show me the drugs they had obtained, I used to advise them which was advantageous for the patient's current condition. And, although they said that the patient had become more acutely ill through the drug I advised and that, for this reason, they feared to use it, now at least after I urged them on and after they were persuaded by me to use it, I have shown them and you that each of two things Herophilus said is true: for, if you say that drugs alone *per se* are nothing, you will make an appropriate statement, since they are nothing if they do not have a person who employs them correctly; and again, if you say drugs are just like the hands of the gods, this, too, will be a correct statement. For they effect great things if they have as their utilizer a person who is trained in the 'rationalist' method and, along with this, is also intelligent by nature.

250 Galenus, *De compositione medicamentorum secundum locos* 3.1 (XII, p. 613K)

Ἡροφίλου τοίνυν οὕτως ἐπαινοῦντος τοὺς διορισμοὺς (sc. τῶν φαρμάκων) ὡς οὐκ οἶδ' εἴ τις ἄλλος, αὐτοῦ τε τοῦ Ἀπολλωνίου τὰ τῆς κεφαλαλγίας φάρμακα μετὰ διορισμῶν γράψαντος, ἔτι μᾶλλον θαυμάζω τὸ κατὰ τὰς ὠταλγίας ἀδιόριστον αὐτοῦ.
5 (*Vid. infra AM.17.*)

250 So, since I do not know of any other person who recommended differentiations [between remedies, according to the causes and exact nature of the affection,] as much as Herophilus, and since Apollonius himself, too, recorded the drugs for headaches with such differentiations, I am all the more amazed at Apollonius' lack of differentiation in cases of ear-aches. (*See Chapter* XXIII *below, AM.17.*)

251 A. Cornelius Celsus, *Medicina* 5 (*Artes* 10), prohoem. 1 (*CML* I, p. 190 Marx)

dixi de is malis corporis, quibus victus ratio maxime subvenit: nunc transeundum est ad eam medicinae partem, quae magis medicamentis pugnat. his multum antiqui auctores tribuerunt, et Erasistratus et ii, qui se empiricos nominarunt, praecipue
5 tamen Herophilus deductique ab illo viro, adeo ut nullum morbi genus sine his curarent. multaque etiam de facultatibus medicamentorum memoriae ⟨prodiderunt⟩, qualia sunt vel Zenonis vel Andriae vel Apolloni qui Mys cognominatus est.

4 empericos *J*   5 viri *F³*   7 prodiderunt *add. J: om. F*

251 I have spoken of those afflictions of the body for which the regulation of diet is most useful; now I must pass on to that part of medicine which combats them more by drugs. The ancient authors attributed much to these [sc. to drugs]; both Erasistratus and those who call themselves Empiricists did so, but especially Herophilus and those descended from this famous man, so much so that they did not treat any kind of disease without drugs. They also transmitted many things about the powers of drugs to later traditions, as in the works of Zeno or Andreas or Apollonius surnamed 'Mys'. (*Cf. Chapters* XI, *An. 22;* XV, *Zn. 3;* XXIII, *AM. 9.*)

252 Galenus, *De simplicium medicamentorum temperamentis et facultatibus* 6, prooemium (XI, p. 795K)

ἡ δὲ πλείστη τῶν φαρμάκων χρῆσις ἐν αὐταῖς ταῖς θεραπευτικ-
αῖς πραγματείαις ὑπό τε τῶν παλαιῶν γέγραπται καὶ προσέτι
τῶν νεωτέρων ἀπάντων σχεδόν· καὶ γὰρ πρὸς Ἱπποκράτους
εἴρηται πολλὰ καὶ πρὸς Εὐρυφῶντος καὶ Διεύχους καὶ Διοκ-
5 λέους καὶ Πλειστονίκου καὶ Πραξαγόρου καὶ Ἡροφίλου καὶ οὐκ
ἔστιν οὐδεὶς ἀνὴρ παλαιός, ὃς οὐ συνεβάλλετό τι τῇ τέχνῃ
μεῖ3ον ἢ μεῖον εἰς ἐπιστήμην φαρμάκων . . .(*Cf. An.24 infra.*)

252 In the therapeutic treatises written both by the ancients and by
almost all the more recent authors, most of the uses of drugs are
recorded. For, many were mentioned by Hippocrates, Euryphon,
Dieuches, Diocles, Plistonicus, Praxagoras, and Herophilus. In fact,
there is no ancient author who did not make a greater or lesser
contribution to the knowledge of drugs . . . (*See Chapter* XI *infra,
An.24.*)

253 Galenus, *De simplicium medicamentorum temperamentis et facultatibus* 1.29 (XI, p. 433K)

φασὶ γὰρ ἕνεκα τῆς τῶν συνθέτων φαρμάκων κατασκευῆς τε καὶ
χρήσεως ἐπισκέπτεσθαι τῶν ἁπλῶν τὰς δυνάμεις καὶ τούτων
μάρτυρας ἐπικαλοῦνται σχεδὸν ἅπαντας τοὺς παλαιούς, Ἐρασίστρατον, Ἡρόφιλον, Φυλότιμον, Διοκλέα, Πραξαγόραν καὶ
5 αὐτὸν Ἱπποκράτην.

253 They say that one must examine the powers of simple drugs in
order to prepare and use compound drugs. As their witnesses for
simple drugs they call on almost all the ancient physicians: Erasistratus, Herophilus, Phylotimus, Diocles, Praxagoras, and Hippocrates
himself.

254 C. Plinius Secundus, *Naturalis historia* 25.5.15

inde et plerosque ita video existimare, nihil non herbarum vi
effici posse, sed plurimarum vires esse incognitas, quorum in

numero fuit Herophilus clarus medicina, a quo ferunt dictum
quasdam fortassis etiam calcatas prodesse. observatum certe est,
5 iam sanari vulnera ac morbos superventu eorum, qui pedibus
iter confecerint.

1 vim *E*   3 in quo *E*   4 calcatis *V¹*   5 iam sanari *coni.*
Warmington (*vel* minus inflammari): inflammari *codd.*: vel sanari *coni.*
Ma   earum *Eag*   6 confecerunt *V*

254 Hence I see that most people also have the opinion that there is
nothing which cannot be accomplished by the power of plants, but
that the powers of most plants are unknown. Numbered among
people with this view was Herophilus, famous in medicine, by whom,
they say, it was said that certain plants are perhaps of benefit to one
even if [merely] trodden upon. It certainly has been observed that the
wounds and diseases of those who have made a journey on foot are
already healing upon their arrival.

255 C. Plinius Secundus, *Naturalis historia* 25.23.57–8

sed antiquorum vitium erat quod propter hos metus parcius
dabant (sc. helleborum), cum celerius erumpat quo largius
sumitur. Themison binas, non amplius, drachmas datavit;
sequentes et quaternas dedere claro Herophili praeconio, qui
5 helleborum fortissimi ducis similitudini aequabat; concitatis
enim intus omnibus ipsum in primis exire.

3 thebison *VRdf*   3 dedit *dT*: donavit *vulg. ante Gelenium*
5 similitudine *EagX*   6 omnibus *EagX*: omnium *rell.*   6 in primis
exire *EagX*: *om. rell.*

255 It was a defect of the ancients that they gave rather small doses of
hellebore because of these fears [sc. of its consuming effects], since the
larger the dose taken the faster it passes out. Themison gave doses of
two drachmae, and no more. His successors also gave [doses of] four
[drachmae] because of the famous proclamation by Herophilus, who
used to equate hellebore with the likeness of a very courageous
general: for when it has aroused all inside, it itself marches out in the
vanguard.

256 Ps.-Galenus, *De remediis parabilibus* 2.13 (XIV, p. 444K)

Ἡρόφιλος δὲ ἐπ' αὐτῷ (sc. τῷ φθισικῷ) χωρίς τινος δίδωσι ταρίχους σὺν ἄρτῳ καὶ ἐπιπίνειν ὕδωρ κελεύει, λέγων ὅτι ἐπείπερ ἅλες ἐπὶ ταρίχῳ συστρέφουσι τὴν κοιλίαν, οἶνος δὲ δοθεὶς λύει.

3 οἶνος] *fort.* ὕδωρ

256 For him [sc. for the person suffering from consumption], Herophilus prescribes salted pickled fish and bread without anything [else]. And he orders the patient to drink water afterwards, saying that, since the salt in the fish astringes the abdomen, when wine* is administered it relaxes it.

257 Galenus (e Critone?), *De compositione medicamentorum secundum locos* 5.3 (XII, p. 843K)

Ἡροφίλου χλωρόν· " ♃ ἰοῦ < β'. μάννης < δ'. στέατος μοσχείου < ιβ'. χαλβάνης < γ'. κηροῦ < π'. ῥητίνης < κ'. ὄξους τὸ ἀρκοῦν."

257 Herophilus' green plaster: 'Mix two drachmae verdigris, four drachmae frankincense powder, twelve drachmae calf-fat, three drachmae all-heal juice, eighty drachmae wax, twenty drachmae pine-resin, and an adequate amount of vinegar.'

258 Andromachus Iunior apud Galenum, *De compositione medicamentorum secundum locos* 7.4 (XIII, p. 79K)

ἄλλη (sc. σύνθεσις φαρμάκων) πρὸς αἵματος ἀναγωγήν, ὡς Ἡρόφιλος· " ♃ συμφύτου ῥίζης Ϝ γ', γῆς ἀστέρος Ϝ α', λιβάνου Ϝ β', βαλαυστίου Ϝ α', ὑποκιστίδος χυλοῦ Ϝ α', κρόκου τριώβολον, σμύρνης < β', ὀπίου < α', μίλτου Λημνίας Ϝ γ' καὶ τριώβολον, κόμμεως < α', χυλῷ πολυγόνου ἢ ἀρνογλώσσου ἀναλάμβανε."

3 ὑποκιστίδος *scripsi*: ὑποκυστίδος *edd.*

* For 'wine' perhaps read 'water'.

258 Another [compound of drugs] for the expectoration of blood, according to Herophilus: 'Make up three ounces [*oungiai*] comfrey root, one ounce Samian clay, two ounces frankincense, one ounce wild pomegranate flower, one ounce hypocist juice, three obols saffron, two drachmae myrrh, one drachma opium, three ounces and three obols Lemnian red-ochre, one drachma gum; make it up with the juice of knot-grass or plantain.'

259 Andromachus Iunior apud Galenum, *De compositione medicamentorum secundum locos* 9.6 (XIII, p. 308K)

ἑδρικὴ (sc. σύνθεσις φαρμάκων) ὡς Ἡρόφιλος· " ♃ ῥόδων ξηρῶν ἢ χλωρῶν < β'. ψιμυθίου < β'. πομφόλυγος < β'. κρόκου < β'. λιθαργύρου πεπλυμένου < β'. μελιλώτου < β'. σχοίνου < α'. μηκωνίου < α'. οἰσύπου < α'. ὠοῦ λέκιθον ὀπτὴν
5 α'. ῥοδίνου τὸ ἱκανόν, χυλοῦ ἀρνογλώσσου κυάθους δύο."

259 A [compound of drugs] for the anus, according to Herophilus: 'Mix two drachmae dry or green roses, two drachmae white lead, two drachmae zinc oxide (*pompholyx*), two drachmae saffron, two drachmae washed litharge [lead monoxide (*lithargyros*)], two drachmae melilot, one drachma rush, one drachma opium, one drachma woolgrease, one roasted egg yolk, an adequate amount of rose-oil, two ladles (*kyathoi*) of plantain juice.'

5 *Herophilus' 'On Eyes'**

260 Aëtius Amidenus, *Libri medicinales* 7.48 (*CMG* VIII.2, p. 303 Olivieri)

Ἡρόφιλος δὲ τὸ ἀνάπαλιν ἐν τῷ περὶ ὀφθαλμῶν φησί. "πρὸς τοὺς ἐν ἡμέρα μὴ βλέποντας κόμμι, κροκοδείλου χερσαίου κόπρον, μίσυ, χολὴν ὑαίνης λείαν, μετὰ μέλιτος ὑπόχριε δὶς τῆς ἡμέρας, καὶ ἐσθίειν δίδου νήστει ἧπαρ τράγου."
5 ἐγὼ δὲ τεκμαίρομαι τοῦτο ποιεῖν μᾶλλον τοῖς νυκτὸς μὴ ὁρῶσιν.

* Cf. Chapters VI (T85–T89) and VII (T140) for ophthalmological testimonia which may also belong to *On Eyes*. See also Appendix, III–IV, and Chapter XXVIII.

2 κόμμι] τάδε οἶον κώμεως C: κρόμειον Q   2 post χερσαίου add. ἢ ω
3 κόπρον] κόπρου Lᵃ: κόπρος AQω   3 μίσυος χολὴ (-ῆς C) CAQ
3 λεῖα Cχψ   4 νήστει] νήστης C: νῆστιν χω: om. DP   4 τράγιον
C   5 νύκτωρ APω

260 Herophilus says the reverse in his work *On Eyes*: 'For those who
cannot see in the daytime, twice daily rub on an ointment [composed
of] gum, the manure of a land-crocodile, vitriolic copper, and the bile
[gall] of a hyena made smooth with honey; and give the patient goat-
liver to eat on an empty stomach.'

But my guess is that one should rather do this to people who cannot
see at night.

C · COMMENTS

T231 In the first part of this testimonium Herophilus seems to be mentioned
only with immediate contemporaries. Like Herophilus, **Xenophon** was a
pupil of Praxagoras of Cos and possibly active in Alexandria too (cf. Cod.
Laurent. Lat. 73.1, published by Wellmann, 1900a: 370); see Steckerl, 1958:
127–9. Cf. also Kudlien, 1967b. Like Erasistratus and Herophilus, **Dionysius** perhaps belongs to the generation after Chrysippus (Erasistratus'
teacher?); cf. Pliny, *Natural History* 20.113; Rufus of Ephesus, *Names of the
Parts* 205 (p. 162 D/R). There are, however, a number of other physicians
called Dionysius (cf. Wellmann, 1905a: no. 132), and absolute certainty
about the identity of the one in T231 is at present unattainable.

T235 The 'little boy' Galen discusses is perhaps the same as the young boy
referred to in *On Anatomical Procedures* 7.12–13 (II, pp. 631–3K) as the *pais*
('boy'; 'slave'?) of Marullus, a writer of mimes (cf. Kroll, 1930). Galen's
procedure for exposing the heart is discussed *op. cit.*, 7.12 (II, pp. 626–31K),
and his view of the pericardial membrane, 7.2–3 (II, pp. 593, 595K). The
details of Herophilus' views on the dangers involved in lesions or incisions of
the pericardium are not known.

T252 This list of authors who wrote on therapeutics covers a broader
chronological spectrum than that of T231, and by placing Plistonicus before
Praxagoras, it does not adhere to the usual chronological sequence. Apart
from its confirmation that Herophilus wrote on therapeutics, its main value
accordingly lies (a) in its evidence about his prescription of drugs, and (b) in
the illustrious therapeutic rank accorded Herophilus. In antiquity **Euryphon** was often considered Hippocrates' most distinguished rival. (The
common attribution of the book *Knidiai gnomai* to Euryphon might, however,
be erroneous; cf. Jouanna, 1974: 13 n. 5). Cf. also Testimonia 3–9, 13, 15–16,

19–24, and 27–34 in Grensemann, 1975. Equally distinguished were the other figures with whom Herophilus is ranked here. On Dieuches' therapeutic fragments cf. Bertier, 1972: 26ff.and fr. 6–19. See also Diocles, fr. 5 Wellmann; Plistonicus, pp. 124–6 (especially fr. 6) Steckerl; and Praxagoras, fr. 4 (cf. fr. 96–120) Steckerl.

T257 Vinegar was well known in Greek antiquity as a therapeutic and hygienic substance: Hp., *Acut.* 61 (16L); Hp., *Reg.* 2.52; Dieuches, fr. 15.61 and 63, fr. 18.10 Bertier; Diocles of Carystus, fr. 83 Wellmann (against epilepsy), and, for regimen in health, frs. 138 and 141 (p. 185.3) Wellmann; Rufus of Ephesus in Oribasius 5.11; Celsus 2.18.11 (but cf. 2.21). See Dsc. 5.13, 5.17, 5.43, and 5.44; Galen, *De simplicium medicamentorum temperamentis ac facultatibus* 1.19 (XI, pp. 413f.K). Cf. Chapter I, n. 45.

T259 While better known as an unguent (Hipponax 58 West) and a perfume (Theophrastus, *De odoribus* 5.25), rose-oil frequently also served medicinal purposes in antiquity. Cf. the extensive description in Dsc. 1.43.

T260 While the fragment from *On Eyes* offers only pharmacological information, it seems possible, on the basis of T84–T89 (Chapter VI) and T140 (Chapter VII), that Herophilus also discussed the anatomy and physiology of the eye in this treatise. See also Appendix, IV.

cannot see in the daytime: Aëtius may be dependent on Demosthenes Philalethes for this fragment (see Chapter XXVIII), especially since Demosthenes also dealt with day- and night-blindness (cf. *DP.* 16). On day- and night-blindness (the same word, *nyktalōps*, often was used for both), cf. the rest of this chapter (7.48) in Aëtius; Hp., *Prorrhetic* 2.33 (IX, pp. 64–6L); Aristotle, *On the Generation of Animals* 5.1.780a16; Oribasius, *Synopsis ad Eustathium* 8.48 (*CMG* VI.3, p. 266 Raeder); ps.-Galen, *Definitiones medicae* 343 (XIX, p. 435K), and the passages mentioned below s.v. 'goat-liver'. Cf. also Hirschberg, 1899: especially pp. 98–107; Magnus, 1901: 297–8, 565–6, 164–5; Gourevitch, 1980.

manure of crocodile: Excrement was widely used in ancient Greek medicine, and also in early Egyptian medicine (see Chapter I); for a parallel from Graeco-Roman antiquity (perhaps derived from Herophilus) cf. Pliny, *Natural History* 28.28.107–11. Crocodile dung later became such a prized ingredient that counterfeit versions found their way into the drug trade; cf. Dsc. 2.80.6; Chapter I, n. 70 *supra*; Horace, *Epodes* 13.11.

bile (gall) of a hyena: With this recommendation Herophilus initiated a belief in the efficacy of hyena bile (as an ingredient in eye salves) that endured until the Byzantine period. Cf., for example, Oribasius, *Ad Eunapium* 4.24.11 (*CMG* VI.3, p. 447, line 28, Raeder), where it again is mixed with honey; Dsc. 2.78; Pliny, *Natural History* 28.27.94–5; Galen, *De* *compositione medicamentorum secundum locos* 4.9 (XII, p. 800K); Scribonius Largus 38; Galen, *De simplicium medic. temp. ac. facult.* 10.2.13 (XII, pp. 276–7K).

goat-liver: A felicitous recommendation, and one which was accepted by many physicians after Herophilus. See, for example, Galen, *De compositione medicamentorum secundum locos* 4.9 (XII, pp. 802–3K); ps.-Galen(?), *De remediis parabilibus* 1.5 (XIV, p. 350K); Dioscurides, *De simplicibus medicamentis* 1.43; Oribasius, *Ad Eunapium* 4.18 (*CMG* VI.3, pp. 445–6 Raeder); Paul of Aegina 3.22.29 (*CMG* IX.1, p. 184 Heiberg) – all of whom recommend goat-liver in cases of νυκτάλωψ, i.e. day- or night-blindness. Cf. also Galen, *De simpl. med.* 11.1.11 (XII, p. 336 K); Dsc. 2.45 for the value attached to the goat, perhaps because it had a reputation for having extraordinary night vision. See Magnus, 1901: 319–20; Chapter I, n. 71 *supra*.

IX · HIPPOCRATIC
EXEGESIS; VARIA

A · INTRODUCTION

Continuity and discontinuity, tradition and innovation, the old medicine and the new – nowhere is the relation between the two made more explicit than in the comments the innovators and discoverers make about precursor texts. While the subterranean acceptance and rejection of the old by the new might often be more telling than their surface relations, and while open resistance at times is perhaps less revealing than the veiled agon between old and new, the texts presented in this chapter offer a measure of the public posture which Herophilus' 'new' Alexandrian medicine assumed toward the 'old' pre-Hellenistic medicine of the Hippocratics.

Often celebrated as a radically innovative scientist, Herophilus emerged in the preceding two chapters as a physician who in crucial respects had not emancipated himself from the Hippocratic tradition. But here, in his public comments on Hippocratic texts, the posture in significant respects is one of resistance, revision, and rejection. Modern discussions of these texts[1] have focused almost exclusively on a question already raised above (Chapter III.A): whether Herophilus initiated the Alexandrian tradition of Hippocratic exegesis. But this focus has been maintained at the expense of a larger issue, viz. the role and status of Hippocratic medicine in early Alexandria.

Even if one disregards the controversial evidence (see Chapter III) concerning Herophilus' commentary on the *Aphorisms*[2] and his explanation of unusual Hippocratic words[3], there cannot be much

---

[1] Cf. Chapter III, especially nn. 20–4.

[2] T271 = Chapter III, T34; cf. Cobet's conjecture (critical apparatus).

[3] T270; see the critical apparatus, *ad loc.*, for Cobet's emendation, which has rendered this text of dubious value for Herophilus: ὁ Ἡροφίλειος ἐποίησε Βακχεῖος for ὁ Ἡρόφιλος ἐποίησε καὶ Βακχεῖος.

doubt that the shadow of Hippocrates loomed large in Alexandria too, and that the early Ptolemies actively acquired Hippocratic texts for the Royal Library.[4] Herophilus might have lived too early to benefit as fully from these Ptolemaic acquisitions as did his pupil Bacchius (*c.* 275–200 B.C.), who compiled one of the more influential Hippocratic lexica of all times.[5] But having been trained by a physician from Cos – Praxagoras – Herophilus undoubtedly was familiar with some Hippocratic texts, especially with the *Prognostic* and *Epidemics* VI. (As I pointed out above, he also was acquainted with Hippocratic theories not developed in these two works.)

Herophilus' explicit responses to these texts are striking for their unorthodoxy. Unlike the Alexandrian Empiricists and numerous other ancient physicians, both early and late (including Galen), Herophilus did not succumb to the temptation to invoke the sanction of 'Hippocrates' to legitimate his own views. Instead, he faced the spell of the Hippocratic tradition squarely, if not always successfully. Two ancient sources, Caelius Aurelianus and Galen,[6] confirm that Herophilus developed arguments in opposition to views expressed in the Hippocratic *Prognostic* and, as I suggested above,[7] these anti-Hippocratic arguments may well have been presented in the form of an entire treatise devoted to polemics against – or even to a polemical exegesis of – the Hippocratic work. This perhaps is the Herophilean work to which Galen refers in his *Commentary on Hippocrates' Prognostic* when he discusses the place of earlier commentators in his own commentary: 'I have also postponed examining all the things written so poorly by Herophilus against Hippocrates' prognoses' (προγνώ-σεις).[8] Ludwig Edelstein and Wesley Smith admittedly doubted that Herophilus ever wrote such an anti-Hippocratic work,[9] but no one has doubted the critical and polemical nature of Herophilus' public response (in whatever form it was presented) to the revered Hippocratic treatise.

---

[4] Cf. Chapter XIV, *Ba.*7; Chapter XV, *Zn.*5–6; Wellmann, 1929; Fraser, 1972: vol. I, pp. 325–30, 364–5, vol. II, p. 540 nn. 243–5; Edelstein, 1935a: cols. 1310–12; W. D. Smith, 1979: 199ff.; Nutton, 1975: 5. See also Galen, *In Hp. De nat. hom. comm.* 1.4, 2 prooem. (*CMG* v.9.1, pp. 55.6–14 and 57.12–16 Mewaldt).

[5] See Chapter XIV.A, and *Ba.* 12–76.   [6] T261, T264.

[7] Chapter III. A. 2, 'Genuine and spurious works'.

[8] T266 = Chapter III, T33.

[9] Edelstein, 1935a: col. 1309. For Smith's views see *Comments*, T261–T266. Cf. also Chapter III.A.2 above.

Contentious though the Greeks were, Herophilus' polemics represent an unprecedented step in the history of ancient medicine. Previous physicians had abandoned individual Hippocratic positions silently and implicitly, but no one had confronted the Father of Medicine with open criticism. The absence of traditional inhibitions, along with the spirit of scientific frontiersmanship in a new city, Alexandria, may have emboldened Herophilus to risk open confrontation, to question the dominant authority, and thus to clarify and enhance his own status as the initiator of a new tradition.

Herophilus' work on Hippocratic texts was, however, not indiscriminately polemical. He also initiated, even if only in inchoate fashion and not single-handedly,[10] the great Alexandrian tradition of interpreting and elucidating Hippocratic words. If Kühn's text is accepted, two testimonia from Galen suggest (a) that Herophilus interpreted obscure and rare Hippocratic words (*glōttai*),[11] and, as mentioned earlier, (b) that he wrote a commentary on the Hippocratic *Aphorisms*.[12] Both testimonia are, however, of dubious value and have been emended plausibly in such a way as to represent a statement about the Herophilean Bacchius, not about Herophilus himself.[13] Yet, even if these emendations are accepted, there are still at least eight other texts which seem to confirm that Herophilus tried to elucidate the meaning of certain Hippocratic words. Seven of these are culled from ancient commentaries on Hippocratic treatises,[14] and the remaining one occurs in a famous Hippocratic lexicon of the Neronian period.[15] This suggests that Herophilus' explanations of the relevant words were presented in the course of commenting – in whatever form – upon Hippocratic texts, and not in a context entirely independent of 'Hippocrates'.

[10] 'Not single-handedly', because Xenocritus of Cos is said by Erotian to have been the earliest Hippocratic glossographer, and he was probably a contemporary of Herophilus (but certainty about his date is unattainable). Cf. Chapter xiv, *Ba*.13; Chapter xiii, *Cm*.7; Fuhrmann, 1967; Erotian, *Vocum Hippocraticarum collectio*, pp. 4.24 and 12.7 (Nachmanson). Herophilus' explanation of Hippocratic words might, however, predate formal glossography of the kind apparently initiated by Xenocritus.

[11] T270: ... τὰς γλώττας ἂν ἐξηγήσαιτο μόνας ... On the distinction between γλῶτται and λέξεις see Pfeiffer, 1968: 198.

[12] T271 (= Chapter iii, T34).

[13] In both T270 and T271 the emendations are those of C. G. Cobet (later suggested – apparently independently – by J. Klein); see critical apparatus, T270 and T34. These emendations are eminently plausible.

[14] T262–T265, T267a, T267b, T268.   [15] From Erotian, T269.

Three of the eight testimonia – one from Galen, one from John of Alexandria, one from Palladius (but all three ultimately dependent on the Empiricist Zeuxis)[16] – concern the meaning of *nēpios* (usually 'infant') in a passage from Book VI of the Hippocratic *Epidemics* dealing with puberty: αἱ τῶν νηπίων ἐκλάμψιες ἅμα ἥβῃ ἔστιν οἷσι μεταβολὰς ἴσχουσι καὶ ἄλλας, 'in some cases the sudden blooming of *nēpia* in the prime of youth [i.e. at puberty?] involves other changes too'.[17] Although the use of *nēpia* to refer to pre-pubescent youths rather than to infants is rare, Herophilus apparently found this usage legitimate and retained it himself, saying of the characteristics of youth up to puberty that seed production, lactation, menstruation, conception, and baldness do not occur in *nēpia*.[18] Herophilus' pupil Callimachus,[19] mistaking this use of *nēpia* to mean 'infants', ridiculed Herophilus for 'merely stating the obvious' (i.e. that seed, etc. do not occur in infants), but Zeuxis firmly defended Herophilus' interpretation and use of the term – a rare though not unique[20] case of an Empiricist coming to the defence of Herophilus.

A further testimonium is provided by an author of the Neronian period, Erotian, perhaps the most famous Hippocratic lexicographer of antiquity. Having taken Herophilus' student Bacchius to task for misinterpreting *alysmos* ('anguished distraction, disquiet'), a word from the Hippocratic *Prognostic*, Erotian absolves Bacchius from sole culpability by tracing the pupil's error to the master: Herophilus, he says, erroneously equated ἀλύειν, 'to be distraught', with πλανᾶσθαι, 'to wander about aimlessly'.[21] Again, the context of Herophilus' observation seems to have been Hippocratic exegesis, and the fact

---

[16] T267a (Galen), T267b (John of Alexandria), and T268 (Palladius). Palladius and John of Alexandria apparently depended on Galen for their information, and Galen in turn explicitly ackowledges the early Empiricist Zeuxis as his source. Cf. Deichgräber, 1965: fr. 351.

[17] Hp., *Epidemics* 6.1.4. (V, p. 268, lines 1–2, L).

[18] T267a, T267b. On other ancient and modern interpretations of the Hippocratic passage (as well as possible emendations) cf. W. Bräutigam, 1908: 7–8.

[19] Cf. Chapter XIII, *Cm.*9.

[20] Another (but perhaps not equally conclusive) example is provided in Chapter XIV, *Ba.*13: when the Empiricist (and renegade Herophilean – see Chapter XVIII, Mantias) Heraclides of Tarentum wrote a treatise in three books against the Hippocratic lexicon of the Herophilean Bacchius, another Empiricist, Apollonius of Citium, responded with a treatise in no less than eighteen books (against Heraclides' attack on Bacchius). Cf. Deichgräber, 1965: fr. 311.

[21] T269. The lemma ἀλυσμός occurs in Hp., *Prognostic* 3 (I, p. 81.19Kw); *Epidemics* 4.46 (V, p. 188L); *Diseases of Women* 1.11 (VIII, p. 44L); and in several other

that Erotian refers to it in his discussion of a word from the Hippocratic *Prognostic* strongly suggests that Herophilus' work against this Hippocratic treatise may have been in the form of partially polemical exegesis rather than a general *Streitschrift*.

Further confirmation of this view seems to be offered by the remaining four testimonia, all of which concern the distinction between *prognōsis* and *prorrhēsis*. Both words are used in the Hippocratic *Prognostic*, and Herophilus was not the only ancient commentator puzzled by the relation of 'prognosis' to 'prediction'. Herophilus' solution is straightforward but overly subtle and not acceptable to subsequent commentators: *pro-gnōsis* ('fore-*knowledge*'), he says, is accompanied by firm certainty, whereas *pro-rhēsis* ('fore-*telling*') is not.[22] Stephanus of Athens, who depended on Galen, gives a different and perhaps less authentic version of Herophilus' distinction in his commentary on the *Prognostic*: *prognōsis* takes place 'whenever one recognizes something in advance but does not mention it to anyone', whereas *prorrhēsis* occurs 'whenever, having recognized something in advance, I *mention* that which has been recognized'.[23] The distinction is not attributed to Herophilus in this form by Galen, and since Stephanus does not seem to have had independent access to any of Herophilus' works, his account does not inspire great confidence.

In all these cases of textual interpretation, the elucidation of individual words seems to have been Herophilus' main purpose. This suggests that even if the Galenic statement in Kühn's text that Herophilus 'interpreted the [unusual or problematic] *words*' of Hippocrates[24] is emended out of existence, as several scholars wish,[25] we still have strong evidence that Herophilus initiated a long Alexandrian tradition of explicating Hippocratic texts. Many of his followers, from Bacchius, Callimachus, and Zeno to Heraclides of Erythrae,[26] continued the founder's interest in interpreting Hippoc-

Hippocratic works, but not in any extant part of the *Aphorisms*. Cf. Chapter xiv, *Ba*. 14.

[22] T262, T264.   [23] T265.   [24] T270.
[25] Cf. Chapter iii.A. 2, 'Genuine and spurious works': Cobet, Klein, Wellmann, and Fraser are among those who are convinced that T270 requires a textual emendation that would eliminate Herophilus from the ranks of Hippocratic lexicographers. While I doubt that Herophilus engaged in systematic lexicography, his explanations of Hippocratic words are amply attested.
[26] See below, Chapters xiii, xiv, xv, xxiv. Cf. also Chapter vii, T185, on the Herophileans' 'literary learning'.

ratic texts – albeit perhaps without the polemics against 'Hippocrates' that had characterized some of Herophilus' comments – and became famous for their commentaries and lexicographic contributions. (The other prominent medical school in Alexandria, the Empiricists, likewise engaged extensively in Hippocratic exegesis,[27] beginning with Herophilus' apostate pupil Philinus, who wrote a polemical work in six books against Bacchius' famous Hippocratic lexicon.[28])

The rapid, sustained development of Hippocratic exegesis and lexicography within the Alexandrian medical schools was probably encouraged – and perhaps in part inspired – by the broad, intense scholarly preoccupation with precursor texts in Alexandria. Like the poets, the physicians could not resist the Sirens of philology. The consequences for the transmission of Hippocratic texts and words were of considerable historical significance, as shown in Part 2. Perhaps equally important, focusing philological attention on medical terms may have encouraged the development of new terms (especially of a new anatomical terminology, to which Herophilus made a rich contribution) and may have aided the struggle toward terminological standardization, neither of which can be separated from the advance of medicine itself.[29]

B · TEXTS

1 *Hippocratic exegesis*

261 Caelius Aurelianus, *Tardae passiones* 4.8.113

Herophilus vero libro quem ad Hippocratis Prognosticum scripsit sive vivos sive mortuos (sc. lumbricos) excludi negat incongruum.

261 In the book he wrote against Hippocrates' *Prognostic* Herophilus

---

[27] Cf. Deichgräber, 1965: fr. 309–65 and pp. 317–22.
[28] Cf. Chapter XIV, *Ba*.13.
[29] On the relevance of terminology to the development of science see Lloyd, 1983: 149–67.

in fact says the passing of intestinal worms, whether alive or dead, is not a sign of disorder.

262 Galenus, *In Hippocratis Prorrheticum* I. *Comment.* I, prooemium (*CMG* v.9.2, p. 3 Diels)

οὐ μὴν οὐδὲ τὴν Ἡροφίλου νομοθεσίαν ἀποδεκτέον, ἐπιχειροῦντος διωρίσθαι πρόγνωσιν προρρήσεως τῷ βεβαίῳ τε καὶ οὐ βεβαίῳ.

1–2 ἐπιχειρῦντος] πῶς χειροῦντοσ *T*   2 διωρίσθαι *R*: διαιερῖσθαι *LT*

262 One should certainly not accept Herophilus' legislation when he attempts to distinguish prognosis (*prognōsis*) from prediction (*prorrhēsis*) by means of the certain and the uncertain.

263 Galenus, *In Hippocratis Prognosticum* I. *Comment.* 1.4 (ad Hp. II, p. 112.10–11 L) (*CMG* v.9.2, p. 203 Heeg)

ἃ δ' οἱ περὶ τὸν Ἡρόφιλον εἰρήκασιν διορίζοντες τὴν πρόγνωσιν τῆς προρρήσεως οὐ μόνον ἄχρηστά ἐστιν ἢ ἀνοίκεια τὰ σημαινόμενα, ἀλλὰ καὶ σοφιστικὰ καὶ ψευδῆ. καίτοι δοκοῦσί γε διαφορὰς πραγμάτων διδάσκειν, οὐ σημαινόμενα νομοθετεῖν,
5 ἁμαρτάνοντες ἐν αὐτῷ τούτῳ πρῶτον, ὅτι ἀγνοοῦσι περὶ σημαινομένων ποιούμενοι τὸν λόγον, οὐ περὶ πραγμάτων φύσεως ἰατρικῇ χρησίμων.

3 γε *om. P*   7 ἰατρικῆς *P*

263 What Herophilus and his followers said when distinguishing prognosis (*prognōsis*) from prediction (*prorrhēsis*) not only is useless or has significations that are alien to these words, but is also sophistic and false. Although they do seem to give instruction about differences in real things and not merely to legislate meanings, they are mistaken, first in this very respect, namely that they do not recognize that they are making their argument about meanings [sc. 'certain' *prognōsis* vs. 'uncertain' *prorrhēsis*], not about the nature of things that are useful to the art of medicine.

264 Galenus, *In Hippocratis Prognosticum 1. comment.* 1.4 (ad Hp. II, p. 112.10ff.L) (*CMG* v.9.2, pp. 204–5 Heeg)

οἱ δὲ περὶ τὸν Ἡρόφιλον ἡγοῦνται τὴν μὲν πρόγνωσιν τὸ βέβαιον ἔχειν, τὴν πρόρρησιν δὲ οὐκέτι· πολλὰ γὰρ τῶν προρρηθέντων οὐ γίνεσθαί φασιν, ὥσπερ δυναμένου τινὸς προειπεῖν ἄνευ τοῦ προγνῶναι. ἢ ἄλλο τι τὸ διὰ τῆς φωνῆς
5 ἑρμηνευόμενον, ὅτι μὴ τὸ κατὰ τὴν ψυχὴν γινωσκόμενον; εἰ δ' οὐ γινωσκόμενον ἐθέλοιεν ὀνομάζειν αὐτό, πάντως γε δοξαζόμενον ἐροῦσιν, ὡς προηγήσασθαι κατὰ τὴν ψυχὴν τοῦ προλέγοντος εἰ καὶ μὴ πρόγνωσιν, ἀλλὰ προδόξασιν. οὐ μὴν ὀνομάζουσί γε προδόξασιν οἱ Ἕλληνες, ὥσπερ οὐδ' οἱ περὶ τὸν Ἡρόφιλον
10 αὐτοί, καίτοι πλεῖστα βαρβαρίζοντες.

ἢ γοῦν νομοθετείτωσαν λέγεσθαί [τι] προδόξασιν ἕτερόν τι τῆς προγνώσεως ἅμα τῷ καὶ τοὺς ἀνθρώπους πεῖσαι παραδέξασθαι τὴν νομοθεσίαν αὐτῶν, ἢ τοῦτο πρᾶξαι μὴ δυνάμενοι τὰ σημαινόμενα τῶν ὀνομάτων ὡς εἴθισται νοείτωσαν. εἴθισται δὲ
15 καὶ τὴν ὡς τὸ πολὺ περὶ τῶν μελλόντων ἔσεσθαι ἐλπίδα καὶ τὴν ἀσφαλῆ καλεῖσθαι πρόγνωσιν . . .

ἴσως δὲ κακῶς ἐποίησα τὴν ἀρχὴν μνημονεύσας τῶν περὶ τὸν Ἡρόφιλον· ἄμεινον γάρ ἐστιν δηλοῦν τάληθῆ ὅτι τάχιστα τοῖς σπεύδουσιν ἐπὶ τὰ τῆς τέχνης ἔργα . . . κάλλιον οὖν μοι δοκεῖ
20 διὰ τῶνδε τῶν ὑπομνημάτων αὐτὰ τὰ χρήσιμα μόνα διεξελθεῖν, ἐξετάσαι δὲ αὖθις ἐπὶ σχολῆς πλείονος ἐν ἑτέρᾳ πραγματείᾳ καὶ διασκέψασθαι περὶ τῶν ὑπὸ Ἡροφίλου πρὸς τὸ Προγνωστικὸν Ἱπποκράτους ἀντειρημένων.

5 *post* ἑρμηνευόμενον *habet* ὃν F¹   9 οἱ *om.* F¹   10 αὐτὸν F¹   11 γοῦν P: *om. cett.* (*qui ante* λέγεσθαι *habent* οὖν ἢ)   νομοθετήτωσαν F¹ *edd. vett.*   τι *del.* Heeg: τινα *coni.* De Lacy   17 μνημονεύσας τὴν ἀρχὴν P   20 διελθεῖν *Ald Bas. Charterius*   22 ὑπὸ *om.* RP
23 ἀντειρημένον F

264 Herophilus and his followers believe that prognosis (*pro-gnōsis* (fore-knowledge)) possesses firm certainty, whereas foretelling (*pro-rhēsis*) does not. For, they say, many of the things that have been foretold do not come about – as if anyone is able to foretell without foreknowing (*pro-gnōnai*). Or is anything else expressed by this word [sc. *pro-gnōsis*] that isn't that which is 'known' by the soul? But if they do not want to call it 'known', surely they will have to call it 'opined' (*doxazomenon*); for, if indeed the antecedent in the soul of a person who foretells is not 'fore-knowledge' (*pro-gnōsis*), it [must], on the contrary, be 'fore-opinion' (*pro-doxasis*). The Greeks in fact do not give it the name 'fore-opinion', nor do Herophilus and his followers themselves do so, even though they commit very many barbarisms.

Let them, then, either legislate that 'fore-opinion' means something other than 'prognosis', and at the same time persuade people to accept their legislation, or, if they are unable to do this, let them understand the significations of words in their customary usage. It is in accord with such usage that both the expectation 'for the most part' concerning the future and the firm expectation concerning the future are called 'prognosis' . . .

But perhaps I made a poor start by mentioning Herophilus and his followers, for it is better to make clear the truth as rapidly as possible to those who have an eager attitude to the tasks of our art . . . It therefore seems better to me to expound through these commentaries only the details that are actually useful, but subsequently, at a time of greater leisure, to examine and scrutinize again in another treatise the things said by Herophilus in opposition to Hippocrates' *Prognostic*.

265 Stephanus Philosophus, *In Hippocratis prognosticum* 1 *Comm.* 1.4 (ad Hp. II, p. 110.3L) (*CMG* XI.1.2, p. 40 Duffy)

'Ηρόφιλος ἐξηγήσατο ἄλλο εἶναι πρόγνωσιν καὶ ἄλλο πρόρρησιν. "καὶ πρόγνωσις μέν", φησίν, "ὅταν προγνῶ, μὴ εἴπω δέ
τινι. πρόρρησις δέ ἐστιν ὅταν προεγνωκὼς εἴπω τὸ προεγνωσ-
μένον." καὶ αὕτη μὲν ἡ 'Ηροφίλου ἐξήγησις καταγέλαστος
5 οὖσα, ἰστέον τοίνυν ὅτι πρόγνωσις καὶ πρόρρησις οὐδὲν
διαφέρει, πλὴν κατὰ τὴν ἕξιν τοῦ ἰατροῦ καὶ τοῦ νοσοῦντος.

2 πρόγνωσιν *codd.*: *corr. Duffy*   φησιν] φασιν *L*   4 αὕτη μὲν ἡ
'Ηροφίλου] περὶ (παρὰ *VY*) μὲν ἡροφίλω *MPVY*

265 Herophilus explained that 'prognosis' (*prognōsis*) is one thing and 'prediction' (*prorrhēsis*) another: ' "Prognosis" is whenever I recognize something beforehand but do not mention it to anyone, whereas "prediction" is whenever, having recognized something beforehand, I mention that which has been recognized'. And since this interpretation of Herophilus' is ridiculous, one should, of course, know that prognosis and prediction differ in no respect except the respective dispositions [sc. epistemological?] of physician and patient.

436 HEROPHILUS

266 Galenus, *In Hippocratis Prognosticum comment.* 1.4 (*CMG* v.9.2, p. 207 Heeg)

See Chapter ii, *T33 supra.*

267a Zeuxis apud Galenum, *In Hippocratis Epidemiarum 6.1.4 comment. 1.5* (ad. vol. v, p. 268.1–2L) (*CMG* v.10.2.2, pp. 20–1 Wenkebach)

ὁ δ' αὐτὸς οὗτος Ζεῦξις "νήπια", φησίν, "εἴρηται πάντα τὰ παιδία, καθότι καὶ Ἡρόφιλος ὠνόμασεν αὐτὰ οὕτως." καὶ γὰρ περὶ τούτου γράφει τόνδε τὸν τρόπον διὰ ταύτης τῆς λέξεως·
"φαίνεται νήπια λέγων ὁ Ἱπποκράτης τὰ ἕως ἥβης καὶ οὐχὶ
5 τὰ νεογνὰ μέχρι τῶν πέντε ἢ ἐξ ἐτῶν, ὡς νῦν οἱ πλεῖστοι λέγουσιν. ἥρκει δὲ καὶ ὁ Ἡρόφιλος τὰ τηλικαῦτα λέγων νήπια, δι' ὧν φησι· 'τοῖς νηπίοις οὐ γίνεται σπέρμα, [με]γάλα, καταμήνια, κύημα, φαλακρότης.'
"οὐ γὰρ τοῖς μέχρι τῆς προειρημένης ἡλικίας παραγινομέ-
10 νοις λέγει μὴ γίνεσθαι ταῦτα, τουτέστιν ἀπὸ τῆς πρώτης εὐθέως γενέσεως, ὅπερ τινὲς δεχόμενοι καταγελῶσιν αὐτοῦ, ὡς τὰ πᾶσι γινωσκόμενα διδάσκοντος, ὧν ἐστι καὶ ὁ Καλλίμαχος, ἀλλὰ τοῖς μέχρις ἥβης, ἐπειδή τινες ὑπέλαβον καὶ ἐν τούτοις ταῦτα γίνεσθαι."
15 ταῦτα μέν σοι καὶ τὰ τοῦ Ζεύξιδος.

1 εἴρηται *Deichgräber*: εἰρῆσθαι *U edd.* 6 τηλικαῦτα *e* τηνικαῦτα *corr. U* 7 σπέρμα, γάλα *H*(*cf. T267b infra*): σπέρμα μεγάλα *U*: σπέρματα μεγάλα *ab Aldo edd.* 10 τουτέστιν *Cornarius Charterius*: hoc est *Crassus*: τουτί *U*

267a This same Zeuxis says: 'All young children (*paidia*) are called infants (*nēpia*), just as Herophilus, too, calls them.' For he [Zeuxis] writes about it [sc. the word *nēpios*] in the following way, in these very words:
'Hippocrates seems to call [children] up to puberty "infants", and not just the newborns up to five or six years, as most people nowadays do. And Herophilus, too, was content to call [children] of such an age [sc. up to puberty] "infants", inasmuch as he says: "In 'infants' (*nēpia*) seed, milk [lactation], menstruation, foetus, and baldness do not occur."
'For, he [Herophilus] does not mean that these things do not occur

in [children] until they reach the aforementioned age, i.e. right from the first moment of their birth, which is exactly the [erroneous] interpretation [of Herophilus' words] that some people – among them Callimachus, too – accept and for which they ridicule Herophilus, as though he were teaching things that are recognized by all. But [Herophilus in fact means] children up to puberty, [and he makes this point] because some people assume that these things occur in them, too.'

So much for the words of Zeuxis. (*Cf. p. 430 supra.*)

267b Iohannes Alexandrinus, *Commentaria in VI. librum Hippocratis Epidemiarum*, Particula 1, 121a.46–52 (pp. 17–18 Pritchet)

'Infantes' dicit Ypocras non solum qui lactant sed qui sunt usque ad pubertatem. et quod hoc sit verum, sic Yrofilus et Xeutippus (sc. Zeuxis) dicunt. ' "infantibus" neque lac fit neque pariunt neque calvi fiunt nisi post pubertatem.' nisi enim
5 dixissent 'infantes' usque ad pubertatem, ridiculosum esset; quod diceretur ab eis quod 'infantes' lactantes neque lac habent neque pariunt neque calvi fiunt. hoc enim et non intelligentes confitentur . . .

1 dicit Ypocras *PBVAEU*²: *om. U*   2 pubertatem] pubertatem intendit *U*   5 dixissent] dixisset *V*

267b Hippocrates uses 'infants' not only of those who are unweaned but also of children up to puberty. And Herophilus and Xeutippus [i.e. Zeuxis] also say that this is true. ' "Infants" do not produce milk, do not give birth, and do not become bald except after puberty.' Now, unless 'infants' meant [children] up to puberty, it would be ridiculous; what would [otherwise] be meant by them is that unweaned 'infants' do not lactate, do not give birth, and do not become bald. But this even those who have no understanding concede . . . (*Cf. p. 430 supra.*)

268 Palladius, *In Hippocratis Epidemiarum 6. commentarius 1.4* (vol. II, p. 12 Dietz)

νήπια λέγει (sc. Ἱπποκράτης) οὐ τὰ ὑποτίτθια, ἀλλὰ τὰ παιδία,

ὥσπερ καὶ Ἡρόφιλος· νήπια οὐ φαλακροῦνται, οὐκ ἀγρυπνοῦ-
σιν, ἀντὶ τοῦ παιδία.

2 ἡρώφυλος *AL*

268 By *nēpia* ('infants') Hippocrates does not mean breastfed babies
but young children (*paidia*), just like Herophilus: *nēpia* are not bald
and do not lie awake; it stands for *paidia*.

269 Erotianus, *Vocum Hippocraticarum collectio* α.1
(p. 10 Nachmanson)

ἀλυσμόν· . . . οἱ γοῦν ἀλύοντες ἄχθονται μὲν ἐν τῷ ὀδυνᾶσθαι,
οὐκ ἀλύουσι δὲ οἱ πλανώμενοι. ἀλλ᾽ ὡς εἰκὸς ἐπλάνησεν αὐτὸν
(sc. Βακχεῖον) Ἡρόφιλος συνώνυμον θεὶς τὸ ἀλύειν τῷ πλανᾶσθαι. κεῖται ἐν τετάρτῳ ἐπιδημιῶν καὶ ἐν α´ γυναικείων καὶ ἐν
5 ἀφορισμοῖς.

269 [On the word] 'distraught state' (*alysmos*): . . . Those, then, who
are 'distraught' are oppressed with grief in their suffering, whereas
those who 'wander aimlessly' are not 'distraught'. But, as it seems,
Herophilus caused him [Bacchius] to 'wander astray' by rendering
'to be distraught' (*aly-ein*) synonymous with 'to wander' (*planasthai*).
It (*alysmos*) occurs in [the Hippocratic] *Epidemics* IV, *Diseases of Women*
I, and in the *Aphorisms. (See n. 21 supra, pp. 430–1.)*

270 Galenus (?), *Explanatio vocum Hippocratis*, prooemium (XIX,
pp. 64–5K)

ταῦτά τε οὖν ἡμεῖς περιίδωμεν καὶ πρὸς τούτοις ἔτι τὸ
διηγεῖσθαι τὴν ἰδέαν ἑκάστου φυτοῦ καὶ βοτάνης καὶ τῶν
μεταλλευομένων, ἤδη δὲ καὶ τῶν ἰχθύων καὶ τῶν ζῴων ὅλων,
ὅσων ἂν ἑκάστοτε τύχῃ μεμνημένος ὁ Ἱπποκράτης, ἅπερ ὁ
5 Διοσκουρίδης οὐκ αἰδεῖται μεταγράφων ἐκ τῶν Νίγρου τε καὶ
Παμφίλου . . . καὶ ἄλλων μυρίων. οὕτως δὲ καὶ πόλεων ὀνόματα
διηγεῖται γνωριμωτάτων καὶ ἄστρων ὁμοίως ἐπιφανεστάτων, ἃ
μηδὲ ἂν παῖς ἀγνοήσειεν. ταῦτα δὲ καὶ ἄλλοι πολλοὶ τῶν
ἐξηγησαμένων ἁμαρτάνουσιν. εἰ τοίνυν ταῦτά τις περιέλοι

10 πάντα, τὰς γλώττας ἂν ἐξηγήσαιτο μόνας, ὥσπερ ὁ Ἡροφίλειος ἐποίησε Βακχεῖος, Ἀριστοφάνους τοῦ γραμματικοῦ τὸ
πλῆθος αὐτῷ τῶν παραδειγμάτων ἀθροίσαντος, ὡς φασιν.
ἡμεῖς δέ, ὡς οἶσθα, πλείω κἀκείνων ἐκλέξαντες ἐν ὑπομνήμασιν
ἔχομεν.

1 περιίδωμεν *LM*: περιίδομεν *edd. vett.*   8 μὴ δὲ *Iunta*   10 γλώσσας
M⁰ D   ἐξηγήσατο *vulg.: corr. Franze*   10–11 ὁ Ἡροφίλειος ἐποίησε
Βακχεῖος *Cobet Klein Wellmann*: ὁ Ἡρόφιλος ἐποίησε καὶ Βακχεῖος
ALMDR: καὶ *om. M⁰ Ald*   11 Ἀριστοφάνους *Klein Ilberg Wellmann*:
Ἀριστάρχου *codd.* (Ἀριχάρχου *D*)   12 φησίν *D*   13 ἐκλέξαντες
scripsi: ἐκλείψαντες *vulg.*: ἐλλείψαντες *DM⁰*

270 Let us then disregard these things and in addition let us pass up a
detailed exposition of the form of each plant, herb, and mineral, also
of fish and altogether of all the animals which Hippocrates happens to
have mentioned on each occasion. All of this is what Dioscorides is not
ashamed to copy from the books by Niger and Pamphilus . . . and
countless others. Thus Dioscorides also gives a detailed exposition of
the names of perfectly well-known cities and similarly of the most
visible stars, of which not even a child could be ignorant. These
mistakes many others who have provided interpretations have also
made. Now, if one were to pass over all of these things, one would
interpret only the rare words, as did the Herophilean Bacchius,* after
Aristophanes, the grammarian, had collected a large number of
examples for him, as they say. And, as you know, I have selected more
even than they and I provide them in my commentaries. (*Cf. Chapter*
XIV.A).

271 Galenus, *In Hippocratis Aphorismos* (7.69) *comment.*7.70 (XVIIIA,
pp. 186–7K)

See Chapter III, *T34 supra.*

2 *Varia*

272 Galenus, *De diebus decretoriis* 2.7 (IX, pp. 874–5K)

διὰ τοῦτο τοίνυν ὁ μέν τις αὐτῶν οὔτε κρίσιμον ἡμέραν οὔθ ὅλως

* C. G. Cobet, J. Klein, and M. Wellmann emend 'Herophilus and Bacchius' to
read 'Bacchius the Herophilean'. This emendation is probably correct. Cf.
Chapter III, T34.

κρίσιν ὑπάρχειν φησίν, ὁ δὲ κρίσιν μὲν εἶναί τινα, οὐ μὴν καὶ
κρισίμους ἡμέρας, ὥσπερ δέον λόγῳ μᾶλλον, ἀλλ᾽ οὐ πείρᾳ τὰς
κρισίμους ἡμέρας καὶ τὰς κρίσεις ἐξευρίσκειν, ἢ φαυλοτέρων
5 ὄντων τῶν ὅσοι διὰ τῆς πείρας ἄμφω μεμαθηκέναι φασίν. ἡμῖν
μὲν τοίνυν ὅσοι μεθ᾽ Ἡρόφιλόν τε καὶ Ξενοφῶντα καὶ Ἀσκληπιάδην ἐγενόμεθα τάχ᾽ ἂν εἴη τις εἰς τοὺς ἄνδρας ἐκείνους ἢ
φθόνος ἢ φιλονεικία. τῷ πρώτως δ᾽ ἀκριβῶς αὐτὰς ἐξευρόντι
διὰ τῆς πείρας, ὡς τὰ τῶν ἐπιδημιῶν ἐνδείκνυται γράμματα,
10 πόθεν ἂν ἐπῆλθε τὸ προγνῶναί τινας ἔσεσθαι ἐξ ὑστέρου
τοιούτους σοφιστάς;

272 It is for this reason then that one of them says there is neither a
critical day [sc. of a disease] nor any critical turning point (*krisis*) at
all, while another says there is a critical turning point but there are
not critical days – as though it were necessary to discover critical days
and critical turning points not by experience but rather by reason, or
as though all persons who say they have learnt of both [sc. of critical
days and of critical turning points] through experience rank among
the worse [sc. physicians]. Indeed, we who were born after Herophilus, Xenophon, and Asclepiades perhaps would experience some
envy of, or rivalry with, those men. But whence could prescience of
the fact that some members of posterity would be such sophists have
come to the man [sc. Hippocrates] who first made an accurate
discovery of critical days and turning points through experience, as
his *Epidemics* indicate?

273 Galenus, *Methodus medendi* 2.5 (x, p. 110K)

. . . τοῖς γὰρ ἀποχωρήσασι μὲν τῶν λογικῶν ἀποδείξεων, ὅτι δ᾽
Ἡρόφιλος οὕτως ἐκέλευσεν ἢ Ἐρασίστρατος, ἀξιοῦσι πισ-
τεύειν, ἀνάγκη πᾶσαν λοιδορίαν καὶ μάχην ἀκολουθῆσαι, τὰ
θαυμαστὰ τῶν νῦν διαλόγων ἄθλα . . . καὶ ἄλλος τις . . . παρ-
5 ελθὼν ὡς μὲν οὐκ ὀρθῶς εἴρηται τῶν εἰρημένων ὁτιοῦν μηδ᾽
ἐπιχειρήσειεν ἀντειπεῖν, μόνον δ᾽ ἐπιτιμῶν ὡς περιττὰ ζητοῦσι,
καὶ μάρτυρα τὸν Ἐρασίστρατον ἢ τὸν Ἡρόφιλον ἐπάγοιτο . . .

273 Every kind of abuse and contention – the wondrous prizes
bestowed upon current discourse – necessarily follows those who have
gone astray from logical proofs and, simply because Herophilus or

Erasistratus gave the order, think one should trust [it] . . . Yet another person might come along and not even try to argue that anything of what was said was said incorrectly, but only censure them for making superfluous investigations, and he would call in Erasistratus and Herophilus as his witnesses . . .

274 Michael Italicus(?), *Epistula ad medicum Lipsioten* (*Anecdota Graeca Oxoniensia*, ed. J. A. Cramer, vol. III (1836), pp. 188–9; *Michael Italikos*, ed. P. Gautier, no. 32, pp. 204–5)

φιλοσοφώτατέ μοι καὶ γραμματικώτατε ἰατρῶν· . . . οἶδας γὰρ
καὶ τὰ τοῦ Σωράνου καὶ τὰ τοῦ Ἱπποκράτους· ἐπίστασαι
Γαλήνειά τε καὶ Ἡροφίλεια, καὶ τὰ τοῦ Ἡρωδιανοῦ καὶ τὰ τοῦ
Τρύφωνος καὶ τὰ τοῦ Ἡροδότου καὶ τὰ τοῦ Ἥρωνος· καὶ οὐ
5   μόνον ἀλλὰ καὶ λέγεις αὐτὰ εἰδέναι καὶ οὔτ' εἰρωνεύῃ οὔτ'
ἀλαζονεύῃ τοῖς λόγοις· τὰ μὲν γὰρ οἶδας ὡς ἰατρός, τὰ δὲ ὡς
γραμματικός, τὰ δὲ ὡς μηχανικός.

274 My most philosophical and philological of doctors! . . . For you know the writings of both Soranus and Hippocrates; you are versed in things Galenic and Herophilean, and in the writings of Herodian, Tryphon, Herodotus, and Heron. Not only that, but you also *say* that you know them, and you are neither ironic nor pretentious in what you say. Some of these things you know as a physician, others as a grammarian, still others as an engineer.

275 Galenus, *In Hippocratis Epidemiarum 3.1.1 comment.* 1.4 (ad vol. III, p. 24.4ff. L) (*CMG* v.10.2.1, pp. 21–2 Wenkebach)

καίτοι καὶ τῶν ἐμπειρικῶν ἔνιοι, καθάπερ ἔφην, ὡς ἐν δράματι τὸ
περικείμενον ὑποκρίνονται πρόσωπον, Ἱπποκράτειον μὲν ἐξη-
γούμενοι βιβλίον ὡς Ἱπποκράτειοι, τῶν δ' Ἐρασιστράτου τι καὶ
Ἡροφίλου καὶ Ἀσκληπιάδου καὶ τῶν ἄλλων ⟨ὡς⟩ ἀπ' ἐκείνων
5   ἑκάστου τῆς αἱρέσεως ὄντες.

1 καὶ *om.* O   2 παρακείμενον *VP*   3 τι *O:* τε *L*   4 ὡς *add.*
Wenkebach   4–5 ἀπ' ἐκείνων τῶν αἱρέσεως *V*

275 Admittedly some of the Empiricists, too, as I said, act the part of

the mask they are wearing, as in a play, interpreting a Hippocratic work like Hippocratics, but any of the works of Erasistratus, Herophilus, Asclepiades, and others as though they belong to the school descended from each of these.

C · COMMENTS

T261–T266 W. D. Smith, 1979: 191–3, concedes that 'Galen believed that Herophilus . . . wrote against Hippocratic prognosis', but speculates that 'Galen had blown up a perfectly normal verbal distinction made in a Herophilean work' – probably, in Smith's view, Herophilus' On *Common Opinions* – ' . . . into an imaginary historical quarrel.' Smith also believes that the evidence presented by Caelius Aurelianus is based on a doxographic fiasco: 'first, by a normal error of interpretation, a view about worms which Diocles rejected was attributed to Hippocrates and then specifically to the *Prognostic* . . . Second, a name was made up for the book in which Herophilus wrote of worms . . . That he wrote a book in opposition to Hippocrates' *Prognostic* seems unlikely in the extreme.' However, the cumulative weight of the evidence presented in this chapter supports the view that Herophilus took a strong, active interest in Hippocratic exegesis – an interest sustained and developed by his followers (see below, Chapters x, xiii, xiv, xxiv).

T264 in another treatise: perhaps this refers to Galen's *Commentary on Hippocrates' Prorrhetic*, although his comments there are no more elaborate; see T262.

T267a–b Zeuxis: see Deichgräber, 1965: 25–8; Kudlien, 1972d ('Zeuxis, 7'). For Herophilus' views on stages of life see Chapter vii.A.4, T176–T186, and *Comments*, T176.

Part 2

THE HEROPHILEANS
(*c.* 250 B.C.–A.D. 50)

X · HEROPHILUS
AND THE HEROPHILEANS

A · INTRODUCTION

A problem which surfaced persistently in the preceding chapters –the relation of the old to the new, of the precursor to the successor, of tradition to innovation – enters a new stage with the death of Herophilus. At issue is no longer just the relation of the new Alexandrian medicine to the old medicine of the Hippocratics (or to Aristotelian biology), but the relation of Alexandrian pupils to their Alexandrian master, of Herophileans to Herophilus. It is a relation complicated first by the dynamic nature of the Herophilean school – which, unlike Galenism or Epicureanism, always remained open to changes in emphasis, to doctrinal shifts, and to radical revisions –and, secondly, by the remarkably long history of the school, roughly from 300 B.C. to A.D. 50, through periods in which varying demands and needs exercised frequently changing pressures upon scientists and physicians. Throughout these three and a half centuries the sanction provided by the common label 'follower of Herophilus' was sought and shared by numerous distinguished physicians, but this nominal uniformity cannot conceal the diversity and the fierce, often contentious individualism accommodated within the 'school'.

Perhaps the single most striking development in this context is the retreat from anatomy, the turning away from dissection, which had been Herophilus' most significant and renowned contribution to scientific medicine.[1] Few, if any, activities played a more powerful

---

[1] Many of the views presented in this chapter were developed in von Staden, 1982: 85–95 and 201–6.
For a discussion of the relevant anatomical evidence concerning Herophilus see Chapter VI.A. Among his followers only Andreas, who commented on the relation of marrow and bone (Chapter XI, *An.*5), and Hegetor, who defended anatomy as essential to the discovery of correct surgical procedures (Chapter XVII, *Hg.*3), are

role in the rise of scientific medicine in Alexandria than the dissection – and possibly vivisection – of humans, and apparently few were as completely and as suddenly abandoned by Herophilus' successors. About the reasons for this sudden and almost total surrender of a major tool of scientific medicine, one can only speculate. Several possible causes were suggested above (Chapter VI.A), among them the reassertion of Greek and Egyptian taboos, the fundamental insecurity of science within the social order under almost all but the first two Ptolemies, and the rising popularity of the Alexandrian Empiricists' theory of scientific method (which denied the scientific value and clinical relevance of systematic dissection).[2] But whatever the reasons might be, with one or two notable exceptions (e.g. Hegetor, Chapter XVII below) the followers of Herophilus, from the third century B.C. to the first century A.D., seem to have turned their backs on anatomy – at least if one may generalize on the basis of the roughly three hundred extant texts concerning the followers of Herophilus.

All was, however, not retreat, rebellion, and revision within the school. There are some clear strands of continuity between the founding master and his followers. Perhaps the most striking of these is the sustained interest Herophilus' followers showed in pulse theory, a branch of pathophysiology which assumed immense diagnostic significance in antiquity (and which owes its first thorough investigation to Herophilus himself, as pointed out earlier).[3] From Bacchius (c. 275–200 B.C.) to Demosthenes Philalethes (first century A.D.), the followers of Herophilus kept alive the sphygmological tradition initiated by the founding master of their school. Yet, even within this broad continuity, one is confronted with the independence and innovative ambitions of individual members of the school.

Herophilus' analysis of the pulse was not simply transmitted with piety and reverence from one generation to the next, like an orthodoxy that had become canonical or obligatory. Instead, each Herophilean tried to improve not only on Herophilus' definition but also on those of his immediate predecessors and contemporaries

---

reported to have displayed an active interest in anatomy. Whether Hegetor actively practised dissection, as has recently been claimed, or was only trying to score points in a methodological debate, remains uncertain (see Chapter XVII).

[2] Cf. Kudlien, 1968a: 44–6; Deichgräber, 1965: fr. 66–70; n. 13 infra.

[3] Cf. Chapter VII, especially T144–T188; Chapter VI, T115–T128.

within the school. The result is a striking example of the incessant shuffling and dissent that lurk not too far beneath the homogeneous surface suggested prima facie by the label 'Herophileans':

Herophilus: The pulse is a perceptible motion of the arteries received from the heart; it is born and dies with a living being; it exists naturally and attends us involuntarily at all times, occurring both when the arteries are filled and when they are emptied, i.e. when they dilate and contract.[4]

Bacchius: (a) The pulse is a dilation (*diastolē*) and contraction (*systolē*) occurring simultaneously in all the arteries;[5] (b) the pulse is a distention (*diastasis*) of the artery or of the arterial part of the heart.[6]

Zeno (*c.* 200–150 B.C.): The pulse is an activity of the arterial parts – an activity which is a mixture of contraction and distention.[7]

Chrysermus (mid first century B.C.): The pulse is a distention and contraction of arteries, occurring when the arterial coat, through the agency of a psychic and vital faculty, rises on all sides and then again shrinks together; it is a constant concomitant in both healthy and diseased conditions, and it can be apprehended by sense-perception.[8]

Alexander Philalethes (*c.* 50 B.C.–A.D. 25): Objectively, the pulse is an involuntary contraction of the heart and the arteries, such as can become apparent; subjectively, it is the beat of the continuous, involuntary motion of the arteries against one's touch, and the interval occurring after the beat.[9]

Heraclides of Erythrae (last half of the first century B.C.): The pulse is a contraction and dilation of the arteries and the heart, accomplished through the agency of a vital and psychic faculty which is dominant.[10]

Aristoxenus (first half of the first century A.D.): The pulse is an activity of the heart and the arteries – an activity peculiar to them.[11]

Demosthenes Philalethes (*c.* 20 B.C.–A.D. 50): Objectively, the pulse is a dilation of the heart and the arteries, or their natural contrac-

---

[4] This is a composite description of Herophilus' view, culled from T147–T148, T150, 154–T155, T158–T160. Cf. Kollesch, 1973: 128–38.
[5] Chapter XIV, *Ba.*1.
[6] Chapter XIV, *Ba.*2.   [7] Chapter XV, *Zn.*1.   [8] Chapter XX, *Cr.*1.
[9] Chapter XXII, *AP.*3.   [10] Chapter XXIV, *HE.*2.   [11] Chapter XXV, *Ar.*1.

tion, capable of becoming apparent; subjectively, it is a natural beat of the heart or of the arteries against one's touch and the interval which occurs after the beat.[12]

This selective enumeration of Herophilean pulse definitions provides only one example of that diversity – within a common thematic concern – which became characteristic of the Herophileans. Acutely aware of one another's views, in part through doxographic treatises concerning their own school, each Herophilean strove for a fresh and more viable definition of the essential nature of the pulse, attempting at the same time to meet objections raised to his precursors' formulations. What might, from a modern perspective, look like sophistic quibbling over minor differences concerning a definition, to most of the participants in this revisionary process was anything but a mere exercise in patricidal and fratricidal eristic. Rather, it was a search for a correct understanding of the essential nature of a major diagnostic tool and, simultaneously, a reaffirmation of the value and relevance of theoretical investigations for the clinician.

What unites almost all followers of Herophilus is in fact precisely their interest not only in clinical but also in scientific or 'theoretical' medicine, and this is, of course, also what distinguishes them most sharply from their chief rivals in the early period, the Alexandrian Empiricists, who rejected systematic dissection and physiology as irrelevant for clinical purposes.[13] Even those Herophileans for whom no pulse-lore is attested (for example, Andreas) dealt with physiological questions that were taboo to the Empiricists – taboo, exactly because these questions required forming hypotheses concerning what nature has concealed. Thus Andreas dealt with a question which fascinated many Greek philosophers and physicians, namely the nature and location of the controlling instance in human beings (τὸ ἡγεμονικόν) – again, a question regarded as clinically irrelevant by the Alexandrian Empiricists, but answered by Andreas with an

---

[12] Chapter xxviii, *DP.*1.

[13] Although the Empiricists did engage in anatomical observation when the opportunity afforded itself (cf. Deichgräber, 1965: fr. 66–70), they rejected dissection. Similarly, at least some later Empiricists, notably Heraclides of Tarentum (first century B.C.), were willing to offer empirical descriptions (ὑπογραφαί) – but not definitions – of the pulse in terms of 'beat', but not to acknowledge the validity of concepts such as 'diastole' and 'systole', or to allow the introduction of physiological principles to explain the pulse or to grant great diagnostic significance to pulse theory; cf. Deichgräber, 1965: fr. 71–7.

audacity characteristic of the earliest Herophileans: there is no
supreme, directing faculty of vitality and intelligence that is identifiable with the soul; rather, the soul is a nonentity and the controlling
faculty or what is called 'soul' or 'mind' is nothing but the senses.[14]

With the exception of pulse-lore, the physiological questions which
interested Herophilus do not, however, seem to have preoccupied his
followers more than sporadically. The four faculties or humours,[15]
the nervous system,[16] the problem of respiration,[17] dream theory[18] –
none of these is tackled by any of his followers. Here and there we do
get glimpses of continuity: Herophilus made a major contribution to
the anatomy and physiology of the male and female reproductive
organs,[19] Alexander Philalethes speculates on the origin and nature
of 'seed' (and Andreas on conditions conducive to procreation);[20]
Herophilus developed a theory of digestion and absorption, Alexander Philalethes returns to the same question.[21] But these strands of
continuity tend to be the exception and they are relatively fragile.

A similar pattern of spasmodically emerging affinities between
master and followers is found in pathology. Thus, Herophilus dealt
with various kinds of haemorrhage, and two Herophileans, Bacchius
and Demetrius of Apamea, classify them by cause;[22] Herophilus gave
the concept 'moisture' (or 'humour') a central place in his pathology,
and so apparently does Aristoxenus;[23] Herophilus recognized the
pathological significance of the brain and the meninges, and so does
the Herophilean Gaius.[24] Again, the affinities are there, but they are
occasional and do not reflect sustained continuity.

The same is true of related branches of medicine: Herophilus, who
wrote the first book on midwifery, was interested not only in the
reproductive organs of women but also in gynaecological and
obstetrical problems in general. Thus he dealt with the causes of
difficult labour, and so do the Herophileans Andreas and Demetrius

[14] Chapter xi, *An.*6; cf. Chapter vii, T137–T139 and T136.
[15] Cf. Chapter vii, T130–T134.   [16] *Ibid.*, T140; Chapter vi, T80ff.
[17] Chapter vii, T143a–c.   [18] *Ibid.*, T226a–c.
[19] Chapter vi, T101–T114; Chapter vii, T189–T193, T198–T199, T202.
[20] Chapter xxii, *AP.*9; Chapter xi, *An.*8.
[21] Cf. Chapter vii, T146; Chapter xxii, *AP.*6.
[22] Cf. Chapter viii, T231; Chapter xiv, *Ba.*5; Chapter xvi, *DA.*11.
[23] Cf. Chapter vii, T133: *in umidis omne vitium est*; T205(a): ἐν ὑγροῖς; Chapter xxv,
*Ar.*6: *corruptionem et abundantiam liquoris.* See Chapter vii.a.1.
[24] Cf. Chapter vii, T137–T139; Chapter xxvii, *G.*1. (See also Chapter vi,
T75–T79.)

of Apamea, while Mantias also deals with the problem of afterbirth which is not expelled;[25] Herophilus dealt with the question whether there are diseases peculiar to women, and so do Demetrius, Alexander Philalethes, and Apollonius Mys;[26] Herophilus speculated about the nature and effects of menstruation, and so do Demetrius and Alexander.[27]

To find a part of medicine – other than sphygmology – both nurtured by Herophilus and actively pursued by a majority of his followers, one has to turn to pharmacology. Herophilus had, after all, called drugs 'the hands of the gods'[28] and had made active therapeutic use of them. Not only is his expertise in simple drugs attested, but some of his compound drug prescriptions are also extant. From the earliest generation of Herophileans to the last, this pharmacological part of Herophilus' legacy was honoured and cultivated. Andreas, the court physician who was probably a direct pupil of Herophilus, made a monumental contribution especially to the study of simple drugs, compound drugs, and the toxic effects of certain plants and animals.[29] He is mentioned, and quoted exten- sively, no less than twenty-five times by ancient sources in pharmaco- logical contexts; his views on the deleterious effects of opium, his 'amazing' emollient (as Galen calls it), and the versatile uses to which his drug compounds could be put became renowned throughout antiquity. Perhaps the most famous pharmacologist of antiquity, Pedanius Dioscurides, even dignified Andreas with this characteriza- tion: 'Crateuas the herbalist and Andreas the physician actually seem to have dwelled on this part [of medicine] with greater accuracy than the rest of them, though they passed over many very useful roots . . . Yet, to the credit of these ancients it must be attested that, for all the paucity of what they transmitted, they also contributed accuracy, whereas this cannot be conceded to modern authors . . .'[30]

Similarly, in the first generation of Herophileans, Callimachus and Bacchius displayed an active interest in pharmacology,[31] and in the

---

[25] Cf. Chapter vii, T196–T197(a) and (b); Chapter xi, An.9; Chapter xvi, DA.20–1, 25; Chapter xviii, Ma.12.

[26] See Chapter vii, T193–T194; Chapter xvi, DA.18; Chapter xxii, AP.11; Chapter xxiii, AM.7.

[27] See Chapter vii, T203–T204; Chapter xvi, DA.17; Chapter xxii, AP.10.

[28] Chapter viii, T248–T249. (Cf. also T251–T260.)

[29] Chapter xi, An.18–46.

[30] Ibid., An.23.   [31] Cf. Chapter xiii, Cm.5–6; Chapter xiv, Ba.6.

second century B.C. the Herophilean physicians Zeno, Demetrius, and Mantias again kept this tradition alive.[32] Mantias, in particular, more than once is recognized by Galen as the true father of the compound drug tradition.[33] Mantias apparently was the first to arrange his comprehensive compilations of drug prescriptions not only by kind or *per genera*, κατὰ γένη (e.g. purgatives, clysters, emollients, etc.), but also by place or *secundum locos*, κατὰ τόπους (e.g. prescriptions for headaches, ear-aches, skin conditions, eye ailments, upset stomach, etc.) – a useful taxonomic principle which was also adopted by Galen in his massive and influential pharmacological treatises, and which hence became entrenched for centuries.[34]

In the first century B.C., too, Herophileans did not abandon their pharmacological legacy. Chrysermus, for example, became known both for his views on simple drugs, such as asphodel, and for his compound drug prescriptions,[35] and Chrysermus' pupil Apollonius Mys composed one of the more famous pharmacological treatises of antiquity, *Euporista* or *Readily Accessible Remedies* (also known as *On Common Remedies*), from which Galen quotes liberally, especially in his treatise *On the Composition of Drugs according to Place*.[36] Judging by Galen's accounts, Apollonius adopted one of Mantias' taxonomic principles, namely arranging his common remedies topically (i.e. by place of application, κατὰ τόπους), and the practicality of this arrangement, along with the fact that all the ingredients used by Apollonius were readily accessible, may account for its popularity in the first two centuries A.D. About the state of pharmacology in the last visible generation of the Herophilean school we are less well informed. No relevant evidence concerning Aristoxenus is extant, and it is uncertain whether the drug prescriptions attributed to a certain Demosthenes were in fact the work of the great Herophilean ophthalmologist, Demosthenes Philalethes.[37] (It seems very likely,

---

[32] Cf. Chapter xv, *Zn*.4; Chapter xvi, *DA*.23–4; Chapter xviii, *Ma*.1–11. See also Chapter viii, T248–T260, for evidence concerning Herophilus' contribution.

[33] See Chapter xviii.A, and *Ma*.1–2, *Ma*.6.

[34] Cf. Galen, *De compositione medicamentorum per genera* (xiii, pp. 362–1058K), vs. *De compositione medicamentorum secundum locos* (xii, pp. 378–1007K; xiii, pp 1–361K).

[35] See Chapter xx, *Cr*.5 (the use of asphodel in treating parotid abscesses); *Cr*.6 (a prescription for dropsy and affections of the spleen).

[36] Chapter xxiii, *AM*.11–26 and *AM*.28. See also *AM*.9–10 and *AM*.29–46.

[37] See Chapter xxviii, *DP*.47–8 (included as *Dubia*).

however, that Demosthenes Philalethes did include prescriptions for
eye ointments in his famous *Ophthalmicus*.)

This rapid survey of the pharmacological tradition within the
Herophilean school suggests, then, that pharmacology, like pulse-
lore, represents a strong strand of continuity in the history of the
school. But whereas no spectacular advances over Herophilus' theory
of the pulse were made by his successors, pharmacology was an area
in which the Herophileans grew in strength and knowledge after
Herophilus' death, advancing well beyond his level of expertise.

There is a further significant difference between these two instances
of continuity. Whereas Herophilus' pulse theory was firmly rejected
by the Herophileans' chief rivals – the Alexandrian Empiricists – as a
part of theoretical or speculative medicine and hence irrelevant to
medical practice, the Empiricists embraced pharmacology as an
empirical discipline of unquestionable clinical import. From the time
of Herophilus' heretical pupil, Philinus of Cos (who founded the
Empiricist school), until the first century A.D., Empiricists repeatedly
engaged in pharmacological activity: Philinus, Glaucias, Mantias'
renegade pupil Heraclides of Tarentum, Diodorus, Lycus, and
Zopyrus of Alexandria are examples of Empiricists who actively
affirmed the significance of pharmacology.[38]

Having largely abandoned research in the area which brought
Herophilus his greatest fame, i.e. anatomy, the Herophileans now
seem to have stressed a branch of learning found unobjectionable by
their rivals. The same is true of two further areas in which
Herophileans took a more active interest after Herophilus' death:
surgery and Hippocratic exegesis. This particular constellation –
pharmacology, surgery, and Hippocratic exegesis – renders them
virtually indistinguishable from their Empiricist rivals, and it is
conceivable that the Empiricists' sustained polemics against theoretical medicine in general, and against the Herophilean school in
particular, exercised pressure upon the Herophileans to concentrate
on clinical medicine and the Hippocratic Corpus, perhaps in part at
the expense of anatomical exploration (but even while physiological
speculation, especially concerning the pulse, remained alive in
Herophilean circles).

A few examples of the new-found interest in surgery among

---

[38] Cf. Deichgräber, 1965: fr. 136–9, 157–63, 192–240, 252–5, 259, 262–4, 267–74.

Herophilus' followers might illustrate this tendency. Andreas, perhaps one of Herophilus' earliest students, constructed a famous
instrument for reducing dislocations of the larger joints, apparently
exploiting the new mechanical technology (developed by his contemporaries Archimedes, Ctesibius, and Philo) for its surgical potential.[39] This instrument, still known and highly regarded by Celsus
(early first century A.D.), by Galen (second century A.D.), and by
Oribasius (fourth century A.D.),[40] symbolizes a significant departure
from the rather passive attitude Herophilus seems to have had toward
surgery in general and toward orthopaedic surgery in particular.[41]

A further example of this trend is provided by the Herophilean
Bacchius who, in his Hippocratic lexicon or *Lexeis*, grants a place of
unusual prominence to lemmata from Hippocratic works on orthopaedic surgery, such as *On Joints* and *Instruments of Reductions*,[42], and,
in his classification of causes of haemorrhage, also makes an
apparently clinical reference to fractures.[43] Demetrius of Apamea
likewise refers to orthopaedic matters, in particular to the distinction
between fractures and depressions in the bones of new-born infants.[44]
Finally, Mantias dealt with the problem of the relative merits of the
simple ligations used by Hippocrates, on the one hand, and, on the
other, the complex forms of bandaging employed by more recent
physicians – a context which, along with his procedure for expelling
afterbirth retained *post partum*, perhaps suggests a surgical interest.[45]

Equally striking is the growing interest among Herophileans in
Hippocratic philology. Whereas Herophilus' relation to 'Hippocrates' had been marked by ambivalence, polemics, and the need to
establish himself as the emancipated founder of a new tradition (see
Chapter IX), the later Herophileans, perhaps less burdened by the
need to move visibly out of the long Hippocratic shadow and to
establish themselves as the vanguard of the new, scientific medicine,
could approach Hippocratic texts in a relatively dispassionate,

---

[39] See Chapter XI, *An.*11–17.
[40] Oribasius, though the latest source, gives the fullest descriptions of Andreas'
instrument; see Chapter XI, *An.*14–17. For Celsus and Galen, cf. *An.*11 and *An.*
12–13 respectively. Cf. also Drachmann, 1963: 171–85.
[41] Cf. Chapter VIII.A.
[42] Cf. Chapter XIV, *Ba.*17–19; *Ba.*31, *Ba.*40–3, and *Ba.*55–8 for glosses on lemmata
from *On Joints*; *Ba.*20–2, *Ba.*33–4, *Ba.*46, and *Ba.*62–6 offer glosses on lemmata
from *Instruments of Reduction*. For *On Fractures* see *Ba.*39, *Ba.*54.
[43] *Ibid.*, *Ba.*5.   [44] See Chapter XVI, *DA.*9.   [45] Cf. Chapter XVIII, *Ma.*14.

critical manner. Neither polemics nor an effort to legitimate their own views through an appeal to the sanction of the father of medicine marks their treatment of the Hippocratic texts. But there is a further significant dimension to their interest in Hippocratic exegesis.

The emergence of philology and criticism as a major, and highly respected, research activity in Alexandria by the mid third century B.C. must be understood in a larger Alexandrian context. While Philo of Byzantium in his work *On Artillery* (c. 200 B.C.) still reports a royal interest in applied science,[46] and while scientists like Archimedes continued being invited to Alexandria,[47] the scholars who increasingly dominated Alexandrian intellectual life and, judging by some anecdotes which survive,[48] had the most intimate contact with the Ptolemaic court, were no longer philosopher-scientists like Strato of Lampsacus, and certainly not physician-scientists like Herophilus, but the philologists and poet-critics like Zenodotus, Apollonius, Aristophanes of Byzantium, and Aristarchus. In a world in which the learned librarian or the learned poet, such as Callimachus, apparently became more revered than the medical research scientists, it is perhaps not surprising that physicians, too, turned to new sources of respect and status: exegesis and lexicography.

Not that Herophilus had shown no critical interest in Hippocratic texts; as I pointed out in the previous chapter, Herophilus offered exegetical and lexical observations. But Hippocratic criticism still played a relatively subsidiary role in Herophilus' activity as a physician and scientist, whereas it seems to have vied strongly with theoretical medicine and, in some cases, even with clinical medicine for a position of dominance in the works of some of his followers.

Already in the first generation of Herophileans this tendency

---

[46] Philo, *Belopoeica* 3 (50.24–6 Wescher; p. 108 Marsden): 'The craftsmen in Alexandria were the first to have provided this [sc. the calibrating formulae for constructing war engines], because they had obtained large subsidies (μεγάλην- ... χορηγίαν) since they had ambitious kings who encouraged technology [or: craftsmanship].'

[47] Cf. Diodorus' claim that the Archimedean screw was invented by Archimedes 'when he went to Egypt': *Bibl.*5.37.3. Cf. Heiberg, 1879: 5; Heath, 1912: xvi; Hultsch, 1896; Mugler, 1970–2: vol. I, p. viii; Dijksterhuis, 1956: 21–3 ('*The Cochlias*').

[48] Eratosthenes and a Stoic philosopher, Sphaerus of Borysthenes, are also among the intellectuals depicted as spending time in the company of the royal family. Cf. Athenaeus, *Deipnosophistae* 7.2.276A–C (= *FGrH* 241F16); D.L. 7.177; Plutarch, *De cohibenda ira* 458A–B. See also Zuntz, 1959: 35 n.3.

becomes clear. The Herophilean physician Callimachus provided glosses on Hippocratic words,[49] and the *Lexeis* of his contemporary Bacchius became the most influential Hippocratic lexicon of the Hellenistic period. More than sixty testimonia and fragments from Bacchius' lexicon are still extant,[50] and the range of Hippocratic works it covered – at least eighteen[51] – was unprecedented in the history of Alexandrian philology. But Bacchius was not only a lexicographer; he also edited the Hippocratic treatise *Epidemics* III (and possibly other Hippocratic works), and wrote commentaries on the Hippocratic *Aphorisms*, on *Epidemics* VI, and on *In the Surgery*.[52] Not much later the Herophilean Zeno provided further glosses on Hippocratic words[53] and apparently triggered the protracted Alexandrian debate about the authenticity and meaning of obscure letter-symbols found in an Alexandrian copy of *Epidemics* III.[54] In the first century B.C. two Herophileans continued this tradition: Dioscurides Phacas – apparently a prominent counsellor and ambassador of Cleopatra, of her father, and of her brother – composed a Hippocratic lexicon in seven books,[55] and Heraclides of Erythrae not only wrote a commentary on *Epidemics* II, III, and VI but also resumed, and perhaps terminated, the controversy concerning the provenance and significance of the letter-symbols in *Epidemics* III.[56] Cydias, too, seems to have engaged in Hippocratic exegesis.[57]

This Herophilean trend can, therefore, be documented richly. Also significant is the fact that Hippocratic philology gained a prominent position in the school of the Alexandrian Empiricists, too. From the founder of the school, Philinus of Cos, who wrote a polemical work against Bacchius' Hippocratic lexicon, to Apollonius of Citium and Heraclides of Tarentum in the first century B.C., Empiricists engaged as actively as Herophileans in exegesis and lexicography.[58] That this similar but not identical movement of two arch-rivals, Empiricists and Herophileans, away from scientific research into philology,

---

[49] Chapter XIII, *Cm.*7–9.   [50] Chapter XIV, *Ba.*12–76.

[51] Enumerated in the Introduction to Chapter XIV, *infra*.

[52] Chapter XIV, *Ba.*7–10; cf. also *Ba.*11, which suggests that Bacchius may have written a commentary of *Epidemics* II as well.

[53] Chapter XV, *Zn.*7–9.   [54] *Ibid.*, *Zn.*5–6.   [55] Chapter XIX, *Ds.*4–7.

[56] Chapter XXIV, *HE.*5. Cf. also *HE.*4 and *HE.*6–10, which confirm that Heraclides wrote commentaries on Hp., *Epidemics* II and VI.

[57] Chapter XXVI, *Cy.*1. See also Chapter VII, T185 *supra*.

[58] Cf. Deichgräber, 1965: fr. 309–65 and pp. 317–22.

cannot be attributed to a diminution of royal patronage has been argued above. On the contrary, there are indications that this development was encouraged, directly or indirectly, by at least some of the Ptolemies. Thus Apollonius of Citium, author of the only work of Hellenistic medicine to have survived intact, states in the introduction of his commentary on the Hippocratic work *On Joints* that he undertook the exegetical task on the king's orders and now offers the finished product to him for approval.[59] The Ptolemy in question is probably Cleopatra's father Auletes (*c.* 112–51 B.C.),[60] and hence this is relatively late evidence, but it does reveal, as P. M. Fraser has argued,[61] 'the direct' – but, I would add, not always scientifically fruitful – 'stimulus that writers received from a royal patron'. It also vividly suggests the power of the patron to coax a physician away from scientific medicine by prescribing his exegetical tasks for him, although, as suggested above (Chapter IX.A), the development of a more precise, standardized medical terminology might have been a useful product of Herophilean and Empiricist philology.

Perhaps closely related to the burgeoning critical interest in precursor texts is another movement away from anatomical and physiological research, namely the growing importance of doxography within the Herophilean school. As in the case of Hippocratic exegesis, the Herophileans could perhaps appeal to the example of Herophilus – who had written a treatise with a doxographic thrust – to legitimate their own doxographic efforts. But here, too, there is a significant difference, namely the increasingly self-centred nature of Herophilean doxography. While Herophilus and Andreas were still primarily concerned with going on the offensive in their doxographic efforts – Herophilus wrote *Against Common Opinions*,[62] Andreas *On*

---

[59] Apollonius Citiensis, *In Hippocratis De articulis commentarius* I (*CMG* XI.1.1, p. 10 Kollesch/Kudlien): '*I* see, King Ptolemy, that *you* are interested in medicine, while *you* see that *I* eagerly execute your orders ... [and I have explicated the inventions of the most divine Hippocrates concerning instruments for helping men], which you ordered me to communicate to you at present.' The same king is likewise addressed in the prefaces to Books II and III of Apollonius' commentary (pp. 38, 64 Kollesch/Kudlien).

[60] Cf. Deichgräber, 1965: 206: Apollonius' floruit is roughly 70 B.C.

[61] Fraser, 1972: vol. I, p. 312.

[62] Cf. Chapter VII, T203; T204 perhaps belongs to the same treatise – a suggestion based on the thematic affinities between T204 and T203.

False Beliefs and *On the Genealogy of Physicians*[63] – Bacchius set in motion a long Herophilean tradition of writing about, or in defence of, the opinions or *doxai* held by various members of one's own school. This trend reaches its culmination in the last years of the school's visible existence with treatises entitled *On the School of Herophilus* written by no less than three different Herophileans: Apollonius Mys, Heraclides of Erythrae, and Aristoxenus.[64]

This sudden accumulation of works with an apologetic and protreptic purpose in the final stages of the history of the school might well, as I shall argue below, reflect the growing insecurity of the followers of Herophilus in the midst of new challenges. Whereas they were reasonably successful in surviving the Empiricist challenge, in part, as suggested above, by distinguishing themselves in branches of medicine highly valued by the Empiricists themselves (pharmacology, surgery, semiotics or symptomatology,[65] Hippocratic philology), the last generations of Herophileans faced the challenge not only of the Empiricists but also of new eclectic 'dogmatists' or 'rationalists' and of sceptics who were rapidly gaining in popularity: the 'Pneumatic' and 'Methodist' schools of medicine.[66]

Herophileans no longer had the appeal of novelty or the strength of anatomical and physiological excellence; with the exception of their sphygmological and gynaecological persistence, the concerns of most Herophileans had become virtually indistinguishable from those of their Empiricist rivals. Furthermore, the rebellious and individualistic strain that marked the long, rich history of the school, from the time when Herophilus was abandoned by one pupil and ridiculed by another[67] down to Aristoxenus' sharp censure of almost all his Herophilean predecessors and contemporaries in the first century A.D.,[68] might paradoxically have hampered its chances of surviving the fresh challenges. Herophilean polemics became increasingly

---

[63] Chaper xi, *An*.47 and *An*.45.
[64] Chapter xxiii, *AM*.4; Chapter xxiv, *HE*.3; Chapter xxv, *Ar*.3. Cf. Chapter xxii, *AP*. 3: Alexander's *Opinions*.
[65] Callimachus (Chapter xiii, *Cm*.3) and Demetrius of Apamea both dealt explicitly with signs; Demetrius wrote a book entitled *Signs* or *Semiotics* (*DA*.1–3).
[66] See Chapter xxiii n. 22 for references to literature on the rise of the 'Pneumatic' and 'Methodist' schools of medicine.
[67] Cf. Chapter ii, T1; Chapter xiii, *Cm*.9; Deichgräber, 1965: fr. 6, fr. 351.
[68] See Chapter xxv.A.

fratricidal in nature – Herophilean pitted against Herophilean – and the self-centred doxography referred to earlier became its vehicle.

Yet even at the moment of its last visible gasps the school of Herophilus displayed some of the ambiguity and tenacity that characterized much of its history: while one of the last representatives of the school, Aristoxenus, was engaging in sophistic censure of his fellow-Herophileans, another, Demosthenes Philalethes, made enduring, if not always original, contributions to the pathology and therapy of eye ailments, contributions whose general impact upon ancient and medieval medicine was matched by those of no other Herophilean except Herophilus himself.[69]

Self-destructive scrutiny and heuristic triumph, looking over one's shoulder and looking ahead, preoccupation with the words of predecessors and aggressive discovery – these are some of the ambivalent dimensions of the history of Herophilus' school, and they persist from its inception to its apparent death in the first century A.D.

This raises a final question that must be dealt with here: the institutional history of the school of Herophilus. In most parts of this work, 'school' is used in a loose, broad sense, because there is no clear evidence that Herophilus or his followers were organized institutionally in the first two hundred or two hundred and fifty years of the existence of this group of physicians. As pointed out in the first chapter, there is no evidence that Herophilus, or any representative of scientific medicine, was associated with the Alexandrian Museum. Rather, the general system of medical apprenticeship characterized in Chapter II probably also prevailed in Alexandria, and Bacchius' use of the phrase 'those from the *house* of Herophilus' to refer to early Herophileans[70] might well be an indication of the informal and non-institutional – but not necessarily unrigorous – nature of medical apprenticeships in Alexandria.

Despite – or perhaps in part because of – this apparent absence of formalization and institutionalization of the 'school', despite the individualism and dissent that marked relations between 'members' of the school, and despite the political and social vicissitudes which buffeted science and scholarship in Ptolemaic Alexandria (such as the expulsion of a large number of intellectuals, including physicians,

---

[69] See Chapter xxvIII.
[70] Cf. Chapter xIV, *Ba.* 78. See also pp. 478–9, 482 on this use of *oikia*; cf. Glucker, 1978: 166–206.

from Alexandria in 145/144 B.C.),[71] Herophilean medicine survived without noticeable interruption as a prominent force in Alexandrian life at least until the late first century B.C.; there is no century in the history of Ptolemaic Alexandria in which Herophileans failed to assert their presence in the royal capital. Thus we find the Herophilean physicians Andreas, Callimachus, and Bacchius in Alexandria in the third century B.C.; Zeno, Demetrius, Hegetor, and Mantias in the second century B.C.; Dioscurides Phacas, Chrysermus, Apollonius Mys, and Heraclides of Erythrae in the first century B.C.

A novel phase in the institutional development of the school seems to have been reached, however, with the expansion of the school into Asia Minor in the mid or later first century B.C., after it had been associated exclusively with Alexandria for at least two hundred years. Founded by Zeuxis 'Philalethes' or 'Truth-Lover' (a reverential title traditionally reserved for Hippocrates) at the famous temple of the moon god Men Karou, in the vicinity of the Phrygian city Laodicea on the great Eastern trade route, this branch of the school apparently had a more institutional character than the 'school' in Alexandria. Several factors seem to support this conclusion. First, Strabo calls it a 'large place of instruction' or 'great school' (διδασκαλεῖον μέγα).[72] διδασκαλεῖον is an expression rarely used of the Alexandrian 'school' of Herophileans – or, for that matter, of any other medical 'school'; indeed, the word usually is reserved for the kind of formal institution attended by schoolchildren and run by rhetoricians and grammarians and is almost never applied to the apprenticeship arrangements that were characteristic of medical education in classical and Hellenistic Greece.[73] Secondly, the association of the school with a cult centre also suggests an institutionalization of the kind well known from the Alexandrian Museum (but nowhere attested for the Herophilean 'school' in Alexandria): in the Museum a group of scientists and scholars were joined together not only as researchers

---

[71] Cf. Chapter III.A for a description by Menecles of Barca of the far-ranging effects of this expulsion order; see also Chapter III n.2.

[72] Chapter XXII, AP.1. See also Chapters XXI.A, XXV.A, and XXVIII.A.

[73] Cf. Epicurus, fr. 20.2 Arrighetti (= fr. 50 Usener); Plato, Laws 764c8; Thucydides 7.29.5; Hyperides, In Defence of Euxenippus 22 (col. 34); Aeschines, Against Timarchus 9. But cf. also Antiphon, On the Choreutes 11, of a training room or practice room fitted out by the choregus in his own house. T278, in which Galen refers to the Herophilean and Erasistratean 'schools' as didaskaleia, represents an exception.

sharing patronage and meals, but also as members of a cult association presided over by a priest.[74] A similar arrangement probably prevailed at the Museion in Ephesus, which was famous for its συνέδριον of physicians and its annual 'medical Olympics'.[75] While the Herophilean school at the temple of the Men Karou might not have shared all these characteristics with the Alexandrian Museum and similar institutions, its association with a cult is suggestive. Furthermore, the *Lex Iulia de collegiis* might have stipulated, among the conditions for establishing medical or other formal associations (*synodoi*, *collegia*), that cult worship must be fostered by such an association or institution.[76] It is conceivable that the Herophilean school at Men Karou was constituted as just such a *collegium*.

The history of the Herophilean school in Asia Minor extends roughly one century or three generations, from about 40 B.C. to A.D. 50. The successive leaders of the school were Zeuxis Philalethes, Alexander Philalethes, and Demosthenes Philalethes. Another influential member of the school was a student of Alexander Philalethes, Aristoxenus, whose sharp criticism of a number of Alexandrian Herophileans might be indicative of rivalry, or at any rate of disharmonious relations, between the Alexandrian mother school and her Asian offspring.

It has been argued persuasively, but not conclusively, that there are two further prominent Herophileans from Asia Minor: Menemachus Philalethes and Tiberius Claudius Athenodotus Philalethes.[77] The former is known only through a single coin of the Augustan

---

[74] Cf. Strabo, *Geography* 17.1.8 (793–4C): 'The [Alexandrian] Museum is also part of the royal quarters; it has a covered walk (*peripatos*), an arcade (*exedra*), and a large house, in which the common meal of the men of learning (*philologoi*) who share the Museum [is provided]. For this association there exist common funds and a priest supervising the Museum, who in those days was appointed by the kings [sc. Ptolemies], but now by Caesar.' See also Müller-Graupa, 1933; Rostovtzeff, 1953: vol. I, pp. 1084–5, vol. II, p. 1596 n. 39.

[75] On Ephesus see Keil, 1905; Wolters, 1906. On the Mouseion in Smyrna see Robert, 1937: 146–8. The evidence concerning the Mouseion in Athens remains controversial; cf. J. D. Oliver, 1934, vs. Graindor, 1938. Cf. also the general discussion in Fraser, 1972: Vol. I, pp. 312ff.

[76] Cf. Herzog, 1935: 967ff., 981 (also, pp. 1005–6, on Mouseia outside Alexandria). On Men and Men Karou cf. McMinn, 1956 (esp. 206); and *infra* Chapter XXI, *Zx*.1. See also Pohl, 1905: 79–91.

[77] Benedum, 1974: especially 226ff. See also *infra*, pp. 582–3, on Aglaias.

period from the town of Acmonea; the latter only through an inscription from Eumeneia in Phrygia. It is indeed striking that both bear the honorific 'Philalethes', which was shared by all known leaders of the Herophilean school at Men Karou. But neither Menemachus nor Tiberius Claudius Athenodotus is identified as a physician, let alone as an Herophilean. Furthermore, the honorific 'Truth-Lover' was not the exclusive property of Herophileans, as pointed out earlier. A slightly more plausible case can perhaps be made for Menemachus: according to the pseudo-Galenic treatise *Introductio sive medicus*, a certain Menemachus of Aphrodisias (a town not too far from Laodicea and Acmonea) started out as a 'Methodist' physician but turned apostate. Did he convert to Herophileanism, as Benedum suggests? The mere honorific 'Philalethes' seems too weak a link on which to build a confident positive answer, although the circumstantial evidence marshalled by Benedum is very suggestive.[78]

The evidence concerning Tiberius Claudius Athenodotus is equally flimsy but tantalizing. The inscription from Eumeneia not only grants him the honorific 'Philalethes', but also identifies him as a priest of Apollo Propylaeus. And Apollo Propylaeus is apparently the Greek name for the Phrygian god Men, who was worshipped as 'Men Karou' in the Carian-Phrygian border area. Since there was a famous temple of Apollo Propylaeus in Attanassus, near Eumeneia, Benedum concludes that yet a further branch of the Herophilean school was established at Apollo's temple in Attanassus – a school modelled after the branch at Men Karou and presided over by none other than Tiberius Claudius Athenodotus, who, argues Benedum, lived from A.D. 20 to A.D. 80[79] This imaginative and carefully argued conclusion has much appeal, but it is, of course, purely speculative inference. The only firm knowledge we have concerning this figure is offered by the inscription, which does not even identify him as a physician: 'Tiberius Claudius Athenodotus Philalethes, son of Tryphon, priest of Apollo Propylaeus'.[80]

Equally appealing, but perhaps no more plausible, is the suggestion that a notorious earthquake which struck the area around Laodicea during the reign of Nero, in A.D. 60, coincided with the end

---

[78] Benedum, 1974: 226–8.
[79] Benedum, 1974: 231; *id*., 1978: 307–8.
[80] Ramsay, 1895–7: vol. II, p. 374, no. 196: Τιβέριον Κλαύδιον Τρύφωνος υἱὸν Ἀθηνόδοτον Φιλαλήθη ἱερέα Προπυλαίου Ἀπόλλωνος.

of the Herophilean school.[81] Other factors mentioned above should, however, not be ignored in favour of a cataclysmic hypothesis. The Herophileans' disputes with the Empiricists and with each other became internecine; the partial usurpation of Herophilus' emphasis on anatomy and physiology by Hippocratic philology and doxography left many Herophileans vulnerable at a theoretical level (as did the restriction of physiology to pulse-lore, at least by a majority of Herophileans); and the rising popularity and influence of new schools of medicine with vociferous claims to sweeping theoretical innovation exercised strong pressures upon Herophileans who, by now, were at home mainly in pharmacology, pulse-lore, and, to a lesser extent, in gynaecology. The Herophileans' long days of prominence and glory were counted, and their last agonized gasps came in the mid first century A.D. But even then one of the *morituri*, Demosthenes, saw to it that his gasp reverberated loudly at least until the thirteenth century.[82]

B · TEXTS

276 Galenus, *De pulsuum dignotione* 4.2 (VIII, pp. 929–30K)

Ἡρόφιλος μὲν οὖν ὅσα γε τὰ τῆς αἰσθήσεως πάθη γράφων, οὐδαμῇ πληρότητος (sc. τοῦ σφυγμοῦ) ἐμνημόνευσεν, ἧς οὐδεπώποτε ᾔσθετο. οἱ δ' ἀπ' αὐτοῦ μὲν κληθέντες Ἡροφίλειοι πάντα μᾶλλον δόντες ἢ τοῦτο λέγεσθαι βούλονται σοφισταὶ καὶ
5 πολυλόγοι γενόμενοι σχεδὸν ἅπαντες, οὔτ' ἄλλο τι τῶν Ἡροφι-λείων θεωρημάτων ἐπ' αὐτῶν τῶν ἔργων τῆς τέχνης προύθυμήθησαν ἀσκῆσαι. καὶ πρὸς ἄλλοις πολλοῖς οἷς ἐλυμήναντο τὴν τέχνην, ἔτι τε καὶ τὸν πλήρη σφυγμὸν ἡμῖν ἐπεισήγαγον ταῖς διαγνώσεσιν, ἵνα δηλαδὴ μικρᾶς οὔσης τῆς τέχνης ἔχωμεν
10 ἡμεῖς νῦν ὃ πράττωμεν. οὔτε γὰρ παρελθεῖν οἷόν τε σφυγμὸν ὑπ' ἀνδρῶν οὕτως ἐνδόξων πεπιστευμένον οὔθ' ὃν οὐδεπώποτε

---

[81] Benedum, 1974: 231–2. On the earthquake see Tacitus, *Annales* 14.27. An earlier earthquake at Laodicea, in the reign of Tiberius, is reported by Suetonius, *Tiberius* 8. Cf. also Ramsay 1895–7: vol. I, p. 38, and *Oracula Sibyllina* 4.106–8.

[82] The preceding observations introduce Chapters x–xxviii, but the texts included in this chapter are confined to those that are not attributable to an *individual* Herophilean; they are not representative of the history of the Herophilean school, for which the reader will have to turn instead to Chapters xi–xxviii.

εὕρομεν ἐπὶ τῶν ἔργων διαγνῶναι προχείρως ἡμῖν θετέον, ἀλλοτρίαις ἀκολουθήσασιν ἀποφάσεσιν. ἀλλ’ ἀνάγκη δεῖξαι πρῶτον μὲν ὅτι μέχρι τῆς ἐννοίας ὁ σφυγμὸς οὗτος πρόεισιν,
15 ἔπειτα ὡς οὐδ’ Ἡρόφιλος αὐτὸν αἰσθήσει διεγίνωσκεν. εἰ μὲν οὖν μὴ συγκεχύκεσαν αὐτοὶ τὸ σημαινόμενον τοῦ ὀνόματος, ἤδη εἶχόν τι κἀγὼ λέγειν . . .

1 ὅσα γε conieci: ὡς ἂν vulg.

276 Herophilus, then, to the extent that he writes about the affections of sense-perception, nowhere mentions 'fullness' (*plērotes*) [of the pulse], which he never perceived. But those called 'Herophileans' after him, almost all of whom were loquacious sophists, granted everything rather than wanting this to be stated. Nor did they show any eagerness to put any other Herophilean theory to a practical test against the actual facts of the art of medicine. And in addition to the many other outrages that they inflicted upon the art, they also introduced the 'full pulse' for our use in diagnoses, so that we now may have something to do, since our art so 'clearly' is paltry. For, neither can one skip over a pulse believed in by such 'reputable' authors, nor must I follow the assertions of others and postulate that a pulse which I have never actually discovered in my work can be discerned readily. Rather, it is necessary to show, first, that this pulse does proceed as far as its concept [sc. 'fullness'] does, then that not even Herophilus discerned it by means of sense-perception. If, then, they themselves had not confounded the meaning of the word, I, too, would have had something to say . . . (*See Chapter* VII, *T162 supra*.)

277 Galenus (ex Aristoxeno?), *De pulsuum differentiis* 4.2 (VIII, p. 704K)

. . . ὥστε τοῖς Ἐρασιστρατείοις οὕτως ὁριστέον ἐστίν (sc. τὸν σφυγμόν), ὡς ἐνδείκνυσθαι τὸ ἴδιον ἐξ Ἐρασιστράτου δόγμα περὶ τῆς τῶν σφυγμῶν οὐσίας, τοῖς δ’ Ἡροφιλείοις, ὡς τὸ ἴδιον Ἡροφίλῳ, καὶ τοῖς ἄλλοις ἅπασιν ὡσαύτως οἰκεῖον ἑκάστοις
5 ἐστὶν ὅρον ποιητέον τῷ σφετέρῳ δόγματι . . .

277 Consequently the Erasistrateans must define [the pulse] in such a way that their own distinctive teaching – derived from Erasistra-

tus – concerning the essence of pulses is demonstrated, whereas the Herophileans must define it so that the teaching distinctive of Herophilus is demonstrated, and all the others likewise must compose a definition appropriate to their own respective teachings . . .

278 Galenus (ex Aristoxeno?), *De pulsuum differentiis* 4.2 (VIII, pp. 714–15K)

ἀνάλογον δὲ τοῖς ὅροις τοῖσδε καὶ οἱ ἀπὸ τῶν ἄλλων αἱρέσεων ὁριοῦνται τὸν σφυγμόν, ἕκαστος δηλονότι κατὰ τὰς οἰκείας ὑποθέσεις. ἐὰν μὲν οὖν τελέως ὁρίζωνται, συμφωνήσουσιν ἀλλήλοις· ἐὰν δὲ ἐλλιπῶς ἢ περιττῶς ἢ κατά τι μοχθηρῶς,
5 διενεχθήσονται. τούτου δέ σοι πίστις μεγίστη τὸ τοὺς Ἡροφι- λείους, οἵπερ δὴ καὶ πρῶτοι τὸν σφυγμὸν ἐπεχείρησαν ὁρίζεσ- θαι, διενεχθῆναι πρὸς ἀλλήλους, ἀντιπαρεξάγοντας δὲ αὐτοῖς καὶ τοὺς Ἐρασιστρατείους – ἤκμασε γὰρ ἄμφω ταῦτα τὰ διδασκαλεῖα μετὰ τὸν Ἡροφίλου θάνατον – ἑτέρως πάλιν καὶ
10 αὐτοὺς ποιεῖσθαι τὸν ὅρον τοῦ σφυγμοῦ, διαφωνοῦντας ἀλλή- λοις τε καὶ τοῖς Ἡροφιλείοις.

278 The descendants of the different schools [of medicine] will define the pulse in a manner analogous to these definitions, each person obviously in accordance with his own [school's] hypotheses [sc. concerning physiology, pathology, and anatomy]. If they produce perfect definitions, they will be in agreement, but if they define it too narrowly or redundantly or poorly in some respect, they will be in disagreement. Your greatest proof of this is that the Herophileans, who indeed were also the first to try their hand at defining the pulse, disagree among themselves, and secondly that the Erasistrateans parade arguments against the Herophileans – both these schools flourished after Herophilus' death – and that they too [sc. the individual Erasistrateans] compose their definitions of the pulse in different ways, [thus] disagreeing both among themselves and with the Herophileans.

279 Galenus, *De pulsuum differentiis* 4.2 (VIII, p. 719K)

λέγωμεν οὖν αὖθις ἀναλαβόντες ὑπὲρ τοῦ κατὰ τὸν σφυγμὸν

ὅρου, μνημονεύοντες ὀνομαστὶ τῶν δοξάντων αὐτὸν ὡρίσθαι καλῶς. ἤρξαντο μὲν οὖν, ὡς ἔφην, τῆς τοιαύτης περιεργίας οἱ Ἡροφίλειοι, διεδέξαντο δ᾿ αὐτοὺς ἔνιοι τῶν Ἐρασιστρατείων, 5 εἶθ᾿ οἵ τε πνευματικοὶ καλούμενοι καί τινες τῶν μεθοδικῶν.

279 Let me then resume and speak again concerning the definition of the pulse, mentioning by name those who seem to have defined it correctly. The Herophileans, as I said, actually started this kind of elaboration, and some of the Erasistrateans became their successors, then those called 'Pneumatics' and some of the Methodists.

280 Galenus, *De plenitudine* 3 (VII, pp. 525-8K). (Cf. *SVF* II, 439-40.)

καὶ γὰρ οἱ μάλιστα εἰσηγησάμενοι τὴν συνεκτικὴν δύναμιν, ὡς οἱ Στωϊκοί, τὸ μὲν συνέχον ἕτερον ποιοῦσι, τὸ συνεχόμενον δὲ ἄλλο· τὴν μὲν γὰρ πνευματικὴν οὐσίαν τὸ συνέχον, τὴν δὲ ὑλικὴν τὸ συνεχόμενον· ὅθεν ἀέρα μὲν καὶ πῦρ συνέχειν φασί, γῆν δὲ καὶ 5 ὕδωρ συνέχεσθαι. καίτοι γε ἔνιοι τῶν νῦν Ἡροφιλείους ἑαυτοὺς ὀνομαζόντων, οὐδ᾿ ὄναρ ἀκηκοότες ταῦτα, τολμηρῶς ἀποφαίνονται περὶ τῆς συνεκτικῆς δυνάμεως, εἰ μὲν ἀὴρ ἢ πῦρ ἢ τὸ συναμφότερόν ἐστι τὸ συνέχον τοὺς λίθους τε καὶ τὰ ξύλα καὶ τἆλλα ὅσα τοιαῦτα μὴ γινώσκειν ὁμολογοῦντες, ἀποφαινόμενοι 10 δὲ ἁπλῶς ὅτι δύναμίς τίς ἐστιν ἡ συνέχουσα τὰ τοιαῦτα πάντα, διαλυθῆναι γὰρ ἂν καὶ διαρρυῆναι, μηδενὸς αὐτὰ συνάγοντός τε καὶ σφίγγοντος.

εἶτ᾿ ἐρωτηθέντες εἰ καὶ τοιούτῳ τινὶ τολμῶσιν ἀξιώματι χρήσασθαι κατὰ τὸν λόγον, ὡς ἅπαντα τὰ ὄντα δεῖται τοῦ 15 συνέχοντος, ἢ μή, παραχρῆμα μὲν ἑτοίμως ἀποφαίνονταί τε καὶ καταφάσκουσι τὴν ἐρώτησιν. ἀπαχθέντες δ᾿ ἐντεῦθεν ἐπ᾿ ἄτοπον, ἀνατίθενται εἰς τὰ εἰρημένα, καὶ ἀγανακτοῦσι τοῖς ἐρωτῶσιν ὡς περιέργοις τε καὶ σοφισταῖς . . .

ὅπως τοίνυν ἀναγκαῖόν ἐστιν εἰς ἄτοπον τὸν λόγον ἀχθῆναι, 20 θεμένων ἡμῶν ἅπαν τὸ ὂν δεῖσθαι συνεκτικῆς αἰτίας, ἤδη σοι δίειμι· τὴν συνεκτικὴν αἰτίαν, ἥτις ποτ᾿ ἐστίν, οὐ γὰρ ὁμολογοῦσιν αὐτὴν οἱ Ἡροφίλειοι γιγνώσκειν. ἆρά γε ἐκ τῶν ὄντων τι καὶ αὐτοὶ ὑπολαμβάνουσιν ἢ τῶν οὐκ ὄντων; εἰ μὲν γὰρ τῶν οὐκ ὄντων τι, θαυμάζω τὴν σοφίαν τῶν ἀνδρῶν, εἰ καὶ τῶν ὄντων

25 ἕκαστον δεῖσθαί φασι τῶν οὐκ ὄντων τινός· εἰ δὲ τῶν ὄντων
τίθενται τὴν συνεκτικὴν αἰτίαν, ἀναμνησθήτωσαν ὡς ἅπαν τὸ
ὂν ἔφασαν αἰτίας δεῖσθαι συνεκτικῆς εἰς τὸ εἶναι. συμβήσεται
γὰρ οὕτως καὶ αὐτὴν τὴν αἰτίαν αἰτίας ἑτέρας, ἵνα ὑπάρχῃ,
δεηθῆναι, κἀκείνην αὖθις ἄλλης, καὶ τοῦτο εἰς ἄπειρον . . .
30 οὐδὲ γὰρ οὐδ' οἱ πολλοὶ τῶν Ἡροφιλείων οὐδ' οἱ νεώτεροι
Στωϊκοὶ λέγουσί τινα ἀπόδειξιν τοῦ τὸ μὲν πνεῦμα καὶ τὸ πῦρ
συνέχειν ἑαυτό τε καὶ τὰ ἄλλα, τὸ δὲ ὕδωρ καὶ τὴν γῆν ἑτέρου
δεῖσθαι τοῦ συνέχοντος . . .
πρὸς μὲν δὴ τὴν τῶν Στωϊκῶν ὑπόθεσιν ἑτέρωθι λέλεκται διὰ
35 πλειόνων, ἐπὶ δὲ τοὺς Ἡροφιλείους ἐπάνειμι, καὶ πρὸς τούτους
ἀρκέσει μοι κατά γε τὸ παρὸν εἰπεῖν ὡς προστάτης αὐτῶν
ἐναντιώτατα πέπονθεν, ἀπορῶν μὲν ἐν παμπόλλοις ἀποδείξεις
προχείρους ἔχουσιν, ἀποφαινόμενος δὲ ἐν ἄλλοις, ὧν αἵ τ'
ἀποδείξεις ἀδύνατοι ἤ θ' ὑπόθεσις ψευδής.

19 τὸν coni. von Arnim. (SVF II, 440): τι vulg.   21 post δίειμι non
interpunxit Kühn   22 αὐτὴν fort. delendum est (vid. Comment. ad T280 infra)

280 It is especially those who, like the Stoics, introduce 'the faculty
which can hold [things] together' [sc. the cohesive faculty], that make
what causes cohesion one thing, and what is held together [i.e., the
cohesive matter] another. For, [in their view] the pneumatic
substance is that which causes cohesion, while the material substance
is that which is held together [made cohesive], so that they say air and
fire make [things] cohesive while earth and water are made cohesive.
Yet some of those who nowadays call themselves Herophileans,
although they have not listened to these things, not even in a dream,
confidently make pronouncements concerning 'the faculty which
causes cohesion'. While they concede that they do not know whether
that which 'holds together' [renders cohesive] stones, wood, and all
other such things is air or fire or both together, they nevertheless
pronounce unreservedly that 'what holds together all such things is a
certain faculty'; for, they say, all things would be dissolved and
disintegrate if nothing drew them together and bound them together.
    Next, when asked whether or not they dare to use an axiom of the
following kind, too, in their argument, viz. 'all things which exist
require that which makes them cohesive', they immediately and
readily give their decision and answer the question in the affirmative.
Then, when refuted by a *reductio ad absurdum*, they refer back to what

was said before and become annoyed with their questioners, as though these were hyper-subtle sophists , . .

I shall now explain how it is therefore necessary, once we have postulated that everything which exists requires a cause that can make it cohesive, to reduce the argument to the absurd. You see, the Herophileans concede that they do not know what 'the cause which can make [it] cohesive' is. Do they assume that it is one of the things which exist or one of the non-existents? For, if it is one of the non-existents, I am astonished at the wisdom of these men, if they are saying that each of the existing things also requires one of the non-existents. But if they make 'the cause which can make [it] cohesive' one of the existing things, let them recall that they said everything that exists, in order to exist, requires a cause which makes it cohesive. You see, it will thus follow that the cause itself, too, requires another cause in order to exist, and this cause in turn another, and this *ad infinitum* . . .

Neither most of the Herophileans nor the more recent Stoics mention any proof that pneuma and fire make both themselves and other things cohere, whereas water and earth require [something] other [than themselves] to make them cohere . . .

Against the Stoics' hypothesis I have spoken at length elsewhere; but I return to the Herophileans, and against them I find it sufficient, for the present at least, to say that their leader's experience was the exact contrary of theirs: he remained in doubt concerning many matters of which 'proofs' are readily at hand, whereas he made pronouncements in other matters in which proofs are impossible and the hypothesis false.

281 A. Cornelius Celsus, *Medicina* 3 (*Artes* 8).9.3–4 (*CML* 1, p. 116 Marx)

> si . . . febre liberaverat, protinus suillam assam et vinum homini dabat (sc. Petro); si non liberaverat, decoquebat aquam sale adiecto eamque bibere cogebat, ut movendo ventrem purgaret. et intra haec omnis eius medicina erat: eaque non minus grata
> 5 fuit is, quos Hippocratis successores non refecerant, quam nunc est is, quos Herophili vel Erasistrati aemuli diu tractos non adiuverunt. (*Vid. T234.*)

2 liberabat *J*   4 eaque *JF*²: eaqueve *V*: aque *F*   7 adiuverunt *FV*: expedierunt *J*

281 If [Petro] . . . had freed the patient from fever, he at once used to give him roast pork and wine. If he had not freed the patient from it, he boiled water with salt and forced the patient to drink it, in order to purge the stomach by moving [the bowels]. And his entire medical art existed within these boundaries. Yet this was no less welcome to those whom Hippocrates' successors had not restored to health, than it is nowadays to those whom the disciples of Herophilus or Erasistratus have not helped although they treated them for a long time. (*See Chapter* VIII, *T234.*)

282 Caelius Aurelianus, *Celeres vel acutae passiones* 2.38.218–19

antiquorum plurimi cardiacorum curationem tacuerunt, aliqui vero memoraverunt, ut Serapionis atque Heraclidis sectatores et quidam Herophili, item Asclepiades et Themison, parvissime quidem, at iisdem deceptionibus implicati. phlebotomant enim
5 et clysteres adhibent acerrimos, et ob calefaciendum articulorum frigus pannos applicant calidos et lanas oleo infusas ac sulfure fumigatas. terunt etiam oleo veteri ac sicyonio cum pipere sulfur et cachry et ammoniaci guttam et laserpicium cum bulbis. cataplasmant praeterea ex lasere et bulbis, sympasmati-
10 bus utentes, quae nos aspergines dixerimus, item ex calce cum pipere; cibis acribus utentes atque edacibus, alio, salsamento, et lasere. et per totum diem atque noctem vino usque ad ebrietatem replerunt. alii vero in acquam frigidam aegros deposuerunt.

10 *post* dixerimus *add.* ex faecibus *Wellmann coll. 2.38.223 (1913: p. 85 adn. 2)* ex *Wellmann (l.c.):* et G 11 allio *coni. Drabkin (coll. 2.38.224):* alii G

282 Most of the ancients remained silent about the treatment of patients with cardiac diseases, but some did mention it, like the followers of Serapion and Heraclides, some followers of Herophilus, and likewise Asclepiades and Themison. They say very little, but they are entangled in the same deceptions. For they use phlebotomy and apply very harsh clysters; and to warm up the patient's chilled limbs they apply warm rags and wool that has been steeped in olive-oil and smoked with sulphur. In old Sicyonian olive-oil they also grind up sulphur with pepper, parched barley, gum ammoniac, and silphium

with bulbs. In addition, they apply poultices of silphium and bulbs, using sprinkling powders (*sympasmata*), which we might call 'sprays' (*aspergines*), also made of limestone with pepper. And they use acrid and pungent foods: garlic, salted and pickled food, and silphium. And throughout the entire day and night they filled [the patient] with wine to the point of intoxication. Others, however, put their patients into cold water.

283 Caelius Aurelianus, *Tardae passiones* 5.2.50–1

> specialiter autem veterum pertransiendo errores vanum puto atque prolixum quod de podagricis scripserunt, et propterea fastidiosum maxime cum sufficiat communis materiarum memoratio suprascripta, tacitis dominis qui nunc dicentur:
> 5 Diocles libris quos de passionibus atque causis et curationibus scripsit: Praxagoras tertio libro de morbis: Erasistratus libro quo de podagra scripsit, . . . item Herophili sectatores multi . . .

283 In surveying the mistakes of the ancient physicians, however, I think what they wrote about cases of podagra is particularly vacuous and long-winded. And this is especially disagreeable because general mention of the substances used in remedies, as described above, would have sufficed. Yet the masters whom I will now mention remained silent [about these substances]: Diocles in his books *On Diseases and their Causes and their Treatment*, Praxagoras in Book III of his *On Diseases*, Erasistratus in the book he wrote *On Podagra*, . . . likewise many followers of Herophilus . . .

284 Soranus, *Gynaecia* 4.5[57].4 (*CMG* IV, pp. 134–5 Ilberg)

> τούτων οὖν ῥηθέντων τῶν αἰτίων οὐδείς ἐστιν ὁ ἀντερείσας αὐτῷ καὶ ἀντειπών, ἀλλὰ καὶ μαρτυρήσας καὶ στηρίξας αὐτὸν ὡς ἀληθῶς [ἄρα καὶ] λέγοντα· εἰ μὴ ἄρα καὶ δικαίως ἐν τούτῳ μεμψαίμεθα τοὺς Ἡροφιλείους, ἐπεὶ δυνάμεις ἐπιτελεστικάς
> 5 φαμεν ἐν τῷ περὶ νοσημάτων τόπῳ ὑπόστασιν μὴ ἔχειν. οὐδὲ γὰρ αὐτοὶ τὴν οὐσίαν αὐτῶν ὁμολογοῦσιν. (*Vid. DA.21 et DA.24 infra.*)

1 ἀντέρεισας sive ἀντερίσας Herwerden: ἀντερρήσας P   2 αὐτῷ del.
Rose   αὐτόν] αὐτά Rose   3 ἆρα καὶ del. Ermerins   λέγοιτο P: corr.
Dietz   4 ἐπιτελεστικάς Ilberg: ἐπιτεθειναι P: ἐπιλεληθυίας Rose:
ὑποθετικάς Ermerins: ἐπιθετικάς Kalbfleisch

284 These, then, are the causes [of difficult labour] which he [sc. Demetrius?] mentioned, and no one has offered resistance or spoken in opposition to him, but rather [everyone] has both confirmed and buttressed him as one who speaks the truth. Except that here, too, we might justly reproach the Herophileans, since we assert that faculties capable of bringing things to fulfilment do not have any fundamental place in a discussion of diseases. In fact, they themselves [sc. the Herophileans] do not even agree with regard to the true nature of these faculties. (See Chapter XVI, DA.21 and DA.24 infra.)

285 Galenus, *In Hippocratis Epidemiarum 6.4.19 comment.*4.26 (ad vol. v, p. 312.7–8L) (*CMG* v.10.2.2, p. 239 Wenkebach)

ἀλλὰ ταύτης γε τῆς θερμασίας (sc. ἐμφύτου) τὴν διαφορὰν οὔτε Λύκος οὔτ' ἄλλος τις ἢ 'Ερασιστράτειος ἢ 'Ηροφίλειος ἢ ἐμπειρικὸς ἐγίνωσκε καὶ διὰ τοῦτο κακῶς ἐξηγήσαντο πάμπολλα τῶν ὑφ' 'Ιπποκράτους γεγραμμένων.

1–3 has duas species non dignoscunt *Hunaini versio Arabica, fort. recte*

285 But the distinct difference of this [innate] heat neither Lycus nor any other person recognized, whether Erasistratean or Herophilean or Empiricist. And for this reason they interpreted poorly many of the things written by Hippocrates.

286 Galenus, *De experientia medica* 24.8–9 (translated from the Arabic version of the lost Greek text by Richard Walzer, p. 135)

When, therefore, anyone attempts to decide between people who hold diverse opinions with regard to invisible things, only two possibilities are open to him: either . . . he remains suspended, showing no inclination or partisanship, or else he is one of those people who hold a decided opinion . . . For there are some people amongst them, who are led to do so by their inclination to the sort of thing that would carry conviction to Erasistratos; and so they praise Erasistratos' view and reject the views of all other people, calling themselves for this reason Erasistrateans and band themselves together like capable soldiers who are led by a single leader. Other people, again, assert Praxagoras' view to be good and right . . . Then you will find a third army, the disciples of Asclepiades, and you will find other people who have made Herophilos their leader, master, and director in all affairs, others again accord Hippocrates this position.

287 Georgius Choeroboscus(?), *De quantitate*, ed. J. A. Cramer, in *Anecdota Graeca e codd. manuscriptis Bibliothecarum Oxoniensium*, vol. II (Oxford, 1835), pp. 285–6

τὰ ἐπὶ αἱρέσεων κτητικὰ διὰ τῆς ει διφθόγγου γράφεται, οἷον Ἡροφίλειος ⟨Ἡροφίλου⟩ αἱρέσεως.

2 Ἡροφίλου *suppl. R. Schneider, 'Bodleiana' (Lipsiae, 1887), p. 29* αἱρέσιος *cod.: corr. Schneider*

287 In the case of schools of thought ['sects'] the possessives are written with the diphthong *ei*; for example, 'Herophil*ei*os' [i.e., 'Herophilean'] of the school of Herophilus.

C · COMMENTS

T280 In T280.21–3 von Arnim (*SVF* II, 440) punctuates as follows: τὴν συνεκτικὴν αἰτίαν, ἥτις ποτ᾽ ἐστίν (οὐ γὰρ ὁμολογοῦσιν αὐτὴν οἱ Ἡροφίλειοι γιγνώσκειν), ἆρά γε ἐκ τῶν ὄντων τι καὶ αὐτοὶ ὑπολαμβάνουσιν ἢ τῶν οὐκ ὄντων; This has its obvious appeal but is somewhat problematic since interrogative ἆρα in prose 'almost always stands first in the sentence' (LSJ, s.v. ἆρα, B). When it does not stand first, it occurs after only a few other introductory words (e.g. Plato, *Gorgias* 467E6–7; Julian, *Oration* 3(2).61c). The relatively late position to which von Arnim assigns ἆρα – locating it after two complete subordinate clauses and after the direct object of the main clause – renders the alternative of taking τὴν συνεκτικὴν αἰτίαν etc., as the object of ὁμολογοῦσιν (perhaps with deletion of αὐτήν, which then would be somewhat redundant) attractive. Galen, unlike Plato and the dramatists, does not postpone interrogative ἆρα freely. Cf. Blomquist, 1969: 128–9; Denniston, 1954: 48–50; Ch. VII, nn. 52–3 *supra*.

For Herophilus' views on causes see above, Chapter V.

XI · ANDREAS

(*An.*)

A · INTRODUCTION

Andreas and Dioscurides 'Phacas' are the only Herophilean physicians explicitly identified with the Ptolemaic court. Andreas was the personal physician of Ptolemy IV Philopator (*c.* 244–205 B.C.), while Dioscurides seems to have been associated with the court in the first century, during the reigns of Auletes, Ptolemy XIII, and Cleopatra.[1] Polybius provides a vivid account of Andreas' death in the course of the Fourth Syrian War: the Aetolian traitor Theodotus, conspiring with Antiochus III, burst into Ptolemy's tent at early dawn and, not finding the king there, killed his physician Andreas.[2] The murder occurred in 217 B.C., on the eve of the battle of Raphia,[3] and this indicates that Andreas was one of Herophilus' earliest pupils. Rough confirmation of his date is provided by the charge of his illustrious contemporary Eratosthenes that Andreas was a 'literary Aegisthus' who had committed plagiarism (the work or works with which Andreas committed the illicit intimacy were presumably Eratosthenes' own).[4] Eratosthenes' date is *c.* 275–194 B.C.; given the premature nature of Andreas' death, they may well have been approximately the same age.[5]

While more is known about the social status Andreas achieved, his

---

[1] See Chapter XIX.A and *Ds.*1–2. On Egyptian court physicians in the third century B.C. cf. Gorteman, 1957 (331–2 on Andreas).

[2] *An.*1. The Fourth Syrian War, launched by Philopator against Antiochus III ('the Great') is described by Polybius, *Hist.* 5.58–87.

[3] Polybius 5.82.1–5.86.6. Cf. Walbank, 1957–79: vol. I, pp. 607–15; Rostovtzeff, 1953: vol. I, pp. 49, 327, 332, 414–15, 497, and vol. II, pp. 624, 646, 710, 713, 720, 727–8; Droysen, 1952–3: vol. III, p. 43 (n. 32); Fraser, 1972: vol. I, pp. 60, 75, 179, 222 (with notes).

[4] *An.*2.

[5] Cf. also *An.*29: the Empiricist Serapion (fl. 200 B.C.) quoted Andreas.

social and ethnic background remains relatively unknown. His father's name was perhaps Chrysareus,[6] and he probably came from the same city as the famous fourth-century B.C. physician Diocles, i.e from Carystus, one of the four largest cities on the island of Euboea.[7] But even knowledge of these details depends on the assumption that 'Andreas of Carystus', 'Andreas the son of Chrysareus' and 'Andreas the Herophilean' are all identical – an assumption here made only tentatively, in the absence of evidence to the contrary and in view of the infrequency with which physicians called 'Andreas' occur in ancient medical literature.

As pointed out in Chapter I (pp. 24–5), it was exceedingly rare in Alexandria not only for a Herophilean physician to become a court physician, but also for a court physician to be a person of literary and scientific distinction. Judging by the almost fifty ancient texts concerning Andreas that are extant, he represented just such a rare combination. Although the bulk of the evidence is about his pharmacological expertise (*An.*21–42) and his famous instrument for reducing dislocated limbs (*An.*11–17), his interests extended beyond drugs and surgery. Among his books the ancient sources mention not only (1) *Narthex* ('Casket'), a work on drug remedies or cosmetics (*An.*25), but also (2) an epistolographic work, *To Sosibius* (*An.*9) – i.e. dedicated to Ptolemy Philopator's eminent minister – which dealt *inter alia* with obstetrics; (3) *On the Genealogy of Physicians* (*An.*47), apparently a medico-historical work; (4) *On Poisonous Animals* (a very popular topic throughout the Hellenistic period), in which Andreas also prescribed antidotes (*An.*18); (5) *On False Beliefs*, perhaps also – like *On the Genealogy of Physicians* – a work with a doxographic thrust (*An.*45), but directed primarily against the beliefs recorded by paradoxographers. He is also reported to have dealt with hydrophobia (*An.*20), 'pantophobia' (i.e. fear of all things – an extreme form of paranoia?) (*An.*10), and the sexual habits conducive to procreation (*An.*8). The fact that Heraclides of Tarentum mentions Andreas in the context of Hippocratic exegesis (*An.*7) suggests that Andreas may also have produced a commentary, although this remains uncertain in the absence of any further evidence. All of this points to the wide-ranging interests that had been characteristic of

[6] *An.*38.
[7] *An.*5. But Wellmann, 1891: 818 n. 238 does not ascribe *An.* 5 and *An.* 47 to the Herophilean.

the founder of the school too: physiology, pathology, perhaps Hippocratic exegesis, surgery and pharmacology.

Andreas' works had an immediate and continuous, if limited, impact in antiquity. Thus the Empiricist leader Serapion (fl. 200 B.C.) approvingly quotes at least one of Andreas' drug remedies (*An.*29), and in the next century the poet Nicander (*Theriaca* 826–7) seems to allude to Andreas' attack on the popular view, first advanced by the Alexandrian Archelaus in his *Idiophyeis* (fr. 9 Giannini, fr. XI Westermann), that sea eels go ashore to mate with vipers (*An.*45, *An.*46, from *On False Beliefs*). In the first century B.C. the Empiricist Heraclides of Tarentum and the Pneumatist Athenaeus deem Andreas' views on reproduction worthy of discussion (*An.*7, *An.*8), and in the next century Dioscurides introduces his *Materia medica* by characterizing Andreas as one of the two most accurate writers on medicinal roots and plants (*An.*23). Celsus also singles out Andreas as one of three writers who have transmitted much about the powers of drugs (*An.*22), and Pliny mentions Andreas as a source for no less than fourteen books of his *Natural History* (*An.*4), although it is likely that their knowledge of Andreas was mediated by a pharmacological source such as Sextius Niger. Subsequently Soranus, Galen, Athenaeus (author of the *Deipnosophistae*, probably end of the second century A.D.), and, in the early third century, Tertullian likewise contributed to the transmission of Andreas' views. As late as the time of the Emperor Julian we find rich indications of respect for Andreas' achievements. It is worth noting that our latest ancient source, Oribasius (fourth century A.D.), offers extensive and invaluable, if problematic, descriptions of Andreas' famous instrument of reduction – a device which seems to have depended in part on the discoveries of Alexandrian mechanical technology.

Yet the absence in the testimonia concerning Andreas of any mention of anatomy (except in passing[8]) and sphygmology – which seem to have been Herophilus' two main preoccupations (or at least the main spheres of his subsequent impact upon ancient medicine) – is striking. The re-emergence of the traditional opposition to the dissection of humans[9] might have been one reason for Andreas' apparent shift of emphasis from anatomy to surgery and pharma-

---

[8] E.g., *An.*5, on the anatomical relation of marrow to bone.
[9] Cf. Chapter VI.A.

cology (which Herophilus had, after all, sanctioned by calling drugs
'the hands of the gods'[10]) but it would not in itself account for an
abandonment of pulse theory. Another factor might have been the
growing strength of the Empiricist school of medicine. As pointed out
above, the Empiricists were opposed to both dissection and physiology – and hence also to sphygmology – but laid great store by
pharmacology and surgery. It is not inconceivable that a physician
dependent on the favour of the Ptolemaic court did not wish
unnecessarily to antagonize the medical trend-setters of the day, who
were engaging in sharp polemics against the Herophileans, and that
he therefore concentrated instead on the more clinical aspects of
medicine. Clinical expertise and efficacy might, in any case, have
made a greater impression on his royal patrons and patients than
theoretical contributions to physiology or anatomy.[11]

B · TEXTS

*An.*1   Polybius, *Historiae* 5.81.1–7 (II, pp. 204–5 Büttner-Wobst; V, p. 141
        Pédech)

*An.*2a *Etymologicum Magnum* 198.19–21, s.v. *Bibliaigisthos* (col.570 Gais-
        ford)

*An.*2b *Lexica Segueriana* 5: *Lexeis Rhetorikai*, s.v. *Bibliaigisthos* (Immanuel
        Bekker, *Anecdota Graeca* I (Berlin, 1814), p. 226)

*An.*3   Anonymus Laurentianus: Codex Laurentianus 73.1 (s.XI), fol.
        143r, col. 1 (*Hermes* 35 (1900), 370 Wellmann)

*An.*4   C. Plinius Secundus, *Naturalis historia* I (on the sources of Books XX–
        XXVIII, XXXI–XXXV)

*An.*5   Cassius Iatrosophista, *Problemata* 58 (*Physici et medici Graeci minores*,
        vol. I, p. 161 Ideler)

*An.*6   Tertullianus, *De anima* 15.2 (p. 19 Waszink). (See Chapter VII,
        T139.)

*An.*7   Heraclides Tarentinus apud Galenum, *In Hippocratis Epidemiarum
        2.2.20 comment. 2* (ad vol. V, p. 92.8–12L). From Ḥunain's Arabic
        translation of the lost original; *CMG* v.10.1, p. 232 Pfaff. (See also
        below, Chapter XIV, *Ba.*11 and *Ba.*37)

---

[10] Chapter VIII, T248–T249.
[11] It is conceivable that Andreas is identical with the 'Andreas' of the Septuagint
      story, particularly given the Herophilean's close association with the Ptolemaic
      court. See Josephus, *Jewish Antiquities* XII.18,24,50,58; *id.*, *Against Apion* 2.46; ps.-
      Aristeas 12, 19, 40, 43, 123, 173.

An.8   Athenaeus apud Oribasium, *Collectiones medicae, lib. incert.* 23.2–3 (*CMG* VI.2.2 = vol. IV, p. 116 Raeder)

An.9   Soranus, *Gynaecia* 4.1 [53].6 (*CMG* IV, p. 131 Ilberg). (See also Chapter VII above, T196)[12]

An.10   Caelius Aurelianus, *Acutae passiones* 3.12.108

An.11   A. Cornelius Celsus, *Medicina* 8 (*Artes* 13).20.4 (*CML* I, p. 407 Marx)

An.12a   Galenus, *In Hippocratis De articulis comment.* 4.47 (XVIIIA, p. 747K)

An.12b   Oribasius, *Collectiones medicae* 49.6 (*CMG* VI.2.2 = vol. IV, p. 12 Raeder)

An.13   Galenus, *In Hippocratis De articulis comment.* 1.18 (XVIIIA, pp. 338–9K)

An.14   Oribasius, *Collectiones medicae* 49.4.8–13 (*CMG* VI.2.2 = vol. IV, p. 6 Raeder)

An.15   Oribasius, *op.cit.* 49.4.19–20 (IV, p. 7 Raeder)

An.16   Oribasius, *op.cit.* 49.4.45–50 (IV, p. 9 Raeder)

An.17   Oribasius, *op.cit.* 49.5.1–5 (IV, p. 10 Raeder)

An.18   Athenaeus, *Deipnosophistae* 7.90.312D

An.19   Galenus, *De antidotis* 2.13 (XIV, p. 180K)

An.20   Caelius Aurelianus, *Acutae passiones* 3.9.98. (See Chapter XXVII.A below)

An.21   Scholium in Nicandri *Alexipharmaca* 537 (p. 217 Bussemaker; pp. 185–6 Geymonat)

An.22   A. Cornelius Celsus, *Medicina* 5 (*Artes* 10), prohoemium 1 (*CML* I, p. 190 Marx). (See also Chapter VIII above, T251; and below Chapter XV, *Zn*.3; Chapter XXIII, *AM*.9)

An.23   Pedanius Dioscurides, *De materia medica*, praefatio 1 (I, p. 1 Wellmann)

An. 24   Galenus, *De simplicium medicamentorum temperamentis ac facultatibus* 6 , prooemium (XI, pp. 795–6K). (See above Chapter VIII, T252)

An.25   Scholium in Nicandri *Theriaca* 684 (p. 193 Bussemaker; p. 253 Crugnola)

An.26   Celsus, *op. cit.* 5 (*Artes* 10).18.13–14 (*CML* I, p. 197 Marx)

An.27   Celsus, *op. cit.* 6 (*Artes* 11).6.16A–C (*CML* I, pp. 267–8 Marx)

An.28   Celsus, *op.cit.* 5 (*Artes* 10).18.7 (*CML* I, p. 196 Marx)

An.29   Asclepiades Iunior apud Galenum, *De compositione medicamentorum secundum locos* 10.1 (XIII, pp. 343–4K)

An.30   Andromachus Iunior apud Galenum, *De compositione medicamentorum per genera* 7.7 (XIII, pp. 982–3K)

An.31   Asclepiades Iunior apud Galenum, *De compositione medicamentorum per genera* 4.13 (XIII, p. 735K)

---

[12] Reading Σωσίβιον for Σώβιον.

An.32   Asclepiades Iunior apud Galenum, *De compositione medicamentorum secundum locos* 4.8 (XII, pp. 765–6K)

An.33   C. Plinius Secundus, *Naturalis historia* 32.27.87

An.34   C. Plinius Secundus, *op.cit.* 20.76.200

An.35   Pedanius Dioscurides, *De materia medica* 4.64.6 (II, p. 221 Wellmann)

An.36   C. Plinius Secundus, *Naturalis historia* 22.49.102

An.37   Pedanius Dioscurides, *op.cit.* 3.126–7 (II, pp. 136–7 Wellmann)

An.38   Galenus(?), *Explanatio vocum Hippocratis*, s.v. 'Indikon' (XIX, p. 105K)

An.39   Pedanius Dioscurides, *op.cit.* 4.118 (II, p. 268 Wellmann)

An.40   Pedanius Dioscurides, *op.cit.* 4.33 (II, p. 194 Wellmann)

An.41   Athenaeus, *Deipnosophistae* 3.83.115E

An.42   Scholium in Nicandri *Alexipharmaca* 611 (p. 219 Bussemaker; p. 207 Geymonat)

An.43   Philonides apud Athenaeum, *Deipnosophistae* 15.17.675A–C

An.44   Scholium in Aristophanis *Aves* 266 (pp. 62–5 White)

An.45   Athenaeus, *Deipnosophistae* 7.90.312E

An.46   Scholium in Nicandri *Theriaca* 823 (p. 198 Bussemaker; p. 290 Crugnola)

An.47   Soranus(?), *Vita Hippocratis* 4 (*CMG* IV, p. 175 Ilberg)

An.48   Asclepiades apud Galenum, *De compositione medicamentorum secundum locos* 9.2 (XIII, p. 242K)

Dubium

An.49   Aëtius Amidenus, *Libri medicinales* 12.68 (p. 125 Costomiris)

XII · CALLIANAX
(*Cn.*)

A · INTRODUCTION

Our knowledge of Callianax at present is confined essentially to the first text listed below (*Cn.*1). The other two testimonia are both derived from the first – directly or indirectly – and are consequently of little evidential value. The suggestive implication of Hans Gossen and Max Wellmann[1] that the *Quaestiones medicinales* of Rufus of Ephesus provides further information about Callianax, and that Callianax wrote a treatise similar to that of Rufus (i.e. a work on the questions a physician should ask his patients) is, to my knowledge, without foundation.

The best indication of Callianax' date is the fact that Bacchius, in his *Memoirs on Herophilus and the Members of his 'House'*, mentioned the tactless wit with which Callianax responded to his patients' fear of death (*Cn.*1.). If Bacchius lived approximately from 275 to 200 B.C., as I argue below (Chapter XIV), Callianax must have achieved his notoriety no later than the latter part of the third century B.C. Wellmann's claim[2] that Callianax was at his prime much earlier, about 280 B.C., remains unsubstantiated but cannot be excluded with certainty. If Wellmann's hypothesis is correct, Callianax would be a contemporary, rather than a successor, of Herophilus – a theory which is perhaps plausible in the light of the use of 'Herophilus' House' (*oikia*), and not the more common 'school' or 'sect' (*hairesis*), in the title of Bacchius' above-mentioned treatise. P. M. Fraser has argued that 'house' always 'refers to a particularly close relationship between master and pupil, and not merely to an adherent of this or that particular school'.[3] The great reluctance with which ancient

---

[1] Gossen, 1919; Wellmann, 1900a:383.   [2] Wellmann, *ibid.*
[3] Fraser, 1972: vol. I, p. 357. See above, p. 458.

sources use the word 'house' to refer to a master–pupil relationship or to a 'school' context,[4] and the absence of *oikia* in all references to Herophileans later than Callianax and Callimachus, seem to lend some – but by no means conclusive – support to this interpretation. If Herophilus died about 255–250 B.C., as I argued earlier, and if Callianax was indeed a direct pupil of Herophilus, Callianax would be a figure of the mid third century B.C.

Callianax' use of fatalistic quotes from Homer and Greek tragedy to 'reassure' those patients who feared death that only being immortal could possibly save them from death (or that heroes, too, have had to die – 'witness Patroclus') is perhaps not only illustrative of the psychological ineptitude and callousness which Galen here so firmly rejects. It might also be indicative of a growing emphasis on high literacy and philology within the Herophilean school – a trend to which Pliny later attributes the decline of the Herophilean school: 'Deserta deinde et haec secta (sc. Herophili) est, quoniam necesse erat in ea litteras scire' (*Natural History* 29.5.6; Chapter VII, T185 *supra*).

B · TEXTS

Cn.1 Zeuxis apud Galenum, *In Hippocratis Epidemiarum 6.4.7 comment.* 4.10 (ad vol v, p. 308.15–16L); *CMG* v.10.2.2, p. 203 Wenkebach

Cn.2 Palladius, *In Hp. Epidemiarum 6.4.7 comment.* 4.8 (II, pp. 111–12 Dietz)

Cn.3 Iohannes Alexandrinus, *Commentaria in VI. librum Hippocratis Epidemiarum*, Particula 4, fol. 134a.52–6, p. 202 Pritchet

---

[4] In addition to *Cn.* 1 Erotian, *Vocum Hippocraticarum collectio*, praef. (p. 4 Nachmanson = Callimachus, T7) and Galen, *De venae sectione adversus Erasistrateos Romae degentes* 2 (XI, p. 197K; perhaps not an exact parallel) have come to my attention. Cf. also Antiphon, *On the choreutes* 11. See Ch. X, p. 458 *supra*.

XIII · CALLIMACHUS
(*Cm.*)

A · INTRODUCTION

If the testimonia concerning Callimachus provide a representative indication of the nature of his research – and if all the testimonia refer to the same Callimachus – he provides a further example of a trend characteristic of the Herophilean 'school' after Herophilus' death: the usurpation of Herophilus' best known interests, anatomy and physiology, by subjects also stressed by the Empiricists, viz. clinical medicine, pharmacology, and Hippocratic exegesis. Thus Callimachus' emphasis on the study of symptoms or signs (*sēmeia, Cm.*3), his work on the toxic effects of wreaths (*Cm.*4–5), his study of specific drugs (*Cm.*6), and his interest in the interpretation of Hippocratic words (*Cm.*7–9) stand squarely in an emerging Herophilean tradition which, while reasserting the 'rationalist' need for theory, in most other respects resembled the practice of the Herophileans' Empiricist rivals.

The Hellenistic historian Polybius apparently considered Callimachus a figure of such influence and consequence that he referred to him as one of two eponymous founders – the other being Herophilus – of a 'Rationalist'[1] or 'Theoretical' school of medicine in Alexandria (*Cm.* 1). Polybius' assessment of Callimachus' significance might be coloured by his use of an Empiricist source.[2] If this is the case, not only Polybius but also the chief Alexandrian rivals of the

---

[1] On the problematic nature of the label 'rationalist,' see Chapter II, *Comments*, Herophilus T1. In *Cm.* 1, Ἡροφ. καὶ Καλλιμ., καὶ could be epexegetical, but this is less likely.

[2] Cf. Deichgräber, 1965: 269 n.1 and 324–5; Walbank, 1957–79: vol. II, pp. 388–91. On Polybius' comparison of historiography with medicine, see also Chapter V, T56, and Wunderer, 1898–1909: pt 3, pp. 62ff.

Herophilean school apparently regarded Callimachus and his followers as formidable 'theoretical' opponents of empiricism.

It is, however, striking that most other ancient authors do not seem
to have shared Polybius' judgment. Only Rufus of Ephesus, probably
writing about A.D. 100, seems to lend some (but not entirely
unambiguous) support to Polybius' characterization, saying that
Callimachus is 'among our predecessors – at least among those of
whom one would even make mention' (Cm. 3). In view of Rufus'
polemical posture toward some Alexandrians,[3] this concession is not
incommensurate with Polybius' attribution of considerable importance to Callimachus. Yet Celsus, in his historical survey of famous
'rationalists', does not mention Callimachus. Galen mentions him
only once in passing – but, perhaps significantly, citing the Empiricist
Zeuxis as his source (Cm.9) – while Soranus and his Latin 'translator',
Caelius Aurelianus, do not mention him even once. The Byzantine
medical encyclopaedists (Oribasius, Paul of Aegina, and Aëtius of
Amida) likewise maintain silence about Callimachus. No authors
after Rufus therefore seem to have had direct knowledge of Callimachus, and among the earlier sources only the Empiricist Zeuxis (early
second century B.C.;[4] Cm.9), Erotian (first century A.D.; Cm.8), and
the elder Pliny (c. A.D. 23–79; Cm.4–6) seem to have had access to
details of Callimachus' views.

Callimachus' exact date is uncertain but three considerations seem
to point to the last half of the third century B.C. (and perhaps the early
years of the second century B.C.). First, the reference to 'Callimacheans' by Polybius (c. 200–120 B.C.) provides a firm terminus ante
quem. Secondly, Erotian's insertion of Callimachus' name between
those of Bacchius (floruit c. 230 B.C.[5]) and the founder of the
Empiricist school, Philinus (c. 280–210 B.C.[6]), suggests that he might
have been a contemporary of both Bacchius and Philinus, especially
in light of Erotian's tendency to use chronological clusters in his

[3] E.g. Rufus, De nominatione partium hominis 133 (p. 151 Daremberg/Ruelle), where
the attack on 'Egyptians who speak Greek poorly' is, however, confined to their
anatomical nomenclature.

[4] CMG v.10.2.2, pp. 131, 401, 451; v.9.2, p. 73. Deichgräber's assumption (1965:
263) that Zeuxis lived in the first half of the first century A.D. seems to be without
foundation. See also Kollesch, 1975b, and Kudlien, 1972d, on Zeuxis. The
Empiricist Zeuxis is not to be confused with the Herophilean discussed in Ch. XXI
infra.

[5] See Chapter XIV.A.   [6] Cf. Deichgräber, 1965: 163–64, 254–5.

enumerations of the pioneers of Hippocratic exegesis (*Cm*.8). (Less
clear is whether or not Erotian actually refers to Callimachus as one of
the two first interpreters of difficult Hippocratic words, *Cm.* 7.) A
third factor is the Empiricist Zeuxis' reference to Callimachus (*Cm*.9).
Since Galen numbers Zeuxis among the earliest Alexandrian Empiricists, it seems likely that Zeuxis became influential no later than the
late third or early second century B.C.[7] Zeuxis' mention of Callimachus would accordingly place the Herophilean in the immediate
chronological vicinity of Bacchius and other early Herophileans.

A date of roughly 275–205 B.C. would not only be compatible with
the probable date of Zeuxis.[8] It would also explain why Polybius
implies that Callimachus was a founder of the Alexandrian 'rationalist' school, why Erotian lumps him together with Bacchius and
Philinus, and perhaps why he is referred to (*Cm*.7) as a member of the
'house' (*oikia*) of Herophilus (on the possible significance of *oikia* see
Chapter XII: 'Callianax', A).

Only the anonymous author of a catalogue of famous medical
writers in a Florentine codex of the eleventh century seems to refer to
Callimachus' birthplace, Bithynia (*Cm*.2). On the face of it, this text
would seem to be a relatively late onomastic pastiche and hence not
particularly trustworthy, but Wellmann's analysis has shown that on
the whole it is in fact fairly accurate.[9] The value of the testimonium is,
however, seriously compromised by textual uncertainty: the MS
reads *Scomachus bitinius*, and only if Wellmann's audacious emendation *Callimachus Bithynius* is correct does the text have any claim to
inclusion in this chapter. If Callimachus' birthplace was indeed
Bithynia, he would be the only third-century Herophilean to go to
Alexandria from the same remote area as Herophilus,[10] and this
might be of significance for evaluating Erotian's testimony that he
was accepted into the 'house' of Herophilus (*Cm*.7).

If Callimachus was a pupil of Herophilus (as Erotian says), and if

---

[7] See n. 4.
[8] Gärtner (1962: 65) suggests the first half of the second century B.C., but the other
considerations raised here point to an even earlier date. Wellmann, 1900a: 382, is
on the right track: 'es ist nicht unmöglich, dass er noch dem Ausgange des 3.
Jahrhunderts angehört . . .'.
[9] Wellmann, 1900a: 367–84.
[10] Herophilus was from Chalcedon; cf. Chapter II: Life (A). Demetrius of Apamea
was from Bithynia too, but his date is considerably later (*c.* 100 B.C.? Cf. Chapter
XVI). On 'house' (*oikia*) see pp. 458, 478–9.

Polybius' testimonium refers to the same Callimachus (as I have assumed tentatively in the absence of suggestions to the contrary in the ancient sources), why does Polybius explicitly distinguish between 'the Herophileans' and 'the Callimacheans', as though being a Callimachean is not the same as being a follower of Herophilus? A partial answer might lurk in *Cm.*9: 'Some people, among them Callimachus too . . . have ridiculed Herophilus as though he were teaching things known to all.' The highly critical and even heretical pupil is of course not just a modern phenomenon (Aristotle's repudiation of Plato, despite the almost twenty years he spent in Plato's school, might be the earliest significant example), and Callimachus may have been such a recalcitrant pupil too. Yet, although Callimachus staked out his independence from the master in some questions, perhaps in response to the Empiricists' influential attacks on Herophilus, Polybius' attack on Callimachus' 'rationalism' makes clear that Callimachus – unlike other renegade Herophileans – never went so far as to cross the boundary into the Empiricist camp. This relative independence might explain not only why Polybius regards Callimachus and his followers as a group of 'rationalists' quite distinct from the other chief representatives of 'rationalism', i.e. the Herophileans, but also why Erotian alone among the ancient sources actually refers to Callimachus' association with Herophilus' school (*Cm.*7).

B · TEXTS

*Cm.*1   Polybius, *Historiae* 12.25d4. (See also above, Chapter v, T56)

*Cm.*2   Anonymus Laurentianus: Codex Laurentianus 73.1 (s.XI), fol. 143r, col.2 (*Hermes* 35 (1900), 370 Wellmann)

*Cm.*3   Rufus Ephesius, *Quaestiones medicinales* 3.21 (pp. 5–6 Gärtner, ed. Teubn.)

*Cm.*4   C. Plinius Secundus, *Naturalis historia* 1 (on his sources for Books XXI–XXVII; perhaps also XXXI)

*Cm.*5   C. Plinius Secundus, *Naturalis historia* 21.9.12

*Cm.*6   C. Plinius Secundus, *Naturalis historia* 25.106.167–8

*Cm.*7   Erotianus, *Vocum Hippocraticarum collectio*, praefatio (p. 4 Nachmanson)

*Cm.*8   Erotianus, *Fragmentum* 33 (Scholia R[H], C[H], U[H], ad Hp., *Morb. Sacr.* 1; p. 108 Nachmanson): θειοτέρη

*Cm.*9   Zeuxis apud Galenum, *In Hippocratis Epidemiarum 6.1.4 comment.* 1.5 (ad vol. v, p. 268.1–2L; *CMG* v.10.2.2, p. 21 Wenkebach). (See also above, Chapter IX, T267a)

XIV · BACCHIUS
(*Ba.*)

A · INTRODUCTION

Originally from the flourishing Boeotian city of Tanagra,[1] Bacchius was one of relatively few immigrants from central Greece to achieve prominence in early Alexandria. While the North African city Cyrene, remote Bithynian and Aetolian towns, the Sicilian city Syracuse, and islands such as Cos, Samos, and Rhodes made considerable contributions to the brilliant intellectual life of Alexandria, central Greece – including Athens – kept its distance, perhaps in part because of lingering anti-Macedonian sentiments harboured against the 'New World' successors of Philip and Alexander. The occasional Boeotian or Athenian does turn up among Ptolemaic officials,[2] but Bacchius, Euclid (if he was in fact an Athenian[3]) and Demetrius of Phaleron are the only intellectuals from central Greece to rise to fame in Alexandria in the third century B.C.

Bacchius' presence and prominence in Alexandria is not only exceptional for a Boeotian; it is also evidence of the extent to which Alexandria had encroached upon the hegemony of traditional centres of medical learning such as Cos, Cnidus, and Sicily. Herophilus came from the Bosporus, his pupil Callimachus likewise came from

---

[1] On Tanagra, the most important town in south-eastern Boeotia, see Pausanias, *Description of Greece* 9.20.1–9.22.4; D. B. Thompson, 1966: 590–5 (with further references). Cf. also Heraclides 1.8–10 (in Pfister, 1951: 76–8).

[2] Cf. Fraser, 1972: vol. I, pp. 66–7, 69, 101, 222 (with notes) on Boeotians and Athenians in Ptolemaic administrations.

[3] Euclid's relation to Athens remains controversial. No ancient source identifies him as an Athenian, and the only ground for inferring that he studied in Athens is Proclus' references to Platonic influences on Euclid's life and thought (*In primum Euclidis Elementorum comm.*, pp. 68–9 Friedlein). Cf. Heiberg, 1882: Pt. II (pp. 22–8); Loria, 1914: 193–4, 203 n.1; Heath, vol. I, pp. 2–3. See also Fraser, 1972: vol. I, p. 387.

Bithynia, Bacchius from Boeotia, Demetrius from Apamea, and so on – and they all were attracted to Alexandria, not to Cos or Cnidus. Several physicians, among them Herophilus' renegade pupil Philinus, even left Cos for Alexandria. Whether patronage was a significant factor in the attractiveness of Alexandria is unknown (but doubtful, as I argued above (Chapter 1)). There is no evidence that Bacchius, for example, ever was subsidized by the Crown. Instead, the fresh opportunities for relatively uninhibited research, the general Ptolemaic encouragement of scholarship, at least in the third century B.C., the renown of the immigrant intelligentsia, and the extraordinary level of scientific medicine attained by Herophilus as early as the reign of the first Ptolemy, in all likelihood were the leading factors in Alexandria's usurpation of previous centres of medical learning.

Bacchius probably lived from about 275 B.C. to 200 B.C., and was therefore at his prime during the reigns of Euergetes (246–221 B.C.) and Philopator (221–205 B.C.). This date is suggested, first by Erotian's report that the Empiricist Philinus was Bacchius' contemporary (*Ba.*13), and secondly, by Galen's report that Philinus had been a direct pupil of Herophilus before he broke away from Herophilus' school to found the Empiricist school.[4] Deichgräber sets Philinus' floruit at 250 B.C., and this seems plausible.

Not all scholars accept the date I have assigned to Bacchius. One scholar, for example, believes that Bacchius' prime lies about 200 B.C.,[5] perhaps because a Galenic text – if it has been emended correctly – claims that Bacchius in his famous Hippocratic lexicon made use of a collection of words compiled by the grammarian Aristophanes of Byzantium (*Ba.*12), who succeeded Eratosthenes as head of the Alexandrian Library only about 194 B.C. Aristophanes' date is, however, approximately 257–180 B.C., and, though a younger contemporary of Bacchius, he might well have composed his major lexicographic work (*Lexeis*) in the third century, enabling Bacchius to borrow examples from this work for his own Hippocratic lexicon[6] well before Aristophanes became Librarian at the age of sixty-two.

---

[4] On Philinus' relation to Herophilus cf. Deichgräber, 1965: fr. 6 and pp. 254–5.
[5] Kudlien, 1964a.
[6] It was in particular the references to poetic texts (with which Erotian (*Ba.*13) says that Bacchius filled his lexicon) that were borrowed from Aristophanes' *Lexeis*. On Aristophanes' lexicographic activity cf. Pfeiffer, 1968: 197ff., 135; Erbse, 1950: *passim*.

Although most famous for his Hippocratic lexicon (*Lexeis*) – it is referred to more than sixty times in ancient texts (*Ba*.12–76) – Bacchius was a versatile physician and scholar. He pursued Herophilus' interest in pulse theory (*Ba*.1–4), contributed to pathology (*Ba*.5) and pharmacology (*Ba*.6), produced an edition of Book III of the Hippocratic treatise *Epidemics* (and perhaps of other Hippocratic treatises as well (*Ba*.7)), wrote commentaries on *In the Surgery* (*Ba*.8), on the *Aphorisms* (*Ba*.9), on *Epidemics* VI (*Ba*.10) – and perhaps on *Epidemics* II (*Ba*.11) – and on other 'difficult' Hippocratic works (*Ba*.8); furthermore, he composed an influential doxographic work, *Memoirs on Herophilus and the members of his 'House'* (*Ba*.78). Conspicuously absent from the testimonia concerning Bacchius is, however, the area of Herophilus' greatest scientific achievement, anatomy. Whether the Empiricists' attacks on systematic anatomy, the apparent abandonment of human dissection after Herophilus' death, or the Alexandrian intelligentsia's increasing preoccupation with philology played a role in Bacchius' shift of the central focus from anatomy to Hippocratic scholarship, is unknown, but in all likelihood these were significant contributory factors.

Bacchius' lexicographic work on Hippocratic words (*Lexeis*) is of immense significance not only because it is a richly documented sample of the methods and aims of Alexandrian philology, but also because it provides evidence concerning the Hippocratic works accessible to Alexandrians in the third century B.C. Furthermore, it contains a number of textual variants not recorded elsewhere,[7] and hence provides valuable insight into the state of some Hippocratic texts in third-century Alexandria.

Bacchius' *Lexeis* were divided into three books or sections (συντά-ξεις[8]). The Hippocratic words listed in it were apparently not arranged alphabetically – a task first undertaken by Epicles of Crete in the first century B.C. in his abridged, revised edition of Bacchius' glossary[9] – but instead in the sequence in which they appeared in those Hippocratic works covered in each of the three sections.

---

[7] For a summary of these see Wellmann, 1931: 3–14; Nachmanson, 1917: Chapter VI (especially pp. 499–523).

[8] *Ba*.13. Cf. W. D. Smith, 1979: 202–4.

[9] Erotian, *Vocum Hippocraticarum collectio*, p. 7 (Nachmanson): ... Ἐπικλῆς μὲν ὁ κατὰ στοιχεῖον ποιησάμενος τὴν ἀναγραφήν, ματαίου συντομίας ἐγένετο ʒηλωτής. See also *Ba*.13.

The first part contains glosses on words from the Hippocratic treatises *Prognostic, On the Sacred Disease, On Joints, Instruments of Reduction* and *Epidemics* I and VI.[10] In Book II Hippocratic words from the treatises *Prognostic, Prorrhetic* I, *On Joints, In the Surgery, Instruments of Reduction, Regimen in Acute Diseases*, and *Epidemics* II are explained.[11] Book III offers glosses on words from what later became known as *On the Nature of Bones*, from *On Fractures, On Joints, In the Surgery, On Places in Humans*, and perhaps *Epidemics* V.[12] In addition, there are glosses which are not attributed to a specific book of Bacchius' *Lexeis*. These are on words from *Prognostic, Prorrhetic* I, *On Fractures, On Joints, On Wounds in the Head, In the Surgery, Instruments of Reduction, On Diseases* I, *On Places in Humans, On the Use of Liquids, Aphorisms*, and *Epidemics* I, II, III and V.[13] The glosses concerning the *Aphorisms* and *Epidemics* III may also have been provided in Bacchius' commentary on, or edition of, these works.[14]

At least eighteen Hippocratic treatises therefore seem to have been known to Bacchius as 'Hippocratic', and it is worth noting that the so-called 'Coan' treatises dominate the list at the expense of 'Cnidian' treatises. If the distinction between the 'Cnidian' and 'Coan' works of the Hippocratic Corpus has any merit,[15] the early contact between the Herophilean school and Cos, as well as the lively and significant contact between the Ptolemaic court and this island,[16] might explain this preponderance of 'Coan' treatises in Bacchius' work.

It is striking that words from *Prognostic* as well as *Instruments of*

---

[10] *Ba.* 14–25.   [11] *Ba.*26–37.   [12] *Ba.*38–48.   [13] *Ba.*49–76.

[14] For evidence of such commentaries see *Ba.*9 and *Ba.*7.

[15] A distinction recently challenged by W. D. Smith, 1973. Even those who accept the distinction do not agree on which treatises are 'Cnidian' and which 'Coan'. Thus Ilberg, 1924, identifies twelve Hippocratic treatises as Cnidian, including the gynaecological ones, while Edelstein found only three 'Cnidian' treatises in the Corpus (1931b: 159 with n.) and Bourgey (1953) only two, viz. *On Diseases* II and *On Internal Affections* (Edelstein had added *On Regimen in Acute Diseases* and *Sp.*). Lonie (1965b) and Jouanna (1974) deal only with those 'Cnidian' works which may have used the Κνίδιαι Γνῶμαι as their common stock (Jouanna especially *On Diseases* II A and B, *On Diseases* III, *On Internal Affections*, Lonie with these as well as *On Diseases* I and *On Affections*), whereas H. Grensemann, 1975, taking a more comprehensive view, also discusses the gynaecological works emphasized by Ilberg (*Women's Diseases, On the Nature of Woman*) and *On Seed, On Sterility, On the Nature of the Child*. See also Lonie, 1978 (a palinode); Thivel, 1981: ch. 2.

[16] See Chapter II.A.1, and Fraser, 1972: vol. I, p. 307.

Reduction are treated in both Book I and Book II of Bacchius' *Lexeis*,[17] and that lemmata from *On Joints* occur in all three parts.[18] This suggests that Bacchius did not consider what appears to be his general principle – grouping together the lemmata from each Hippocratic work – inviolable, and that other considerations, for example, thematic or semantic affinities, at times caused him to explain words from one and the same Hippocratic work in different books of his lexicon. (That Bacchius' work in fact offered identification of the works to which the lemmata pertain is indicated by Erotian's statement that Epicles the Cretan not only alphabetized his abridgment of Bacchius' *Lexeis* but also dropped the identification of the Hippocratic works.[19])

If Bacchius did arrange his lemmata by the Hippocratic treatises from which they are drawn, what was the principle of determining the sequence of these treatises? The once popular notion that Bacchius in his *Glossary* used the same sequence in which the Hippocratic works were ordered in his edition of the 'Corpus' – an *editio princeps* in the influential view of Wellmann[20] – is untenable in the absence of proof that Bacchius in fact edited any Hippocratic treatises other than *Epidemics* III.[21] Nor can it be claimed with any confidence (*pace* Wellmann)[22] that Bacchius arranged the Hippocra-

[17] *Ba.*14–15 and 26 (cf. also *Ba.*49–51); *Ba.*20–2 and 33–4 (cf. also *Ba.*62–6, not identified by book).

[18] *Ba.*17–19 (Book I of Bacchius' *Lexeis*), *Ba.*31 (Book II), *Ba.*40–3 (Book III). Also from *On Joints* are the lemmata in *Ba.*55–8, but the source (Erotian) does not attribute them to a specific part of Bacchius' *Lexeis*.

[19] Erotian, *Vocum Hippocraticarum collectio*, p. 8 (Nachmanson): πρὸς τῷ γὰρ μὴ πάσας (sc. λέξεις) ἐξηγήσασθαι, ἔτι καὶ τὰ συντάγματα, ἐν οἷς αὐτῶν ἑκάστη κατεγέγραπτο, σιωπῆς ἱκανῆς αἴτιον ἐγένετο τοῖς ἀναγινώσκουσι.

[20] Cf. Wellmann, 1931: 11: 'Geordnet waren die Glossen nicht nach dem Alphabet ... sondern nach der Reihenfolge der hippokratischen Schriften in seiner Ausgabe ähnlich wie in dem Urglossar Erotians', and p. 85: '[Bakcheios] machte die erste Ausgabe der hippokratischen Schriften.' Cf. Chapter III, n. 25 *supra*.

[21] Cf. *Ba.*7 and Chapter III, T34 (= *Ba.* 9).

[22] Wellmann, 1931: 2: 'Was die Anordnung der Schriften [in der Hippokratesausgabe des Bakcheios] angeht, so ist es sehr wahrscheinlich, dass ihre Einteilung nach dem von Erotian in seiner Praefatio ... angegebenen Schema in semiotische, physiologisch-ätiologische und therapeutische Schriften von ihm [Bakcheios] herrührt.' Wellmann bases his argument primarily on two factors: (a) Bacchius' *Lexeis* consisted of three parts (*Ba.*13); and (b) according to *Ba.*77 Bacchius mentioned that 'Hippocrates' composed *On the Nature of the Child* after the *Aphorisms*, i.e. in the same sequence in which Erotian treats these two works in his

tic texts according to the classification used by Erotian (without specific reference to its origin) in his enumeration of genuine Hippocratic works: first semiotic works, then physiological-aetiological works, third therapeutic works, fourth a mixed class, and finally 'those pertaining to the Art', such as the *Oath*, *On the Art*, the *Law*, and *On Ancient Medicine*.[23] Erotian's work itself, even before a redactor produced the roughly alphabetized version we now have, did not adhere strictly to this classificatory sequence, and the distribution of Hippocratic works among the three parts or volumes of Bacchius' *Glossary* is perhaps even less in accordance with this scheme.

Part one of Bacchius' work, for example, treats not only semiotic works (*Prognostic*), but also works from the second class (*On the Sacred Disease*), from the third or 'therapeutic' class (*On Joints, Instruments of Reduction*) and from the 'mixed' class (*Epidemics* I and VI).[24]

Similarly, Book II of Bacchius' *Glossary* explains words from semiotic works (*Prognostic, Prorrhetic* I), from therapeutic works (*On Joints, Instruments of Reduction, Regimen in Acute Diseases*), and from the 'mixed' class of works (*Epidemics* II).[25]

Book III, by contrast, chiefly treats lemmata from works classified as 'therapeutic' (*On Fractures, On Joints, In the Surgery, On Places in Man*) although the compilation later known as *On the Nature of Bones* also seems to be represented.[26] The notion that the first part of Bacchius' *Lexeis* treated lemmata from semiotic works, and the second those from physiological or 'aetiological' Hippocratic treatises, is therefore untenable, whereas there is more support for the identification of Book III – but not Book III alone – with therapeutic works.

The exact organizational principles of Bacchius' lexicon therefore remain considerably more elusive than has generally been thought.

glossary. But as pointed out below, (a) the three parts of Bacchius' *Lexeis* do not correspond to the semiotic–aetiological–therapeutic sequence, and (b) *Ba.*77 is inconclusive.

[23] Erotian, *Vocum Hippocraticarum collectio*, p. 9 Nachmanson.

[24] 'Semiotic' representatives in Bacchius, *Lexeis* I, are *Ba.*14–15; 'physiological–aetiological' *Ba.*16; 'therapeutic' *Ba.*17–22; fourth or 'mixed' class *Ba.*23–5.

[25] Glosses on lemmata from 'semiotic' works in Bacchius, *Lexeis* II, are *Ba.*26–30; from 'therapeutic' works *Ba.*31–6; from the 'mixed' class *Ba.*37.

[26] Lemmata from 'therapeutic' works in *Lexeis* III are *Ba.*39–47. *On the Nature of Bones* (from which the lemma in *Ba.*38 is drawn) is primarily an anatomical and physiological compilation dealing with the vascular system in a doxographic manner. If my identification of the lemma in *Ba.*48 as being from *Epidemics* 5.1 is correct, a work from the 'mixed' class would also be represented in *Lexeis* III.

As I mentioned earlier, Erotian too does not abide strictly by the sequence suggested in the classificatory scheme depicted in his preface, but seems to have treated the fourth class, i.e. 'mixed' works (*Epidemics* I–VI, *Aphorisms*), right after the first class (semiotic works), and to have started his treatment of therapeutic works with the *Law*, a work of the fifth class.[27] Nevertheless the tripartite sequence – semiotic, physiological, therapeutic works – in general was observed in the original version of Erotian's glossary, and it is conceivable, though by no means certain, that Bacchius or an early Empiricist had previously developed this classificatory scheme without putting it to unadulterated, sustained use for lexicographic purposes.[28]

In the collection of Bacchius' glosses that follows (*Ba*.14–76) only limited use has been made of the tripartite sequence, first, because of the uncertainty concerning its authorship, and secondly, because of Bacchius' habit of explaining words from one treatise in more than one book of his *Glossary*. Slightly more than half the glosses are explicitly identified as belonging to a specific book of Bacchius' *Glossary*: twelve from Book I (*Ba*.14–25), twelve from Book II (*Ba*.26–37), and eleven from Book III (*Ba*.38–48). These are followed by a fourth group of glosses, numbering twenty-eight, which are not explicitly attributed to a specific book of the *Glossary* (*Ba*.49–76). In each of these four groups the lemmata from each Hippocratic work represented are clustered together, and, for want of a closer knowledge of Bacchius' method, the classificatory sequence found in Erotian's preface is then adopted to determine the sequence of Hippocratic works in each group. It is tempting to assign some glosses in the fourth group to specific books of the *Lexeis*. Based on the distribution of the glosses identified by book, it seems likely that the unidentified ones from *Prorrhetic* I (*Ba*.52–3) and *Epidemics* I (*Ba*.73) belong to Book II, the ones from *On Fractures* (*Ba*.54), *On Places in Man* (*Ba*.68–9), and *Epidemics* V (*Ba*.75) to Book III, and the ones from *Epidemics* I (*Ba*.72) and *Prognostic* (*Ba*.49–51) to Book I. But in the light of Bacchius' unequivocally attested practice of explaining words from

---

[27] Cf. Ilberg, 1893: 141–2; Nachmanson, 1917: 26off., 329.

[28] Philinus and Glaucias were apparently the earliest lexicographers of the Empiricist school; later Heraclides of Tarentum and Apollonius of Citium also contributed Hippocratic glossaries. Cf. *Ba*.13 and *Ds*.5; Deichgräber, 1965: fr. 311, 311a.

a given Hippocratic treatise in more than one book of his glossary, I considered it sounder to leave these glosses in a separate group.

The identification of the Hippocratic passages from which the lemmata are drawn remains tentative for several reasons. First, the Hippocratic passages to which Erotian's lemmata pertain are not always known (although their identification has been furthered immensely by the meticulous analyses of Nachmanson and others).[29] Thus λάπτει (*Ba*.76) and στερρωθείη (*Ba*.44) have not yet been identified conclusively. Secondly, even when a consensus has been reached concerning the provenance of a lemma in Erotian, the fact that Erotian under a given lemma quotes a gloss by Bacchius does not always mean that Bacchius' gloss pertains to the same word, let alone the same pasage, as Erotian's. A good example is provided by *Ba*.17: in his explanation of περιωτειλοῦται, a word from *Instruments of Reduction* 33 (II, p. 263 Kühlewein), Erotian cites Bacchius, but he is in fact using Bacchius' gloss on ὠτειλαί, a word from *On Joints*. While this is a somewhat exceptional case, it does warn one against assuming that Erotian's glosses always refer to the same passages as Bacchius', and that identifying Erotian's lemmata is tantamount to identifying Bacchius'. A third factor which renders the identification of the passages from which Bacchius' lemmata are drawn a precarious undertaking is, of course, that the same word often occurs in more than one Hippocratic treatise. In such cases it is often easier to determine the provenance of Erotian's lemmata – since the rough sequence in which he used Hippocratic texts has been reconstructed – than it is to assign Bacchius' lemmata to specific Hippocratic texts. The tentative identification of Hippocratic treatises provided in B (infra) is therefore based not only on the general probability that Erotian cites Bacchius on the same passages from which his lemmata are drawn, but also on a consideration of the Hippocratic works known to have been accessible to Bacchius. Thus Erotian's lemma θράσσει (*Ba*.58) might well be drawn from the Hippocratic *Gynaecia*, as Grensemann plausibly argues,[30] but since there is no evidence that Bacchius knew this 'Cnidian' work, whereas his acquaintance with

---

[29] Nachmanson, 1917: *passim* (and in his edition); Grensemann, 1964, and 1968b; Ilberg, 1893, Deichgräber, 1933: 85–6; Wellmann, 1931: *passim*.
[30] Grensemann, 1968b: 188–9.

On Joints is richly attested, I have referred Bacchius' explanation to *On Joints* 46.[31]

The principles of interpretation adopted in Bacchius' lexicon are elusive but seem to have included the following: first, he did not confine himself to rare and obsolete words, as Galen's statement that Bacchius interpreted only γλῶτται (*glōttai*) implies;[32] rather, the more neutral title of Bacchius' work, *Lexeis*, accurately reflects the fact that it included any words peculiar in form and significance, or rare in prose usage, and consequently in need of explanation, whether or not they were still in use. In choice of subject-matter it is therefore closer to the *Lexeis* of Aristophanes of Byzantium than to other works of Hellenistic lexicography, such as the *Glossai* of Philitas, Simias, and Zenodotus, or to the *Local Nomenclature* (Ἐθνικαὶ ὀνομασίαι) of the poet Callimachus.[33] Philitas and Simias had made comprehensive, learned collections of rare and obsolete epic and dialectical words (Philitas' glossary had no systematic arrangement, and is hence also known as Ἄτακτοι γλῶσσαι or Ἄτακτα)[34], Zenodotus produced the first alphabetized glossary of rare epic and lyric words[35], and Callimachus' Onomastikon, of which *Local Nomenclature*[36] was probably only one part, 'listed and disposed *all* the names [of fishes, winds, birds in different localities] he could find for . . . purely literary reasons', i.e. also for reference when writing his own poems.[37] Bacchius, by contrast, neither confined himself to rare and obsolete words nor chose his lemmata only on the basis of thematic coherence, but carefully selected words for their morphological or semantic peculiarity, their obscurity, their infrequent occurrence, their homonymy and the resulting ambivalences, or because of the fact that they were not normally used in prose. To the latter category belongs, for example, a word like ἅλις, 'enough' (*Ba*.32): its inclusion might at

[31] Nachmanson, 1917: 497 (and in his edition, p. 44 – but with the misprint '*De arte*' for '*De articulis*'), and Wellmann, 1931: 5, also assigned this lemma to *On Joints* 46. On the deviation of the lemma from the Hippocratic MSS, see my edition (forthcoming) of the fragments of Bacchius and other Herophileans.

[32] *Ba*.12. On the distinction between γλῶτται and λέξεις cf. Pfeiffer, 1968: 198.

[33] For brief discussions of their lexicographic works see Pfeiffer, 1968: 79, 90ff., 115, 135, 197ff.; cf. also 228.

[34] For Philitas see fr. 29–59, in Kuchenmüller, 1928; for Simias, Fränkel, 1915: fr. 29–32, and Maas, 1927: 156.

[35] Cf. the fragments and testimonia in Pusch, 1890: 191f. See also Erbse, 1953: 180.

[36] Callimachus, fr. 406 Pfeiffer.

[37] Pfeiffer, 1968: 135 (italics added).

first seem uncalled for, since it is a very common word; but it is in fact a poetic word only rarely used in Greek prose,[38] and Bacchius refers the reader to two synonyms, ἀρκεόντως and ἱκανῶς, that were widely used by prose authors (including 'Hippocrates').

A second aspect of Bacchius' method is mentioned by Erotian: Bacchius not only used other Hippocratic treatises to explain a puzzling occurrence of a word in a given treatise, but also 'cited many pieces of evidence from poets'.[39] Much of this poetic evidence was probably drawn from Aristophanes' *Lexeis*, as suggested by Galen's statement that Bacchius interpreted the words of Hippocrates 'after Aristophanes the grammarian had collected a large number of examples for him'.[40] Although most of the corroborating quotations from both Hippocratic and poetic texts in Erotian's *Collection of Hippocratic Words* are not identified as having been drawn from Bacchius' *Lexeis*, it is likely that Bacchius in turn became Erotian's source. In view of the impossibility of sorting out which references and quotations in Erotian's work were taken over from Bacchius, which were provided by other Hippocratic lexicographers, which were taken from Aristophanes' *Lexeis*, and which from Apollodorus' work on etymology,[41] quotations not explicitly attributed to Bacchius by Erotian have in general not been included in the list which follows, in

---

[38] Herodotus (the 'most Homeric' of ancient authors – Longinus) uses it only twice (1.119.5; 9.27.5), once in narrative and once in direct speech, while Thucydides never uses the word. Plato uses it only once, in a rhetorical flourish, to conclude an argument (*Statesman* 287A6). Aristotle uses it more freely, but in a similar manner (*Nicomachean Ethics* 1.3.1096a3, 1.13.1102b11, 10.1.1172b7; *Generation of Animals* 3.6.757a13). (*Nic. Eth.* 9.11.1171b18, a more poetic usage, does not qualify as an instance of its use in prose, since the phrase is probably culled from a tragedian, as Bonitz suggests.)

[39] *Ba.*13.

[40] *Ba.*12. But see Ch. IX, T270.11 (with critical apparatus).

[41] Apollodorus, son of Asclepiades of Athens, was a pupil of the Stoic Diogenes of Seleucia in Athens and of the famous Homeric critic Aristarchus of Samothrace in Alexandria. His *Etymologiae* or *Etymologoumena* built on an earlier glossographic tradition and became very influential with later lexicographers. Cf. *FGrHist* 244, F222–5 (F226–84, although not attributed to specific books of Apollodorus, contain a number of etymologies too). Other sources Erotian may have used include the grammarian Antigonus of Alexandria (of the time of Augustus and Tiberius), in whom Wellmann (1931) sees the primary intermediary between Bacchius and Erotian, Lysimachus of Cos (cf. Chapter XXVI, *Cy.*1 and n. 1), the grammarian Artemidorus of Tarsus (first century B.C.), and Sextius Niger (Augustan period).

accordance with the principles developed in the Introductory Notes
(pp. xvi–xvii).

The results of Bacchius' lexicographic efforts are not always
encouraging. That a medical author of the third century B.C. could
sometimes misunderstand texts that were often barely a hundred
years old, could assign controversial meanings to certain words, and
could be confounded by a large number of Hippocratic words, does
not inspire confidence in the modern reader's ability to unravel all
semantic tangles of ancient medical texts.

Already some of his contemporaries found reason to criticize
Bacchius' lexicon, although the reasons for their criticism remain
unclear. The Empiricist Philinus of Cos,[42] for example, wrote a
polemical treatise in six books against Bacchius' lexicon, from which
Erotian preserves three glosses – all of them, ironically, instances of
substantial or complete agreement between Bacchius and Philinus.[43]
In the first century B.C. two Empiricists, Heraclides of Tarentum and
Apollonius of Citium, again subjected Bacchius' glosses to ridicule.[44]
Apollonius accuses him in particular first, of having collected
occurrences of a word which are useless because they are not
presented in context, and secondly, of not having investigated the
peculiarly Coan usage of the word.[45] Some of their polemics were
undoubtedly justified, others were probably inspired by the school
rivalry between the Empiricists and the Herophileans. These attacks
notwithstanding, Bacchius' lexicon continued to have a considerable
impact on Hippocratic scholarship in antiquity. Thus Epicles of
Crete (also first century B.C.) found Bacchius' work worthy of a
revised, abridged edition, and Erotian, a sensitive and perceptive
grammarian of the Neronian age, found Bacchius' explanations of
Hippocratic terms worth mentioning more than sixty times in his own
Hippocratic glossary. Although he frequently rejects Bacchius'
explanations as incorrect, he seems to be in full or partial agreement
with Bacchius' explanations in about half of the instances he cites,
often explicitly preferring them to those of illustrious ancient
grammarians and commentators.[46] No Hippocratic lexicographer

[42] *Ba.*13; Deichgräber, 1965: fr. 311.
[43] Cf. *Ba.*15, 41, and 49; Deichgräber, 1965: fr. 328, 322, 327.
[44] *Ba.*13 (=Deichgräber, 1965: fr. 311); *Ba.*42; *Ba.*55. Apollonius, however, also
attacked Heraclides' polemics against Bacchius: *Ba.13*
[45] *Ba.*42; *Ba.*55.   [46] Cf., for example, *Ba.*41.

until Erotian had an impact matching Bacchius', and the evidence presented in this chapter strongly suggests that Rudolf Pfeiffer's judgment that the Empiricist Philinus 'became the most influential medical glossographer'[47] of Alexandria must be revised in favour of Bacchius.

B · TEXTS

*Ba.*1a   Galenus (ex Aristoxeno?), *De pulsuum differentiis* 4.6 (VIII, pp. 732–3K)

*Ba.*1b   Marcellinus, *De pulsibus* 3 (p. 457 Schöne)

*Ba.*2   Galenus (ex Aristoxeno?), *De pulsuum differentiis* 4.10 (VIII, pp. 748–9K)

*Ba.*3   Ps.-Galenus, *Definitiones medicae* 220 (XIX, pp. 408–9K). (See also above Chapter VII, T172, and below Chapter XV, *Zn.*2, and Chapter XVII, *Hg.*4)

*Ba.*4   Galenus, *De pulsuum dignotione* 4.3 (VIII, p. 955K). Cf. Chapter VII, T162.

*Ba.*5   Caelius Aurelianus, *Tardae passiones* 2.10.121–2

*Ba.*6   Andromachus Iunior apud Galenum, *De compositione medicamentorum per genera* 7.7 (XIII, p. 987K)

*Ba.*7   Galenus, *In Hippocratis Epidemiarum 3.2.8 comment.* 2.8 (ad vol. III, p. 56.1L; *CMG* v.10.2.1, p. 87 Wenkebach)

*Ba.*8   Galenus, *In Hippocratis De officina medici comment.* 1, praefatio (XVIIIB, pp. 631–2K)

*Ba.*9   Galenus, *In Hippocratis Aphorismos comment.* 7.70 (XVIIIA, pp. 186–7K). (See above Chapter III, T34, with critical apparatus)

*Ba.*10   Galenus, *In Hippocratis Epidemiarum 6. comment.*, prooemium (*CMG* v.10.2.2, pp. 3–4 Wenkebach)

*Ba.*11   Galenus, *In Hippocratis Epidemiarum 2.2.20 comment.* 2 (ad vol. v, p.92.8–12L). From Ḥunain's Arabic translation of the lost original; *CMG* v.10.1, p. 230 Pfaff.

BACCHIUS' HIPPOCRATIC LEXICON

*Ba.*12   Galenus, *Explanatio vocum Hippocratis*, prooemium (XIX, pp. 64–5K). (See above Chapter IX, T270)

*Ba.*13   Erotianus, *Vocum Hippocraticarum collectio*, praefatio (pp. 4–5 Nachmanson)

---

[47] Pfeiffer, 1968: 92, n.2.

BOOK I

1 Hp., *Prognostic*

*Ba.*14   Erotianus, *Vocum Hippocraticarum collectio* α.1 (p. 10 Nachmanson):
          ἀλυσμόν
*Ba.*15   Erotianus, *op.cit.* α.4 (p. 10 Nachmanson): ἀτρεκέως
          See also *Ba.*26, *Ba.*49–51.

2 Hp., *On Sacred Disease*

*Ba.*16   Erotianus, α.47 (p. 17 Nachmanson): ἀλάστορες

3 Hp., *On Joints*

*Ba.*17   Erotianus, Fragmentum 46 (Scholium R^H in Hp. *Mochl.* 33; p. 113
          Nachmanson): ὠτειλαί
*Ba.*18   Erotianus, τ.20 (p. 85 Nachmanson): τύρσις
*Ba.*19   Erotianus, ς.46 (p. 81 Nachmanson): σκεθροτέρης
          The following also seem to be glosses on lemmata from the
          Hippocratic *On Joints*, but they are not attributed to Book I of
          Bacchius' Lexicon: *Ba.*31, *Ba.*40–3, *Ba.*55–8.

4 Hp., *Instruments of Reduction*

*Ba.*20   Erotianus, α.73 (p. 21 Nachmanson): αὐτίκα
*Ba.*21   Erotianus, α.69 (p. 20 Nachmanson): ἀνοκώχησις
*Ba.*22   Erotianus, ε.36 (p. 38 Nachmanson): ἕδος
          The following also seem to be glosses on words from this
          Hippocratic treatise, but they are not attributed to Book I: *Ba.*33–4,
          *Ba.*46, *Ba.*62–6.

5 Hp., *Epidemics* I

*Ba.*23   Erotianus, ς.2 (p. 76 Nachmanson): σπληνὸς κατ' ἴξιν
          Cf. also *Ba.*72, which is a gloss on a lemma from *Epidemics* I; it
          might belong to Book I of Bacchius' *Lexeis*.

6 Hp., *Epidemics* VI

*Ba.*24   Erotianus, Fragmentum 25 (Scholium R^H in Hp. *Epidemiarum* lib.
          6.1.5; p. 106 Nachmanson): ἐλινύειν
*Ba.*25   Erotianus, γ.8 (p. 30 Nachmanson): γυῖον

BOOK II

1 Hp., *Prognostic*

*Ba.*26   Erotianus, τ.2 (pp. 83–4 Nachmanson): τρύζειν
          Other glosses on expressions from this Hippocratic treatise occur
          in *Ba.*14–15 and *Ba.*49–51 (none of which are ascribed to Book II of
          Bacchius' lexicon by our ancient sources).

2 Hp., *Prorrhetic* I

Ba.27   Erotianus, α.8 (p. 13 Nachmanson): ἀπολελαμμένοι
Ba.28   Erotianus, λ.7 (p. 57 Nachmanson): λαπῶδες
Ba.29   Erotianus, Fragmentum 6 (Scholia R^H et U^H ad Hp. *Prorrheticum* 1.100; p. 100 Nachmanson): γριφώμενα
Ba.30   Erotianus, ε.5 (p. 35 Nachmanson): ἐκχλοιούμενα

3 Hp., *On Joints*

Ba.31   Erotianus, α.107 (p. 24 Nachmanson): ἀγάλλεται
         See also *Ba*.17–19, *Ba*.40–3, *Ba*.55–8.

4 Hp., *In the Surgery*

Ba.32   Erotianus, α.68 (p. 20 Nachmanson): ἅλις
         See also *Ba*.44–5 and 60–1 for lemmata from *In the Surgery*.

5 Hp., *Instruments of Reduction*

Ba.33   Erotianus, Fragmentum 40 (Scholium R^H ad Hp. *Mochl.* 1; p. 111 Nachmanson): ἐπιμυλίδα
Ba.34   Erotianus, ε.35 (p. 38 Nachmanson): ἐσματτευόμενον
         Ba.20–2, *Ba*.46, *Ba*.62–6.

6 Hp., *Regimen in Acute Diseases*

Ba.35   Erotianus, π.54 (p. 73 Nachmanson): ποταίνια
Ba.36   Erotianus, π.55 (p. 73 Nachmanson): πυθμενόθεν

7 Hp. *Epidemics* II

Ba.37   Heraclides Tarentinus apud Galenum, *In Hippocratis Epidemiarum 2.2.20 comment.* 2 (ad vol. v, p. 92.8–12L). From Ḥunain's Arabic translation of the lost original; *CMG* v.10.1, pp. 232–3 Pfaff (on πρὸς τἀφροδίσια αἱ οὐραὶ ἔβλεπον). See also *Ba*.73.

BOOK III

1 Hp., *On the Nature of Bones*

Ba.38   Erotianus, ε.39 (p. 38 Nachmanson): ἐνεφλεβοτόμησε

2 Hp., *On Fractures*

Ba.39   Erotianus, μ.18 (p. 60 Nachmanson): μετεξέτεροι
         See also *Ba*.54.

3 Hp., *On Joints*

Ba.40   Erotianus, α.101 (p. 23 Nachmanson): ἀνάγκη
Ba.41   Erotianus, α.103 (p. 23 Nachmanson): ἄμβην. See also Chapter xv, *Zn*.7.

Ba.42 Apollonius Citiensis, *In Hippocratis De articulis comment.* 1 (*CMG* XI.1.1, p. 28 Kollesch/Kudlien): ἄμβην
Ba.43 Erotianus, ς.41 (p. 80 Nachmanson): στερρωθείη
For further lemmata from *On Joints* see *Ba*.17–19, 31, 55–8.

4 Hp., *In the Surgery*

Ba.44 Erotianus, ε.30 (p. 37 Nachmanson): ἕδρη
Ba.45 Erotianus, ε.32 (p. 38 Nachmanson): ἐξαρύεται
For further lemmata from *In the Surgery* see *Ba*.32, 60–1.

5 Hp., *Instruments of Reduction*

Ba.46 Erotianus, Fragmentum 45 (Scholium R^H in Hp. *Mochl.* 30, p. 113 Nachmanson): λυγγώδεες. See also *Ba*.20–2, 33–4, 62–6.

6 Hp., *On Places in Humans*

Ba.47 Erotianus, α.58 (p. 19 Nachmanson): ἀορτέων. See also *Ba*.68–9.

7 Hp., *Epidemics* v

Ba.48 Erotianus, ς.1 (p.76 Nachmanson): συχνόν. See also *Ba*.75.

FROM UNIDENTIFIED BOOKS OF BACCHIUS' LEXICON

1 Hp., *Prognostic*

Ba.49 Erotianus, Fragmentum 33 (p. 108 Nachmanson): θειοτέρη. See Chapter XIII above, *Cm*.8.
Ba.50 Erotianus, ν.1 (p. 62 Nachmanson): νείαιρα γαστήρ
Ba.51a Erotianus, α.5 (p. 12 Nachmanson): ἀλλοφάσσοντες
Ba.51b Erotianus, Fragmentum 1 (Scholium R^H ad *Prognosticum* 20; p. 99 Nachmanson): ἀλλοφάσσοντες
For further lemmata from *Prognostic* see Ba.14–15, 26.

2 Hp., *Prorrhetic* I

Ba.52 Erotianus, κ.6 (pp. 47–8 Nachmanson): κλαγγώδη
Ba.53 Erotianus, α.6 (p. 12 Nachmanson): ἀραιά
For other lemmata from *Prorrhetic* see Ba.27–30.

3 Hp., *On Fractures* (?)

Ba.54 Erotianus, π.45 (p. 72 Nachmanson): πηχέδεον. See also *Ba*.39.

4 Hp., *On Joints*

Ba.55 Apollonius Citiensis, *In Hippocratis De articulis comment.* 1 (*CMG* XI.1.1, pp. 16–18 Kollesch/Kudlien): ἀμφισφάλλουσι τὸ ἄρθρον
Ba.56 Erotianus, ο.32 (p. 66 Nachmanson): ὄκρις
Ba.57 Erotianus, ο.33 (p. 67 Nachmanson): ὅπλα

Ba.58   Erotianus, θ.5 (p. 44 Nachmanson): θράσσει
         For further glosses on lemmata from *On Joints* see *Ba.*17–19, 31,
         40–3.

                         5 Hp., *On Wounds in the Head*

Ba.59   Erotianus, β.8 (p. 28 Nachmanson): βλιχῶδες (πλιχ-)

                         6 Hp., *In the Surgery*

Ba.60   Erotianus, Fragmenta 37 et 61 (Scholia R^H et B^H2 ad Hp. *De officina
         medici* 2; pp. 110 et 117 Nachmanson): ἄρμενα
Ba.61   Erotianus, α.66 (p. 20 Nachmanson): ἀθέλγεται
         For further glosses on words from *In the Surgery* see *Ba.*32, 44–5.

                         7 Hp., *Instruments of Reduction*

Ba.62   Erotianus, Fragmentum 42 (Scholium R^H ad Hp. *Mochl.* 1; p. 112
         Nachmanson): βαλβιδῶδες
Ba.63   Erotianus, λ.19 (p. 58 Nachmanson): λελυγισμένα
Ba.64   Erotianus, ο.17 (p. 65 Nachmanson): ὀκχῇ
Ba.65   Erotianus, Fragmentum 43 (Scholium R^H ad Hp. *Mochl.* 22; p. 112
         Nachmanson): ῥοικοὶ μηροί
Ba.66   Erotianus, Fragmentum 44 (Scholium R^H ad Hp. *Mochl.* 26; p. 112
         Nachmanson): γαυσότεροι
         For further glosses on words from *Instruments of Reduction* see *Ba.*
         20–2, 33–4, 46.

                         8 Hp., *On Diseases* 1

Ba.67   Erotianus, ε.65 (p. 40 Nachmanson): ἔμπηροι

                         9 Hp., *On Places in Humans*

Ba.68   Erotianus, κ.28 (p. 50 Nachmanson): κυβίτῳ
Ba.69   Erotianus, μ.9 (p. 60 Nachmanson): μάσσον
         Ba. 47 also offers a gloss on a word from *On Places in Humans.*

                         10 Hp., *On the Use of Liquids*

Ba.70   Erotianus, α.48 (p. 18 Nachmanson): αἰόνησις

                         11 Hp., *Aphorisms*

Ba.71   Erotianus, α.31 (p. 15 Nachmanson): ἀμφιδέξιος

                         12 Hp., *Epidemics* 1

Ba.72   Erotianus, Fragmentum 14 (Scholium R^H ad Hp. *Epidemiarum* lib. 1.
         β'; p. 102 Nachmanson): βλησTρισμός
         For another gloss on a word from *Epidemics* 1 see *Ba.* 23.

13　Hp., *Epidemics* II

*Ba.*73　Erotianus, ε.13 (p. 36 Nachmanson): ἐκθύματα
　　　　See also *Ba.*37.

14　Hp., *Epidemics* III

*Ba.*74　Erotianus, φ.5 (p. 91 Nachmanson): φωναὶ κατείλλουσαι

15　Hp., *Epidemics* V

*Ba.*75　Erotianus, Fragmentum 18 (Scholium R^{H} ad Hp. *Epidemiarum* lib.
　　　　5.15; p. 104 Nachmanson): ἐσφακέλισε
　　　　See also *Ba.*48 for a lemma from *Epidemics* V.

Unidentified lemmata

*Ba.*76　Erotianus, λ.16 (p. 57 Nachmanson): λάπτει
*Ba.*77　Anonymus Bruxellensis, *Vita Hippocratis* (ed. H. Schöne, *RhM* N.F.
　　　　58 (1903), 59): νήπιον
*Ba.*78　Zeuxis apud Galenum, *In Hippocratis Epidemiarum 6.4.7 comment.* 4.10
　　　　(ad vol. v, p. 308.15–16L). (*CMG* v.10.2.2, p. 203 Wenkebach)
　　　　See Chapter XII above, *Cn.*1.

Dubium

*Ba.*79　Soranus, *Gynaecia* 1.12.3 (*CMG* IV, p. 9 Ilberg).
　　　　See Chapter VI, T106 (app. crit., Rose's conjecture).

XV · ZENO

(*Zn.*)

A · INTRODUCTION

One of the more bizarre learned controversies in Ptolemaic Alexandria concerned the provenance and meaning of certain marks or symbols (*charaktēres*) in Alexandrian copies of Book III of the Hippocratic *Epidemics*.[1] Entered in clusters of four or five at the conclusion of individual case histories in *Epidemics* III, these symbols – usually Greek letter symbols, such as E, H and Y, or combinatory derivations from letter symbols, e.g. ⊓ and Ɗ – were attributed to Hippocrates himself by the Herophilean physician Zeno.[2] This attribution unleashed a protracted controversy which apparently occupied much of the second half of the second century B.C. and continued well into the first: after Zeno had made his views public, the Empiricist Apollonius the Elder of Antioch wrote a polemical reply to Zeno's theory, opposing the notion that Hippocratic authorship of the symbols could be established. Zeno responded with a counter-attack, only for another Empiricist, Apollonius 'the Bookworm' (Byblas), also from Antioch, to join the fray – although Zeno was no longer alive – with what Galen characterizes as a 'super-refutation' of the Herophilean's views.[3] But neither Zeno's death nor such an elaborate refutation could end the dispute. Perhaps because of the continuing influence of Zeno's views (according to Galen he had an army of followers),[4] or perhaps simply because any later

---

[1] The only extensive account is provided by Galen in his commentary on Hp., *Epidemics* III (*CMG* v.10.2.1, ed. E. Wenkebach, pp. 75–95). Cf. Wenkebach, 1920; *id.*, 1925; Ilberg, 1895: 30–53; Littré, *Oeuvres complètes d'Hippocrate* III (Paris, 1841), 28–33; Kind, 1920; Deichgräber, 1965: fr. 341–6 and p. 257; Wellmann ap. Susemihl, 1891–2: vol. I, p. 823; W. D. Smith, 1979: 199–201.

[2] *Zn.*5–6.

[3] Cf. *Zn.*6: τὸν καλούμενον παρεξέλεγχον (*CMG* v.10.2.1, p. 87.5).

[4] Cf. *Zn.*6 (= *CMG* v.10.2.1, p. 93.10): τῶν ἐκ τοῦ Ζηνωνείου στρατοπέδου.

Empiricist worth his salt still had to engage 'in contentious rivalry' with the Herophilean, as Galen suggests,[5] yet another Empiricist, Heraclides of Tarentum, entered the controversy in the first century B.C. with subtle (and suspect) arguments both against Zeno's interpretation of the symbols and against his view of their origin.[6] The conflict finally simmered down when an Herophilean, Heraclides of Erythrae, agreed with the Empiricists' contention that the symbols were interpolated.[7]

Against Zeno's theory that Hippocrates himself was responsible for entering the symbols in *Epidemics* III the Empiricists, in particular Apollonius Byblas, argued that an obscure Pamphylian physician, Mnemon of Side, entered them anonymously and surreptitiously as a kind of short-hand summary of essential aspects of each case history, perhaps for mnemotechnical purposes.[8] Too little is known about Mnemon to judge the accuracy of these claims, but there is a prima facie likelihood that these signs were invented in the context of the new Alexandrian philology rather than in the course of a Coan's clinical activity, especialy since they were apparently not used in any other books of the *Epidemics*.

While Zeno and the Empiricists disagreed both on the authorship and on the meaning of the symbols, they were in agreement on the acrostic principles underlying their use: each symbol constitutes the initial letter or letters of a key word. Thus in Zeno's decipherment of the symbols used in *Epidemics* III, Case History 7,[9] ΠΙ is a sign for Π I, the first syllable of πιθανόν; Δ is a sign for Δ I, the first syllable of διαχωρημάτων; Ε stands for ἐπίσχεσις, Η for η′ (the 'eighth' [day]) and Θ for θάνατος, so that the sequence   ΠΙ Δ Ε Η Θ means 'It is plausible that the patient died on the eighth day because of blockage of the stool.' Similarly, in Case History 8, Zeno explains the sequence

---

[5] Cf. *Zn*.6 (= *CMG* v.10.2.1, p. 89.22–3), of Heraclides of Tarentum: φιλοτιμούμε-
νος πρὸς τὸν Ζήνωνα μᾶλλον ἢ ἀκριβῶς ἐξετάζων τὸ πρᾶγμα . . .
[6] *Zn*.6 (*CMG* v.10.2.1, pp. 87.13–89.23); Deichgräber, 1965: fr. 342–3.
[7] See Chapter XXIV, *HE*.5 (*CMG* v.10.2.1, p. 80).
[8] On Mnemon of Side cf. Raeder, Deichgräber & Kroll, 1932; Wellmann ap.
Susemihl, 1891–2: vol. I, pp. 814–15 and vol. II, pp. 681–2. The Hippocratic case
histories, widely interpreted in antiquity as valuable because of their typicality,
were recognized as a challenge to the memory. Some ancient authors, for example,
interpreted Hippocrates' mention of the exact location of the residence of each
patient discussed in the *Epidemics* as a mnemotechnical device resembling the
Aristotelian place system.
[9] Cf. *Zn*.5.

ΠΞΖΘ as πιθανόν, ξενόν, ζ' (the 'seventh' [day]), θάνατος, meaning 'It is plausible that the patient died on the seventh day because something strange [unaccustomed] had happened to him.'[10] The first sign in the sequence therefore always introduces a statement of what seems likely or plausible, the final sign signifies the outcome ('death' or 'health'), the penultimate sign the number of days the patient was ill, while the sign or signs between the first and the penultimate signify the cause of the disease.

The Empiricists agreed that these were the essential mechanisms of the system – i.e. that each letter symbol is the first letter of the word for which it stands – but they disagreed with Zeno on the words for which each symbol stands, taking care to refer to Hippocratic usage in order to refute Zeno's identification of certain words with the symbols. They furthermore charged that Zeno altered these – inauthentic – symbols whenever he could not give a plausible account of their original version, in order to facilitate his system of interpretation. It is difficult, if not impossible, to verify this charge, but Apollonius 'the Bookworm's' statement that he could not find Zeno's version of the signs appended to *Epidemics* III, Case History 8, in any copy of *Epidemics* III, 'neither [in] the one found in the Royal Library nor [in] the one from the merchant-ships nor [in] the one in the "edition" made by Bacchius'[11] could, if true, be evidence of Zeno's manipulation of his evidence.

Zeno's interest in Hippocratic texts extended beyond the signs in *Epidemics* III. The Neronian lexicographer Erotian and Galen also cite his glosses on controversial words from the Hippocratic works *On Joints* and *On Places in Humans*.[12] It is therefore conceivable that Zeno followed in the lexicographic footsteps of his Herophilean predecessor Bacchius (whose definition of the pulse had a decisive influence on Zeno's pulse theory).

Although Zeno became most famous for his interpretation of the symbols in *Epidemics* III, he was also an accomplished and versatile physician in the broad Herophilean tradition. Galen, who dignifies him with the characterization 'a man second to none among the Herophileans', gives an extensive and, on the whole, positive account

---

[10] *Zn*.6.
[11] *Zn*.6 (*CMG* v.10.2.1, p. 87.9–12); cf. Chapter XIV, *Ba*.7, and Deichgräber, 1965: fr. 342 (p. 236).
[12] *Zn*.7–9.

of Zeno's pulse theory,[13] conceding, however, that some of Aristoxe-nus' criticisms,[14] especially of redundancies in Zeno's definition of the pulse, are justified. A relatively orthodox Herophilean in essential tenets of his sphygmology – the pulse, Zeno said, is an activity of 'the arterial parts', a mixture of contraction and distention, having the same sequence in all its parts, whether the activity is completed in equal or unequal time-units – Zeno did stake out his independence from the founding master, not only by joining Bacchius in using 'distention' (*diastasis*) rather than 'dilation' (*diastolē*) of the artery, but also by his elaborations upon the Herophilean definition and, more significantly, as Galen notes, by his omission of explicit mention of the heart in his definition of the pulse. This omission was however, not prompted by a total disregard of the function of the heart in pulsation, but rather by an acceptance of Bacchius' use[15] of the term 'arterial parts' to refer to both the arteries and to the left ventricle of the heart – a modification which might have been a response to some of the Erasistratean criticisms of Herophilus' pulse theory.[16]

In addition to sphygmology and Hippocratic philology, Zeno was also known in antiquity for his pharmacological effort, although relatively little is known about this aspect of his work.[17] Tempting though it would be to identify him with the famous pharmacologist Zeno of Laodicea (several of whose prescriptions for drug compounds are extant[18]), especially since Laodicea was very close to the site of a renowned and active Herophilean school of medicine, there is nothing in the ancient evidence to link these two Zenos. In accordance with the criteria for inclusion texts concerning the Laodicean pharmacologist are therefore not included below under B.[19]

---

[13] *Zn.*1. [14] *Zn.*1. Cf. Chapter xxv, *Ar.*1.

[15] Chapter xiv, *Ba.*2. (While the use of 'distention' [*diastasis*] is also attributed to Bacchius in *Ba.*2, 'dilation' [*diastolē*] is used in *Ba.*1.)

[16] Cf. pp. 464–5.

[17] The only evidence is contained in *Zn.*4 and *Zn.*3; *Zn.*11 is of dubious value, since (a) the Zeno it mentions is not explicitly identified as the Herophilean, and (b) there are at least two other ancient physicians called Zeno: Zeno of Laodicea (see n. 19 below) and Zeno of Cyprus (on whom see Julian, *Letters* 58 (Bidez); Eunapius, *Lives of the Sophists* 19–22, pp. 497–9 Didot; pp. 87–7, 89 Giangrande).

[18] Cf., for example, Philumenus, *De venenatis animalibus* 10.6–9 (*CMG* x.1.1, pp. 14–15 Wellmann); Galen, *De compositione medicamentorum per genera* 4.5 (xiii, pp. 691–2K); Galen, *De antidotis* 2.10 (xiv, p. 163K) and 2.11 (xiv, p. 171K).

[19] Kudlien distinguishes Zeno of Laodicea from the Herophilean treated in this

About Zeno's exact date there is no direct evidence, but the indirect evidence provided by his dispute with the Empiricists, notably with the two Apollonii from Antioch, suggests the first half of the second century B.C.[20] – a date which would also be consonant with the influence Bacchius apparently exercised upon his work.

B · TEXTS

*Zn.*1   Galenus (ex Aristoxeno?), *De pulsuum differentiis* 4.8 (VIII, pp. 736–41 K)

*Zn.*2   Ps.-Galenus, *Definitiones medicae* 220 (XIX, p. 409K)

*Zn.*3   A. Cornelius Celsus, *Medicina* 5 (= *Artes* 10), prohoemium 1 (*CML* 1, p. 190 Marx). See Chapter VIII, T251.

*Zn.*4   Galenus, *De simplicium medicamentorum temperamentis et facultatibus* 1.29 (XI, p. 432K)

*Zn.*5   Galenus, *In Hippocratis Epidemiarum 3.3′ comment.* 2.4 (ad Hp., vol. III, pp. 52.11–54.7L) (*CMG* V.10.2.1, pp. 75–7 Wenkebach)

*Zn.*6   Galenus, *In Hippocratis Epidemiarum 3. comment.* 2.8–9 (*CMG* V.10.2.1, pp. 86–94 Wenkebach)

*Zn.*7   Erotianus, *Vocum Hippocraticarum collectio* α.103 (p. 23 Nachmanson): ἄμβην

*Zn.*8   Erotianus, κ.31 (p. 51 Nachmanson): καμμάρῳ

*Zn.*9   Galenus (?), *Explanatio vocum Hippocratis*, s.v. *kammoron* (XIX, p. 108K)

*Zn.*10   Diogenes Laertius, *Vitae philosophorum* 7.35

Dubia

*Zn.*11   Caelius Aurelianus, *Tardae passiones* 4.7.99

*Zn.*12   C. Plinius Secundus, *Naturalis historia* 22.44.90

*Zn.*13   Alexander Aphrodisiensis (?), *De febribus* 1 (p. 3 Passow)

chapter, but identifies both as Herophileans (1972c). Jutta Kollesch has, however, reverted to a more traditional view, pointing out that nothing in the ancient evidence links the Laodicean with the Herophilean school: 1975a (Wellmann ap. Susemihl, 1891–2: vol. I, p. 824, does not exhibit appropriate caution). The fact that the pharmacologist was from Laodicea, and that there was a Herophilean school at Men Karou, near Laodicea (see below, Chapters XXI, XXII, XXVIII), is not conclusive evidence that Zeno the pharmacologist belonged to the Herophilean school, let alone that the pharmacologist is identical with the Herophilean treated in this chapter (as Sprengel, 1846: 545f., assumed while conceding that uncertainties remain).

[20] On the dates of the Apollonius the Elder (*c.* 175 B.C.) and Apollonius Byblas (*c.* 150 B.C.), see Deichgräber, 1965: 171–2.

XVI · DEMETRIUS
OF APAMEA (*DA.*)

A · INTRODUCTION

While his predecessors Bacchius and Zeno became best known for their exegetical work on Hippocratic texts,[1] few Herophileans were as well known in antiquity for a broad interest in general pathology as Demetrius of Apamea. Mania, priapism, satyriasis, phrenitis, hydrophobia, lethargy, dropsy, 'diabetes', pneumonia, pleurisy, cardiac disorders, and haemorrhage are among the conditions whose symptoms and causes Demetrius discussed.[2] Both of his treatises known by title – *On Affections* or *On Diseases*, in at least twelve books,[3] and *Signs* or *Semiotics*[4] – are devoted to pathology and to a closely related subject, symptomatology, and among the testimonia concerning Demetrius very few do not offer pathological theories and observations.

Despite the relative wealth of evidence concerning Demetrius' general pathology, the aetiological principles underlying his observations on individual diseases are not clear. Whether he was a humoral pathologist, a plethorist, or an 'atomist' – like Asclepiades, with whom he is sometimes mentioned – is not revealed by the ancient sources, but his adherence to the Herophilean rather than the Empiricist school suggests, first, that he did have a general pathological theory, and secondly, that it most likely was a humoral theory. It is also possible that the Empiricists' influential polemics against theorizing and, in particular, against causal hypotheses,[5] caused Demetrius to emphasize his individual clinical observations at the expense of a generalizable causal theory.

[1] See Chapter XIV, *Ba.*7–77, and Chapter XV, *Zn.*5–9.
[2] Cf. *DA.* 1–16.
[3] In *DA.*6 Caelius Aurelianus refers to Book XII of Demetrius' *On Affections*.
[4] See *DA.*1–3.   [5] See Chapter V.A.

Demetrius continued the gynaecological tradition initiated by Herophilus.[6] Like Herophilus, he devoted particular attention to the causes of difficult childbirth, attributing some cases to the parturient, others to the foetus, and still others to 'the passage through which birth occurs'.[7] Also extant are his views on inflammation of the uterus,[8] his differentiation between six kinds of vaginal discharge experienced by women,[9] and, on a heatedly debated topic, his statement that there are diseases peculiar to women.[10] The latter view is, of course, in direct contradiction to the assertion of Herophilus – and other Herophileans – that there are no diseases unique to women.[11] (As was suggested above, this is not the only instance of disagreement between Herophilus and his followers. Thus one of Herophilus' earliest pupils, Callimachus, ridiculed his explanation of a Hippocratic passage[12], and Herophilus' pulse theory was repeatedly modified and elaborated upon by subsequent Herophileans.[13])

It is striking that Demetrius' pathological interest seems to dominate the gynaecological texts, too,[14] whereas Herophilus had devoted at least as much attention to the anatomy of the female reproductive organs.

Along with the testimonia concerning Demetrius' views on the causes of abnormally difficult childbirth, on vaginal discharge, and on menstruation, his descriptions of priapism and satyriasis suggest that Demetrius followed the example of Herophilus and paid particular attention to the pathophysiology of the reproductive system. Priapism and satyriasis are both depicted as pathological

---

[6] For Herophilus' gynaecological views cf. above Chapter VI, Fr61 and T105–T114; Chapter VII, T193–T204 (see also Chapter VIII, T247).

[7] DA.21. Cf. also Chapter VII, T196, and Chapter XI, An.9, for the views of Herophilus and Andreas on difficult childbirth.

[8] DA.19.   [9] DA.17.   [10] DA.18.

[11] Chapter VII, T194. In agreement with Herophilus, and hence in disagreement with Demetrius, were two later Herophileans: Apollonius Mys and Alexander Philalethes. See Chapter XXII, AP.11, and Chapter XXIII, AM.7.

[12] Chapter XIII, Cm.9.

[13] For example, by Bacchius (Ba.2–3), Zeno (Zn.1–2), Chrysermus (Cr.1–2), Alexander Philalethes (AP.3–4), Heraclides of Erythrae (HE.2), Aristoxenus (Ar.1–2), and Apollonius Mys (AM.2). See pp. 446–8 supra.

[14] His observations are, as was pointed out above, on pathological conditions: inflammation of the uterus, six kinds of vaginal discharge (i.e. not only normal menstruation), abnormally difficult childbirth, and so on. Cf. DA.17–22.

states observed in older male patients; they are marked by 'a goading desire for sexual gratification' and by sustained, numb erections of the penis, lasting several months, from which no relief could be gained by masturbation.[15] While Herophilus seems to have been more interested in the anatomy and physiology of the sexual and reproductive organs than in their pathology, Demetrius does represent a significant continuation of this early Herophilean tradition.

A further emphasis emerges from the testimonia concerning Demetrius: therapeutics. Caelius Aurelianus from Numidia, a physician of the fifth century A.D. (who is, however, dependent on a much earlier Greek source, Soranus (c. A.D. 100)), is our main source for Demetrius, and he also provides the main therapeutic testimonium (concerning the treatment of sciatica and affections of the psoas by cauterization, plasters, and so on).[16] The treatment mentioned in the testimonium is, however, ascribed to 'the followers of Demetrius' (*Demetrii sectatores*) – perhaps Caelius Aurelianus' translation of an ambiguous Greek phrase such as οἱ περὶ Δημήτριον or οἱ ἀπὸ Δημητρίου – and it is possible that Demetrius himself was not the author of this treatment.

Another therapeutic testimonium is offered by Galen: Demetrius of Bithynia, he says, recommended applying borax, made up with hot wax, to persistent sores.[17] The qualifier 'of Bithynia' does not necessarily contradict the identification of the Herophilean with Demetrius of Apamea (see below), since there was a well known town called Apamea in Bithynia[18] (although Apamea on the Orontes river in Syria is better known). Other early Herophileans, e.g. Herophilus[19] and Callimachus,[20] came from Bithynia too, and if Galen's testimonium does in fact refer to the Herophilean, it would provide evidence that Herophilus' native region continued to contribute prominent medical scientists to the Herophilean school in Alexandria after the first generation.

That 'Demetrius the Herophilean' is identical with 'Demetrius of Apamea' seems assured by the fact that Caelius Aurelianus alterna-

---

[15] See *DA*.1–2.   [16] *DA*.23.   [17] *DA*. 24..
[18] On Apamea on the Propontis in Bithynia see Strabo, *Geography* 12.4.3 (563–4C); Pliny, *Natural History* 5.42.149; Appian, *Mithradatic Wars* 77 (= *Roman History* 12.11.77); *CIG* 3710–16; *CIL* III, 334–42; LeBas & Waddington, 1870: nos. 1124–39 (vol. III, part 1, pp. 290–1; vol. III, part 2, pp. 278–9).
[19] Cf. Chapter II, T1–3.   [20] Cf. Chapter XIII, Cm.2.

tely refers to Demetrius as a follower of Herophilus and as a native of Apamea. Thus, in his discussion of dropsy, Aurelianus first refers to him as 'sectator Herophili', only to revert to 'Demetrius Apameus' a few lines later, as though for the sake of *variatio*.[21] In his *Gynaecology*, Soranus likewise vacillates between 'Demetrius the Herophilean' and 'Demetrius of Apamea', and Caelius Aurelianus' variations undoubtedly go back at least to Soranus. (Despite the strong case that can be made for the identity of the Herophilean with the Apamean, it remains striking, however, that all three references to Demetrius' book *On Affections* or *On Diseases* (*De passionibus* or περὶ παθῶν) refer to the author only as 'the follower of Herophilus' or 'the Herophilean', not as 'the Apamean',[22] whereas the author of *Signs* or *Semiotics* (*Signa* or Σημειωτικόν) is identified exclusively as 'Demetrius of *Apamea*' – or simply as 'Demetrius' – but not as a Herophilean;[23] perhaps a faint doubt about equating the two would be appropriate.)

Demetrius' date can be determined only within very rough boundaries. Soranus implies that he lived after his Herophilean predecessor Andreas (who died in 217 B.C.).[24] If Galen's reference to 'Demetrius of Bithynia'[25] is in fact to the Herophilean, it would provide evidence that he lived before the Empiricist Heraclides of Tarentum (*floruit c.* A.D. 75[26]), inasmuch as Galen's source, Heraclides, quoted Demetrius.[27] This points roughly to some time between the later third century B.C. and the early first century B.C. as the period of Demetrius' literary activity.

B · TEXTS

1 Demetrius' *Signs* or *Semiotics*

DA.1   Caelius Aurelianus, *Tardae passiones* 5.9.89

---

[21] See *DA*.5 and *DA*.8, both drawn from the same continuous passage.
[22] Cf. *DA*.4–6.   [23] See *DA*.1–3.
[24] Soranus, *Gynaecia* 4.1[53].6–2[54].1 (*CMG* IV, p. 131 Ilberg): ὁ δὲ Ἀνδρέας ἐν τῷ Πρὸς Σωσίβιον . . . τοῖς ἀπὸ Ἡροφίλου συντίθεται μόνον προσθεὶς τὸ παραλελυμένον ἔμβρυον καὶ ἰσχνόν· . . . ὁ δὲ Ἡροφίλειος Δημήτριος ἀντιδιαστέλλεται τοῖς ῥηθεῖσι λέγων τὰ αἴτια τῆς δυστοκίας τὰ μὲν παρ' αὐτὴν εἶναι . . . Cf. Chapter XI, *An*.9; *DA*.21, *DA*.25.
[25] *DA*.24.
[26] On Heraclides, a renegade pupil of the Herophilean Mantias, see Deichgräber, 1965: fr. 168–248 and pp. 258–62.
[27] *DA*.24.

DA.2   Caelius Aurelianus, *Celeres vel acutae passiones* 3.18.178–9
DA.3   Soranus, *Gynaecia* 2.55[124].1 (*CMG* IV, p. 91 Ilberg); cf. M.F. and
         I.E. Drabkin, 1951: 61

2 *General Pathology*

(a) *On Diseases*

DA.4   Caelius Aurelianus, *Celeres vel acutae passiones* 1, praef. 4–5.
         See above, Chapter VII, T211.
DA.5   Caelius Aurelianus, *Tardae passiones* 3.8.99
DA.6   Caelius Aurelianus, *Cel. vel acut.* 2.25.141

(b) From unidentified work(s)

DA.7   Caelius Aurelianus, *Cel. vel acut.* 3.5.55
DA.8   Caelius Aurelianus, *Tardae passiones* 3.8.102
DA.9   Soranus, *De signis fracturarum* 9 (*CMG* IV, p. 156 Ilberg)
DA.10 Caelius Aurelianus, *Cel. vel acut.* 2.33.173
DA.11 Caelius Aurelianus, *Tardae passiones* 2.10.122–3
DA.12 Caelius Aurelianus, *Cel. vel acut.* 2.1.4
DA.13 Caelius Aurelianus, *Cel. vel acut.* 3.11.106
DA.14 Caelius Aurelianus, *Tardae passiones* 1.5.150
DA.15 Caelius Aurelianus, *Cel. vel acut.* 3.7.71–72
DA.16 Caelius Aurelianus, *Tardae passiones* 2.2.64

3 *Gynaecology*

DA.17 Soranus, *Gynaecia* 3.43 (*CMG* IV, p. 122 Ilberg). Cf. Drabkin, 1951:
         87–8; Chapter VII, T203–T204 *supra*
DA.18 Soranus, *Gynaecia* 3.2 (*CMG* IV, p. 94 Ilberg)
         See above, Chapter VII, T193–T195.
DA.19 Soranus, *Gynaecia* 3.19 (*CMG* IV, p. 106 Ilberg)
DA.20 Soranus, *Gynaecia* 4.1[53] (*CMG* IV, p. 129 Ilberg)
DA.21 Soranus, *Gynaecia* 4.2[54] (*CMG* IV, pp. 131.8–132.4 Ilberg). Cf.
         DA.25.
DA.22 Papyrus Coll. Goleniščev (Pack² 2347), col. III 3–5 (see Bäck-
         ström, 1906; Marganne, 1981: 61–2)

4 *Therapeutics*

DA.23 Caelius Aurelianus, *Tardae passiones* 5.1.21–2
DA.24 Heraclides Tarentinus apud Galenum, *De compositione medicamen-*
         torum per genera 4.7 (XIII, p. 722K)

Dubia

DA.25   Soranus, *Gynaecia* 4.2[54]–5[57] (*CMG* IV, pp. 132.4–134.26
         Ilberg)
DA.26   Erotianus, *Vocum Hippocraticarum collectio*, praefatio (p. 5 Nachman-
         son)
DA.27   *Pap. Enteux.* 69.1 (Guéraud, 1931–2: 171)

XVII · HEGETOR
(*Hg.*)

A · INTRODUCTION

Only three undisputed, unequivocal ancient references to the Herophilean Hegetor are extant: Marcellinus' quotation of Hegetor's definition of the pulse; Galen's passing allusion to Hegetor's pulse theory; and an intriguing quotation from Hegetor's treatise *On Causes*, preserved by an Alexandrian Empiricist, Apollonius of Citium. Apollonius' lengthy attempt to refute Hegetor[1] does not throw much light on Hegetor's views, but the quotation offered by Apollonius (*Hg*.3) suffices to confirm that a fundamental disagreement between the Alexandrian Empiricists and the followers of Herophilus continued to lie in their theories of scientific method.[2] It also reveals that Hegetor believed that clinical medicine, in particular surgery, could be greatly improved by a knowledge of anatomy. Hegetor is quoted as arguing that the Empiricists could have avoided some of the surgical difficulties they were experiencing if only 'they had understood the cause on the basis of anatomy' (*Hg*.3).

In this context it is important to remember that the Empiricists, at whom Hegetor throws down the gauntlet in *On Causes*, rejected Herophilus' emphasis on dissection and physiology (see above, Chapter x.A). The physician, they argued, needs to know only which treatment is efficacious for each disease, and not why it is efficacious – let alone what caused the disease. The fragment from Hegetor's *On Causes* contains many resonances of this feud. His allusions, in part ironic, to the Empiricists' facile recourse to analogy, to their anti-

---

[1] Apollonius Citiensis, *In Hp. De articulis comment.* 3 (*CMG* xi.1.1, pp. 78–94 Kudlien/ Kollesch).

[2] On the methodological tripod of the Empiricists see von Staden, 1975: Part iii; and Deichgräber, 1965: 291–305. See also Chapter v.A above, and cf. Chapter x.A and Chapter x n.1.

aetiological stance and their consequent failure to discover the causes of particular disorders, to their use of 'what happens more frequently' (i.e. their use of statistical differentiation at the expense of causal theory), and his own insistence that only an understanding of causes (in this case based on anatomy) could resolve certain apparently insoluble problems which beset the practising surgeon – all of these are clear reverberations of this protracted Alexandrian feud between Empiricists and 'rationalists' such as the Herophileans.

About the date of Hegetor we cannot be sure. The earliest of our three sources, Apollonius (first century B.C.), provides a useful *terminus ante quem*. Apollonius' attack on Hegetor does not, however, necessarily guarantee that they were contemporaries or near contemporaries. Furthermore, the fact that Apollonius' other main target, the Empiricist Heraclides of Tarentum (against whose criticisms of an early Herophilean, Bacchius, Apollonius wrote a treatise in eighteen books),[3] was a contemporary of Apollonius, does not provide a firm basis for assuming that Hegetor also must have been his contemporary. Here, too, the chronology of ancient medicine remains shrouded in uncertainty.

Jutta Kollesch has tried to provide a further quotation from Hegetor by emending one of the pseudo-Galenic *Definitions* (*Hg.* 4).[4] The context and content of the pseudo-Galenic passage seem to lend some support to her emendation: first, the quotation she ascribes to Hegetor is a definition of rhythm, a concept of which Herophilus, too, had given a definition in his work *On Pulses*.[5] Second, the definition Dr Kollesch ascribes to Hegetor is preceded by definitions of rhythm unequivocally identified as by other Herophileans (Bacchius and Zeno[6]), and this suggests that the entire chapter (*Definitiones medicae* 220) might have been drawn from a source that enumerated Herophilean definitions of rhythm. Third, Zeno's definition is almost identical with the one assigned to Hegetor (who only substitutes *schesis*, 'relation' or 'condition', for *taxis*, 'order' or 'orderly arrangement'), and such close affinity is more likely to exist between two Herophileans than between Zeno and a non-Herophilean. Further-

---

[3] Erotian, *Vocum Hippocraticarum collectio*, praef. (p. 5 Nachmanson); see Chapter XIV, *Ba.* 13.

[4] Kollesch, 1973: 73, n. 44.

[5] Cf. Chapter VII, T172; Chapter VII n. 134.

[6] Chapter XIV, *Ba.* 3; Chapter XV, *Zn.* 2.

more, it is not uncharacteristic of Herophileans to accept the general outlines of their Herophilean predecessors' definitions while insisting on altering or adding single phrases or words.[7] Finally, Hegetor's interest in pulse lore is independently attested.[8] All in all, then, there is much to support Kollesch's emendation, but insufficient knowledge of the MSS tradition seems to render the inclusion of *Hg*.4 only on a provisional basis (as a *Dubium*) advisable.

B · TEXTS

Hg.1   Marcellinus, *De pulsibus* 3 (p. 457 Schöne)
Hg.2   Galenus, *De pulsuum dignotione* 4.3 (VIII, p. 955K).
         See above, Chapter VII, T162.
Hg.3   Apollonius Citiensis, *In Hippocratis De articulis comment.* 3 (*CMG* XI.1.1, pp. 78–80 et 94 Kollesch/Kudlien)

Dubium

Hg.4   Ps.-Galenus, *Definitiones medicae* 220 (XIX, p. 409K).
         See J. Kollesch, 1973: p. 73 n. 44 and p. 137 n. 183.

[7] See Chapter X.A for examples from Herophilean sphygmology.
[8] *Hg*. 2.

XVIII · MANTIAS

(*Ma.*)

A · INTRODUCTION

Although pharmacological observations predate Mantias (*c.* 165–90 B.C.)[1] by several milennia, he is repeatedly referred to in antiquity as the first great writer on compound drugs.[2] Galen, for example, characterizes him as 'the first person I know of to have recorded compounds of very many drugs that are worth recommending',[3] as 'the first to record many drugs',[4] and also as 'not being among the physicians of little consequence'.[5] Herophilus too had produced prescriptions for compound drugs and had taken a strong interest in clinical medicine (Chapter VIII), thereby providing Mantias' pharmacological activity with the sanction of the founding master.

Mantias' apparent concentration on pharmacology and on clinical problems might render him virtually indistinguishable from his Empiricist rivals, but Galen reports that 'Mantias, who had been a Herophilean from the outset, remained one throughout', whereas

[1] The floruit of his pupil, Heraclides of Tarentum (see *Ma.*1–2), namely *c.* 85–75 B.C. (cf. Deichgräber, 1965: 172, 258ff.), provides a *terminus ante quem*. If Mantias' compound for upset stomachs, known as 'Attalus' remedy' (*Ma.*9), was given this name in honour of Attalus III – a dubious honour, it seems – as Wellmann (1913: 38 n. 1) and Kind (1928) argue, we have a further significant chronological clue: Attalus III (Philometor Euergetes) ruled in Pergamum from 138–133 B.C. A king whose 'short reign was famous only for its dénouement' (G. T. Griffith, *OCD*), Attalus might have been happy to have a prescription for upset stomach named after him. (Cf. also the *Attalium medicamentum* in Celsus, *Medicina* 5.19.11 and 6.6.5 (*CML* I, pp. 202, 262 Marx).) But the views of Wellmann and Kind are purely speculative. P. M. Fraser's suggestion (1972: vol. I, p. 358) that Mantias belongs 'to the *early* part of the second century' B.C. is not compatible with a floruit of *c.* 75 B.C. for his pupil Heraclides of Tarentum.

[2] I stress *compound* drugs, since Galen emphasizes that many *simple* drugs had been recorded before the time of Mantias; cf. *Ma.*8. See also Ch. VIII.A and T248a–T259 *supra.*

[3] *Ma.*1. [4] Cf. *Ma.*6: Mantias *and* his pupils. [5] *Ma.*4.

Mantias' pupil, Heraclides of Tarentum, followed the example of Philinus of Cos, a student of Herophilus, and became an Empiricist.[6] Galen's sharp distinction between Herophilean teacher and Empiricist pupil suggests that Mantias continued adhering to teachings that were distinctively Herophilean, even if these were not given expression in the writings that made him famous.

At least two treatises by Mantias are referred to by title. One is *Dynameis* or *Drug Remedies*,[7] the other *Druggist or In the Physician's Office*.[8] The first is probably the source of most of our information concerning Mantias' pharmacological efforts, although the second also contained drug prescriptions (for example, one for sores which heal with difficulty).[9] Galen also attributes individual pharmacological books 'on purgatives, on draughts, on clysters', and 'on remedies according to place' (i.e. topical drugs) to Mantias.[10] It is unclear whether these are to be understood as two or more entirely distinct treatises[11] or as individual books of the larger treatise called *Dynameis*. The latter view – that they are parts of a larger work – would not necessarily be incompatible with Galen's forceful distinction between Dioscurides' comprehensive collection of all drugs in five books and Mantias' specialized presentations; Galen's point is that Dioscurides' massive treatise differs sharply from the book(s) attributed to Mantias, in so far as Dioscurides does not present remedies according to Mantias' limited classificatory scheme but produces a far more comprehensive collection. Whichever view is correct, Mantias' pharmacological work (or cluster of works) formed the basis of his claim to fame in antiquity. In addition to Galen, the earlier pharmacologists Asclepiades the Younger ('*Pharmakion*') and Heras – both of whom Galen used as sources – found Mantias' drug remedies worthy of transmission.

Mantias' pharmacological work(s) probably did not only offer prescriptions but also contained at least some discussion of the symptoms, and perhaps the causes, of the ailments for which various prescriptions were recommended. This seems to be indicated by

[6] *Ma.*2. On Philinus see Chapter ii, T1; also Deichgräber, 1965: fr. 6 and pp. 163, 254–5.
[7] Cf. *Ma.*9.   [8] Cf. *Ma.*10; *Ma.*15–16.   [9] *Ma.*10.   [10] *Ma.*3.
[11] This seems to be the view of Kind, 1928. Wellmann ap. Susemihl, 1891–2: vol. i, 825) is more explicit: he regards τὰ κατὰ τόπους and περὶ καθαρτικῆς ἢ προποτισμῶν ἢ κλυσμῶν as two – not four – different treatises, a view which reflects Galen's turns of phrase (*Ma.*3) more closely.

Galen's statement, in a pharmacological context, that 'Mantias *explained what kind of affection* inflammation of the uvula is'.[12] But such passages are the exception; as a rule, the emphasis seems to have been on the remedies themselves.

Parts of Mantias' second major treatise, *Druggist or In the Physician's Office*,[13] contained drug prescriptions,[14] but other sections were apparently modelled after the Hippocratic work with roughly the same title, κατ' ἰητρεῖον, perhaps best known in English as *In the Surgery*. Practical advice concerning bandaging and other problems encountered by a general practitioner were probably the subjects dealt with in the 'Hippocratic' section of the work.[15] It is here that Mantias may also have presented his positive views on the value of bloodletting,[16] which had been advocated as a therapeutic measure from the time of the Hippocratic Corpus and was adopted by Herophilus too.

Two further areas interested Mantias: regimen,[17] about which no specific details have survived, and gynaecology. The latter is represented by two texts.[18] One deals with 'hysterical suffocation',[19] i.e. a condition characterized by obstructed respiration, loss of speech, a seizure of the senses, clenching of the teeth, bulging veins on the face, and convulsive contractions of the extremities.[20] It was called 'hysterical' because of the belief that it was caused by an abnormal condition of the uterus (*hystera*), due to premature birth,

---

[12] *Ma.*5. Michler, 1968: 103, suggests that Mantias operated for this illness, but Galen attributes only a description and an explanation of the disease to Mantias.

[13] In view of the discrepancy in title between *Ma.*10 and *Ma.*15–16, there is a possibility that we are dealing with two works by Mantias: (a) *On Things Pertaining to the Physician's Office*, and (b) *The Druggist In The Physician's Office* or, reading Kind's conjecture ἤ for ὁ in *Ma.*10, *Druggist or In The Physician's Office*. (Michler (1968: 103) accepts Kind's emendation, but there do not seem to be compelling reasons for rejecting the traditional reading.) In all likelihood these were not different works, however; confusion and uncertainty about the exact titles of works by no means was rare in antiquity. Cf. C. Fabricius, 1972: 199.

[14] *Ma.*10.

[15] *Ma.*15–16; cf. *Ma.*14, which is, however, from a pseudo-Galenic forgery.

[16] *Ma.*13.

[17] Cf. *Ma.*1: Heraclides imitates Mantias 'also in the part of the art which concerns *regimen*'.

[18] *Ma.*11–12.   [19] *Ma.*11.

[20] For ancient views on hysterical suffocation see, e.g., Soranus, *Gynaecia* 3.4.26–29 (*CMG* IV, pp. 109–13 Ilberg); Hp., *Diseases of Women* 2.123–130 (VIII, pp. 266–78L).

long widowhood, retention of menses, etc.[21] But Mantias, perhaps characteristically, seems to have been less interested in its aetiology and its symptoms than in ways of curing it, and the only details explicitly attributed to him are therapeutic: after an attack he prescribed a drink of castor and bitumen with wine; when an attack of hysterical suffocation was imminent, he ordered the playing of flutes and beating of drums, perhaps in recognition of the psychosomatic nature of the disorder. The other gynaecological-obstetrical testimonium is again therapeutic in emphasis: how to expel afterbirth which, after parturition, has been retained within.[22]

B · TEXTS

Ma.1   Galenus, *De compositione medicamentorum per genera* 2.1 (XIII, p. 462K)

Ma.2   Galenus, *De compositione medicamentorum secundum locos* 6.9 (XII, p. 989K)

Ma.3   Galenus, *De simplicium medicamentorum temperamentis ac facultatibus* 6. prooem. (XI, pp. 794–5K)

Ma.4   Galenus, *De compositione medicamentorum secundum locos* 2.1 (XII, p. 534K)

Ma.5   Galenus, *ibid.*, 6.8 (XII, p. 972K)

Ma.6   Galenus, *De compositione medicamentorum per genera* 2.5 (XIII, p. 502K)

Ma.7   Galenus, *ibid.*, 3.9 (XIII, p. 642K)

Ma.8   Galenus, *De compositione medicamentorum secundum locos* 7.1 (XIII, p. 13K)

Ma.9   Asclepiades Iunior apud Galenum, *ibid.*, 8.3 (XIII, pp. 162–3K)

Ma.10 Heras apud Galenum, *De compositione medicamentorum per genera* 4.14 (XIII, pp. 751–2K)

Ma.11 Soranus, *Gynaecia* 3.4.29 (*CMG* IV, p. 112 Ilberg)

Ma.12 Soranus, *Gynaecia* 4.14[1.71].5 (*CMG* IV, p. 145 Ilberg)

Ma.13 Galenus, *De venae sectione adversus Erasistratum* 5 (XI, p. 163K)

Ma.14 Ps.-Galenus, *De fasciis* 1 (XVIIIA, p. 770K)

Ma.15 Galenus, *In Hippocratis De medici officina comment.* 1, praefatio (XVIIIB, pp. 629–30K)

Ma.16 Galenus, *ibid.*, 1.5 (XVIIIB, p. 666K)

---

[21] Soranus, *ibid.*

[22] *Ma.*12. This is a problem which evoked much discussion in antiquity, e.g. by Euryphon, Euenor, Sostratus, Apollonius of Prusa, Dio, the Erasistratean Strato, and Soranus; cf. Soranus, *Gynaecia* 4.14 [1.71] – 4.16 [1.73] (*CMG* IV, pp. 144–6). On terminological difficulties concerning 'afterbirth' in Greek texts cf. Kudlien, 1964d. See also Michler, 1968: 103.

XIX · DIOSCURIDES PHACAS
(Ds.)

A · INTRODUCTION

The physician Dioscurides (*Ds.*), nicknamed 'Phakas' because of the moles or warts (*phakoi*) on his face,[1] is identified as an adherent of the Herophilean school by Galen.[2] Four ancient sources – Julius Caesar, Galen, Paul of Aegina, and the *Suda* – also refer to a Dioscurides who resided in Alexandria,[3] and one of them – the *Suda* – implies that the Alexandrian Dioscurides is in fact Dioscurides Phacas. The general consensus of modern scholars has been that the other references are to the Herophilean physician as well, and there are good chronological and biographical reasons for accepting this conclusion.[4] Dioscurides therefore provides strong evidence of the continuing presence of the Herophilean school at Alexandria in the first century B.C., and of its remarkable durability amidst the political and social vicissitudes that marked the history of science and scholarship in Alexandria.

There is intriguing evidence that Dioscurides, unlike most Herophilean physicians, developed a close and colourful association with the Ptolemaic court during the reigns of Auletes and his famous but rancorous children, Ptolemy XIII and Cleopatra. The *Suda*, an encyclopedic lexicon of *c.* A.D. 1000, reports that Dioscurides Phacas 'was associated with Cleopatra at the time of Antony',[5] and Caesar characterizes Dioscurides as a very influential adviser and ambassa-

---

[1] *Ds.*1.   [2] *Ds.*3.   [3] *Ds.*2, *Ds.*6, *Ds.*7, *Ds.*1.

[4] Cf. Wellmann, 1905b; *id.*, ap. Susemihl, 1891–2: vol. II, pp. 443–4; Kudlien, 1967c; Fraser, 1972: vol. I, pp. 367 and 372, vol. II, pp. 543 (n. 268) and 547–8 (nn. 303–5). A notable exception is Münzer, 1903, who regards the Dioscurides mentioned by Caesar (*Ds.*2) as an entirely different person. See also the discussion by Heinen, 1966: 103–4. The *Suda* says he is from Anazarbus – a confusion with Pedanius Dsc.? – but places him in Cleopatra's Alexandrian company.

[5] *Ds.*1.

dor of both Auletes and his son Ptolemy XIII.[6] This makes Dioscurides the only Herophilean besides Andreas for whom an association with the Alexandrian court is explicitly attested. For both physicians it was an association which, however, led to violent – and, at least in one case, successful – attempts on their lives.[7]

Although the identification of the 'Dioscurides' mentioned in all the texts which follow with the Herophilean remains only probable at best, the combined weight of the evidence suggests that Dioscurides was active primarily in the first half of the first century B.C. Auletes, whom Dioscurides had represented in Rome at one time, ruled roughly from 80 to 51 B.C., and the disastrous, perhaps fatal, mission which Dioscurides undertook on behalf of Auletes' son Ptolemy XIII[8] probably took place in early November 48 B.C. This points to a floruit no later than the mid first century B.C.

If Caesar's account is interpreted – as it usually is – to imply that Dioscurides was killed in November 48 B.C., while on a mission as Ptolemy XIII's emissary, the *Suda*'s apparent claim that he was a close associate of Cleopatra 'at the time of Antony' becomes problematic, inasmuch as Cleopatra's affair with Antony did not start until 41 B.C. Caesar's depiction of the events of 48 B.C. is, however, open to a different interpretation. Talking about Dioscurides and Serapion, the two representatives whom Ptolemy XIII sent to Achillas, Caesar says: 'One of them, after being wounded, was seized by his own people and carried away *as if* he were dead; the other was killed.'[9] It is therefore possible that Dioscurides survived the attempt on his life. If he did survive, the man whom Caesar describes as 'one of the most influential members of Ptolemy's inner circle' may well have had the political finesse and instinct to re-emerge in an influential role at the court when the relation between Cleopatra and Antony blossomed (41–30 B.C.). In that case, Caesar's evidence would in fact be compatible with the statement in the *Suda*. This conclusion remains predicated, however, upon the uncertain though plausible assumption that Caesar and the *Suda* are both referring to Dioscurides the Herophilean.

Rufus of Ephesus reports that a Posidonius and a Dioscurides were contemporaries,[10] and this statement has naturally tantalized those

---

[6] *Ds.*2.   [7] Cf. Chapter xi, *An.*1; Chapter xx.A.   [8] *Ds.*2.   [9] *Ibid.*
[10] *Ds.*8. Cf. Edelstein & Kidd, 1972: T113; Theiler, 1982: vol. ii, p. 414.

who have sought for clues to the Herophilean's date. Although it would make excellent chronological sense to assert that the Stoic philosopher Posidonius (c. 135–50 B.C.) and the Herophilean physician Dioscurides lived at the same time,[11] Rufus neither identifies Posidonius as the Stoic nor refers to Dioscurides as 'Phacas' or 'the Herophilean'. Furthermore, no ancient testimonium concerning the Herophilean confirms the rest of Rufus' statement, i.e. that Dioscurides and Posidonius both wrote on the 'bubonic' plague which had struck Libya. Tempting though it would be to use this testimonium as confirmation of Dioscurides' date and of his association with North Africa, the uncertainty concerning the identity of both 'Posidonius' and 'Dioscurides' renders advisable the inclusion of this text among the *Dubia*.

With the exception of the *Suda*'s reference to Dioscurides' twenty-four books on medicine,[12] all that is known with certainty about the Herophilean's medical interests is that he, like most Herophileans, engaged in Hippocratic exegesis. Thus the famous Neronian author of an Hippocratic glossary, Erotian, reports that Dioscurides wrote a polemical work in seven books on Hippocratic lexicography and quotes from it one of Dioscurides' glosses.[13] Galen, too, mentions a Hippocratic gloss by 'Dioscurides of Alexandria', and Paul of Aegina, a Byzantine medical encyclopedist of the seventh century, quotes 'Dioscurides the Alexandrian's' explanation of a Hippocratic word which had provoked comment by a number of other ancient commentators as well.[14]

The *Suda*'s mention of Dioscurides' 'twenty-four books, all medical and renowned'[15] clearly implies, however, that the Herophilean did not merely engage in Hippocratic scholarship. The fragment transmitted by Paul of Aegina, though perhaps derived from an exegetical context, also includes therapeutic measures,[16] and if Rufus' problematic testimony is in fact about the Herophilean physician, it would indicate an interest in close clinical observation as well. These interests would be consonant with two of the main emphases which emerged within the Herophilean school soon after Herophilus' death, as pointed out above: Hippocratic exegesis and clinical medicine.

---

[11] Kudlien, 1967c, identifies Posidonius with the Stoic philosopher, and Dioscurides with the Herophilean physician. But cf. *id.*, 1962: especially 428–9, and previous n.

[12] *Ds.*1.   [13] *Ds.*4–5.   [14] See *Ds.*6–7.   [15] *Ds.*1.

[16] *Ds.*7 (terebinth-like swellings *and* their treatment).

B · TEXTS

*Ds.*1   Suda, Δ .1206 (s.v. *Dioskorides*) (II, p. 113 Adler)

*Ds.*2   C. Julius Caesar, *De bello civili* 3.109.3–6

*Ds.*3   Galenus(?), *Explanatio vocum Hippocratis*, prooem. (XIX, p. 63K)

*Ds.*4   Erotianus, *Vocum Hippocraticarum collectio* φ.5 (p. 91 Nachmanson):
φωναὶ κατείλλουσαι

*Ds.*5   Erotianus, *ibid.*, praefatio (p. 5 Nachmanson)

*Ds.*6   Galenus(?), *Explanatio vocum Hippocratis*, s.v. *Indikon* (XIX, p. 105K).
See also above, Chapter XI, *An.*37.

*Ds.*7   Paulus Aegineta, 4.24 (*CMG* IX.1, p. 345 Heiberg)

Dubium

*Ds.*8   Rufus Ephesius, *De externis passionibus*, apud Oribasium, *Collectiones medicae* 44.14.2 (*CMG* VI.2.1 = vol. III, p. 132 Raeder)

XX · CHRYSERMUS

(*Cr.*)

A · INTRODUCTION

The distinguished upper-class Alexandrian family of the Chrysermi, perhaps of Thracian origin,[1] was close to the Ptolemaic court from the third century B.C. onward. They are found in strikingly diverse and influential roles. Thus Plutarch in his account of the Alexandrian sojourn of the idealistic Spartan king Cleomenes III in 222 B.C. describes Ptolemaeus, son of a certain Chrysermus, as a friend of Ptolemy Euergetes I.[2] Another member of the family is listed with an extraordinary accumulation of what appear to be Ptolemaic honours[3] in an inscription of the second century B.C. from the island of Delos:[4] 'Chrysermus of Alexandria, son of Heraclitus, kinsman of

---

[1] An inscription with a list of victors in the βασίλεια from the *chora*, perhaps Heracleopolis, lists a Χρύσερμος Ἀμαδόκου Θρᾶιξ, 'Chrysermus of Thrace, son of Amadocus' (*Tit. Cair. ined.*, of the year 268/7 B.C.). The name Chrysermus and names of similar formation are, however, generally thought to be Ionian; cf. J. & L. Robert, 1965: 203; Daux, 1967: 492 ('très ionienne'). Cf. also Bechtel, 1917: 166, 164; Sittig, 1911: 111–16, on Chrysermus and related 'Hermes names'.

[2] Plutarch, *Life of Cleomenes* 57 (36).2: 'Ptolemaeus, the son of Chrysermus, a friend of the king's, had shown a decent civility to Cleomenes all this time . . .'

[3] Although the inscription suggests a Ptolemaic context, especially with the identification of Chrysermus as an Alexandrian, there were many *mouseia* in the Greek world (cf. Fraser, 1972: vol. I, pp. 312–14). Furthermore, at least two of the titles in this Delian inscription (ἐπὶ τῶν ἰατρῶν and ἐπιστάτης τοῦ Μουσείου) do not occur in any of the Egyptian evidence. See below, nn. 4, 6 and 7.

[4] *Inscriptions de Délos*, ed. P. Roussel and M. Launey (Paris, 1937), no. 1525 (p. 35) = *Orientis Graeci Inscriptiones Selectae*, vol. I (ed. W. Dittenberger (Berlin, 1903), no. 104 (pp. 181–2):
Χρύσερμον Ἡρακλείτου Ἀλεξανδρέα
τὸν συγγενῆ βασιλέως Πτολεμαίου
καὶ ἐξηγητὴν καὶ ἐπὶ τῶν ἰατρῶν
καὶ ἐπιστάτην τοῦ Μουσείου . . .

King Ptolemy, Exegete,[5] Superintendent of Physicians,[6] Administrator of the Museum[7] . . .'. Similarly, a Chrysermus is mentioned in Egyptian papyri of 243 B.C. as holding a high legal office,[8] and another (or possibly the same one) is mentioned, also in Egyptian papyri, as an eponymous commander in 222/1 B.C.[9] Even the children seem to have excelled: in an Egyptian inscription[10] a young Chrysermus – perhaps identical with one of the above mentioned – is listed as the winner of a boxing contest for boys in 268/7 B.C., in games

[5] On the magistracy called that of the 'exegete' cf. Strabo, *Geographica* 17.1.12 (797C): 'Among the local officials of the city are the exegete, who wears a purple robe and possesses hereditary honours and has the responsibility for the public services in the city; the *hypomnematographos* [recorder; scriba publicus?]; the *archidikastēs* [chief judge]; and in the fourth place the night commander. These offices, then also existed in the time of the kings [sc. Ptolemies] . . .' Cf. also *Sammelb.* 2100 (mid-first century B.C.; see Fraser, 1972: vol. II, p. 193 n. 94 for an account of a different view of its date); *Prosopographia Ptolemaica* (Peremans and van't Dack) 5349–50 (= *Sammelb.* 6669). See also Fraser, 1972: vol. I, pp. 96–7.

[6] ἐπὶ τῶν ἰατρῶν. The exact implications of this designation remain unclear. Whether it means that Chrysermus was responsible for all medical services in Ptolemaic Egypt, or only in charge of the doctors in Alexandria, or only in charge of the doctors in the Museum, or of the court physicians, is uncertain. It is also unclear whether he himself was a physician or an administrator without medical qualifications. The relation of the title ἐπὶ τῶν ἰατρῶν to the titles ἀρχιατρός (*archiatros*) and βασιλικὸς ἰατρός, 'Royal Physician', is likewise uncertain. Cf. *Sammelb.* 5216, a papyrus describing the *archiatros* Athenagoras' authority over native Egyptian mummy-dressers and priests of Fâyyum in the question of the release of a body. For 'Royal Physician' see Wilcken, 1927–37: vol. II. 1, no. 162, col. II line 26 (p. 62); Rostovtzeff, 1953: vol. II p. 1093; Sudhoff, 1909: 258. See also Woodhead, 1952: 241 (Chrysermus was 'Minister of Health'); and Rostovtzeff, 1953: vol. II, p. 1091. On later developments in the use of *archiatros* (both for 'royal physician' and for 'civic physician'), see Nutton, 1977. Cf. Ch. XXIII, n. 52.

[7] ἐπιστάτης τοῦ Μουσείου, '*epistatēs* of the Museum', is a title which does not recur in the Egyptian evidence, although Strabo (*Geographica* 17.1.8; 794C) reports there was a ἱερεὺς ὁ ἐπὶ τῷ Μουσείῳ, τεταγμένος τότε μὲν ὑπὸ τῶν βασιλέων ('a priest in charge of the Museum, who in those days was appointed by the kings . . .'). The native temples of Egypt also each had an *epistatēs* or supervisor appointed by the Ptolemaic rulers; they were distinct from the regular priesthood and functioned primarily as administrators (and tax collectors); cf. Otto, 1905–8: vol. I, pp. 38–52 ('Vorsteher der Tempel'); Evans, 1962: 200–3; Cumont, 1937: 114–16; Wilcken, 1927–37: vol. I, pp. 44ff.; Rostovtzeff, 1953: vol. I, p. 282. The *epistatēs* of the Museum might likewise have had primarily administrative functions, as Fraser (1972: vol. I, p. 316) suggests, and is therefore perhaps not identical with the priest mentioned by Strabo.

[8] *P. Cair. Zen.* 59355, lines 107, 114, 124; *ibid.*, 59356, line 9. Cf. *P. Enteux.* 8, line 2.

[9] *P. Enteux.* 8, line 2; cf. *Papiri greci et latini* 513, line 12, of the year 252/1 B.C

[10] *Tit. Cair. Ined.* (268/7 B.C.); cf. n. 1 above. A later example (A.D. 125–6) of a Chrysermus in Egypt is *P. Oxy.* 3557.1–11.

commemorating the birthday of Ptolemy II Philadelphus. It is probably to this accomplished and influential family that the Herophilean physician belonged.

There is, however, no evidence that Chrysermus the Herophilean was also associated with the Ptolemaic court. The above-mentioned Delian inscription, on a statue base set up at Delos to honour a Chrysermus who was 'superintendent' or 'overseer'[11] of the physicians, cannot refer to the Herophilean, since it belongs to the second century B.C.[12], whereas the Herophilean's floruit probably lies no earlier than the mid first century B.C., as I argue below. The only physicians known to have associated closely with the Ptolemaic court in the Herophilean's own time are Zopyrus of Alexandria,[13] Apollonius of Citium[14] (both Empiricists), Dioscurides Phacas the Herophilean (see Chapter XIX, Ds.1–2), and the young medical apprentice Philotas of Amphissa, to whom Plutarch's glittering depiction of Alexandria in his Life of Antony is considerably indebted.[15] Chrysermus the Herophilean is not mentioned in the context of the court by any of the ancient sources, and while arguments from silence are problematic, it seems reasonable to conclude provisionally that he followed the example of most Herophilean physicians and kept his distance from the vicissitudes which rendered life at the Ptolemaic court insecure for many.[16]

The best evidence concerning Chrysermus' date is the fact that he was a teacher of the famous Heraclides of Erythrae (Cr.1), whom Strabo (c. 64 B.C.–23 A.D.) describes as a contemporary.[17] If Strabo

[11] See n. 7 above on epistatēs.

[12] The exact date is uncertain, but it seems to belong to the second half of the second century B.C. P. M. Fraser's vacillation is indicative of the chronological uncertainties: 'c. 125 B.C.' (1972: vol. II, p. 180 n. 31 and p. 192 n. 89); 'about 170 B.C.' (vol. I, p. 105); 'middle or later part of the second century B.C.' (vol. I, p. 316); cf. also vol. II, p. 547 n. 297.

[13] Apollonius of Citium, In Hp. De articulis comm. I (CMG XI.1.1, p. 12 Kollesch/ Kudlien); Celsus, Med. 5.23.2 (CML I, p. 210 Marx).

[14] Ibid., pp. 10, 38, 64 (at the start of each of the three books comprising Apollonius' commentary).

[15] Plutarch, Life of Antony 28.

[16] Cf. the examples of Andreas (Chapter XI, An.1) and Dioscurides (Chapter XIX, Ds.2.)

[17] Strabo, Geographica 14.1.34 (645C) = Chapter XXIV (below), HE 1. Cf. Ch. XXI, n. 13.

can be trusted[18], Chrysermus' floruit probably lies in the mid first century B.C. or slightly later. Strabo also describes Heraclides as a 'fellow-pupil' of another famous Herophilean physician of the latter half of the first century B.C., Apollonius Mys,[19] and it therefore seems sensible to infer Chrysermus was Apollonius' teacher as well. Since Heraclides and Apollonius are the only two prominent Alexandrian Herophileans of the second half of the first century B.C. – the others, notably Alexander and Zeuxis, were associated with the Herophilean school in Laodicea, not with Alexandria – and since both were apparently Chrysermus' students, Chrysermus was probably the leading Herophilean physician, and perhaps the leading physician-scientist, of his generation in Alexandria.[20] Like his fellow-Herophilean Dioscurides Phacas,[21] he would therefore have been an eminent figure of the reigns of Auletes and Cleopatra; but whereas Dioscurides developed close (and, for him, possibly disastrous) ties with the Crown, Chrysermus apparently remained truer to the mainstream of the Herophilean tradition, devoting himself to pedagogic, theoretical, and clinical objectives rather than to political ties and tasks.

Most of the extant details of Chrysermus' medical views concern his pulse theory (Cr. 1–2; cf. Cr.3), an emphasis which is, of course, hardly surprising in the case of an Herophilean. He did not, however, simply receive and transmit the sphygmological views of Herophilus and other earlier Herophileans but, as Galen makes clear (Cr.1–2), amplified and modified previous definitions of the pulse, in particular through his inclusion of the 'psychic and vital faculty' as the agent of pulsation. Unfortunately Chrysermus' arguments for this elaboration (which subsequent Herophileans such as Aristoxenus censured as superfluous) are not extant, and its exact purpose therefore remains shrouded in uncertainty. It might, however, be an elaboration of Herophilus' view that the arteries have their own power or faculty (dynamis) of pulsation, which is not an independent, arterial, physiological tendency but which the arteries receive from the

---

[18] Strabo tends to use the phrase 'in my time' (kath' hēmas) within rather expansive limits. See D. Wyttenbach in Bake, 1810: 263–4, and Mariotti, 1966: 40, 21 ff.

[19] Chapter XXIII (below), AM 1 (= Strabo, loc. cit.).

[20] In addition to the traditional association of the Chrysermi with Alexandria, there is an explicit statement by Galen linking Apollonius to Alexandria (see Chapter XXIII, AM.13).

[21] Chapter XIX, Ds.1–2 (above).

heart.[22] Chrysermus apparently neglected Herophilus' emphasis on the heart, elaborating instead upon Herophilus' use of the notion of *dynamis* or faculty, with the essentially alien help of the Stoic and Erasistratean distinction between 'psychic' and 'vital',[23] which later became a central aspect of Galen's physiology.

In most other respects, however, Chrysermus' pulse theory remains identical with Herophilus': the restriction of pulsation to the arteries as opposed to the veins, the perhaps anti-Erasistratean depiction of the pulse as a constant of physiological behaviour (i.e. independent of disease or health),[24] the emphasis on the arterial coat, and the firm assertion of the perceptibility of the pulse.

In addition to pulse theory, Chrysermus seems to have been interested chiefly in the therapeutic aspects of pharmacology. His treatment of scrofulous tumours and of abscesses of the parotid or salivary glands (reported by Pliny in his discussion of uses of asphodel[25]) as well as his invention of a drug compound in lozenge form (described by Galen[26]) testify to his continuation of the long-standing pharmacological tradition of the Herophilean school.

---

[22] Cf. Galen, *De pulsuum differentiis* 4.2 (VIII, pp. 702–3K) = Chapter VII, T155.

[23] Cf. *SVF* II, 876 (ζωτικὸς τόνος), II, 877 (τὸ ψυχικὸν πνεῦμα); cf. also Galen, *De Hp. et Platonis placitis* 2.8 (*CMG* v.4.1.2, p. 164 DeLacy) on τὸ ψυχικόν and τὸ ζωτικόν. For Erasistratus' view that the air breathed in by the nostrils and the mouth goes to the lungs and the heart, where it is transformed into 'vital spirit' (*zōtikon pneuma*), and from there some reaches the meninges, where it becomes 'psychic spirit' (*psychikon pneuma*), see, e.g., Galen, *ibid.*, *De usu respirationis* 5 (IV, p. 502K), and *An in arteriis sanguis contineatur* (IV, pp. 703–36K; Furley & Wilkie, 1984: 144–83). For Galen see, e.g., *De usu partium* 7.8 (I, pp. 392–4 Helmreich). On Galen's accounts and criticisms of Erasistratus' views, and for Galen's own use of 'vital' and 'psychic', cf. also L. G. Wilson, 1959: 293–314; Temkin, 1951; De Martini, 1964; Harris, 1973: 349–64. While Chrysermus took over 'psychic' and 'vital' from Erasistratus, there is no indication that he follows Erasistratus in the application of these concepts to pneuma.

[24] A significant shift from pre-Herophilean medicine, when the terms 'to pulsate' (σφύζειν) and 'pulse' were used mainly of the perceptible throbbing of inflamed – not healthy – parts of the body, and when 'pulsation' therefore was viewed as a pathological symptom. Since Erasistratus at one time also used 'pulse' in this pathological sense, Chrysermus' emphasis on the pulse as 'a constant concomitant in both healthy and diseased conditions' (*Cr.*1) might well be a rejection of the ancient view of pulse as well as an anti-Erasistratean statement. Cf. Galen, *De pulsuum differentiis* 4.2 (VIII, pp. 716–17K) and *Quod animi mores corporis temperamenta sequantur* 8 (Scr. Min. II, pp. 62–3). See p. 268 *supra*.

[25] See *Cr.*5.

[26] See *Cr.*6.

B · TEXTS

*Cr.*1   Galenus (ex Aristoxeno?), *De pulsuum differentiis* 4.8–10 (VIII, pp. 741–3K)

*Cr.*2   Galenus (ex Aristoxeno?), *De pulsuum differentiis* 4.10 (VIII, pp. 744–6K). See T156, p. 331 *supra.*

*Cr.*3   Galenus, *De pulsuum dignotione* 4.3 (VIII, p. 955K). See Chapter VII, T162.

*Cr.*4   C. Plinius Secundus, *Naturalis historia* 1 (on his sources for Book XXII)

*Cr.*5   C. Plinius Secundus, *Naturalis historia* 22.32.71

*Cr.*6   Asclepiades Iunior apud Galenum, *De compositione medicamentorum secundum locos* 9.2 (XIII, pp. 243–4K)

*Cr.*7   Sextus Empiricus, *Hypotyposes Pyrrhoneae* 1.84

XXI · ZEUXIS

$(\mathcal{Z}x.)$

A · INTRODUCTION

With Zeuxis and Alexander Philalethes we reach a novel stage in the history of the Herophilean school of medicine: its expansion from Hellenized Egypt into Asia Minor. In the Phrygian region of Asia Minor near the major trading and banking centre Laodicea on the Lycus river, first Zeuxis and later Alexander became leaders of a school apparently associated with (or located at) the temple of Men Karou ($\mathcal{Z}x$. 1). The association of a medical school with a shrine might have been inspired by the formal cultic organization within which activities at the Alexandrian Museum were carried on, and it might also have been encouraged by the Roman authorities in this province. By the late Republican period, for example, the association of institutions of higher learning with a cult might have been encouraged by law.[1]

The brutal expulsion of the intelligentsia from Alexandria in 145/144 B.C. by the eighth Ptolemy, Euergetes II,[2] might have contributed to the dispersion of the Herophilean school. Yet, by the time that Zeuxis' school became renowned in the later first century B.C., other followers of Herophilus had again reasserted the scientific presence of Herophileanism in Alexandria itself. One of them, Dioscurides Phacas, had even gained considerable influence with Cleopatra, with her father Auletes, and with her brother, Ptolemy XIII.[3] Zeuxis and his followers accordingly represent only one of two centres of the school in the first century B.C., but it was a centre of

---

[1] For a fuller discussion see above, pp. 459–60 (see also Chapter x, nn. 73–81).
[2] Cf. the account in Athenaeus, *Deipnosophistae* 4.184B–C, quoted above in Chapter III (A.1). See also Chapter III, n.2.
[3] Chapter XIX, *Ds*.1–2. See also the Introduction to Chapter XIX.

considerable significance. Not only was it near Laodicea, a thriving commercial centre and one of the 'illustres urbes Asiae' (as Tacitus later called it);[4] Strabo also reports that the school itself was a 'great' or 'large' place of instruction (διδασκαλεῖον Ἡροφιλείων ἰατρῶν μέγα).[5] Several considerations seem to confirm Strabo's characterization. One is the appearance of the legend 'Zeuxis Philalethes' on the reverse side of two bronze coins from Laodicea, both bearing the head of Augustus (with the customary Greek translation of his title, ΣΕΒΑΣΤΟΣ) on the obverse.[6] One of these coins also has a caduceus on the reverse,[7] and this, along with the traditional association of the title 'Philalethes', 'Truth-Lover,' with the head of the Herophilean school in Laodicea – e.g. Alexander Philalethes,[8] Demosthenes Philalethes[9] – strongly suggests that the Zeuxis honoured on these coins from Laodicea is none other than the leader of the Herophilean centre.

Another measure of the significance of the school at Men Karou seems to be that it endured for at least three generations. It is not absolutely clear from Strabo's account whether Zeuxis was the founder, but the phrase συνέστη . . . ὑπὸ Ζεύξιδος can be interpreted to mean 'it was established . . . by Zeuxis'. The next leader of the school was Alexander Philalethes, followed in turn by Demosthenes Philalethes, a Herophilean who probably lived at least until the mid-first century A.D. (After Demosthenes there is no longer any firm evidence of an active Herophilean school either in Asia Minor or in Alexandria, although there is a tantalizing inscription, mentioned above,[10] which could be interpreted as evidence of the continuation of the 'Philalethes' branch of Herophileanism beyond the time of Demosthenes Philalethes.)

[4] Cf. Ramsay, 1895–7: vol. I, pp. 40ff., 104, 168–9ff. Cicero, who resided in Laodicea from February to May, 50 B.C., in his capacity as proconsul of Cilicia, confirms in his letters that it was a major trading and banking centre; cf. Ad Atticum 5.21, 6.1, 6.2; Ad familiares 3.7, 3.9–10, etc. Laodicea became exceptionally influential not only because it lay on the main road from Ephesus to the East, but also because it was on the Lycus river, and especially because it cultivated close relations with Rome at least until the time of the Second Sophistic, when Antonius Polemo (A.D. 88–143) from Laodicea, known as 'the Phrygian Demosthenes', influenced the Emperor Hadrian to bestow favours on his native city and on Smyrna. Cf. Tacitus, Annales 14.27.1.
[5] Zx.1.
[6] Zx.2–3. Cf. Benedum, 1974 and 1978.
[7] The caduceus is, however, in itself no proof that a physician is intended, since it is often associated with Hermes.
[8] Cf. Chapter XXII.   [9] Cf. Chapter XXVIII.   [10] Chapter X, pp. 460–1.

The date of Zeuxis can only be determined approximately, but we have several good indications. First, in his *Geography*, Strabo (*c.* 64 B.C.–A.D. 23) characterizes himself as a contemporary of Zeuxis and Alexander Philalethes.[11] Secondly, at the time Strabo wrote, Alexander apparently had already succeeded Zeuxis as head of the school.[12] Since Strabo completed his *Geography* by 7 B.C.[13], Alexander must have become the school leader before 7 B.C. Third, the two coins are from a period after 27 B.C. (Octavian accepted the title Σεβαστός or 'Augustus' on 16 January 27 B.C.). Together these factors point to a date of roughly 85/75–10 B.C. for Zeuxis, and a date perhaps between 45 B.C. and 30 B.C. for the founding of the school.

About Zeuxis' contributions to scientific and clinical medicine nothing is known, although the contributions of the other Herophileans from his school (Alexander and Demosthenes) suggest that the wide-ranging interests of the Alexandrian Herophileans – sphygmology, gynaecology, reproductive physiology, pharmacology – were sustained in the Phrygian outpost. But all the more informative ancient references to 'Zeuxis the physician' either refer to the early Empiricist called Zeuxis or are too vague and uncertain to be claimed for the Herophilean.[14] We are therefore left with one laconic geographer and two four-word bronze coins as our only sources for Zeuxis the Herophilean.

B · TEXTS

Zx.1   Strabo, *Geographica* 12.8.20 (580C)
Zx.2   *Sylloge Nummorum Graecorum* (Sammlung H. von Aulock), fasc. 9 (Berlin, 1964), Plate 125, no. 3836/7
Zx.3   *Sylloge Nummorum Graecorum* (Sammlung H. von Aulock), fasc. 9, Plate 125, no. 3855

---

[11] Cf. *Zx*.1: καθ' ἡμᾶς. But cf. Ch. xx, n. 18.
[12] *Ibid.*: ὑπὸ Ζεύξιδος, καὶ μετὰ ταῦτα Ἀλεξάνδρου Φιλαλήθους.
[13] See Pais, 1922: especially 275–91. Pais' conclusions about the date of composition have been accepted by most later scholars; cf., e.g., Aly, 1931: col. 90: 'Wir wissen nur, dass sie [Strabons *Geographie*] um 7 v. Chr. zum grössten Teil abgeschlossen vorlag.'
[14] For the evidence concerning Zeuxis the Empiricist see Deichgräber, 1965: 209, 409–10, 412–13, 417–18, 263. Kudlien (1972d) suggests that the prescription for mentagra attributed to a certain Zeuxis by Galen (*De compositione medicamentorum secundum locos* 5.3 (XII, p. 834K)) might be the Herophilean's, but in view of the fact that the only Zeuxis ever mentioned elsewhere by Galen is the Empiricist – to whom Galen refers quite often – it seems more likely that the Empiricist is meant.

XXII · ALEXANDER
PHILALETHES (*AP.*)

A · INTRODUCTION

One of the more intriguing later Herophileans, Alexander Philalethes ('the Truth-Lover') seems to have lived roughly from 50 B.C. to A.D. 25.[1] No later than 7 B.C. he apparently succeeded Zeuxis[2] as leader of the famous Herophilean school at the temple of Men Karou, near Laodicea (in present-day Turkey) on the great Eastern trade-route, and he soon attracted pupils who became distinguished Herophileans, among them Aristoxenus[3] and Demosthenes Philalethes.[4]

Alexander himself was, however, not trained in the Herophilean school – either in Alexandria or in Asia Minor – but at first was a follower of Asclepiades of Prusias-on-Sea, a Bithynian 'atomist' who also practised medicine in Rome.[5] With the obvious exception of Herophilus, who was trained under the Coan physician Praxagoras,[6] no other Herophilean is known to have joined the ranks of the Herophileans, let alone become their leader, after being trained by an outsider. Yet there seems little doubt that Alexander not only had

---

[1] Strabo (*c.* A.D. 64–23) refers to both Alexander and the latter's predecessor Zeuxis as his own contemporaries (*AP.*1), and this might indicate that Alexander was a younger contemporary. On 'Philalethes' see D.L. 1.17; Benedum, 1978.

[2] Strabo, who completed most of his *Geography* by 7 B.C., reports that Alexander had already succeeded Zeuxis as leader of the school at the time of writing. Cf. Chapter XXI.A and Ch. XXI n. 13.

[3] *AP.*2 Chapter XXV, *Ar.*3.

[4] Cf. *AP.*3, and Chapter XXVIII, *DP.*1 and *DP.*3.

[5] On Asclepiades of Bithynia, on whom Wellmann, 1896a, initially passed harsh judgment ('In der Geschichte der ärztlichen Charlatanerie nimmt Asklepiades eine hervorragende Stelle ein'), see above Chapter II, n.47, and Scarborough, 1975; Dilthey, 1922: 247ff.; Heidel, 1911: 111–72; Ueberweg & Praechter, 1926: Appendix p. 138*; Lonie, 1965a: 126–43; G. Harig in Mette & Winter, 1968: 78–81; Allbutt, 1921: 177–91; Rawson, 1982. Cf. Ch. II, T1, T16.

[6] Chapter II, T9–T11.

been a student of Asclepiades but also remained strongly under his influence after assuming the leadership of the Herophilean school, at least if Alexander's surviving views may be used as a yardstick. Vindician (or whoever wrote the tantalizing fragment *De semine* in the twelfth-century Codex Bruxellensis 1348–59) reports that Alexander 'amator veri appellatus', i.e. Philalethes, was a student (*discipulus*) of Asclepiades,[7] and even if one were inclined to interpret this statement metaphorically – not that Vindician is liberal or licentious with his metaphors – there is enough evidence to suggest a close relationship. Caelius Aurelianus, for example, implies that Alexander and Asclepiades held identical views on lethargy,[8] and the author of a famous papyrus in the British Museum, best known as Anonymus Londinensis, states that they had an identical theory of digestion.[9] Furthermore, the Anonymus introduces 'the followers of Asclepiades and Alexander Philalethes' as though these were all adherents of the same school of thought.[10]

Although crucial parts of the papyrus are riddled with lacunae and virtually illegible, two passages even seem to suggest that Alexander in physiological contexts used the same kinds of arguments that the atomists had used. While Asclepiades was not an orthodox atomist, he was a corpuscular materialist who apparently substituted for 'atoms' the notion of corpuscles or molecules (ὄγκοι) as the ultimate, discrete (but perhaps not indivisible) constituents of all bodies[11] – a

[7] *AP*. 9.
[8] *AP*.12. Caelius Aurelianus' reference to Alexander as 'Alexander of Laodicea in Asia' [sc. Minor] does not necessarily imply that Alexander was born in Laodicea, but could instead be a reference to his position as leader of the Herophilean school near Laodicea.
[9] *AP*. 6. Some critics have argued that Alexander's *Opinions* (τὰ ἀρέσκοντα), a work in at least five books (see *AP*.3), was used as a direct source by Anonymus Londinensis, and while it cannot be demonstrated conclusively, a good case can be made for this hypothesis. Cf. Diels, 1893b and 1893a: 111–12. A doxographic orientation has also been attributed to Alexander's treatise *On Seed* (*AP*.9), but the sequence *dixit . . . dicunt*, etc. (see Chapter VII, T191) does not confirm beyond doubt that Vindician's [?] entire report is ultimately derived from Alexander's *On Seed*. See Diels, *DG*, pp. 185ff.
[10] *AP*.7: οἱ περὶ Ἀσκληπιάδη καὶ Ἀλέξανδρον τὸν Φιλαλήθη. The text is, however, mutilated and 'Asclepiades' is the conjecture of F. Kenyon (accepted by Hermann Diels and W. H. S. Jones).
[11] Cf. S.E., *P* 3.32 (ἄναρμοι ὄγκοι) and *M* 10.318 (= *Adv. Phys.* 2.318); ps.-Galen, *De historia philosopha* 18 (*DG*, p. 610, lines 21ff.); ps.-Galen, *Introductio sive medicus* 9 (XIV, pp. 698–9K); Galen, *Ad Pisonem de theriaca* 11 (XIV, pp. 250ff.): εἰ μὲν γὰρ ἐξ

notion previously advanced by Heraclides of Pontus[12] – but in some respects he remained close to Epicureanism. One of the crucial distinctions Epicurus had employed in his 'Canon' or theory of method and knowledge is the one between visible and invisible reality, or between what is perceptible by the senses (e.g. sweet, bitter), and what is apprehensible by reason alone (e.g. atoms, void). Although the basic distinction goes back to the Presocratics, some of the terminology – especially λόγῳ θεωρητόν or διὰ λόγου θεωρητόν – is specifically Epicurean.[13] The same distinction, with the same Epicurean terminology, seems to have been expropriated by Asclepiades and then used by Alexander. Thus they use a theory of invisible passages (poroi), 'apprehensible only by reason', through which invisible corporeal emanations and intromissions – presumably of molecules or subsensory molecular clusters – take place.[14] One of the arguments advanced to substantiate this theory concerning invisible passages is also of Epicurean provenance: body cannot pass through body.[15] In function and legitimation the invisible poroi accordingly correspond closely to Epicurus' and Democritus' notion of the void. Unfortunately no further details survive concerning the specific physiological uses to which Alexander put these principles, but their provenance seems clear.

ἀτόμου καὶ τοῦ κενοῦ κατὰ τὸν 'Επικούρου τε καὶ Δημοκρίτου λόγον συνειστήκει τὰ πάντα, ἢ ἔκ τινων ὄγκων καὶ πόρων κατὰ τὸν Ιατρὸν 'Ασκληπιάδην . . .
For a somewhat different use of ὄγκος by the atomists themselves, cf. Democritus 68A1 (D.L. 9.44), 68A37DK; Epicurus, Letter to Herodotus 52–54, 56–7, 69; Letter to Pythocles 105; fr. 21.3, 30.24, 34.14 Arrighetti (2nd ed).

12 On Heraclides Ponticus, see S.E., locc. citt. (n. 11); fr. 118–23 Wehrli (vol. 7). Although it has often been argued that Heraclides took over his theory from the Pythagorean Ecphantus, there is no evidence that Ecphantus, though he used atomistic notions, introduced the concept ὄγκος (cf. 51A1–4DK). Furthermore, while Heraclides' 'molecules' are capable of being affected – i.e. perhaps, as some have argued, divisible – and exhibit qualitative differentiation, the 'atoms' introduced by Ecphantus are explicitly said to be 'indivisible bodies' (51A1–2 and A4DK) – an expression used by Ecphantus, says the doxographer Aëtius (Placita 1.3.19; DG, p. 286), to designate 'the Pythagorean corporeal units [monads]'. Cf. Lonie, 1965a; Burkert, 1962: 38, 319 n.17; Wehrli, 1967–9: vol. vII, pp. 101–3; Tannery, 1898. See also Thesleff, 1965: 6, line 1, and p. 23, note on line 22. Cf. Gottschalk, 1980: 37–57.

13 Cf. Epicurus, Letter to Herodotus 47 and 62 (pp. 43, 57 Arrighetti); id., Kyriai Doxai 1 (= Gnomologium Vaticanum 1), p. 121 Arrighetti. On Epicurus' use of θεωρούμενον see Furley, 1971: 615.

14 AP.5 and AP.7.   15 AP.5.

Whereas some Herophileans had become interested mainly in Hippocratic philology and in pharmacology,[16] thereby emphasizing the same areas of inquiry as their Empiricist rivals, Alexander was primarily interested in physiology and gynaecology (at least if the extant testimonia allow any such generalization). Not only the general adaptation for physiological purposes of the principles of ὄγκοι and πόροι or corpuscules and invisible passages – in a manner corresponding to atoms and void – and the theory of visible as well as invisible emanations from the body, but also a strong interest in a traditional Herophilean stronghold, pulse theory, is attested for Alexander. He produced two definitions of the pulse, called 'objective' and 'subjective' respectively. His so-called 'objective' definition – 'the pulse is an involuntary contraction and distention of the heart and the arteries, such as can become apparent'[17] – represents an orthodox Herophilean position. First, relatively early in the history of pulse lore, the Herophileans Bacchius and Zeno had already introduced 'distention' (diastasis) as an alternative to Herophilus' use of 'dilation' (diastolē),[18] and second, the emphasis on the responsibility of both the arteries and the heart for pulsation dates back to Herophilus himself.[19] Third, Alexander's phrase 'such as can become apparent' is apparently a reply to those who had questioned whether all 'parts' of the pulse are perceptible by our tactile sense, and Alexander seems to elaborate upon this issue in his second or so-called 'subjective' definition of the pulse: 'The pulse is the beat of the continuous, involuntary motion of the arteries against one's touch, and the interval occurring after the beat.'[20] Here, too, Alexander is solidly in the Herophilean camp: the Herophilean Chrysermus also found it necessary to emphasize in his definition of the pulse that it 'can be apprehended by sense-perception', perhaps in answer to the charge that Herophilus had not been explicit on this point.[21] If

---

[16] Cf., for example, Chapters XI (Andreas), XIV (Bacchius), XV (Zeno), XXIII (Apollonius Mys).

[17] AP.3.

[18] Cf. Chapter XIV, Ba.2. Bacchius, is, however, not consistently reported to have used diastasis instead of diastolē. In another passage, Galen attributes the use of diastolē, not diastasis, to Bacchius; cf. Ba.1. For Zeno's usage see Chapter XV, Zn.1 (and cf. Zn.2: the arteries 'are distended', διίστανται).

[19] Chapter VII, T148, T153–T155.   [20] AP.3.

[21] Chapter XX, Cr.1. Chrysermus' pupil, Heraclides of Erythrae, apparently no longer found perceptibility a controversial issue and jettisoned this part of

Alexander shared the sensualistic epistemology of his teacher Asclepiades, this particular elaboration upon Herophilus' definition might have been of special significance. The addition of '*and* the interval' is a pointed departure from Herophilus (cf. Ch. VII.A.4, p. 277).

Other physiological problems which interested Alexander include digestion and nutrition: 'In the belly nutriment is merely cut up and made into juice, and a certain predisposition is effected in it but definitely not an assimilation to what is akin'[22] – a view opposed to that of the Anonymus Londinensis[23] and numerous other ancient authors, including Aristotle (who taught that the heat in the stomach also sets the important process of concoction in motion).[24]

Alexander's approach to the nature of blood again reveals the sensualistic confidence of the materialist: 'Whatever blood is *in appearance*, of such a kind it is also in its faculties, viz. something simple and uniform.'[25] Despite his theory that blood is a mixture of the elements earth and water (with air sometimes listed as a third ingredient), Aristotle had, of course, classified blood among the *homoiomerē* (things having parts like each other and like the whole), and Alexander's emphasis on its 'uniform' nature might be a corpuscular theorist's version of the Aristotelian emphasis on its homoeomerous or 'uniform' character.[26]

A closely related problem to which Alexander Philalethes turned his attention is the origin and nature of male 'seed'. Like Aristotle, Herophilus, and physicians of the Pneumatic school of medicine (especially Athenaeus), Alexander accepted the theory of the haematogenous origin of 'seed': 'The essence of seed is the froth of the blood.'[27] This theory put him squarely in opposition to the atomists,

---

Chrysermus' definition; see Chapter XXIV, *HE*.2. Cf. also Chapter VII, T160–T161, where Herophilus' views (on arterial motions perceptible to one's touch) in fact seem to be expressed clearly.

[22] *AP*.6.   [23] *Ibid.*

[24] Cf., for example, Aristotle, *De anima* 2.4.416b2–30; *Parts of Animals* 2.3.650a2–2.4.651a19 and 3.14.674a9–676a5; *On Respiration* 8.474a25–8. (See also *Meteorologica* 4.2.379b12–4.3.381b22.) For the role of concoction in reproduction cf. *Generation of Animals* 3.2.753a18ff. (cf. also 4.1.765b15ff., 5.6.786a17ff.).

[25] *AP*.8.

[26] Cf. Aristotle, *Parts of Animals* 2.2.647b10–648a23, and 2.3.649b20–2.6.652a23.

[27] A testimonium concerning Book I of Alexander's treatise *On Seed* (*AP*.9). How many books this work comprised is unknown, but Vindician's [?] mention of Book I suggests that there were at least two.

because Epicurus had revived the pangenesis theory shared by Democritus and some Hippocratics[28] – i.e. the theory that all parts of the body contribute substantively to the formation of 'seed'. Here, as in his sphygmology, Alexander's Herophilean loyalties seem to dominate, whereas in most other areas his sympathies with Asclepiades' corpuscular physics seem to have gained the upper hand in the contest between teacher and pupil.

In his work *Gynaecology* – a treatise in at least two books[29] – Alexander addressed himself to problems discussed both by Asclepiades and by some Herophileans. Thus, on the controversial question whether there are any diseases peculiar to women, his negative answer lines him up on the side not only of Herophilus[30] and the Herophilean Apollonius Mys[31] but also of Asclepiades[32] (and hence on the opposite side of the Herophilean Demetrius of Apamea[33] and the Asclepiadean Lucius[34]). On another question, however, viz. the nature of 'the female flux', he apparently took over Demetrius' definition, but with a restrictive modification.[35]

It remains unclear whether the Alexander to whom Galen ascribes several remedies – two compounds for headaches, one a *euporiston* for catarrh and coughing – is in fact Philalethes, and I have therefore listed them among the *Dubia*.[36] In view of a slightly later Herophilean's strong therapeutic interest both in headaches and in *euporista* or

---

[28] Cf. Lesky, 1950: 1294–1343 (= pp. 70–119); Ch. VII.A.5 *supra*.
[29] Soranus mentions Book I of Alexander's *Gynaecia*, implying that it consisted of at least two books (*AP.*10).
[30] *AP.* 11. See Chapter VII, T193–T194.
[31] Chapter XXIII, *AM.*7.
[32] Soranus, *Gynaecia* 3.2 (*CMG* IV, pp. 94–5 Ilberg) = *AP.*11.
[33] Chapter XVI, *DA.*18.
[34] Soranus, *loc. cit.* This Lucius (Λούκιος Ilberg: ἐλαιούσιος P) is probably not identical with the famous pharmacologist Lucius or 'Leukios' (ὁ καθηγητής) with whom Asclepiades Pharmacion studied (cf. Galen, *De compositione medicamentorum per genera* 3.9 (XIII, p. 648K); Kind, 1927a), but rather the Lucius or 'Lisius' whom Caelius Aurelianus quotes in his *Chronic Diseases* 2.1.59, 2.7.111, 4.3.78–9. Cf. also Wellmann, 1900a: 369; Kind, 1927b.
[35] For Demetrius of Apamea's definition, see Chapter XVI, *DA.*17. Whereas Demetrius had defined the 'female flux' as 'a flow of *fluid matter* through the uterus over an extended period of time' (*DA.*17), subsuming under 'fluid matter' vaginal discharges of four different colours and with two different kinds of effects, Alexander seems to restrict his definition of 'female flux' to menstruation by substituting 'a greater amount of blood' for 'fluid matter'.
[36] *AP.*14a, *AP.*14b, *AP.*15.

common remedies,[37] it is tempting to suggest that Philalethes, too, wrote on these problems and that these three drug prescriptions are his work. But this argument remains too speculative to emancipate them from their uncertain status.

Finally, Alexander's work *Opinions*, in at least five books (*AP*.3), is a further link in a doxographic chain that seems to stretch back to Herophilus himself.

The picture which emerges from the few extant testimonia is therefore that of an eclectic physician with strong theoretical interests who represented an amalgam of the principles of Asclepiades' corpuscular theory and Herophilus' pulse theory, but who nevertheless inspired the continuation of a relatively orthodox Herophilean school in Asia Minor for at least a further generation.

B · TEXTS

AP.1   Strabo, *Geographica* 12.8.20 (580c). See also Appendix, III, *infra*.

AP.2   Galenus (ex Aristoxeno?), *De pulsuum differentiis* 4.10 (VIII, p. 746K)

AP.3   Galenus (ex Aristoxeno?), *De pulsuum differentiis* 4.4–5 (VIII, pp. 725–7, 731K).
See below, Chapter XXVIII, *DP*.1.

AP.4   Galenus (ex Aristoxeno?), *De pulsuum differentiis* 4.10 (VIII, p. 744K)

AP.5   Papyrus Londinensis 137 (=Anonymus Londinensis, *Iatrica Menonia*), 38.58–39.13 (*Supplementum Aristotelicum* III.1, p. 73 Diels)

AP.6   Papyrus Londinensis 137 (Anon.Lond.), 24.27–35 (p. 44 Diels)

AP.7   Papyrus Londinensis 137 (Anon.Lond.), 35.21–9 (p. 65 Diels)

AP.8   Papyrus Londinensis 137 (Anon.Lond.), 35.53–36.2 (p. 66 Diels)

AP.9   Vindicianus (?), *De semine fragmentum Bruxellense* (Wellman, 1901: p.208; Jaeger, 1938a: 191).
See above, Chapter VII, T191.

AP.10   Soranus, *Gynaecia* 3.43 (*CMG* IV, p. 122 Ilberg). See Chapter VII, T203–T204; cf. Drabkin, 1951: 87.

AP.11   Soranus, *Gynaecia* 3.2 (*CMG* IV, pp. 94–5). See above Chapter VII, T193–T195.

AP.12   Caelius Aurelianus, *Celeres vel acutae passiones* 2.1.5–6

AP.13   Galenus, *De pulsuum differentiis* 4.16 (VIII, p. 758K)

---

[37] Apollonius Mys; see Chapter XXIII, *AM*.10–47.

Dubia

AP.14a Asclepiades Iunior apud Galenum, *De compositione medicamentorum secundum locos* 2.1 (XII, p. 557K)

AP.14b Asclepiades Iunior apud Galenum, *De compositione medicamentorum secundum locos* 2.2 (XII, p. 580K)

AP.15   Ps.-Galenus, *De remediis parabilibus* 3 (XIV, p. 510K)

AP.16   Codex lat. Vendôme 109 (s.XI), fol. 58r. (Wickersheimer, 1966: 176–7)

AP.17   Iohannes Alexandrinus, *Commentaria in librum De sectis Galeni*, proem. 2ra5–8 (p. 14 Pritchet)

AP.18   Agnellus Ravennas(?), *In Galeni De sectis comm.* 4 (p. 22 S.U.N.Y., Arethusa Monogr. 8)

XXIII · APOLLONIUS MYS
(AM.)

A · INTRODUCTION

Whether his graceless nickname 'Mys' means 'Mouse', 'Muscle', or 'Mussel' – or is intentionally ambiguous – is unclear,[1] but the Herophilean physician Apollonius was a figure of considerable stature both in his own lifetime and in subsequent centuries. A contemporary of Strabo,[2] Apollonius lived in Alexandria[3] in the latter half of the first century B.C., and perhaps well into the first century A.D. He is mentioned or quoted not only by Strabo[4] but also by Soranus and Caelius Aurelianus[5] (who was heavily dependent upon Soranus), by Asclepiades the Younger,[6] by Athenaeus,[7] by Celsus,[8] by Plutarch,[9] by the Hippocratic commentators John of Alexandria and Palladius,[10] by the elder Pliny,[11] by Philumenus,[12] and – in about twenty-five continuous passages, possibly in as many as forty passages – by Galen,[13] who gives extensive but not always uncritical

---

[1] Apollonius' nickname 'Mys' is well attested: cf. *AM.*1,2,5,7,9, 30–2, 34; that 'Apollonius Mys' is identical with 'Apollonius the Herophilean' is established unequivocally by *AM.*1. In all likelihood *Mys* means 'mouse'. Using animal names for human beings was a widespread custom in ancient Greece, and Fick and Bechtel observe that *mys*, as a name for humans, was 'alt und weit verbreitet'; cf. Fick & Bechtel, 1894: 317. On the uses of animal names for humans see Fick & Bechtel, pp. 314–25, and Bechtel, 1902: 86–100.

[2] Cf. *AM.*1.   [3] See *AM.*13.   [4] *AM.*1.

[5] *AM.*7 and *AM.*5–6; cf. also *AM.*48a (*Dubium*).

[6] *AM.*30. *AM.*31 is perhaps also excerpted from Asclepiades. Cf. C. Fabricius, 1972: 198, and *AM.*70.

[7] *AM.*8.   [8] *AM.*9; cf. also *AM.*48b (*Dubium*).

[9] *AM.*33.   [10] *AM.*32; *AM.*36.   [11] *AM.*34–5.   [12] *AM.*38–45.

[13] *AM.*2–4. 10–26, 28–31, 46–47. Cf. also *AM.*49–66, the authenticity of which is in doubt; see my discussion (*infra*) of the 'Apollonius' quoted in Galen's excerpts from Andromachus the Younger.

accounts, replete with lengthy quotations, of Apollonius' 'common remedies' for common ailments.

Three of Apollonius' works are known by title. One of these, *On the School of Herophilus*, is mentioned by Galen, Soranus, and Caelius Aurelianus.[14] It consisted of at least twenty-nine books and seems to have been a comprehensive work, covering especially physiological and pathological theories. It was not confined to a doxographic account of the theories of his Herophilean predecessors. In the first and third books, for example, Apollonius provided some of his own gynaecological views,[15] in Book XXVIII he offered his own account of pleurisy[16] and probably of pneumonia, and in Book XXIX he apparently added a defence of his own definition of the pulse to his account of definitions of the pulse by other authors.[17]

Apollonius' *On the School of Herophilus* represents a significant link in a Herophilean tradition that goes back to the third century B.C. Starting with Bacchius, who composed a treatise known as *Memoirs of Herophilus and his School*,[18] a number of Herophileans wrote doxographic works in defence of their own school. At no time in the history of the school was there, however, such a heavy concentration of works of this kind as at the end of the first century B.C. and the beginning of the first century A.D. Apollonius' fellow-student, Heraclides of Erythrae, also wrote a work with the title *On the School of Herophilus*,[19] and so did their younger contemporary Aristoxenus.[20]

As I suggested earlier,[21] the heavy concentration of such doxographic works, with their dual purpose of apologetics and protreptic, in the last generation of the history of the Herophilean school probably reflects the growing insecurity of this school within the world of medicine – an insecurity due in part to the challenges Herophileans had to face, no longer just from their Empiricist rivals in Alexandria, but also from the popularity of the burgeoning 'Pneumatic' and 'Methodist' schools of medicine.[22] Although Apollonius, Heraclides of Erythrae, Aristoxenus, and Demosthenes Philalethes – the last known generation of Herophileans – were not rigidly

---

[14] Cf. *AM*.4–5 and *AM*.7.   [15] *AM*.7.   [16] *AM*.5; cf. *AM*.6.

[17] *AM*.4.   [18] See Chapter XIV, *Ba*.78.   [19] Chapter XXIV, *HE*.3.

[20] Chapter XXV.A. Alexander's *Opinions* (Ch. XXII, *AP*.3) perhaps was not only on Herophileans.

[21] See Chapter X.A.

[22] On the rise of the Pneumatic school of medicine, beginning with Athenaeus of Attalia in the mid first century B.C., see Kudlien, 1968d, and Wellmann, 1895a.

orthodox, unproductive defenders of an obsolescent medical system, but energetic contributors to both theoretical and clinical medicine, they were too practised in interpreting signs to miss the Pneumatic and Methodist writing on the wall. Hence the sudden flourish of doxographic defence on behalf of their school.

The pulse theory Apollonius advocates in *On the School of Herophilus* seems to be in agreement with that of his fellow-student Heraclides of Erythrae. To the statement of their teacher Chrysermus[23] that the pulse arises 'through the agency of a vital and psychic faculty', both Apollonius and Heraclides added '[this faculty] being dominant' (πλειστοδυναμούσης).[24] Their critic and fellow-Herophilean Aristoxenus subsequently dismissed this elaboration as redundant, since, in his view, the 'dominance' of the psychic and vital faculty is not peculiar to pulsation but common to all natural activities of the body.[25] More significant is, however, that essential features of Chrysermus' view of the pulse were retained by Apollonius.

A second work by Apollonius Mys, *On Perfumes and Unguents*, is quoted at length in Athenaeus' polyhistoric treatise of *c.* A.D. 200, *Deipnosophistae*.[26] With this work Apollonius perhaps resumed a Herophilean interest in cosmetics that might date back to Andreas' *Narthex* or *Unguent Casket* (third century B.C.).[27] While cosmetics never became as popular within the Herophilean school as did pharmacology,[28] these two disciplines were closely related at least in

On the Methodist school cf. Meyer-Steineg, 1916; Edelstein, 1935b; *id.*, 1967: 173–91; Deichgräber, 1934a; Allbutt, 1921: 192–201; G. Harig in Mette & Winter, 1968: 81–3; Phillips, 1973: 163–8; Diepgen, 1949: 103–10; Lloyd, 1983: 182–200, Frede, 1982: 1–23. (See also above, Chapter II with nn. 18, 41, on the Methodist Thessalus.)

23 No ancient text explicitly identifies Chrysermus as Apollonius' teacher. But (a) Heraclides of Erythrae is unequivocally called a 'fellow-pupil' (συσχολαστής) of Apollonius Mys by Strabo (*AM.*1), and (b) Heraclides is known to have been the pupil of only one teacher: Chrysermus (cf. Chapter XXIV, *HE.*2a). The inference that Apollonius, too, was a pupil of Chrysermus therefore seems reasonable.

24 *AM.*2; cf. Chapter XXIV, *HE.*2a–b.

25 *AM.*2; cf. Chapter XXV, *Ar.*2.

26 *AM.*8.

27 Cf. Chapter XI above, *An.*25. But Andreas' *Narthex* may have been limited to drug remedies. Cf. *An.*18.

28 Herophilus, Andreas, Callimachus, Zeno, Demetrius, Mantias, Chrysermus, Apollonius, and Demosthenes Philalethes were among the Herophileans who displayed an active interest in pharmacology. (See Chapter X, nn. 28–37 for references.)

so far as the cosmetician and the pharmacologist often had to be familiar with the qualities and effects of the same substances: saffron, rose oil, olive oil, vinegar, spikenard, dropwort, galbanum, bitter almond oil, fenugreek, frankincense, and purslane are examples of the numerous ingredients used both for cosmetic and for pharmacological purposes. It is therefore not surprising that a physician who, like Apollonius Mys, became renowned for his pharmacological expertise, also took an active interest in cosmetic substances.

The bulk of the ancient evidence (*AM*.10–46) concerns a third work by Apollonius, *Euporista* or *Readily Accessible Remedies* (in modern times better known as *On Common Remedies*). In this popular treatise, which consisted of at least two books,[29] Apollonius offered numerous detailed prescriptions for common ailments such as headaches, earaches, toothaches, oral infections, dandruff, and skin irritations. Some of the ingredients used in his prescriptions might strike a modern ear as somewhat esoteric, for example, birthwort, hyssop, iris oil, myrtle oil, camel urine, fenugreek, lupine, purslane, laserwort, nose smart, goose fat, mountain rue leaves, brimstone, wild marjoram, nightshade, fleabane, galingale, hartshorn, Nile milfoil, knotgrass, catnip juice, Cyrenaic juice, chaste tree seeds, myrrh, wormwood, darnel, and pennyroyal. But most of them were readily accessible in the pharmacological market-places of the Hellenistic world, and in particular in Alexandria.

Only once does Galen, to whom we owe our knowledge of most of these remedies, object to one of Apollonius' ingredients on grounds of impracticability or 'troublesomeness', viz. when Apollonius prescribes the use of tortoise blood to combat dandruff.[30] On other occasions too Galen admittedly objects to some of Apollonius' ingredients, but on aesthetic or therapeutic grounds rather than on grounds of inaccessibility. Thus, after reporting that Apollonius prescribed wiping the scalp with the urine of a bull or of a camel for several successive days in order to get rid of dandruff, Galen adds: 'But I would say in reply to Apollonius that not "for many days" but "for no single day" could a clean person bear to have the urine of any such animal poured over his head, especially in the case of an affection that is minor and can be cured easily . . .'[31] Similarly, after quoting one of Apollonius' remedies for a sore throat – viz. drinking as much

[29] Cf. *AM*.11–12, 28 etc.: 'in the *first* book of Apollonius' *Euporista*'.
[30] *AM*.11.   [31] *Ibid.*; cf. *AM*.25.

hot donkey urine as possible – Galen adds: 'I am astonished . . . I myself know that all but very few people would sooner want to die than to drink donkey urine.'[32]

Elsewhere Galen criticizes Apollonius for recommending remedies for certain generic diseases 'without proper differentiation' of their individual causes and symptoms, warning that Apollonius' remedies could 'effect very great harm unless someone knew how to apply the indiscriminately described powers of each prescription at the appropriate moment'.[33] Apollonius did, as Galen concedes, provide adequate differentiation in his account of remedies for headaches – distinguishing between headaches caused by heatstroke and those caused by chills, by intoxication in general, by drinking unmixed wine in particular, by a blow to the head, by falling, and finally, headaches that have no manifest cause[34] – but Galen's chief objection is that Apollonius failed to produce such causal differentiations with consistency in his discussions of remedies for other diseases.

While the existence of Galenic criticisms such as the above cannot be taken lightly, our sources for Apollonius' *Readily Accessible Drugs* – mainly Galen, Philumenus, and Oribasius[35] – in general seem to take for granted not only the accessibility of the ingredients prescribed by Apollonius but also their therapeutic efficacy, and this undoubtedly accounts in part for the circulation Apollonius' *Euporista* achieved.

In addition to the subjects covered in these three works, Apollonius seems to have taken an interest in regimen. Plutarch's statement that Apollonius prescribed a diet of pickled and salty food in cases of malnutrition[36] leaves unresolved, however, whether such dietary prescriptions were accommodated within Apollonius' *Euporista* or were part of a different work. It also remains unclear whether Apollonius wrote only on the therapeutic uses of regimen or on preventive care through regimen as well.

Five characteristic problems presented by the ancient evidence about

[32] *AM*.25.
[33] *AM*.25. Cf. also *AM*.17 ('with reference to ear-aches he offered no . . . differentiations'), *AM*.26 ('astringent, styptic, and discutient remedies are . . . incorrectly mixed together with dispersant and pungent remedies, [all] recorded without differentiation'), and *AM*.29.
[34] *AM*.12–16; see also *AM*.17.
[35] *AM*.10–26, 28–31, 37, 38–45.
[36] *AM*.33.

Apollonius deserve mention:[37] (i) the theory that a treatise *On Simple Remedies*, usually attributed to the famous army physician and pharmacologist Pedanius Dioscurides, is a significant indirect source for Apollonius Mys; (ii) the identity of an 'Apollonius' mentioned in Galen's extensive pharmacological excerpts from Andromachus the Younger; (iii) the identity of an 'Apollonius' quoted more than once by a court physician of Julian the Apostate, Oribasius; (iv) the identity of an 'Apollonius' from whom Alexander of Tralles (a physician of the sixth century A.D.) quotes two fragments; (v) the authorship of Papyrus Oxyrhynchus 234, an anonymous pharmacological text that has been attributed to Apollonius Mys.

(i) Max Wellmann claimed to have found notable similarities between no less than thirty passages of the Dioscuridean work *On Simple Remedies* and the fragments of Apollonius.[38] In at least eighteen

[37] In accordance with the principles developed at the outset, texts in indirect sources are not listed in this chapter; some are mentioned in the *Introduction* and nn. A vexing issue is the identity of the various physicians called 'Apollonius', especially when they are introduced without any further qualification. On this problem cf. Michler, 1968: 119–22; Deichgräber, 1965: 170–2, 256–7, 262–3; Wellmann ap. Susemihl, 1891–2: vol. I, pp. 816f., 821, 824 and II, pp. 440f., 442f.; *id.*, 1895c; *id.*, 1892b: 677–8; *id.*, 1888; C. Fabricius, 1972: 180–2; Harless, 1816: especially pp. 17–19; J. A. Fabricius, 1716–54: vol. XIII, pp. 74–6; Mola, 1962; von Christ, Stählin, & Schmid, 1912–24: vol. II.1, p. 450; Kühn, 1826: 5–8. None of these discussions resolves the problem of the identity of the various Apollonii, and the most extensive analysis – Harless' – is very misleading; he even equates the Herophilean, Apollonius Mys, with the Empiricist, Apollonius of Citium, although no ancient source provides any justification for such an equation. Wellmann's four contributions (*supra*) to the subject are marred by misreadings and unsubstantiated speculation, and Deichgräber by and large accepted Wellmann's findings. Michler's discussion (1968: 82) is more discerning, but he finds only four 'allgemeinchirurgische Zeugnisse' concerning the Herophilean, namely *AM*.8, 22, 28, and 49. But this (a) ignores *AM*.10–21, 23–6. 29–33, 35–6, and 38–47, and (b) fails to recognize that *AM*.49, being an excerpt from Andromachus, cannot be ascribed to the Herophilean with certainty, as pointed out below. Cajus Fabricius' analysis is very helpful but unfortunately is confined largely to the evidence presented by Galen's pharmacological treatises.

[38] Cf. the 'source apparatus' in Wellmann's edition of Dioscurides Pedanius' *De simplicibus*, v. III (Berlin, 1914), *re* pp. 160.13, 170.13, 173.6, 174.5, 174.15, 175.17, 189.8, 202.17, 209.11, 232.14, 303.19, 305.21, 308.4, 309.9, 310.6, 310.18, 311.5, 311.11, 312.1, 312.6, 312.15, 313.3, 313.8, 313.17, 314.7, 315.3, 315.9, 315.17, 316.8, 316.11, 316.16. C. Fabricius, 1972: 182 (with n. 5) seems to indicate his agreement with Wellmann's findings: 'Wellmann verrät . . . in seinen späteren Arbeiten' (e.g. Dsc., vol. III, p. 173), 'dass er den Sachverhalt kannte' (sc. that there are verbatim excerpts from Apollonius in Galen's pharmacological works?). But, as indicated below, Wellmann's findings are erroneous in part and have only tenuous value.

of these instances,[39] however, Wellmann mistakes fragments from
Asclepiades the Younger, also known as Asclepiades 'Pharmacion',[40]
for those of Apollonius. In ten other cases there do seem to be partial,
though rarely extensive or impressive, parallels between Apollonius'
fragments and *On Simple Remedies*.[41] The limited and haphazard
nature of these parallels would not, however, justify the claim that the
Dioscuridean work is a valuable indirect source for Apollonius. It is
not even clear whether the author of the Dioscuridean work drew
directly on Apollonius' *Euporista*, or whether – as seems more likely –
they both relied on common sources, such as Mantias,[42] Heraclides of
Tarentum,[43] Crateuas,[44] or even Apollodorus.[45] What is indisputable,
however, is that Dioscurides never mentions Apollonius Mys by
name; the parallels therefore are not included below (pp. 552–4).

(ii) The identity of an 'Apollonius' whose pharmacological prescriptions
for a wide range of disorders are mentioned or quoted at least
seventeen times in Galen's excerpts from Andromachus the Younger
(*floruit c.* A.D. 70–80) remains an unresolved problem.[46] Most of these
excerpts from Andromachus occur in the same pharmacological work
as Galen's own excerpts from Apollonius Mys, i.e. in Galen's *De
compositione medicamentorum secundum locos* (vols. XII–XIIIK).[47] Nowhere
in this work does Galen distinguish between the Apollonius on whom
he himself draws – i.e. the Herophilean – and the Apollonius cited by
Andromachus. It is therefore tempting to conclude that Androma-

---

[39] Dsc., vol. III, pp. 309–16 (source apparatus). These 'parallel passages' all occur in
      Galen's *On Antidotes* 2.7 (XIV, pp. 138–43K), a passage drawn from Asclepiades,
      not from Apollonius Mys, although Asclepiades twice in this passage seems to
      have referred to Apollonius' remedies; cf. *AM.*30–1.
[40] Cf. Wellmann, 1896b; C. Fabricius, 1972: 192–8.
[41] Dsc., vol. III, pp. 160.13, 170.13, 173.6, 174.5, 175.15, 175.17, 189.8, 209.11,
      303.19, 305.21. See *AM.*11, 14, 18–20, 22, 28, 40, and 43–4.
[42] See above, Chapter XVIII (especially *Ma.*1–2 and *Ma.*6) on Mantias' pharmacological
      achievements. Cf. also C. Fabricius, 1972: 199.
[43] Cf. Deichgräber, 1965: fr. 192–233 (see also *ibid.*, fr. 106–10), and C. Fabricius,
      1972: 200.
[44] On Crateuas and his influence see Wellmann, 1897.
[45] Cf. Wellmann, 1898.
[46] On Andromachus see C. Fabricius, 1972: 185–9; Wellmann, 1894.
[47] Excerpts from Andromachus are scattered throughout *De comp. medic. sec. locos*; for
      example, 3.1 (XII, pp. 625–33K), 3.3 (XII, p. 695), 5.5 (XII, pp. 877–80K), 6.6–6.7
      (XII, pp. 929–59K), 6.9 (XII, pp. 990–1K), 7.2–7.6 (XIII, pp. 15–115K; not
      continuous excerpts), 8.2 (XIII, pp. 126–39), 8.5 (XIII, pp. 186–7K). For a more
      complete account see C. Fabricius, 1972: 185–9.

chus, too, is quoting the Herophilean and that the Andromachean excerpts must be treated as a significant source for Apollonius Mys. At the very least it seems likely that *Galen thought* that Andromachus' references to 'Apollonius' were to the Herophilean.

One element in favour of this hypothesis is that no other 'Apollonius' could lay claim to the place of honour held in the Greek pharmacological tradition by the Herophilean, and that the first 'Apollonius' to come to mind in pharmacological contexts accordingly would be 'Mys'. Moreover, Asclepiades the Younger (fl. *c.* A.D. 100), who drew on Andromachus for some of his pharmacological prescriptions,[48] at least once explicitly identifies the 'Apollonius' whom he quotes as Apollonius Mys.[49] Finally, both Andromachus the Younger and Asclepiades the Younger display considerable familiarity with the pharmacological tradition of the Herophilean school. Thus they quote or refer to Herophilean physicians ranging from Andreas, Bacchius, Mantias, and Chrysermus to Alexander Philalethes and Gaius.[50] It is not inconceivable that their unusual knowledge of this branch of Herophilean medicine is due to their direct use of Apollonius Mys' work *Euporista* (and possibly of his more doxographically oriented work, *On the School of Herophilus* (*AM*.4–5), as well).

Two considerations nevertheless render this hypothesis vulnerable. First, unlike Galen and Asclepiades, Andromachus in the extant excerpts never identifies his 'Apollonius' as 'Apollonius Mys' or as 'the Herophilean'. Only in a single instance, perhaps wishing to make clear that – for once? – a different Apollonius is being introduced, does Andromachus seem to provide closer identification of his

---

[48] Galen, *De compositione medicamentorum secundum locos* 7.2 (XIII, pp. 47–56K) provides a lengthy excerpt from Asclepiades, in which Asclepiades in turn quotes Andromachus (XIII, pp. 53–4K).

[49] Cf. *AM*.30; see also *AM*.31. In some of Galen's other excerpts from Asclepiades further 'Apollonii' seem to surface. Thus 'Claudius Apollonius' is quoted in Galen's excerpt from Asclepiades in *De antidotis* 2.11 (XIV, pp. 171–2), and 'Apollonius Organicus' ('the surgeon?') is mentioned in *De compositione medicamentorum per genera* 5.15 (XIII, p. 856K), while an unidentified 'Apollonius' is mentioned twice in *AM*.70, i.e. in *De compositione medicamentorum secundum locos* 4.8 (XII, p. 776K). (That the latter passage actually occurs in an extensive excerpt from Asclepiades is suggested by XII, p. 730 and 742K; cf. C. Fabricius, 1972: 195.)

[50] Cf. Chapter XI, *An*.29–32; Chapter XIV, *Ba*.6; Chapter XVIII, *Ma*.9; Chapter XX, *Cr*.6; Chapter XXII, *AP*.14a–b (*Dubia*); Chapter XXVII, *G.* 2–4 (*Dubia*). See also Chapter XXVIII, *DP*.43 (*Dubium*), and Chapter VIII, T258–T259 (Herophilus).

'Apollonius': in his *De externorum remediis*, quoted by Galen, Andromachus mentions a multi-purpose lozenge invented by Apollonius 'the chief physician' (*archiatros*)[51] – a title that was not very common in Alexandria.[52] But nothing else is known about 'Apollonius the chief physician',[53] and there is no independent evidence that Apollonius Mys ever held the title *archiatros*. This testimonium accordingly does not contribute to a resolution of the problem. Secondly, and again unlike Galen, Andromachus never identifies Apollonius' work as the *Euporista* or *Readily Accessible Drugs*, but only as τὰ 'Απολλωνίου, 'the [writings] of Apollonius'.[54] At least some uncertainty about the identity of Andromachus' 'Apollonius' therefore remains, and those pharmacological fragments and testimonia concerning 'Apollonius' that depend directly on Andromachus the Younger accordingly are enumerated below among the *Dubia* (*AM.49–66*).

(iii) The name Apollonius occurs at least seven times in Oribasius' extant works,[55] and Raeder suggests that Apollonius of Pergamum – an otherwise virtually unknown physician – is meant in each of these instances.[56] But only twice does Oribasius in fact identify an

[51] Galen, *De compositione medicamentorum per genera* 5.12 (XIII, p. 835K). On the apparent corruption 'Αρχιστράτορος see Wellmann, 1892b: 677–8; *id.*, 1895b: col. 150, s.vv. '(105) Claudius A[pollonios]'.

[52] Cf. *Sammelb.* 5216 (from the Fâyyum, first century B.C.): 'Αθηναγόρας ὁ ἀρχιατρὸς τοῖς ἱερεῦσι τῶν ἐν τῶι Λαβυρίνθωι στολιστῶν καὶ τοῖς στολισταῖς χαίρειν . . . (the issue is the release of a corpse). For non-Alexandrian uses of *archiatros* cf. Dittenberger, 1903–5: vol. I, p. 416, no. 256.5 (in a dedication to Antiochus VIII, from Delos, *c.* 125–96 B.C.); Galen, *De antidotis* 1.1 (XIV, p. 2K): . . . 'Ανδρόμαχος ὁ Νέρωνος ἀρχιατρός . . . Cf. also Rostovtzeff, 1953: vol. II, pp. 1092–3; Fraser, 1972: vol. I, p. 373; and Chapter XX (*supra*), nn. 4 and 6 (on ἐπὶ τῶν ἰατρῶν). See also Nutton, 1977.

[53] There is no conclusive support in the ancient evidence for Wellmann's efforts (1892b, and 1895b: col. 150) to identify him with Claudius Apollonius and to date him before Andromachus and after Alcimion.

[54] Cf. *AM.49–50*, 54, 57.

[55] Oribasius, *Collectiones medicae* 7.19 (*CMG* VI.1.1, p. 218 Raeder), 44.30 (*CMG* VI.2.1, p. 158), 48.41 (*ibid.*, p. 282); *Synopsis ad Eustathium* 1.14 (*CMG* VI.3, p. 12) and 8.12.7 (*ibid.*, p. 252); *Ad Eunapium, praef.* (*CMG* VI.3, p. 318) and 1.9.7 (*ibid.*, p. 325).

[56] Joh. Raeder (ed.), *Oribasii collectionum medicarum reliquiae*, vol. 4 (*CMG* VI.2.2), p. 312, col. 1, s.vv. 'Apollonius (Pergamenus)'. Wellmann's claim that more is known about Apollonius of Pergamum (1895b: col. 150, n. 104) is based (a) on the erroneous identification of the Pergamene with what appears to be Apollonius of Citium in a passage from Alexander of Tralles (see below), and, more plausibly, (b) on a parallel between a short passage on scarification in Galen and *AM.68–9*. *AM.68–9* are not explicitly attributed to the Pergamene Apollonius by Oribasius, but they probably are excerpted from one of his works. See n. 63.

Apollonius as 'Apollonius of Pergamum'.[57] In a third instance the reference is to 'Apollonius the Beast' (*Thēr*),[58] who also was known in antiquity in the context of Hippocratic lexicography.[59]

In four other passages[60] Oribasius simply refers to 'Apollonius' without further identification, and in at least one instance the reference almost certainly is to the Herophilean. In his preface to *Ad Eunapium* Oribasius mentions an 'Apollonius' among the authors who recorded *euporista pharmaka* or 'readily accessible remedies'.[61] Only one Apollonius – the Herophilean or 'Mys' – was famous in antiquity for a work on common remedies (*Euporista*), and this reference in all likelihood, therefore, is to the Herophilean. Although Oribasius' subsequent reference, in his *Ad Eunapium*, to the Pergamene Apollonius[62] might suggest either that Oribasius himself failed to distinguish between the Pergamene and the Herophilean or that the two actually were identical, there is no direct evidence that the Pergamene ever wrote on common remedies. Nor do the ancient sources indicate that Apollonius the Herophilean came from, or practised in, Pergamum, whereas his presence in Alexandria is confirmed unequivocally (*AM*.13).

Oribasius' three remaining excerpts from 'Apollonius' do not contain material that can be shown to be drawn from Apollonius Mys, but a plausible case can be made for ascribing two of them to Apollonius of Pergamum, as the following observations suggest: (1) In *Ad Eunapium* (1.9.7) Oribasius mentions in passing that Apollonius of Pergamum recommended scarification on the lower leg. (2) In two partially identical passages in *Synopsis ad Eustathium* and *Collectiones medicae*, Oribasius quotes an 'Apollonius' on scarification.[63] (3) In both excerpts on scarification, Apollonius recommends scarifying the legs. (4) In the excerpts on scarification offered in *Collectiones medicae*, the author refers to his personal experience of a plague that struck

---

[57] *Synopsis ad Eustathium* 8.12.7 (*CMG* VI.3, p. 252 Raeder); *Ad Eunapium* 1.9.7 (*ibid.*, p. 325).

[58] *Collectiones medicae* 48.41 (*CMG* VI.2.1, p. 282). Might 'Mouse' and 'Beast' be identical?

[59] See Erotian, *Vocum Hippocraticarum collectio* α.103 (p. 23.17 Nachmanson).

[60] *Coll. med.* 7.19 and 44.30; *Synopsis ad Eust.* 1.14; *Ad. Eunap., praef.* (see n. 55 *supra*).

[61] *AM*.37.

[62] *Ad Eunapium* 1.9.7 (*CMG* VI.3, p. 325 Raeder).

[63] *AM*.68–69. One part of both excerpts is identical with Galen (*De hirudinibus* 4; XI, p. 322), to whom Aëtius Amid. 3.21; *CMG* VIII.1, p. 277) attributes all of *AM*.68.

550 THE HEROPHILEANS

'Asia' and to his successful effort to cure himself by means of scarification: ὑποπεσὼν κἀγὼ τῇ νόσῳ ... κατακνισθεὶς τὸ σκέλος ὡς δύο λίτρας αἵματος ἀπέκρουσα καὶ διὰ τοῦτο τὸν κίνδυνον ἀπέφυγον. The reference to personal clinical experience in 'Asia' would perhaps come more naturally from a Pergamene physician than from an Alexandrian. Oribasius himself was, of course, also from Pergamum, and it is uncertain whether *ego* refers to the author of the excerpt – i.e. to Apollonius – rather than to the excerptor (Oribasius). Nevertheless, the two passages on scarification should probably be ascribed to Apollonius of Pergamum, and since Apollonius of Pergamum cannot be shown to be identical with Apollonius Mys, the fragments on scarification probably do not belong in this chapter. Since some doubt remains, they are, however, listed among the *Dubia* (*AM*.68–9).

This leaves us with one excerpt of undetermined authorship: a passage from an 'Apollonius' on remedies for boils – a common ailment for which Apollonius Mys very well might have prescribed 'common remedies' in his *Euporista*. This passage is included below, but again among the *Dubia* (*AM*.67). Not included is, however, a passage on remedies for sprains and bruises from Oribasius' *Synopsis ad Eustathium* which, in the opinion of Max Wellmann, was drawn from Apollonius;[64] but Oribasius does not even mention Apollonius in this context, and there is no persuasive indirect evidence that Apollonius is the author of this passage.

(iv) Alexander of Tralles twice refers to 'Apollonius'.[65] In one of these passages the word *euporiston* – so frequently associated with Apollonius Mys – occurs, but the reference in fact is not to a remedy, but to a diagnostic problem.[66] In both instances Alexander is giving an account of the views of 'Apollonius' on epilepsy. The only 'Apollonius' attested to have written on epilepsy is neither the Herophilean

64 *Syn. ad Eust.* 7.16 (*CMG* VI.3, pp. 221–2 Raeder); Wellmann (ed.), *Dsc.*, vol. III, p. 232–14 (see 'source apparatus').
65 Puschmann, 1878–9: vol. I, *Therapeutica* 1.15, pp. 559 and 561.
66 *Ibid.*, p. 559: ἐκ τῶν Ἀπολλωνίου εὐπόριστον εἴπερ ἰάσιμός ἐστιν ὁ ἐπιληπτικός ... A variant in a Venetian manuscript – Marcianus gr. 295 (= *Mf*) – suggests that at least one copyist thought that *euporiston* referred to the Herophilean's famous pharmacological treatise: ἐν δὲ τῷ Ἀπολλωνίου εὐπορίστῳ εὗρον οὕτως, εἴπερ ἰάσιμος ... It is uncertain whether Apollonius Mys dealt with the diagnosis of diseases in his *Euporista*, but the prescription of thyme and blood is in keeping with his 'common remedies'.

nor (as Wellmann suggested)[67] Apollonius of Pergamum, but the Empiricist, Apollonius of Citium. In his work *Chronic Diseases*, Caelius Aurelianus refers to 'the account of therapeutic treatments by Apollonius of Citium in Book II [where he deals] with epileptics . . .'[68] It therefore seems likely that Alexander's references are to the Empiricist, not to the Herophilean.

(v) Two of the six prescriptions ascribed to Apollonius' *Euporista* by Galen in *AM*.17 recur anonymously in Papyrus Oxyrhynchus 234.[69] Max Wellmann was the first to recognize this correspondence (although he states incorrectly that P. Oxy. 234 parallels Galen XII, p. 646K).[70] But Wellmann's conclusion that, just because there is a close correspondence between thirteen lines of the papyrus fragment (col. II.1–13) and two short prescriptions attributed to Apollonius by Galen (*De compositione medicamentorum secundum locos* 3.1, vol. XII, pp. 616.18.–617.2 and 617.9–11K), the papyrus fragment *in its entirety* (i.e. col. II.1–50) must be from Apollonius' *Euporista*, seems precipitate. The possibility that col. II is part of a compilation of remedies for ear aches from several different sources cannot be precluded (a) in the absence of decisive correspondence between col. II.14–50 and the testimonia and fragments of Apollonius Mys, and (b) in the absence of any explicit identification of Apollonius as the source of any of these prescriptions. In accordance with the criteria for inclusion the papyrus text is not included among the testimonia and fragments of Apollonius.

Physiology, pathology, gynaecology, pharmacology, and medical history: these broad interests of Apollonius Mys are characteristic of the Herophilean school from its earliest beginnings. But once again, as in the case of most of Herophilus' followers, the discipline in which Herophilus himself achieved the greatest distinction – human anatomy – is signally lacking from the substantial list of Apollonius' contributions.

---

[67] Wellmann, 1895b: col. 150, no. 104.
[68] Caelius Aurelianus, *Tardae passiones* 1.4.140 (correctly recognized by Puschmann, 1878–9: I, p. 558 n. 2); Deichgräber, 1965: fr. 278 (p. 208).
[69] *The Oxyrhynchus Papyri*, ed. B. P. Grenfell and A. S. Hunt, II (London, 1899), pp. 135–6.
[70] Wellmann, 1910: 469.

B · TEXTS

AM.1 Strabo, *Geographica* 14.1.34 (645C)

AM.2 Galenus (ex Aristoxeno?), *De pulsuum differentiis* 4.10 (VIII, pp. 744–5K)

AM.3 Galenus, *De pulsuum dignotione* 4.3 (VIII, p. 955K). See Ch. VII, T162.

AM.4 Galenus (ex Aristoxeno?), *De pulsuum differentiis* 4.10 (VIII, p. 746K)

AM.5 Caelius Aurelianus, *Celeres vel acutae passiones* 2.13.88–9

AM.6 Caelius Aurelianus, *Celeres vel acutae passiones* 2.28.147

AM.7 Soranus, *Gynaecia* 3.2 (*CMG* IV, pp. 94–5 Ilberg).
       See also Chapter VII, T193–T195; Chapter XVI, *DA*.18; Chapter XXII, *AP*.11.

AM.8 Athenaeus, *Deipnosophistae* 15.38.688E–689B

AM.9 A. Cornelius Celsus, *Medicina* 5 (= *Artes* 10), prohoem. 1 (*CML* I, p. 190 Marx). See also above, Chapter XI, *An*.22; Ch. VIII, T251.

AM.10 Galenus, *De simplicium medicamentorum temperamentis ac facultatibus* 6, prooemium (XI, pp. 794–5K). See also above, Chapter XVIII, *Ma*.3.

AM.11 Galenus, *De compositione medicamentorum secundum locos* 1.8 (XII, pp. 475–82K). Cf. Theodorus Priscianus, *Euporista* 1.15.

AM.12 Galenus, *De compositione medicamentorum secundum locos* 2.1 (XII, pp. 502–4K)

AM.13 Galenus, *ibid.*, 2.1 (XII, pp. 509–10K)

AM.14 Galenus, *ibid.* (XII, pp. 514–15, 519–20K)

AM.15 Galenus, *ibid.* (XII, pp. 520–8K)

AM.16 Galenus, *ibid.* (XII, pp. 528–33K)

AM.17 Galenus, *ibid.*, 3.1 (XII, pp. 611–19K). Cf. Chapter VIII, T250.

AM.18 Galenus, *ibid.*, 3.1 (XII, pp. 646–50K)

AM.19 Galenus, *ibid.* (XII, pp. 651–5K)

AM.20 Galenus, *ibid.* (XII, pp. 658–9K)

AM.21 Galenus, *ibid.* (XII, pp. 662–4K)

AM.22 Galenus, *ibid.*, 3.3 (XII, pp. 686–8K)

AM.23 Galenus, *ibid.*, 5.5 (XII, pp. 858–9K)

AM.24a Galenus, *ibid.*, 2.2 (XII, p. 582K)

AM.24b Galenus, *ibid.*, 5.5 (XII, pp. 864–6K)

AM.25 Galenus, *ibid.*, 6.8 (XII, pp. 979–83K)

AM.26 Galenus, *ibid.*, 6.9 (XII, pp. 995–1000K)

AM.27 Codex Parisinus graecus 2286 (s.XIV), fol. 94 (*Anecdota Graeca e codd. manuscriptis Bibliothecae Regiae Parisiensis*, ed. J. A. Cramer, I (Oxford, 1839), p. 395)

AM.28 Galenus, *De medicamentorum secundum locos* 5.1 (XII, pp. 814–16K)

AM.29 Galenus, *In Hippocratis Epidemiarum 2.1.11 comment.* 1 (ad vol. v, p. 82.12–14L). From Ḥunain's Arabic translation of the lost original (*CMG* v.10.1, p. 194 Pfaff).

AM.30 Asclepiades Iunior apud Galenum, *De antidotis* 2.7 (XIV, p. 143K)

AM.31 Galenus (ex Asclepiade?), *De antidotis* 2.8 (XIV, pp. 146–7K)

AM.32 Palladius, *In Hippocratis Epidemiarum librum 6. comment.* 3.22 (II, p. 98 Dietz)

AM.33 Plutarchus, *Quaestiones naturales* 3 (Moralia 912D–E)

AM.34 C. Plinius Secundus, *Naturalis historia* 1 (on his sources for Book XXVIII)

AM.35 C. Plinius Secundus, *Naturalis historia* 28.2.7

AM.36 Iohannes Alexandrinus, *Commentaria in VI. librum Hippocratis Epidemiarum*, Particula 3, 132.b30–33 (p. 176 Pritchet)

AM.37 Oribasius, *Ad Eunapium*, praefatio (*CMG* VI.3; vol. V, pp. 317–18 Raeder)

AM.38 Philumenus, *De venenatis animalibus eorumque remediis* 5.5–6 (*CMG* X.1.1, p. 10 Wellmann)

AM.39 Philumenus, *De venenatis* 17.10–11 (*CMG* X.1.1, p. 24 Wellmann)

AM.40 Philumenus, *De venenatis* 19.1–2 (*CMG* X.1.1, p. 26 Wellmann)

AM.41 Philumenus, *De venenatis* 20.3 (*CMG* X.1.1, pp. 26–7 Wellmann)

AM.42 Philumenus, *De venenatis* 23.3 (*CMG* X.1.1, p. 30 Wellmann)

AM.43 Philumenus, *De venenatis* 32.3 (*CMG* X.1.1, p. 36 Wellmann)

AM.44 Philumenus, *De venenatis* 33.5–6 (*CMG* X.1.1, p. 37 Wellmann)

AM.45 Philumenus, *De venenatis* 35.3–4 (*CMG* X.1.1, p. 38 Wellmann)

AM.46 Galenus, *De compositione medicamentorum secundum locos* 5.2 (XII, p. 820–1K)

AM.47 Galenus, *De simplicium medicamentorum temperamentis ac facultatibus* 11.49 (XII, pp. 366–7K)

Dubia

AM.48a Caelius Aurelianus, *Tardae passiones* 1.5.151

AM.48b A. Cornelius Celsus, *Medicina* 7 (= *Artes* 12), prohoemium 1–3 (*CML* I, p. 301 Marx)

Excerpts from Andromachus (*AM*.49–66)

AM.49 Andromachus Iunior apud Galenum, *De compositione medicamentorum secundum locos* 3.1 (XII, p. 633K)

AM.50 Andromachus apud Galenum, *ibid.*, 7.2 (XIII, p. 31K)

AM.51 Andromachus apud Galenum, *ibid.*, 7.3 (XIII, p. 65K)

AM.52 Andromachus apud Galenum, *ibid.*, 7.3 (XIII, pp. 67–8K)

AM.53 Andromachus apud Galenum, *ibid.*, 7.3 (XIII, p. 70K)

AM.54 Andromachus apud Galenum, *ibid.*, 7.3 (XIII, p. 70K)

AM.55 Andromachus apud Galenum, *ibid.*, 7.3 (XIII, p. 72K)

AM.56 Andromachus apud Galenum, *ibid.*, 7.4 (XIII, p. 76K)

AM.57 Andromachus apud Galenum, *ibid.*, 7.4 (XIII, p. 78K)

AM.58 Andromachus apud Galenum, *ibid.*, 7.6 (XIII, p. 114K)

AM.59 Andromachus apud Galenum, *ibid.*, 8.2 (XIII, p. 136–7K)

AM.60 Andromachus apud Galenum, *ibid.*, 9.1 (XIII, p. 231K)

AM.61 Andromachus apud Galenum, *ibid.*, 9.4 (XIII, p. 279K)

AM.62 Andromachus apud Galenum, *ibid.*, 9.4 (XIII, p. 281K)

AM.63 Andromachus apud Galenum, *ibid.*, 9.5 (XIII, p. 295K)

AM.64 Andromachus apud Galenum, *ibid.*, 9.6 (XIII, p. 308K)

AM.65 Andromachus apud Galenum, *ibid.*, 10.1 (XIII, p. 326K)

AM.66 Andromachus apud Galenum, *De compositione medicamentorum per genera* 7.7 (XIII, p. 981K)

Oribasius' references to an unidentified 'Apollonius' (AM.67–9)

AM.67 Oribasius, *Collectiones medicae* 44.30 (*CMG* VI.2.1; vol. III, p. 158 Raeder)

AM.68 Oribasius, *Synopsis ad Eustathium* 1.14 (*CMG* VI.3; vol. V, pp. 12–13 Raeder)

AM.69 Oribasius, *Collectiones medicae* 7.19–20 (*CMG* VI.1.1; vol. I, pp. 218–9 Raeder)

AM.70 Asclepiades Iunior apud Galenum, *De compositione medicamentorum secundum locos* 4.8 (XII, p. 776K)

AM.71 'Caelius Aurelianus', *Gynaecia* 2.113 (Drabkin, 1951: 113)

AM.72 Mustio (?), in *Sorani Gynaeciorum vetus translatio latina* 2.26 (Rose, 1882: 106)

AM.73 Aëtius Amidenus, *Libri medicinales* 7.101 (*CMG* VIII.1, p. 353 Olivieri)

AM.74 Aëtius Amidenus, *Libri medicinales* 7.45 (*CMG* VIII.1, p. 299 Olivieri)

XXIV · HERACLIDES
OF ERYTHRAE (*HE.*)

A · INTRODUCTION

A physician of the latter half of the first century B.C., Heraclides of Erythrae was a contemporary of Strabo[1] and Alexander Philalethes,[2] and a pupil of the Herophilean Chrysermus.[3] He probably belonged to the Alexandrian rather than to the Asia Minor branch of the Herophilean school. While the Asian school at Men Karou, near Laodicea, continued the tradition of maintaining a broad theoretical and clinical expertise[4] – a tradition initiated by Herophilus himself – its leaders (Zeuxis Philalethes, Alexander Philalethes, Demosthenes Philalethes) do not seem to have followed the Alexandrian example of also engaging in Hippocratic philology. Heraclides of Erythrae, by contrast, energetically continued the Alexandrian tradition of Hippocratic exegesis represented within the Herophilean school above all by Bacchius[5] and Zeno.[6]

Most of the evidence concerning Heraclides refers to his commentaries on Books II, III, and VI of the Hippocratic *Epidemics*.[7] Galen explicitly states that Heraclides, unlike the Herophilean Bacchius and the Empiricist Glaucias, did not compose a Hippocratic glossary, but wrote commentaries on Hippocratic works, following the example of, among others, Bacchius and the Empiricists Zeuxis and

---

[1] See *HE*.1. Strabo lived from about 64 B.C. until at least A.D. 23, but, as pointed out above (Chapter XXI, with n. 13), his *Geography* had been largely completed by 7 B.C., and the reference to Heraclides as his contemporary is therefore made in the context of the last or penultimate decade of the first century B.C.

[2] Alexander lived roughly 50 B.C.–A.D. 25 (see Chapter XXII).

[3] See *Introduction* to Chapter XX and *Cr*.1.

[4] See Chapters XXII and XXVIII.

[5] Chapter XIV, especially *Ba*.7–78.

[6] Chapter XV, *Zn*.5–9. See also Chapter XIII, *Cm*.7–9.

[7] *HE*.4–10.

66

THE HEROPHILEANS

Heraclides of Tarentum.[8] In his commentary on *Epidemics* III, Heraclides of Erythrae apparently brought to a close the protracted feud between the Empiricists and the Herophileans concerning the authenticity of the acronymic letter-symbols attached to the case histories in *Epidemics* III.[9] Abandoning the position of the Herophilean Zeno and of Zeno's followers, Heraclides agreed with the Empiricists that these letter-symbols had not been introduced by Hippocrates himself but were later interpolations.[10] Whether Heraclides, like the Empiricists, attributed them to Mnemon[11] remains unclear, but Galen seems to imply that he did, thereby assigning them to the early Hellenistic period.

The bulk of the ancient evidence concerns Heraclides' commentary on *Epidemics* VI.[12] In his own commentary on this work Galen lists Heraclides as one 'of those who first interpreted this book' and refers to the Herophilean's commentary no less than five times – though not always in a complimentary manner. Galen accuses him of introducing inappropriate explanations[13] and of 'padding his commentary with drivel and inaccuracies'.[14] But even at his most polemical Galen concedes that 'it is not normally Heraclides' habit to talk drivel'.[15] Unfortunately too little of Heraclides' commentary survives to judge its interpretative quality, but the few comments transmitted by Galen are not immensely encouraging.

While Galen makes numerous other references to a 'Heraclides', both in this Hippocratic commentary and elsewhere, it is commonly assumed that all passages which mention 'Heraclides' without the ethnic 'of Erythrae' refer to the Empiricist, Heraclides of Tarentum.[16] I have found no firm criteria for salvaging any of these testimonia for the Herophilean.

In keeping with the broad medical tradition represented by Herophilus and other early Herophileans, Heraclides did not,

---

[8] *HE*.4. Zeuxis and Heraclides Tarentum: see Deichgräber, 1965: fr. 337, and pp. 209ff., 172ff. For Bacchius see Ch. XIV, *Ba.* 8–10; cf. *Ba.* 11.
[9] See *Introduction* to Chapter XV and *Zn*.5–6.   [10] *HE*.5.
[11] Cf. Chapter XV; Deichgräber, 1965: fr. 341–343.
[12] *HE*.6–10.   [13] *HE*.9; cf. *HE*.8.   [14] *HE*.10.   [15] *Ibid.*
[16] Cf., e.g., Deichgräber, 1965: fr. 170, 176, 190, 196, 199, 224, 225, 227–8, 230–2, 336. In none of these texts is Heraclides identified as the Empiricist (or as being from Tarentum), although Deichgräber presents indirect evidence that makes the expropriation of most of these texts for the Empiricist reasonable. But fr. 170 (= *HE*.13) almost certainly concerns the Herophilean.

however, confine himself to explicating Hippocratic texts. He contributed actively to pulse theory, perhaps in his doxographic treatise *On the School of Herophilus*, which consisted of at least seven books.[17] In his theory of the pulse, Heraclides staked out his independence from his teacher Chrysermus (but developed a pulse definition which agreed in all essential respects with that of his contemporary Apollonius Mys). Whereas Chrysermus uses 'distention' (*diastasis*) to designate diastole,[18] Heraclides reverts to 'dilation' (*diastolē*). Furthermore, whereas Chrysermus talks only of a 'distention and contraction of the arteries', Heraclides and Apollonius Mys add 'and of the heart'; whereas Chrysermus says the pulse arises 'through the agency of a psychic and vital faculty', Heraclides adds to the description of this faculty 'it being dominant' (πλειστοδυναμούσης).[19] Finally, Heraclides completely omits three phrases in Chrysermus' definition as redundant: (a) pulse occurs 'when the arterial coat rises and again collapses into itself'; (b) the pulsating distention and contraction are 'a constant concomitant of both healthy and diseased conditions'; and (c) it is 'apprehensible by sense-perception'. Heraclides' rebellion against his teacher could not have been more pointed, especially since a central issue of Herophilean physiology – pulse theory – is at stake. But, as suggested earlier,[20] his sharp challenge to his teacher does not render him an atypical Herophilean.

B · TEXTS

HE.1   Strabo, *Geographica* 14.1.34 (645c). See above, Chapter xxiii, *AM*.1.

HE.2a   Galenus (ex Aristoxeno?), *De pulsuum differentiis* 4.10 (viii, pp. 743–5K). Cf. Chapter vii, T156.

HE.2b   Marcellinus, *De pulsibus* 3 (p. 457 Schöne)

HE.2c   Marcellinus, *De pulsibus* 1 (p. 455 Schöne)

HE.3   Galenus (ex Aristoxeno?), *De pulsuum differentiis* 4.10 (viii, p. 746K)

---

[17] This treatise is referred to only in a sphygmological context: see *HE*.3.

[18] Chapter xx, *Cr*.1, vs. *HE*.2a. But, if Marcellinus' account (*HE*.2b) is accurate, Heraclides might have vacillated between *diastasis* and *diastolē*.

[19] Compare *Cr*.1–2 with *HE*.2; cf. also Chapter xxiii, *AM*.2. Schöne, 1893: 11–15, provides a useful summary of these and other modifications introduced by successive generations of Herophilean physicians. See also pp. 446–8 *supra*.

[20] See Chapter x.a.

HE.4   Galenus, *In Hippocratis Epidemiarum 2.2.20 comment.* 2 (ad vol. v, p. 92.8–12L). From Ḥunain's Arabic translation of the lost original (*CMG* v.10.1, p. 230 Pfaff).

HE.5   Galenus, *In Hippocratis Epidemiarum 3.2.7 comment.* 2.4 (ad vol. III, p. 52.10L) (*CMG* v.10.2.1, p. 80 Wenkebach)

HE.6   Galenus, *In Hippocratis Epidemiarum 6. comment.*, prooemium (*CMG* v.10.2.2, pp. 3–4 Wenkebach). See also above, Chapter XIV, *Ba*.10.

HE.7   Galenus, *In Hippocratis Epidemiarum 6.4.8 comment.* 4.11 (ad vol. v, p. 308.17–18L). From Ḥunain's Arabic translation of the lost original (*CMG* v.10.2.2, p. 212 Pfaff).

HE.8   Galenus, *In Hippocratis Epidemiarum 6.4.20 comment.* 4.27 (ad v, p. 312.9L). From Ḥunain's translation (*CMG* v.10.2.2, p. 243 Pfaff).

HE.9   Galenus, *In Hp. Epidemiarum 6.5.15 comment.* 5.26 (ad v, p. 320.4L) (*CMG* v.10.2.2, pp. 304, 306 Wenkebach/Pfaff).

HE.10   Galenus, *In Hp. Epidemiarum 6.6.14 comment.6* (ad v, p. 330.3–7L). From Ḥunain's translation (*CMG* v.10.2.2, p. 378 Pfaff).

HE.11   Galenus, *Ars medica*, prooem. (I, pp. 305–6K). See Chapter IV.A.2.

HE.12   Agnellus Ravennas(?), *In Galeni De sectis comm.* 4 (p. 22 S.U.N.Y., Arethusa Monogr. 8)

Dubia

HE.13   Galenus, *De pulsuum dignotione* 4.3 (VIII, p. 955K)
          See Chapter VII, T162.Cf. n. 16 and Deichgräber, 1965: fr. 170.

HE.14   Agnellus Ravennas(?), *In Galeni De sectis comm.* 5 (p. 26 S.U.N.Y., Arethusa Monogr. 8)

XXV · ARISTOXENUS
(Ar.)

A · INTRODUCTION

Even from the limited passages listed below the lively contours emerge of a contentious, eristic author with stronger but not necessarily better philosophical instincts than most Herophileans. A pupil of the physician Alexander Philalethes[1] – and hence trained in the 'Asian' branch of the Herophilean school at Men Karou, near Laodicea – Aristoxenus in his treatise *On Herophilus and his School*[2] apparently took on all comers, not even sparing some of the more illustrious members of his own school. Bacchius, Zeno, Chrysermus, Apollonius Mys, Heraclides of Erythrae – these fellow-Herophileans are among the targets of his censure.[3] While revisionism had been an essential aspect of the history of the Herophilean school almost from its inception,[4] no adherent of the school seems to have criticized the views of his precursors as freely as Aristoxenus. As a member of the last generation of Herophileans – he probably belongs to the first half of the first century A.D.[5] – Aristoxenus' polemics might reflect the

---

[1] Cf. *Ar.*3. On Alexander Philalethes see Chapter xxii.

[2] *Ar.*3.

[3] *Ar.*1–5. Cf. Chapter xiv, *Ba.*1 with *Ar.*1; Chapter xv, *Zn.*1; Chapter xx, *Cr.*2; Chapter xxiii, *AM.*2; Chapter xxiv, *HE.*2a.

[4] Philinus rebelled against Herophilus and founded the Empiricist school in Alexandria (cf. Deichgräber, 1965: fr.6; above, Chapter ii, T1); Bacchius apparently criticized the Herophilean Callianax (cf. Chapter xii, *Cn.*1) and developed a pulse definition which diverged from Herophilus'; Callimachus ridiculed Herophilus (Chapter xiii, *Cm.*9); Mantias' pupil Heraclides of Tarentum left the Herophilean school to become an Empiricist (Chapter xviii, *Ma.*2); Heraclides of Erythrae rejected Zeno's theory concerning the letter-symbols in Hp., *Epidemics* iii; and almost every Herophilean surfaced with a new definition of the pulse.

[5] The best chronological clues are: (a) Aristoxenus' teacher, Alexander, became head of the Herophilean school at Men Karou no later than 7 B.C. (see Chapter

growing insecurity of an Herophilean amid the burgeoning popularity of new rival schools. His contemporary Demosthenes Philalethes, also a pupil of Alexander Philalethes,[6] did not engage in
extensive polemics of this kind and made positive contributions to
medical science (with the result that his impact endured until the late
Middle Ages[7] and, in certain respects, was matched by that of no
other Herophilean except Herophilus). The censorious Aristoxenus,
by contrast, does not seem to have influenced scientific medicine
significantly, but to have served as a rich source for doxography.

A plausible but not conclusive case has been made for the
hypothesis that Book XIII of Aristoxenus' treatise *On Herophilus and his
School* served as the source of substantial sections of one of Galen's
major treatises on pulse theory.[8] The Galenic passages in question,
which yield unusually rich information concerning various Herophileans,[9] are *De pulsuum differentiis* 4.2 (VIII, pp. 699–715K) and 4.3–10
(VIII, pp. 720–49K). While it is clear that Galen had a copy of
Aristoxenus' work within easy reach when composing much of the
fourth book of *De pulsuum differentiis*, he only rarely makes explicit
reference to Aristoxenus. In keeping with the criteria for inclusion
developed earlier,[10] the texts listed in this chapter are confined to
these explicit references.

The targets of Aristoxenus' criticism range from the earliest
Herophileans (for example, Bacchius and Zeno) to his older contemporaries (Apollonius Mys, Heraclides of Erythrae), but it seems to

---

XXII.A) and probably lived at least until the early years of the first century A.D.; (b)
Aristoxenus mentioned Apollonius Mys and Heraclides of Erythrae – both
apparently pupils of Chrysermus and residents of Alexandria in the latter part of
the first century B.C. – in Book XIII of his *On the School of Herophilus* (cf. *Ar*.2–3). If
Schöne's (1893) reconstruction is correct, the pulse theory of Demosthenes
Philalethes, who perhaps lived *c*. 20 B.C.–A.D. 50, was also discussed by
Aristoxenus. But this is an unconfirmed inference and can therefore not be used to
determine Aristoxenus' date.
[6] Cf. Chapter XXVIII, *DP*.1 and *DP*.3.
[7] See Chapter XXVIII.A on the esteem in which Demosthenes Philalethes was held in
the tenth and thirteenth centuries by a pope and a papal physician respectively.
[8] Schöne, 1893: 1–29. See *Ar*. 3 on Book XII of Aristoxenus' work.
[9] See Chapter VII, T144, T150, 155–7 (and cf. T162); Chapter XIV, *Ba*. 1–2;
Chapter XV, *Zn*.1; Chapter XX, *Cr*.1–2; Chapter XXII, *AP*.2–4; Chapter XXIII,
AM.2 and 4; Chapter XXIV, *HE*.2a–3; *Ar*. 1–3, 5; Chapter XXVIII, *DP*.1–2.
[10] See *Note on text, arrangement and translation*, pp. xvi–xvii.

have been directed mainly at Alexandrian Herophileans.[11] All the extant criticisms concern their pulse theories (and are hence derived from Book XIII of Aristoxenus' *On the School of Herophilus*). Aristoxenus' own definition of the pulse – 'pulse is an activity of the heart and arteries that is peculiar to them'[12] – contains the felicitous reference to the notion that pulsation is uniquely present in the arteries and in the heart, but in other respects his definition is not intrinsically superior to some of those he criticizes. His insistence on starting the definition of any term with its genus before proceeding to its differentiae is also commendable but, as Galen remarks, 'he wishes to argue dialectically but he does not even observe the laws of dialectic himself'.[13]

Hermann Schöne argues that Aristoxenus' analysis of pulse theories was divided into two parts,[14] the first corresponding closely to Galen's *De pulsuum differentiis* 4.2 (VIII, pp. 699–715K), the second to Book 4.3–10 (VIII, pp. 720–49K) of the Galenic treatise. In the first part of Aristoxenus' work, the idea that there are two kinds of definitions is said to have been developed: (a) 'definitions proper' or 'substantial definitions' (ὅροι οὐσιώδεις), and (b) 'conceptual' (ἐννοηματικοί) or 'subjective' (ὡς ἐν ἐπισκέψει) definitions, also described as 'descriptive outlines' (ὑποτυπώσεις or ὑπογραφαί). Aristoxenus subdivided each of these two groups into four, starting with the 'descriptive outlines', and explained how definitions could arise from 'descriptive outlines'. This taxonomic structure was then given doxographic application in the second part of Aristoxenus' analysis, according to Schöne: a critical review of the pulse definitions proposed by one renegade Herophilean (the Empiricist Heraclides of Tarentum) and by eight loyal Herophileans accorded Aristoxenus an opportunity to sort them out into 'descriptive outlines' and 'definitions proper'.[15]

---

[11] The Herophileans explicitly identified as the victims of Aristoxenus' censure – Bacchius, Zeno, Chrysermus, Apollonius, Heraclides – all seem to have practised in Alexandria, but if Schöne's reconstruction is correct, Alexander and Demosthenes Philalethes were also critized by Aristoxenus.Galen, however, nowhere attributes criticism of his fellow-'Laodiceans' to Aristoxenus.

[12] Cf. *Ar.*1–3.   [13] *Ar.*1.

[14] Schöne, 1893: especially pp. 17–24.

[15] According to Schöne (1893: 13–14), Aristoxenus used the same sequence employed by Galen in *De pulsuum differentiis* 4.3–10 (VIII, pp. 720–44K): first Heraclides of Tarentum (included although he was an Empiricist because – argues Schöne – he had been a pupil of the Herophilean Mantias); then

These conclusions have their appeal, but they rest squarely on an assumption which remains open to doubt: that Galen religiously and unswervingly employed the systematizing devices supposedly developed by Aristoxenus. As the testimonia and fragments listed below demonstrate, this is pure, if ingenious, conjecture. Nowhere is the distinction between 'proper definitions' and 'descriptive outlines' – a distinction which perhaps goes back to the Stoics[16] – explicitly attributed to Aristoxenus. Nor, for that matter, are other distinctions which Galen used in the relevant passages, e.g. the distinction between 'conceptual' and 'substantial' definitions (e.g. in *Cr.*1), said to have originated with Aristoxenus. Even the distinction between 'objective' and 'subjective' definitions that had been introduced by Aristoxenus' teacher Alexander (*AP.*3) and was accepted by his contemporary Demosthenes Philalethes (*DP.*1) is never attributed to Aristoxenus, despite Schöne's implications to the contary. Schöne[17] confidently identifies 'subjective definitions' – ὅροι ὡς ἐν ἐπισκέψει – with Aristoxenus' putative ὑποτυπώσεις or 'descriptive outlines' but for this, too, there is no firm basis in the texts. The closest Aristoxenus is explicitly attested to have come to these distinctions is his insistence on starting every definition with the genus.

Galen undoubtedly made use of Aristoxenus' sophisticated work, as the texts listed below suggest, but any attempt to reconstruct the Herophilean's treatise in precise detail is forced to place too much faith in the value of hypothetical indirect testimonia – all of which fail to mention Aristoxenus by name. How problematic and questionable systematic reconstructions based mainly on indirect sources can be has been demonstrated repeatedly, and the veil Galen drew over his own use of source material is often no more penetrable or transparent than the Mayan veils which continue to confound the use of indirect testimonies for reconstructing, for example, aspects of Gnosticism, Stoicism, and Cynicism.

Alexander Philalethes, Demosthenes Philalethes, Bacchius, Aristoxenus himself, Zeno, Chrysermus, Heraclides of Erythrae, and Apollonius Mys. The failure to use a chronological sequence is seen by Schöne as proof that another ordering principle was employed.

[16] I say 'perhaps' because it is not clear that *SVF* II, 227 and 229 (pp. 75–6) are actually attributable to the Stoics.

[17] Schöne, 1893: 18.

For all Aristoxenus' preoccupation with fratricidal polemics and with the problem of the genus of the term pulse and its division, he seems to have devoted time to clinical problems as well. In his discussion of hydrophobia – defined as a simultaneous fear of water and craving for water – Caelius Aurelianus (fifth century A.D.) reports that Aristoxenus prescribed potions and purgative or tempering clysters for all patients.[18] Caelius, moreover, apparently suggests that these prescriptions were motivated by Aristoxenus' adherence to some version of humoral pathology: because Aristoxenus 'is concerned about decay and excess of *liquid*' ('corruptionem atque abundantiam liquoris'), he resorts to remedies with a purgative or tempering power. *Liquor* is, however, too vague and ambivalent a term to allow any exact determination of how closely Aristoxenus' pathological principles resembled those of Herophilus.[19]

The balance sheet seems clear: while we may owe most of our knowledge of the pulse theories of later Herophileans to Aristoxenus' treatise *On the School of Herophilus*, his unquestionable significance as a source and his argumentative subtlety should not be allowed to veil his apparent insignificance as a scientist and a physician.

B · TEXTS

*Ar.*1   Galenus, *De pulsuum differentiis* 4.7 (VIII, pp. 734–5K)
*Ar.*2   Galenus, *De pulsuum differentiis* 4.10 (VIII, pp. 744–5K)
*Ar.*3   Galenus, *De pulsuum differentiis* 4.10 (VIII, pp. 746–7K). Cf. Chapter VII, T157.
*Ar.*4   Galenus, *De pulsuum dignotione* 4.3 (VIII, p. 955K)
         See above, Chapter VII, T162.
*Ar.*5   Galenus, *De pulsuum differentiis* 4.8 (VIII, pp. 738–40K)
*Ar.*6   Caelius Aurelianus, *Celeres vel acutae passiones* 3.16.134
         See also the texts listed in n. 9.

[18] *Ar.*6. Caelius Aurelianus, as mentioned above, is directly dependent on Soranus, so that this is not as late a source as suggested prima facie. Although Caelius does not identify Aristoxenus as a Herophilean, no other physician by this name is known, and Wellmann's suggestion (1895c) that the Herophilean is meant seems reasonable. On hydrophobia see Ch. XXVII.A (with nn. 8–16).

[19] On Herophilus' general pathological principles see Chapter VII, especially T130–T135 and T205ff.

XXVI · CYDIAS

(*Cy.*)

A · INTRODUCTION

Only one testimonium about Cydias seems to have survived. It implies that Cydias followed the example of a number of early Herophileans, including Bacchius and Zeno, and engaged either in Hippocratic lexicography or in some form of Hippocratic criticism: in the context of Hippocratic lexicography it mentions an attack on a work by Cydias. The author who, according to the famous glossographer Erotian, criticized Cydias, was a Hellenistic physician, Lysimachus of Cos. Since Lysimachus' date is uncertain – except, of course, that our source, Erotian (Neronian period), provides a *terminus ante quem* – the date of Cydias remains in doubt too. (But if Lysimachus is, as some have suggested, identical with the pharmacologist whom Varro, Pliny, Hesychius, and others mention, the *terminus ante quem* would have to be much earlier – approximately 60 B.C. – in order to accommodate Varro's mention of Lysimachus. The identification of the lexicographer Lysimachus with this pharmacologist, let alone with an Empiricist,[1] is, however, quite uncertain.) Other than his work(s) concerning Hippocrates, nothing is known about Cydias.[2]

If Lysimachus' 'Coan' epithet indicates a personal connection with

---

[1] Kudlien, 1969b, suggests that the combination of Hippocratic exegesis with pharmacology points to an adherent of the Empiricist school. While such a possibility cannot be excluded, adherents of several other schools – for example, the Herophilean – likewise engaged in both kinds of activity. See Ch. X.A.

[2] The name is unlikely to be a corruption; it was common enough in Greek antiquity. Thus Pliny mentions a painter by this name, a contemporary of Euphranor (*Naturalis historia* 35.40.130), who is perhaps the same as the one to whom Theophrastus attributes a ruddle substitute (*On Stones* 53). Aristotle also refers to an Athenian orator of the fourth century B.C. called Cydias (*Rhetoric* 2.6.1384b32ff.). Cf. also *Poetae melici Graeci*, ed. D. L. Page (Oxford 1962), fr. 714–15.

(or loyalty to) the Hippocratic tradition, the clash between him and the Herophilean, Cydias, would be interesting evidence of a continuing rivalry between the 'old' medicine of Cos and the 'new' medicine of Alexandria. Despite his apprenticeship with Praxagoras of Cos, Herophilus had firmly asserted his independence from the Hippocratic and Coan tradition, among other things by openly criticizing Hippocrates' *Prognostic*. His pupils and later followers, free from any Coan connection or burden to begin with (with the possible exception of the rebel Philinus), perhaps had less of an urge and need to emancipate themselves from the Hippocratic tradition. But they never seem to have sought to sanction their activities or views by proclaiming themselves the true heirs of the Hippocratic tradition either – as did the Empiricists. While the contest with the Empiricists was heated and sustained, the contest with 'The Physician' or 'The Man' (as Hippocrates is often referred to) was muted. It was, however, no less real.

B · TEXTS

*Cy.*1   Erotianus, *Vocum Hippocraticarum collectio*, praefatio (p. 5 Nachmanson)

XXVII · GAIUS

(G.)

A · INTRODUCTION

In his monumental therapeutic work, *On Chronic and Acute Diseases*, Caelius Aurelianus (fifth century A.D.) provides the only firm evidence about Gaius. While Caelius Aurelianus' Greek source, Soranus (*c.* A.D. 100), provides a *terminus ante quem* for Gaius, it is impossible to determine his date more exactly. The use of the name 'Gaius' seems to point to a Roman physician. Although 'Gaios' (Γάιος) was a name disseminated in the Greek world as early as the third century B.C.,[1] it tended to be used only of Romans – so much so, in fact, that the praenomina 'Gaius' and Gaia' came to be used as generic terms for Romans.[2] If the Herophilean was a Roman, he is unlikely to have been among the earliest adherents of this school. Although a number of Romans had been in Ptolemaic service relatively early,[3] and although Roman philosophers had been in

---

[1] *Inscriptiones Graecae* XII.1.161 (Rhodes, second or first century B.C.): τῶν σὺν Γαί[ω]ι; *ibid.*, XII.3.7 (Syme, slightly later): Γάιος ʽΡωμαῖ[ος]; *Supplementum Epigraphicum Graecum* XX.509: βασιλεῖ/Πτολεμαίωι/Γάιος καὶ οἱ ἱππεῖς. Cf. also 'Gaius the Roman' in Book IV of Callimachus' *Aetia* (frr. 106–7 Pfeiffer); unfortunately only the lemma with the diegesis is extant. Cf. Pfeiffer, 1949: vol. I *ad loc.* and vol. II, p. 114 for various explanations of the identity of this Gaius; De Sanctis, 1935: 289ff. (Gaios = Horatius Cocles); Della Corte, 1941: 276–82; Andor, 1951–2: 121–5 (Gaios = Spurius Carvilius); Fraser, 1972: vol. I, pp. 767–8, and vol. II, pp. 1073–5 (nn. 359–65). See also Fraser, 1960: 145–6, on the Greek dedication to a 'king Ptolemy' by 'Gaius and the *hippeis*,' found in Kom Turuga, south-east of Alexandria (quoted above).

[2] Cf. Plutarch of the generic usage in the Roman marriage ceremony too: *Quaestiones Romanae* 30 (*Moralia* 271E). See also Festus, *De verborum significatu*, s.vv. Gaia Caecilia (p. 85 Lindsay); Cicero, *Pro Murena* 12 (27); Quintilian, *Institutiones Oratoriae* 1.7.28.

[3] Fraser, 1972: vol. II, p. 150 (n. 210); vol. I, pp. 89–90; vol. II, pp. 169–70 (nn. 347–8); vol. I, p. 101. Cf. also vol. I, pp. 122 and 159 on Roman residents in Alexandria.

Alexandria in the first half of the first century B.C.,[4] the evidence strongly suggests that significant scholarly and scientific contact between Rome and Alexandria developed only from the time of Caesar onwards. Only after Rome's 'final pacification' of the Near East was there a lively demand for Greek doctors in Rome,[5] and in the Augustan age a number of Alexandrian grammarians and scientists, including physicians, finally did migrate to Rome.[6] But P. M. Fraser has plausibly argued that, with the exception of the grammarian Dionysius Thrax (c. 170–90 B.C.), 'no scholars from Alexandria seem to have migrated to Rome before the middle of the first century B.C.',[7] and conversely no Roman physicians or scientists seem to have gone to Alexandria before this time. Together, these considerations seem to point to a date between 50 B.C. and A.D. 100 for Gaius, also if his affiliation with the Herophileans developed at one of the two known Herophilean centres of medical instruction – Men Karou (near Laodicea) and Alexandria – rather than in Italy.

Gaius' recognition of the importance of the brain and the meninges as centres of the nervous system (*G.*1) is authentically Herophilean, as is his attribution of voluntary motion to the nerves (cf. Herophilus, T81). His attempt, in his work *On hydrophobia*, to explain a deviant psychic condition in terms of physiological and anatomical factors (*G.*1) is also consonant with Herophilus' emphasis on the somatic symptoms and sources of mental disorders.

Explanations of deviant psychic conditions in somatic terms were, however, not confined to the Herophileans. As early as the Hippocratic treatise *On the Sacred Disease* such aetiologies were offered. Similarly, in his discussion of hydrophobia – defined as a powerful craving for, and an irrational fear of, drink[8] – Caelius Aurelianus

---

[4] Lucullus, who held a post similar to proquaestor in Alexandria, was there in company with the Academic philosopher Antiochus of Ascalon no later than 87/86 B.C. Perhaps about 80 B.C. Antiochus returned to Athens to take over the leadership of the Platonic Academy, and subsequently he followed Lucullus to the Second Mithridatic War. Cf. Luck, 1953: 14; Cicero, *Academica priora* [= *Lucullus*] 4.11 (Antiochus, fr. 4 Luck) and 19.61 (Antiochus, fr. 34 Luck). See also *Index Academicorum* XXXIV.3–43 (fr. 33 Luck); Glucker, 1978: 13–21, 90–7.

[5] On the early history of Greek medicine in Rome see Allbutt, 1921: 176ff.; Scarborough, 1969: 38ff.

[6] On the migration of Alexandrian intellectuals to Rome see Fraser, 1972: vol. I, pp. 425, 474–75, 518–19, 809–10.

[7] 1972: vol. I, p. 810.

[8] Caelius Aurelianus, *Celeres vel acutae passiones* 3.10.101: 'Est agnitio hydrophobiae

mentions not only Gaius (G.1) but also numerous previous explanations of its pathology, including Andreas' (An. 20) and Aristoxenus' (Ar. 6), and most of them, too, have recourse to physical causes.[9] (Caelius himself does raise the question whether hydrophobia, which was often associated with rabies,[10] is a disease of the body or of the soul,[11] but he concludes that 'one should not agree with those who assert' that persons who suffer from a pathological fear of water are the victims of a disease of the soul.[12]) Among those who agreed with Gaius that this fear could be traced to somatic causes there was, however, disagreement concerning the part of the body principally affected by the disease. Some argued that the oesophagus was the part affected, others the oesophagus as well as the stomach, still others the diaphragm, and others again argued that several parts were affected individually.[13] Gaius' view – that the brain and its meninges are affected in hydrophobia – comes close to that of the 'atomistic' physician Asclepiades of Bithynia (first century B.C.), who taught that every disease which disorders the mind is centred in its meninges.[14] (This is also the view which Caelius Aurelianus himself generally accepted: 'It is sufficient for the physician to understand that whenever there is any mental derangement [$mens\ alienata$], the head is [physiologically] affected.'[15])

As far as the immediate cause of hydrophobia is concerned, it is not clear whether Gaius agreed with most other physicians that the bite of

$appetentia\ vehemens\ atque\ timor\ potus$ sine ulla ratione ob quandam in corpore passionem.' So too Celsus, $Medicina$ 5.27.2c (CML I, p. 231 Marx): 'simul aeger et siti et aquae metu cruciatur'.

[9] $Op.\ cit.$ 3.13.109–3.16.137.   [10] $Ibid.$, 3.9.99–100; 3.15.121–4.

[11] $Ibid.$, 3.13.109–10 (Caelius uses $anima$ and $animus$ interchangeably of the soul).

[12] $Ibid.$, 3.13.110.   [13] $Ibid.$, 3.14.112–15.

[14] $Ibid.$, 3.14.112. Plutarch, $Quaestiones\ symposiacae$ 8.9 ($Moralia$ 731B) says: 'Elephantiasis and hydrophobia first began to appear in the time of Asclepiades.' But this is a misleading statement, since a discussion of hydrophobia is attributed to a considerably earlier author, Democritus (probably not the Presocratic philosopher, but ps.-Democritus, i.e. Bolus of Mendes in the Egyptian Delta, a third-century B.C. writer on pharmacology, magic, and paradoxography). Cf. Democritus B300.10DK (vol. II, pp. 215–16); Caelius Aurelianus, $op.\ cit.$ 3.14.112, 3.15.120 (confused with the Presocratic), 3.16.132–3. The Herophilean physician Andreas, also third century B.C., likewise discussed hydrophobia.

[15] $Op.\ cit.$ 3.14.115. I say 'generally' because this generalizing statement is later amplified as follows by Caelius Aurelianus: '$prae$patitur enim ea $pars\ quae\ morsu\ fuerit\ vexata$ . . .' (116), and since he refers to 'head', not 'meninges'.

a rabid dog or of other rabid animals (or of a hydrophobic human) is the normal cause.[16] Some physicians had claimed that its immediate cause was unknown, and in the absence of more details concerning Gaius' view, judgment has to be suspended concerning his answer to this question.

In addition to the text which identifies Gaius as an Herophilean (*G.*1), I have included three drug prescriptions attributed to a 'Gaius' by Galen, who once identifies him as an eye-doctor (*G.*2), and once as a Neapolitan (*G.*3). In the absence of any identification of this Gaius with the Herophilean, however, it seemed advisable to include these pharmacological texts under the rubric *Dubia*. The fact that the Herophilean school had not only an anatomical but also a therapeutic interest in the eye from the time of Herophilus (Chapter VIII, T260) until the mid first century A.D. (when Demosthenes Philalethes apparently wrote his *Ophthalmicus*), renders the inclusion of *G.2* among the authentic testimonia tempting, but certainty at present is unattainable.

B · TEXTS

*G.*1   Caelius Aurelianus, *Celeres vel acutae passiones* 3.14.113–14

Dubia

*G.*2   Asclepiades Iunior apud Galenum, *De compositione medicamentorum secundum locos* 4.8 (XII, p. 771K)

*G.*3   Asclepiades Iunior apud Galenum, *De compositione medicamentorum per genera* 5.11 (XIII, p. 830K)

*G.*4   Andromachus Iunior apud Galenum, *De compositione medicamentorum secundum locos* 3.1 (XII, p. 628K)

---

[16] *Ibid.*, 3.9.99–100. The breathing of toxic 'chance emanations' from a mad dog is also listed among the causes of hydrophobia. Cf. also Dsc. 2.47 (I, p. 135 Wellmann); *id.* (?), *Theriaca*, praef. and 3 (*Medicorum Graecorum opera* XXVI, pp. 45, 58, 64 Sprengel); Philumenus' *De venenatis animalibus* 4.5–15 and 1.4 (*CMG* X.1.1, pp. 8–9 and 5 Wellmann); Celsus, *Medicina* 5.27.2A–D (*CML* I, pp. 230–1 Marx); Arrianus, *Epicteti Dissertationes* 4.4.20; Plutarch, *Quaestiones symposiacae* 8.9 (*Moralia* 732A); Cassius, *Problemata* 73 (I, p. 165 Ideler); Galen, *Methodus medendi* 9.5 (X, p. 627K); *id.*, *In Hp. Prorrhet. 1.52 comm.* 2.16 (*CMG* V.9.2, p. 66 Diels). The comedian Menander offered a more colourful explanation of hydrophobia: it is due to wine-drinking (fr. 924 Koerte, from Cael. Aurel., *Cel. vel acut.* 3.15.121).

XXVIII · DEMOSTHENES
PHILALETHES (*DP.*)

A · INTRODUCTION

The structure, workings, and ailments of the human eye fascinated and baffled Greek poets, scientists, and philosophers from Homer to the Byzantine period.[1] Some of the more substantial scientific contributions to an understanding of the eye were made by Herophilus and by one of his last known followers, Demosthenes Philalethes. Herophilus provided remarkably accurate and detailed observations on the coats or tunics of the eye, on the optic nerve, on the optic chiasma, and on the connection of the eye with the brain.[2] In addition, he dealt with defective vision and ways of treating it, as the therapeutic fragment from his work *On Eyes* – one of the earlier purely ophthalmological treatises of Greek antiquity – makes clear.[3] But no ancient author had as durable an impact on ophthalmology as Demosthenes Philalethes.

No more than about forty ancient texts mention Demosthenes by name. But a comparison of the passages which explicitly attest his authorship of certain ophthalmological views and remedies with numerous passages in which Demosthenes is not mentioned by name reveals that more authors of the Roman Imperial, Byzantine, and medieval periods depended on Demosthenes for their knowledge of the eye – and especially for their remedies for eye ailments – than on any other ancient source.[4] Numerous passages in the pseudo-Galenic

---

[1] Cf. Hirschberg, 1899; Magnus, 1878: 1–65; *id.*, 1901; 41–667.

[2] See Chapter VI, T84–T89; Chapter VII, T140.

[3] Chapter VIII, T260. Cf. Ch. 1.5; Hp., *On Vision* (IX, pp. 152–60L). Since the Presocratic era philosophers had written much on vision, but not on eye ailments.

[4] The credit for this discovery belongs above all to Julius Hirschberg, who recognized (1899: 368ff.) that all later ancient writers depended on the same ophthalmological 'canon', and to Max Wellmann, who identified Demosthenes

treatises *Introductio sive medicus* and *Definitiones medicae* (both of which apparently predate Galen), in a work by Rufus of Ephesus (*c.* A.D. 100), in Oribasius' *Collectiones medicae* (fourth century A.D.), in the *Libri medicinales* of Aëtius of Amida (sixth century A.D.), in Paul of Aegina's encyclopedic work on medicine (seventh century), in the *Synopsis iatrikē* of the Byzantine writer Leo (ninth century), and in the anonymous *On Eyes* edited by Theodor Puschmann, depend directly or indirectly on Demosthenes' work *Ophthalmicus*.[5] Many of these passages in fact seem to be verbatim quotations from Demosthenes, even though he is not acknowledged as the source. But in accordance with the principle of severity developed at the outset (pp. xvi–xvii), these anonymous quotations and paraphrases are treated as indirect testimonia and are therefore not included among the fragments and testimonia listed below (pp. 576–8).

Latin authors, too, depended heavily on Demosthenes' treatise. It has been argued that the *Liber ophthalmicus* written by St Augustine's friend Vindician in the fourth century 'was apparently nothing but a Latin translation of Demosthenes' work',[6] and while this might be too confident an assertion, it does seem clear that a manuscript or several manuscripts – all now lost[7] – of a Latin translation of Demosthenes' famous work existed at least from the tenth century A.D. until the end of the thirteenth century. Not only is it listed in a tenth-century catalogue of manuscripts kept in the library of the famous monastery at Bobbio,[8] but when the mathematician and philosopher Gerbert of Aurillac became abbot of the monastery in 982 (by the grace of his

---

Philalethes as the author of the 'canon'; cf. Wellmann, 1903: 546–66. See also Hirschberg, 1919a; Wellmann, 1900b.

[5] On the date of the pseudo-Galenic *Definitiones medicae* see J. Kollesch, 1973: 60–6; she argues persuasively for a date between A.D. 75–100. For the anonymous treatise *On Eyes* see Puschmann, 1886: 134–79.

[6] Wellmann, 1903: 558.

[7] None of the collections in the Vatican contain this MS, and Hermann Diels was unable to list any manuscripts of Demosthenes in his MSS catalogue (Diels, 1905–6: Pt II). Stevenson and other cataloguers of the Vatican MSS were likewise unable to track it down.

[8] Cf. Olleris, 1867: 493: 'Boetii . . . alterum de astronomia, Librum I Demosthenis, Librum M. Victoris de rhetorica'. The Demosthenes MS was apparently no. 399 in the catalogue of MSS at Bobbio. The enumeration of 'Manilius de astrologia, Victorinus de rhetorica, Demosthenis Ophthalmicus' in Gerbert's letter to the monk Rainardus (see below) seems to confirm that this 'Demosthenes' is the physician, not the orator. Cf. n. 10.

former pupil, Emperor Otto II), he wrote to Gisalbert, the abbot of another monastery, requesting him to send over a part missing from the manuscript at Bobbio, viz. the beginning of *Demostenes philosophus'* book *De morbis ac remediis oculorum . . . qui inscribitur Ophthalmicus.*[9] A few years later, when Gerbert fled from Italy and settled in Reims (where, in 991, he became archbishop without Papal sanction), he once more revealed that his interest in Demosthenes' work was neither casual nor fleeting. In a letter to the monk Rainardus he requests copies of three ancient works, apparently with a sense of urgency: 'age ergo et te solo conscio ex tuis sumptibus fac ut mihi scribantur M. Manilius *de astrologia*, Victorinus *de rhetorica*, Demostenis [sic] *Optalmicus.*'[10] Astronomy, rhetoric, and ophthalmology, or Manilius, Victorinus, and Demosthenes: an indication not only of the esteem in which Demosthenes' work was held, but also of the canonicity it had achieved in the Middle Ages as *the* work on the treatment of eye ailments.

When Otto III appointed Gerbert successor to Pope Gregory V in 999, Gerbert – now known as Pope Sylvester II – seems to have had the manuscript of Demosthenes' treatise brought to Rome from his old monastery at Bobbio. Among other things this is suggested by the fact that Simon of Genoa (Simon Ianuensis), the personal physician of Pope Nicholas IV (1288–92), used a manuscript of a Latin translation of Demosthenes' work while residing in Rome and composing his *Synonyma medicinae sive Clavis sanationis*. It is striking that Simon complains that the first part of the manuscript is mutilated. Talking about the *Obtalmicus Demostenis* [sic], Simon says:

Hic liber antiquissimus mihi occurrit, in quo deficiebant de inceptu disputatione de visu plurima et de anatomia oculi. cetera vero aderant . . .[11]

Since Gerbert, too, had apparently missed the first part of the treatise in the copy at Bobbio, as pointed out above, it seems likely that the manuscript from Bobbio – or a copy of it – came to Rome during the papacy of Sylvester II (Gerbert) and that Simon relied on the same manuscript as Gerbert, or on a direct copy of it. In the fourteenth

[9]   The letter to Gisalbert was written in July 983. It is no. 9 in Havet, 1889, and no. 16 in Lattin, 1961. Cf. Picavet, 1897: 85–6.
[10] The letter to Rainard of Bobbio is dated 7 September 988; it is no. 130 in Havet, no. 138 in Lattin. Cf. Leflon, 1946: 47. On the value of Gerbert's letters see also Uhlirz, 1957.
[11] Simon Ianuensis, 1474: praefatio (pages unnumbered).

XXVIII DEMOSTHENES PHILALETHES 573

century Demosthenes is still known in the Latin West: Matthaeus Silvaticus of Mantua quotes Demosthenes five times in his *Liber pandectarum medicinae*.[12] But Silvaticus' quotations might well be derived from Simon rather than from a manuscript. No explicit mention is made of any manuscript of Demosthenes' work after Simon's *Synonyma medicinae sive Clavis sanationis*, and there is apparently no trace of it today – either at Bobbio or in Rome.[13]

Large parts of Book VII of Aëtius of Amida's *Libri medicinales* depend on Demosthenes' *Ophthalmicus*,[14] and if, as has been suggested, Aëtius preserves the organizational principles adopted by Demosthenes, the latter's *Ophthalmicus* may have been arranged as follows: first the anatomy and physiology of the eye were discussed, then the pathology and symptomatology of individual affections of the eye, along with prescriptions for their treatment and discussions of the *materia medica* and surgical interventions applicable in each case, and finally a lengthy treatment of eye-salves. It is not inconceivable that this arrangement dates back to Herophilus' *On Eyes*; but one cannot be sure, first, because the composition of Herophilus' work is not particularly transparent, since only a therapeutic fragment (Fr260) is explicitly attributed to it (although Herophilus was also acutely interested in the anatomy and physiology of the eye; see n. 2), and secondly, because of the fierce independence that characterized the relation of many Herophileans to Herophilus (see Chapter x).

The anatomical and physiological orientation of the first part of Demosthenes' *Ophthalmicus* seems confirmed by Simon's complaint that what is missing from the beginning of his manuscript of the treatise are *de visu plurima et de anatomia oculi*. In the pathological and therapeutic sections which followed (*DP*.3–40) an extraordinary collection of more than forty eye ailments – many still known by the same or similar names, and some perhaps owing their names to Demosthenes – are discussed: among them are myopia, night- and day-blindness, pterygium, glaucoma, ectropion and entropion, amblyopia, marginal cysts, chalazion, paralysis of the eyelid, ptosis, stye, staphyloma, and various other tumours, blisters, abscesses and

---

[12] Silvaticus, 1474.   [13] See n. 7.

[14] Aëtius mentions Demosthenes at least twelve times in Book VII of his *Libri medicinales*; cf. *DP*.5, 7, 12, 14, 18(a)–20, 22, 25(a)–7, 30, 43. In addition, numerous passages depend on Demosthenes even though he is not mentioned by name.

swellings. Poultices, fomenting, simple remedies, minutely described compound eye-salves, dietary regulation, purgatives, and a limited use of blood-letting are among the remedies prescribed. He also records a cataract operation (*DP*.40), and while the operation itself might antedate Demosthenes, this is the earliest mention of the operation by a Greek author.[15]

Like most Herophilean physicians Demosthenes was, however, not a narrow specialist. He also wrote a work in three volumes on pulse theory, aligning himself closely with the sphygmological views of his teacher Alexander Philalethes but without merely repeating Alexander's definition of the pulse. Like Alexander,[16] he offers two pulse definitions, one 'subjective' or from the point of view of the observer's experience, the other 'objective' or from the view of what 'actually happens' in the arteries and in the heart. But, as Galen already pointed out, Demosthenes substitutes 'natural activity' for Alexander's 'involuntary activity' in describing the pulse; he resorts to further minor terminological shifts (πλῆξις for πληγή); and, perhaps more significantly, he makes explicit that the word 'pulse' can be used legitimately of three natural activities: of the pulsating activity of the heart, of the pulsating activity of the arteries, and of the combined activity of the heart and the arteries.[17]

Whether Demosthenes of Massalia (Marseille), to whom Galen

---

[15] The earliest description of the cataract operation is found in Celsus (*Medicina* 7.7.14A–F; *CML* I, pp. 321–2 Marx), a contemporary of Demosthenes Philalethes, but it probably antedates both Celsus and Demosthenes. Aelian (*On the Nature of Animals* 7.14) uses a popular stratagem – 'humans learn by imitating animals' – to explain the origin of the operation: when goats develop poor vision, says Aelian, they go to a thorn bush and push the affected eye into a thorn, thereby curing the cataract. Observing this, physicians transferred the procedure to their cataract operations on humans. For a discussion of the history of this operation see Magnus 1876: 231ff.; *id.*, 1901: 395–7. Less conclusive is the account by Hirschberg, 1899: 329–33. See also Appendix, III, on Aglaias.

Cf. also *DP*.22, where less sophisticated – and less felicitous – measures for treating cataracts are ascribed to Demosthenes. The fact that the earlier of the two sources, Aëtius, fails to ascribe couching to Demosthenes might seem at first to cast doubt on the trustworthiness of our later source, Matthaeus Silvaticus. But the general accuracy of the latter is independently attested, and since surgical couching for cataracts had become known by the time of Celsus, it is not inconceivable that Demosthenes too knew the operation.

[16] See Chapter XXII, *AP*.3.

[17] Cf. *DP*.1 (especially the section on Demosthenes' reasons for using the disjunctive conjunction 'or' instead of the copulative 'and').

says that Asclepiades 'the Younger' (ὁ φαρμακίων) attributes a
remedy for carbuncles,[18] or the Demosthenes whose 'green plaster'
Galen records,[19] is identical with the Herophilean physician is
uncertain. But there cannot be any doubt that the Herophilean,
wherever he was from originally, became associated with the famous
'Asian' branch of the Herophilean school (founded in the late first
century B.C. at the Temple of Men Karou, apparently by Zeuxis
Philalethes). Both Galen and the anonymous introduction to Aglaias'
didactic poem on incipient cataracts confirm that Demosthenes was a
pupil of Zeuxis' successor, i.e. of Alexander Philalethes.[20] And
Demosthenes' honorific, 'the Truth Lover' (Philalethes), strongly
suggests that Demosthenes himself became head of the school,
perhaps as Alexander's successor. If Alexander was the leader of the
school from at least 7 B.C. onward, as suggested above,[21] the main
activity of his pupil Demosthenes probably lies roughly in the first half
of the first century A.D., and certainly no later than the mid first
century A.D.[22]

Demosthenes' achievement and historical impact are all the more
striking because he lived at a time when the school was in its death
throes. He and Aristoxenus represent the last known generation of
Herophileans (See Chapter X.A and Appendix, III). Their contributions could not, however, be more divergent. While Aristoxenus
seems to have expended much of his energy on fratricidal polemics
against other members of his own school and on polemical doxography, Demosthenes was recording keen clinical observations and
making a remarkably enduring contribution to medicine. Undis-

---

[18] DP.48, which is included among the Dubia. It is, however, not excluded only
because DP.10, with its discussion of antrachion, i.e. ἀνθράκιον, seems to confirm
that Demosthenes in fact dealt with carbuncles in his Ophthalmicus. Pace Nutton
(1975: 7, 10; nn. 34, 68), there is no evidence that Demosthenes and other
Herophileans migrated from Men Karou to Marseille.

[19] DP.47 (listed among the Dubia). Cf. Ch. VIII, T257.

[20] DP.1; DP.3; Appendix, III.

[21] See Introduction, Chapter XXII.

[22] There is no firm evidence to support the common assertion that Demosthenes'
main activity occurred as late as Nero's reign, i.e. A.D. 54–68. Cf., for example,
Kudlien, 1964b: 'Berühmter Augenarzt zur Zeit Neros'; Hirschberg, 1919a: 183:
'Demosthenes . . . lebte . . . in den Zeiten von Nero.' If Demosthenes' teacher,
Alexander, became leader of the school no later than 7 B.C., as argued above
(Chapter XXII), Demosthenes' floruit in all likelihood lies before Nero's rule,
although he may have lived beyond the mid-first century A.D. Cf. also Benedum,
1974: 229.

tracted by the rising popularity of rival schools, such as the Pneumatic and Methodist schools of medicine, and unattracted by the subtle and sophistic controversies which apparently lured his contemporary Aristoxenus away both from clinical and from truly scientific medicine, Demosthenes described the cataract operation and defined numerous pathological affections of the eye which are still the subject of intense study in modern medicine. By resisting the allures of the agonistic arena and by concentrating instead on a positive contribution to medical science, Demosthenes 'the Truth Lover' saw to it that the Herophilean school, even at the moment of its death, produced a new canon which was to determine the course of a branch of medicine (ophthalmology) not only in later antiquity but until the end of the Middle Ages. Demosthenes might not have 'burnt and raged against the dying of the light', but he certainly did not walk silently into the night of the Herophilean movement.

B · TEXTS

DP.1   Galenus (ex Aristoxeno?), *De pulsuum differentiis* 4.4–5 (VIII, pp. 726–32K)

DP.2   Galenus (ex Aristoxeno?), *De pulsuum differentiis* 4.10 (VIII, p. 744K). See also above, Chapter XXII, *AP*.4.

DP.3   Aglaias Byzantius, *Supplementum Hellenisticum* 18 (p. 8, adn. Lloyd-Jones/Parsons). See also Appendix, III, *infra*.

DP.4a Oribasius, *Synopsis ad Eustathium* 8.42 (*CMG* VI.3, p. 264 Raeder)

DP.4b Simon Ianuensis, *Synonyma medicinae sive Clavis sanationis* (Padua, 1474), s.v. Chemosis

DP.5   Aëtius Amidenus, *Libri medicinales* 7.14 (*CMG* VIII.2, pp. 265–6 Olivieri)

DP.6   Simon Ianuensis, *Synonyma medicinae sive Clavis sanationis*, s.v. Ydema

DP.7   Aëtius Amidenus, *Libri medicinales* 7.18 (*CMG* VIII.2, p. 269 Olivieri; cf. codd. *CAQω*)

DP.8   Simon Ianuensis, *Clavis*, s.v. Labdion

DP.9   Simon Ianuensis, *Clavis*, s.v. Ypofragma

DP.10 Simon Ianuensis, *Clavis*, s.v. Ulcus

DP.11 Oribasius, *Synopsis ad Eustathium* 8.43 (*CMG* VI.3, p. 264 Raeder; cf. cod. *A*, vers. lat.)

DP.12 Aëtius Amidenus, *Libri medicinales* 7.33 (*CMG* VIII.2, pp. 283–4 Olivieri)

DP.13 Simon Ianuensis, *Clavis*, s.v. Stafiloma
DP.14 Aëtius Amidenus, *Libri medicinales* 7.46 (*CMG* VIII.2, p. 300 Olivieri)
DP.15 Simon Ianuensis, *Clavis*, s.v. Miopie
DP.16 Simon Ianuensis, *Clavis*, s.v. Nictilopa
DP.17a Simon Ianuensis, *Clavis*, s.v. Ambliopia
DP.17b Simon Ianuensis, *Clavis*, s.v. Amplyopia
DP.18a Aëtius Amidenus, *Libri medicinales* 7.50 (*CMG* VIII.2, pp. 304–6 Olivieri; vid. codd. *CAQ*ω)
DP.18b Simon Ianuensis, *Clavis*, s.v. Amaurosis
DP.19 Aëtius Amidenus, *Libri medicinales* 7.51 (*CMG* VIII.2, pp. 306–8 Olivieri)
DP.20 Aëtius Amidenus, *ibid.*, 7.52 (*CMG* VIII.2, p. 308 Olivieri)
DP.21 Simon Ianuensis, *Clavis*, s.v. Glaucoma (*primum*)
DP.22 Aëtius Amidenus, *op.cit.*, 7.53 (*CMG* VIII.2, pp. 308–9 Olivieri)
DP.23 Simon Ianuensis, *Clavis*, s.v. Ptisis
DP.24 Simon Ianuensis, *Clavis*, s.v. Pterigia
DP.25a Aëtius Amidenus, *op.cit.*, 7.73 (*CMG* VIII.2, pp. 322–3 Olivieri)
DP.25b Simon Ianuensis, *Clavis*, s.v. Hectropion
DP.26 Aëtius Amidenus, *op.cit.*, 7.75 (*CMG* VIII.2, pp. 324–45 Olivieri)
DP.27 Aëtius Amidenus, *ibid.*, 7.76 (*CMG* VIII.2, p. 325 Olivieri)
DP.28 Simon Ianuensis, *Clavis*, s.v. Psorotalmia
DP.29 Simon Ianuensis, *Clavis*, s.v. Psori
DP.30 Aëtius Amidenus, *op.cit.*, 7.81 (*CMG* VIII.2, p. 329 Olivieri)
DP.31 Simon Ianuensis, *Clavis*, s.v. Calaza
DP.32 Simon Ianuensis, *Clavis*, s.v. Calasma
DP.33 Simon Ianuensis, *Clavis*, s.v. Chrites
DP.34 Simon Ianuensis, *Clavis*, s.v. Ydatis
DP.35 Simon Ianuensis, *Clavis*, s.v. Dicoriasis
DP.36 Simon Ianuensis, *Clavis*, s.v. Nomas
DP.37 Simon Ianuensis, *Clavis*, s.v. Psilium
DP.38 Simon Ianuensis, *Clavis*, s.v. Ptarmikos
DP.39 Simon Ianuensis, *Clavis*, s.v. Psidraceon
DP.40 Matthaeus Silvaticus, *Liber pandectarum medicinae* (Venice, 1480), s.v. Paracentesis
DP.41 Codex Coislinianus 387 (s.X), fol. 153v (J. A. Fabricius, *Bibliotheca Graeca*, vol. IX (Paris, 1719), pp. 599–602)
DP.42 Codex Bodleianus (olim Meermannus) Auct. T.II.11, fol. 358v (J. A. Cramer, *Anecdota Graeca Parisiensia*, vol. IV (Oxford, 1841), p. 196)
DP.43 Aëtius Amidenus, *Libri medicinales* 7.109 (*CMG* VIII.2, p. 375 Olivieri)
DP.44 Oribasius, *Synopsis ad Eustathium* 3.127 (*CMG* VI.3, p. 100 Raeder)

DP.45   Oribasius, *ibid.*, 3.145 (*CMG* VI.3, p. 104 Raeder)
DP.46   Oribasius, *Collectiones medicae* 49.4.34 (*CMG* VI.2.2; vol. IV, p. 8 Raeder)

Dubia

DP.47   Galenus, *De compositione medicamentorum secundum locos* 5.3 (XII, p. 843K). See Chapter VIII, T257.
DP.48   Asclepiades Iunior apud Galenum, *De compositione medicamentorum per genera* 5.15 (XIII, pp. 855–6K)
DP.49   *Papiri Greci e Latini* (PSI) 12: 1275 verso, ed. M. Manfredi (= Pack² 1011 = Marganne, 1981: no. 165). (Second century A.D.)
DP.50   A. Cornelius Celsus, *Medicinae* 6.6.12 (*CML* I, p. 266 Marx)

APPENDIX

I. It is an interesting measure of Herophilus' stature in later antiquity and in the Middle Ages that the late Latin author of a brief introduction to the art of medicine gave his work the title *Herophilus' Letter to King Antiochus*. Pseudepigrapha were common both in classical and in medieval times,[1] and there are numerous examples of the pseudepigraphic use of a famous name in medical literature too. Galen, for example, complains more than once that numerous falsifications were being sold under his name even during his own lifetime. Herophilus probably became the victim of this pseudepigraphic authorial stratagem because the writer of the 'Letter' harboured hopes that the Alexandrian's name would guarantee his work authority (and hence a reasonable circulation).

The 'letter' is transmitted in at least one Latin manuscript, Bruxellensis 3701–715, fol. 8r–8v (Text XXVI in the MS).[2] In his catalogue of pre-Salernitan medical codices, Augusto Beccaria[3] established that the first part of the manuscript, containing *inter alia* the 'Letter of Herophilus', was written in the ninth century, whereas the second half (fol. 34–65), which contains a commentary on the Hippocratic *Aphorisms*, belongs to the eleventh century. In the first part of the manuscript an excerpt from the *Gynaecology* of Muscio (i.e. Mustio or Moschion[4]), a North African physician of the sixth century A.D., occupies the most prominent place (fol. 15r–31v). Other texts in the older part of the MS include excerpts from Vindician (fol. 1–2), from Isidore of Seville (fol. 6r), and from Oribasius' letters to Eustathius and Eunapius (fol. 7–8), as well as several pseudepigraphic compilations presented with the most basic trappings of the epistolographic genre. There are, for example, some 'letters' by 'Plato' and 'Aristotle' (fol.

---

[1] Cf. Clift, 1945; von Fritz, 1971b.

[2] Cod. Par. lat. 11219 (s. IX) contains a text with close parallels, and there may well be other codices with the same brief text. Vid. de Renzi, 1852–9: vol. IV, pp. 185–292; Beccaria, 1956: 166–73; Wickersheimer, 1966: 112–23; Scherer, 1976.

[3] Beccaria, 1956; cf. also Wiedemann, 1976.

[4] Published in Rose, 1882. For the corresponding Greek text see the edition by F. O. Dewez (Vienna, 1793). Mustio's (or Muscio's) *Gynaecology* consists mostly of a selective, popularizing translation of Soranus' famous gynaecological work.

579

2–4), several 'letters' by 'Hippocrates', and one each by 'Solomon' (fol. 7v), 'Diocles' (fol. 12r), 'Praxagoras' (fol. 10r–10v),[5] and 'Apollo' (fol. 14v). None of these letters exhibits any consistent or distinctive affinity with the teachings of their putative authors, and none corresponds to any extant Greek texts. The occasional implication in these Latin texts that they are translations of Greek originals is nothing but a convention which is well known from medical writings of late antiquity and of the Latin Middle Ages.[6] It is a convention normally intended to guarantee the authenticity of the translation, but it rarely proves the existence of a Greek original.

The letter attributed to Herophilus belongs to this group of epistolographic pseudepigrapha. Like most of them, it does not even do justice to the literary form and fiction claimed by its title. Rather, both its structure and its contents suggest that it belongs to a class of late ancient and early medieval compendia that were intended to introduce the barest 'theoretical' foundations to medicine in summary, schematized form (Cassius Felix served as a model for many of these introductory compendia). The 'letters' in the Brussels MS are not the only examples of the use of an epistolographic framework for such compendia; further instances are the 'Letter of Hippocrates to King Ptolemy', published by Ermerins,[7] and the anonymous 'Letter to Hippocrates' in Codex Parisinus latinus 7028 of the tenth century. A rich tradition of such *epistulae* can be found in Latin medical MSS of the ninth to twelfth centuries.[8]

Letters from physicians to rulers had, however, become an established subgenre well before late antiquity. Thus the letter of 'Hippocrates' to King Demetrius,[9] like the controversial letter to King Antigonus attributed to Diocles (regarded as authentic by Werner Jaeger, but on vulnerable grounds[10]), almost certainly belongs to the Hellenistic period. But the 'Letter of Herophilus to King Antiochus' and the other 'letters' in the codex from Brussels differ sharply from the earlier medical letters. While the earlier authors still attempted to create a semblance of literary and historical authenticity by introducing historically plausible details as well as novelistic

[5] Cf. Schubring, 1962.
[6] Cf., for example, the Epistula Vindiciani in Rose, 1894: 485. See also Beccaria, 1959–71: vol. 2, p. 6; and the 'Epistola' (Practica Petrocelli), in de Renzi, 1852–9: vol. IV, p. 190. Codd. Par. lat. 11218 and 11219 contain several representative examples; see Wickersheimer, 1966: 100–23, and cf. Scherer, 1976; Wiedemann, 1976.
[7] Cf. Ermerins, 1840: 278–97.
[8] Cf., e.g., Vitelli, 1900: 455; Anthimus, *De observatione ciborum ad Theodoricum Regem Francorum epistula*, ed. E. Liechtenhan (*CML* VIII.1, 1963). See also n. 11.
[9] 'Hp.', *Letters* 24 (IX, pp. 398–400L). A very different kind of royal correspondence occurs in *Letters* 1–9; cf. Hanson, 1985: 30–9.
[10] Cf. Heinimann, 1955.

dimensions, the later authors stripped their 'letters' of both personal and historical details, leaving the compilatory, derivative nature – and the didactic purpose–of their 'letters' virtually undisguised.

If the selection of the addressee of the pseudo-Herophilean letter is neither arbitrary nor anachronistic, and if the title is not simply a self-consciously chosen parallel to the famous pseudo-Hippocratic letter to King Antiochus,[11] the 'king' would have to be Antiochus I Soter (c. 324–261 B.C.). (This Antiochus was ruler or co-ruler of the upper satrapies from about 293 B.C.; after the murder of his father, Seleucus I Nicator, by Ptolemy Keraunos at the end of 281 B.C. he became sole ruler of the Seleucid Empire, and it was possibly at his court that Herophilus' distinguished contemporary, Erasistratus, served as physician.) No other Antiochus would be plausible chronologically. But chronological consistency and plausibility rarely played a role in the pseudonymous letters of later antiquity, and these considerations therefore do not merit further examination.

After an introductory definition of 'human being', which singles out his rationality as a differentia specifica, pseudo-Herophilus proceeds to an enumeration of bodily parts, moving from the more general to the more specific. A quaternary division of medicine follows, in which dietetics, despite the subsequent descriptions of its physiological basis, surprisingly is not mentioned (but I suggest *diaeteticus* for *disputatur*). Next the digestive organs, the vascular system, and the anatomy of the nerves are introduced, and finally the conversion of nourishment into blood is depicted. The rest of the 'letter' has not survived; between fol. 8v and fol. 9r several texts are missing. But in the extant parts a number of authentically Herophilean emphases emerge. Unfortunately the Herophilean elements are, however, so intertwined both with popular theories and with non-Herophilean elements that the text is of very limited value for the purposes of this study.

The part of the codex that concerns us (Bruxellensis 3701–15, fol. 1–33) is written in Carolingian minuscule of the ninth century. On the first page is a note in seventeenth-century script: 'Redemi a libris emptis V. Giselinus et secundo P. Crommius.' The references are to the Belgian humanist-physician Viktor Ghyselinck (1543–91) and to the Jesuit professor of theology at Louvain, Adrian Crom (1590–1651). With the exception of these indications, there is no direct evidence concerning either the provenance or the history of the MS.

II. The occasional confusion – modern and ancient – of Herophilus with

---

[11] Edited by M. Niedermann in *Marcelli de medicamentis liber* (*CML* v, 2nd edn E. Liechtenhan, 1968), 18–24; see also Wickersheimer, 1966: 100–23 (further codices with a 'letter from Hippocrates to King Antiochus').

Hierophilus requires only brief comment.[12] Hierophilus 'the Sophist' is a Byzantine author of uncertain date who wrote *On nutriment according to the months* (i.e., the diet appropriate to each of the twelve calendar months) and *On the faculties of nutriment*. In view of the early Alexandrian physician's interest in regimen, and in light of the ancient attribution of the Hippocratic treatise *On nutriment* to him,[13] the confusion is understandable. Hierophilus' treatises are unmistakable products of a much later age: they are replete with Byzantinisms, and one of them is based on the Julian calendar. *On nutriment according to the months* is extant in at least nine manuscripts, and *On the faculties of nutriment* in at least four.[14] Neither treatise yields anything for Herophilus.[15]

Max Wellmann claimed that Hierophilus 'the Sophist' also was the author of an 'excerpt' *On the feverish*, which Hermann Diels had ascribed to Herophilus.[16] The author of this 'excerpt', which Diels listed as being extant in only two manuscripts (Palatinus gr. 400 and Mosquensis 283 Savva = 466 Vladimir) is, however, neither Herophilus nor Hierophilus but Marcellinus, and the title of his text is *On pulses* – a treatise which is extant in at least seven manuscripts[17] and which offers several valuable testimonia concerning Herophilus.[18]

III. A poem by Aglaias of Byzantium (*Supplementum Hellenisticum* 18, pp. 7–8 Lloyd-Jones/Parsons), offering a remedy for incipient cataracts, is preceded in codd. Parisinus gr. 2726 and Marcianus gr. 480 by the following sentence: 'Elegiac verses by Aglaias, most noble of Byzantines, descended from Heracles, pupil of Alexander, fellow-pupil and friend of Demosthenes'. The only known medical teacher–student relationship between an Alexander and a Demosthenes is between the Herophileans discussed above in Chapters XXII and XXVIII, and this seems to suggest that Aglaias belonged to the Herophilean circle at Men Karou. This impression is strengthened by the fact (a) that Aglaias' remedy is for cataracts and (b) Demosthenes is the first Greek author known to have recorded a cataract operation (see Chapter XXVIII, DP.40 and n. 15). It is therefore tempting to include Aglaias' poem

---

[12] Cf., e.g., Chapter VIII, T248a–b (app. crit.).
[13] Cf. Chapter III.A.2 and T35–T36b; Chapter VIII, T230.
[14] See Diels, 1905–6: vol. II, p. 49.
[15] Cf. the editions of *On nutriment according to the months* by Boissonade (1827: 192–273; see also 178) and Ideler (*Physici et medici Graeci minores* I: 409–17). Ideler II: 257–81 appears to be a fragment of Hierophilus' *On the faculties of nutriment* (published by Ideler as 'Anonymus, *On flavours, drinks, and food*').
[16] See Diels, 1905–6: vol. II, p. 48. According to Diels, 1907: 54, Wellmann attributed this text to Hierophilus 'the Sophist'.
[17] Cf. *supra*, pp. xxii–xxiii, and Sigla and Editions, p. xxxvi.
[18] See Chapter VII: T168, T170–T171, T182.

among the Herophilean fragments of the time of the emperors Claudian and Nero. Nowhere is Aglaias, however, explicitly identified as a Herophilean, and there is nothing in the poem – other than its ophthalmological topic – that is distinctively Herophilean. Aëtius of Amida in his *Libri medicinales* (*CMG* VIII.2, pp. 351.19–352.2) attributes a prose version of a very similar remedy for incipient cataracts to an 'Aglaidas', likewise without calling him 'Herophilean'. Also, in view of the documented cases of pupils of Herophileans who did not themselves become members of the 'school', prudence seems to commend excluding both Aëtius' excerpt and Aglaias' poem (with the intriguing Parisian scholia on it) from the corpus of Herophilean texts.

IV. On a fine sard gem of Roman times are cut a contemplative figure of the goddess Roma and the words 'Herophili opob(alsamum)'.[19] It is an oculist's collyrium seal of a kind well known from Roman antiquity. In view of (a) Herophilus' attested interest in ophthalmological materia medica (Chapter VIII, T260), (b) the fact that eye salves, like other drugs, often were named after their inventors, (c) the frequent use of opobalsamum in the Herophilean pharmacological tradition (especially by Apollonius Mys, Chapter XXIII), and (d) the vigorous continuation of the Herophilean ophthalmological tradition in the first century A.D. by Demosthenes Philalethes (Chapter XXVIII) and possibly by Aglaias of Byzantium (Appendix, III), the seal raises interesting possibilities. In all likelihood, however, the seal belonged to a Roman oculist whose real or assumed name was Herophilus. (It is worth noting that another Roman oculist went by the name 'Erasistratus': *CIL* XIII.10021.194, Marcus Vigellus '(H)erasistratus'.) 'Herophilus' is a name well attested not only in Greek communities (see Chapter II, n. 7), but also in Latin inscriptions (e.g., *CIL* XIII.2027). Furthermore, opobalsamum was a favourite substance with Roman oculists, too; see, for example, *CIL* XIII.10021.5, 16, 26, 38, 44, 48, 56, 59, 69, 72, 77, 80, 82, 102–3, 110, 114, 121, 135, 148, 162, 174, 179–80, 183 (opobalsamum for cataracts), and 185. One manuscript tradition of a Roman source, Valerius Maximus, also mentions a Herophilus who was an 'ocularius medicus' of the first century B.C., but it is a contested reading, and the person in question – better known as Amatius or pseudo-Marius – was a notorious, discredited fraud (see Chapter II, n. 7).

Galen, as so often, thickens the plot. In Book IV of his *De compositione medicamentorum secundum locos* (4.8; XII, p. 781K) he attributes a 'most

---

[19] Cf. *Catalogue of the Collection of Assyrian, Babylonian, Egyptian, Greek, Etruscan, Roman, Indian, Peruvian and Mexican Antiquities formed by B. Hertz* (London, 1851), 44; F. Ossan, 'Ein pharmaceutisches Siegel', *Philologus* 8 (1853), 758–64; É. Espérandieu, 'Recueil des cachets oculistes romaines III–V', *Revue archéologique*, 3 série, 24 (1894), 54–64 (especially p. 58: 'vases à collyres' no. 7 – but the Coll. Hertz catalogue gives no indication that it is a vase rather than a signet).

fragrant' drug remedy 'for cataracts, for every (form of) dim-sightedness, and for incipient cataracts' to an otherwise unknown 'Hermophilus'. Among the ingredients is opobalsamum, which is also an ingredient of Aglaias' poetic remedy for incipient cataracts (*Supplementum Hellenisticum* 18, lines 23ff. Lloyd-Jones/Parsons). Especially in view of the Herophilean interest both in cataracts – incipient or not – and in dim-sightedness or *amblyopia* (Chapter XXVIII, *DP*.40, *DP*.17a–b; Appendix, III), it is not inconceivable that 'Hermophilus' is a corruption of 'Herophilus'. This possibility is lent further weight by the prominence of Herophilean drug lore in this Galenic treatise (e.g., T59b, T249–T250, T257–T259; *An*.32, *An*.29, *An*.48; *Ma*.2, *Ma*.8–9; *Cr*.6; *AP*.14a–b; *AM*.11–26, *AM*.28, *AM*.46, *AM*.49–65(?), *AM*.70(?); *G*.2, *G*.4; *DP*.47(?)).

The suggestive nexus Herophilus–ophthalmology–opobalsamum–catar-acts–Aglaias–Demosthenes Philalethes is a further example of the tantalising but not always conclusive harvest Herophilean studies undoubtedly will continue to rake in. Of the powerful presence of Herophilean ophthalmology in the first century A.D. one can be sure, even if it is far from certain that the great Alexandrian's name was carved in sard.

V. It has been suggested that the work *On the Stoic Use of Names* attributed to a Herophilus in cod. Parisinus gr. 1807 (s.X) by Origenes(?) might be by the great Alexandrian scientist, especially given (a) the occasional affinities between Herophilus' views and Stoicism (see, for example, Chapter IV.A) and (b) Herophilus' attested interest in nomenclature and doxography. Two definitions from the treatise are extant, one of *telos*, the other of *theos*: 'They say an end (*telos*) is a category for the sake of which we do other things, but which itself is not for the sake of anything. And what is joined to this, like happiness to being happy, they call the goal (*skopos*), which is the last of the things chosen', and 'most generally they say god is an immortal, rational, living being, in accordance with which every rational soul is god . . .' (see Bernard de Montfaucon, *Origenis Hexaplorum quae supersunt*, vol. I (Paris, 1713), pp. 77–8). Neither definition offers anything that suggests a clear connection with the Herophilean medical tradition, and no Stoic by the name Herophilus is otherwise known. I suspect 'Herophilus' is a corruption of 'Herillus' (the Stoic from Carthage: *SVF* I, 409–21), who also wrote on *telos*. Although no city ethnic appears in the Parisian manuscript, the copyists' frequent confusion of Καρχηδόνιος and Καλχηδόνιος (see Chapter II, T2, app. crit.; *Comments*, T2) might, at an intermediate stage, have contributed to the corruption: from Ἥριλλος ὁ Καρχηδόνιος to Ἡρόφιλος ὁ Καλχηδόνιος. Cf. D.L. 7.165: (Ἥριλλος δ᾽ ὁ) χαλκηδόνιος *codd. BFP*ac *pro* Καρχηδόνιος.

VI. Diogenes Laertius claims that 'there was another Speusippus' – i.e., other than Plato's successor as leader of the Academy – who was 'a Herophilean physician from Alexandria' (4.5). This testimony is neither confirmed nor denied by any other ancient source. About the date and the writings of 'Speusippus the Herophilean' Diogenes remains silent.

ADDENDA

288 Galenus, *Methodus medendi* 1.3 (x, pp. 19–20K)

κἂν γὰρ Ἱπποκράτης καταφρονήσῃ μικρότερον ἑαυτοῦ νομίσας
ἀγωνίσασθαι πρὸς Θεσσαλόν, ἀλλ' ἴσως Ἐρασίστρατος οὐ
καταφρονήσει, καὶ πολύ γε μᾶλλον Ἡρόφιλος, καὶ τούτων ἔτι
μᾶλλον Ἀσκληπιάδης . . .

288 Even if Hippocrates should spurn [taking on Thessalus],
considering it beneath himself to enter into a contest with Thessalus,
perhaps Erasistratus will not spurn it, and much more so Herophilus,
and, even more than these, Asclepiades . . .

289 Galenus, *De praesagitione ex pulsibus* 2.1 (ix, p. 275K)

ἀλλ' ἔνιοι μὲν ἄχρι λόγου πιθανοῦ (sc. τοῦ τε τάχους τῶν
σφυγμῶν καὶ τῆς βραδύτητος) προέρχονται, τεχνολογίας δή
τινας Ἡροφιλείας ὑπὲρ τῶν ἐν τοῖς σφυγμοῖς ῥυθμῶν γράφον-
τες, ἔνιοι δὲ περιλάλησίν τε τὴν τοιαύτην θεωρίαν ἀποκαλοῦσι
5 καὶ τελέως αὐτῆς ἀφίστανται.

289 Some, however, proceed to a plausible account [sc. of quickness
and slowness of pulse], writing systematic accounts of the Herophilean kind about the rhythms in pulses, while others both disparage
such speculation as idle verbosity and distance themselves from it
completely.

290 Galenus, *De pulsuum causis* 3.9 (ix, pp. 138–9K)

εἰ δ' Ἀρχιγένης μὲν πρὸς τοῖς εἰρημένοις καὶ πληρεστάτους
φησὶ φαίνεσθαι τοὺς σφυγμοὺς (sc. κατὰ τοὺς ὕπνους),
Ἀπολλωνίδης δὲ κενωτάτους, οὔ μοι δοκεῖ μηκύνειν ἔτι δεῖν
ἡμᾶς περί γε τῶν τοιούτων, ἱκανῶς ἀποδεδειχότας ἐν ταῖς

5 ἔμπροσθεν πραγματείαις ὡς μάτην τοῦτο τὸ γένος τῶν
σφυγμῶν οἱ μεθ' Ἡρόφιλον ἐπεισήγαγον, ὥσπερ καὶ ἄλλα
πολλά.

290 If, then, Archigenes in addition says that the pulse [in sleep] is
very full, whereas Apollonides says it is very empty, I do not think I
should drag out the discussion, at least not about such matters, since I
have adequately demonstrated in my previous works that those who
came after Herophilus introduced this additional class of pulse, like
many other things, in vain.

291 Galenus, *De difficultate respirationis* 1.21 (VII, p. 812K)

δῆλον δ' ὅτι τὴν αὐτὴν θεωρίαν ὁ τόπος (sc. τῆς ἀναπνοῆς)
ἐκδέξεται τῇ περὶ τῶν ἐν τοῖς σφυγμοῖς ῥυθμῶν ὑφ' Ἡροφίλου
γεγραμμένῃ.

291 It is clear that the same speculation as was recorded by
Herophilus concerning rhythms in the pulse will await this part [sc.
the parts used in respiration, since the respiratory 'rhythms' of
inhalation and exhalation are not unlike the diastolic and systolic
rhythms of the pulse].

292 Galenus, *De pulsuum causis* 1.7 (IX, p. 22K)

ἐπεὶ τοίνυν ἐκεῖνος (sc. ὁ Ἀρχιγένης) αὐτὸ (sc. τὰς ἄλλας
αἰτίας τοῦ τῶν σφυγμῶν τάχους, πλὴν τῆς ῥώμης τῆς
δυνάμεως) παρέλιπε, καίτοι πρόσθεν ὑφ' Ἡροφίλου κεκινημένον,
ἡμεῖς οἷς καλῶς ὅ τε Μάγνος ἔγραψε καὶ ἔτι μᾶλλον ὁ Ἡρόφιλος
5 τὸ λεῖπον προσθέντες τελείαν τὴν διδασκαλίαν τῆς διαγνώσεως
τῶν τὸ τάχος ἐργαζομένων αἰτίων ποιησόμεθα.

292 Since he [sc. Archigenes] omitted it [sc. all the causes of pulse
speed with the exception of the strength of the pulse faculty], even
though this [investigation] had been set in motion previously by
Herophilus, I shall complete my instruction concerning the diagnosis
of the causes that effect pulse speed by adding that which remains
missing to that which Magnus – and even more so Herophilus –
wrote so well.

293 Galenus, *Methodus medendi* 7.2 (x, pp. 461–2K)

οὐ γὰρ δὴ κατὰ φύσιν γε διακείμενον ἀτονεῖ περὶ τὴν οἰκείαν
ἐνέργειαν (sc. τὸ πεπονθὸς μόριον), ἀλλά τι πάντως αὐτῷ παρὰ
φύσιν αἴτιον ἐγγενόμενον ἐξέλυσέ τε καὶ κατέβαλε καὶ νεκρῷ
παραπλήσιον ἀπέφηνεν· ὃ οὔτε Ἐρασίστρατος οὔθ' Ἡρόφιλος
5 οὔτ' ἄλλος οὐδεὶς ἰατρὸς εἶπε τῶν μὴ τολμησάντων ἀποφήνασ-
θαί τι περὶ τῆς τῶν πρώτων σωμάτων φύσεως.

293 After all, it [sc. the affected part] is not lacking in proper tension
when it is in its natural disposition with reference to its own activity,
but when some cause altogether contrary to nature has arisen in it
and has relaxed it, has struck it down, and has made it appear similar
to a dead part. Neither Erasistratus nor Herophilus stated this, nor
any of the other physicians who did not dare declare themselves at all
concerning the nature of the primary bodies.

BIBLIOGRAPHY

For editions of ancient sources, see above, pp. xxviii–xliii. The bibliography lists secondary works (including commentaries and introductions to editions) cited in my text or notes, as well as a few other studies which bear directly on major questions raised. I regret that Dambassis (1968) and Mola (1963) were not available to me. Works published after 1982 could be included only selectively.

Abel, K. (1958) 'Die Lehre vom Blutkreislauf im Corpus Hippocraticum', *Hermes* 86: 192–219; repr. with a 'Retractatio' in Flashar, 1971: 121–64

Ackerknecht, E.H. (1973) *Therapeutics from the Primitives to the Twentieth Century* (London/New York)

Alexanderson, B. (1963) *Die hippokratische Schrift Prognostikon* (Studia Graeca et Latina Gothoburgensia 17)

Allbutt, T.C. (1921) *Greek Medicine in Rome* (London; repr. New York, 1970)

Aly, W. (1931) 'Strabon (3)', *Pauly-Wissowas Realencyclopädie der classischen Altertumswissenschaft* 11.7: cols. 76–155

Amacher, M.P. (1964) 'Galen's experiment on the arterial pulse and the experiment repeated', *Sudhoffs Archiv für Geschichte der Medizin* 48: 177–80

Amundsen, D.W., and Ferngren, G.B. (1978) 'The forensic role of physicians in Ptolemaic and Roman Egypt', *Bulletin of the History of Medicine* 52: 336–53

Andor, J. (1951–2) 'Die römische Episode bei Kallimachos', *Acta Antiqua* 1: 121–5

Arnheim, R. (1974) *Art and Visual Perception*, rev. edn (Berkeley/Los Angeles)

The Athenian Agora (American School of Classical Studies at Athens) (1976) 3rd edn (Athens)

Baader, G. (1974) Review of D. Nickel, ed., *Galen über die Anatomie der Gebärmutter* (Corpus Medicorum Graecorum v.2.1, Berlin, 1971), *Sudhoffs Archiv* 58: 203–4

Bäckström, A. (1906) 'Fragment einer medizinischen Schrift', *Archiv für Papyrusforschung* 3: 158–62

589

Bake, J. (1810) *Posidonii Rhodii reliquiae doctrinae* (Leiden)

Balme, D.M. (1961) 'Aristotle's use of differentiae in zoology', in *Aristote et les problèmes de méthode: Symposium Aristotelicum, 1960*, ed. S. Mansion (Louvain/Paris), 195–212

    (1962) 'ΓΕΝΟΣ and ΕΙΔΟΣ in Aristotle's biology', *Classical Quarterly* N.S. 12: 81–98

Balss, H. (1936) 'Die Zeugungslehre und Embryologie in der Antike', *Quellen und Studien zur Geschichte der Naturwissenschaften und der Medizin* 5.2–3: 1–82 (= 193–274)

Bardong, K. (1951) 'Pleistonikos', *Pauly-Wissowas Realencyclopädie der classischen Altertumswissenschaft* 22.1: cols. 210–12

    (1954) 'Praxagoras', *Pauly-Wissowas Realencyclopädie der classischen Altertumswissenschaft* 22.2: cols. 1735–43

Barnes, J., Brunschwig, J., Burnyeat, M., and Schofield, M., eds. (1982) *Science and Speculation* (Cambridge/Paris)

Barns, J.W.B. (1978) *Egyptians and Greeks* (Papyrologica Bruxellensia 14)

Bauer, K.J. (1870) *Geschichte der Aderlässe* (Munich)

Baumann, E.D. (1937) 'Praxagoras von Kos', *Janus* 41: 167–85

Beccaria, A. (1956) *I codici di medicina del periodo Presalernitano* (Storia e letteratura 53)

    (1959–71) 'Sulle trace di un antico canone latino di Ippocrate e di Galeno, I–III', *Italia medioevale e umanistica* 2: 1–56; 4: 1–75; 14:1–23

Bechtel, F. (1902) *Die attischen Frauennamen* (Göttingen)

    (1917) *Die historischen Personennamen des Griechischen bis zur Kaiserzeit* (Halle)

Behr, C.A. (1968) *Aelius Aristides and the Sacred Tales* (Amsterdam)

Beloch, J. (1904) *Griechische Geschichte*, 4 vols. in 8 (Strassburg/Berlin/ Leipzig; 2nd edn 1927)

Benedum, J. (1974) 'Zeuxis Philalethes und die Schule der Herophileer in Menos Kome', *Gesnerus* 31: 221–36

    (1978) 'Philalethes', *Pauly-Wissowas Realencyclopädie der classischen Altertumswissenschaft*, Suppl. 15: cols. 306–8

Benveniste, E. (1965) 'Termes gréco-latins d' anatomie', *Revue de Philologie* 39: 7–13.

Berg, A. (1942) 'Die Lehre von der Faser als Form- und Funktionselement des Organismus', *Virchows Archiv für pathologische Anatomie und Physiologie und für klinische Medizin* 309: 333–460

Bernand, A. (1966) *Alexandrie la Grande* (Paris)

Bertier, J. (1972) *Mnesithée et Dieuchès* (Leiden)

Bidez, J., and Leboucq, G. (1944) 'Une anatomie antique du coeur humain. Philistion de Locres et le "Timée" de Platon', *Revue des Études Grecques* 57: 7–40

Blankert, S. (1940) *Seneca over natuur en kultuur* (Amsterdam)

Blomquist, J. (1969) *Greek Particles in Hellenistic Prose* (Lund)

Blum, C. (1936) *Studies in the Dream-Book of Artemidorus* (Uppsala)

Boissonade, J.F. (1827) 'Traité alimentaire du médecin Hierophile', in *Notices et extraits des manuscrits de la Bibliothèque du Roi* xi (Paris), 178–80, 192–267

Bonner, C. (1920) 'The Trial of St. Eugenia', *American Journal of Philology* 41: 253–64

Booth, N.B. (1960) 'Empedocles' account of breathing', *Journal of Hellenic Studies* 80: 10–15

Borchardt, L. (1920) *Die altägyptische Zeitmessung* (Berlin)

Boswinkel, E. (1956) 'La médecine et les médecins dans les papyrus Grecs', *Eos* 48.1: 181–90.

Bourgey, L. (1953) *Observation et expérience chez les médecins de la collection hippocratique* (Paris)

Bräutigam, W. (1908) *De Hippocratis Epidemiarum libri sexti commentatoribus* (Diss. phil. Königsberg)

Breasted, J.H. (1930) *The Edwin Smith Surgical Papyrus*, 2 vols. (Chicago)

Brink, K.O. (1946) 'Callimachus and Aristotle: An inquiry into Callimachus' ΠΡΟΣ ΠΡΑΞΙΦΑΝΗΝ', *Classical Quarterly* 40: 11–26

Brumbaugh, R.S. (1966) *Ancient Greek Gadgets and Machines* (New York)

Brunn, H. (1856) *De auctorum indicibus Plinianis* (Bonn)

Buchheim, L. (1958) 'Der "Fleischverband" im alten Ägypten', *Sudhoffs Archiv für Geschichte der Medizin* 42: 97–116

(1960) 'Die Verordnung von "lebendem" Fleisch in altägyptischen Papyri', *Sudhoffs Archiv für Geschichte der Medizin* 44: 97–116

Buess, H. (1968) 'Herophilus und die Geburtshilfe in alexandrinischer Zeit', *Gynäkologische Rundschau* 5: 236–40

Burkert, W. (1962) *Weisheit und Wissenschaft* (Erlanger Beiträge zur Sprach- und Kunstwissenschaft 10, Nürnberg); transl. by E.L. Minar, *Lore and Science in Ancient Pythagoreanism* (Cambridge, Mass., 1972)

(1970) 'Buzyge und Palladion', *Zeitschrift für Religions- und Geistesgeschichte* 22: 356–68

(1972) *Homo Necans* (Berlin)

Bylebyl, J.J., and Pagel, W. (1971) 'The chequered career of Galen's doctrine of the pulmonary vein', *Medical History* 15: 211–29

Capelle, W. (1934) 'Theodas', *Pauly-Wissowas Realencyclopädie der classischen Altertumswissenschaft* II.10: cols. 1713–14

Castiglioni, A. (1947) *History of Medicine*, trans. D.B. Krumbhaar (New York). (Translation of *Storia della Medicina*, 2nd ed., Milan, 1936)

Chassinat, É. (1921) *Un papyrus médical copte* (Mémoires, l'Institut Français d'Archéologie Orientale du Caire 32)

von Christ, W., Stählin, O., Schmid, W. (1912–24) *Geschichte der griechischen*

Literatur, 2 vols. in 3 (Handbuch der Altertumswissenschaft VII.1–2: Munich)

Clarke, E. (1963) 'Aristotelian concepts of the form and function of the brain', *Bulletin of the History of Medicine* 37: 1–14

Clarke, E., and Dewhurst, E. (1972) *An Illustrated History of Brain Function* (Berkeley/Los Angeles, Oxford)

Clarke, E., and O'Malley, C.D. (1968) *The Human Brain and Spinal Cord* (Berkeley/Los Angeles)

Clarke, E., and Stannard, J. (1963) 'Aristotle on the anatomy of the brain', *Journal of the History of Medicine and Allied Sciences* 18: 130–48

Clift, E.H. (1945) *Latin Pseudepigrapha: A Study in Literary Attributions* (Baltimore)

Cockburn, A. and E., eds. (1980) *Mummies, Disease, and Ancient Cultures* (Cambridge)

Cobet, C.G. (1860) 'Ad Galenum', *Mnemosyne* 9: 21–48

Cohn-Haft, L. (1956) *The Public Physicians of Ancient Greece* (Smith College Studies in History 42)

Cole, A.T. (1967) *Democritus and the Sources of Greek Anthropology* (Philological Monographs 25)

Contenau, G. (1940) *La divination chez les Assyriens et les Babyloniens* (Paris)

Crawfurd, R. (1919) 'The Harveian Oration: Forerunners of Harvey in Antiquity', *The British Medical Journal* (1919.2): 551–6

Creutz, R. (1935) '*De optima medicorum secta* im Lichte des XVII. Jahrhunderts', *Medizinische Welt* 9: 775–7

Cumont, F. (1937) *L'Égypte des astrologues* (Brussels)

Dambassis, J.N. (1968) "Ηρόφιλος καὶ 'Ερασίστρατος', Ιατρικὰ Χρόνικα 8: 2: 143–66

Darby, W.J., Ghalioungui, P., and Grivetti, L. (1977) *Food: The Gift of Osiris*, 2 vols. (London/New York/San Francisco)

Daumas, F. (1956) 'Une histoire de la médecine égyptienne antique' (review of G. Lefebvre, *Essai sur la médecine égyptienne*), *Journal des savants* 165–75

Daux, G. (1967) 'Dionysermos, fils d'Anténor, au Louvre', *Bulletin de Correspondance Hellénique* 91: 491–3

Deichgräber, K. (1929) Review of L. Englert, *Untersuchungen zu Galens Schrift Thrasybulos* (1929), in *Deutsche Literaturzeitung* N.F. 6: Heft 37, 1765–8

(1930) 'Marinos', *Pauly-Wissowas Realencyclopädie der classischen Altertumswissenschaft* 14: col. 1796

(1932) 'Mnesitheos (3)', *ibid.* 15.2; cols. 2281–4

(1933) *Die Epidemien und das Corpus Hippocraticum* (Abhandlungen der preussischen Akademie der Wissenschaften, Berlin, phil.-hist. Kl., 1933.3). See below *id.*, 1971

(1934a) 'Themison', *Pauly-Wissowas Realencyclopädie der classischen Altertumswissenschaft* II.10; cols. 1632–8.

(1934b) 'Theophilos (16)', *ibid.*, col. 2148

(1935) *Hippokrates über Entstehung und Aufbau des menschlichen Körpers:* ΠΕΡΙ ΣΑΡΚΩΝ (Leipzig/Berlin)

(1937) 'Pelops (5)', *Pauly-Wissowas Realencyclopädie der classischen Altertumswissenschaft* 19.1: cols. 391–2

(1956) *Galen als Erforscher des menschlichen Pulses* (Sitzungsberichte der Akademie der Wissenschaften, Berlin, phil.-hist. Kl., 1956.3). Repr. in Deichgräber, *Ausgewählte Kleine Schriften* (Hildesheim/Munich,'Zurich, 1984), 288–326

(1961) 'Vindicianus (2)', *Pauly-Wissowas Realencyclopädie der classischen Altertumswissenschaft* II.17: cols. 29–36

(1965) *Die griechische Empirikerschule*, 2nd edn (Berlin/Zurich)

(1971) 'Nachwort und Nachträge', in 2nd edn of (1933): 173–87

(1973) *Pseudhippokrates Über die Nahrung. Eine stoisch-heraklitisierende Schrift aus der Zeit um Christi Geburt* (Abhandlugen, Akademie der Wissenschaften und der Literatur, Mainz, geistes- und sozialwissenschaftliche Kl., 1973.3)

Della Corte, F. (1941) 'Callimaco e i Peucezii: ΔΙΗΓΗΣΕΙΣ v, 26–31', *Aegyptus* 21: 276–82

De Martini, U. (1964) 'Considerazione sulla dottrina della pneuma in Galeno', *Pagine di storia della medicina* 8: 41–7

Denniston, J.D. (1954) *The Greek Particles*, 2nd ed. (Oxford)

de Renzi, S. (1852–9) *Collectio Salernitana*, 5 vols. (Naples)

De Sanctis, G. (1935) 'Callimacho e Orazio Coclite', *Rivista di filologia e d'istruzione classica* 14: 289–301

Diels, H., ed. (1879) *Doxographi Graeci* (Berlin; repr. 1965)

(1893a) *Über das physikalische System des Straton* (Sitzungsberichte der Königlich preussischen Akademie der Wissenschaften, Berlin, 1: 101–27)

(1893b) 'Über die Excerpte von Menons Iatrika in dem Londoner Papyrus 137', *Hermes* 28: 407–34

(1905–6) *Die Handschriften der antiken Ärzte*, Theil I: *Hippokrates und Galenos*; Theil II: *Die übrigen griechischen Ärzte ausser Hippokrates und Galenos* (Abhandlungen der Königlich preussischen Akademie der Wissenschaften, Berlin, phil.-hist. Kl., 1905.3 and 1906.1)

(1907) *Erster Nachtrag zu Handschriften der antiken Ärzte, ibid.* 1907.2

(1914) *Corpus Medicorum Graecorum: Bericht* (Sitzungsberichte der Königlich preussischen Akademie der Wissenschaften, Berlin, 1914.1: 127–30)

(1915) *Über Platons Nachtuhr* (Sitzungsberichte der Königlich preussischen Akademie der Wissenschaften, Berlin, 1915.2: 824–30)

(1920) *Antike Technik*, 2nd edn (Leipzig/Berlin)

Diels, H., and Kranz, W. (1969) *Die Fragmente der Vorsokratiker*, 14th edn, 3 vols. (Zurich/Dublin)

Diepgen, P. (1937) *Die Frauenheilkunde der alten Welt* (Munich)

(1949) *Geschichte der Medizin* I (Berlin)

Dierbach, J.H. (1824) *Die Arzneimittel des Hippokrates* (Heidelberg)

Dietz, F.R. (1834) *Apollonii Citiensis, Stephani, Palladii, Theophili, Meletii, Damascii, Ioannis, aliorum Scholia in Hippocratem et Galenum*, 2 vols. (Königsberg; repr. Amsterdam, 1966)

Dijksterhuis, E.J. (1956), *Archimedes* (Copenhagen)

Diller, H. (1933a) 'Zur Hippokratesauffassung des Galen', *Hermes* 68: 167–81; repr. in Diller, 1973: 3–16

(1933b) Review of L. Edelstein, ΠΕΡΙ ΑΕΡΩΝ *und die Sammlung der hippokratischen Schriften* (1931), in *Gnomon* 9: 65–79; repr. in Diller, 1973: 131–43

(1936a) 'Eine stoisch-pneumatische Schrift im Corpus Hippocraticum', *Sudhoffs Archiv für die Geschichte der Medizin* 29: 178–95; repr. in Diller, 1973: 17–30

(1936b) 'Thessalos (6)', *Pauly-Wissowas Realencyclopädie der classischen Altertumswissenschaft* II.11: cols. 168–82

(1938) 'Philippos (49–51)', *Pauly-Wissowas Realencyclopädie der classischen Altertumswissenschaft* 19.2: cols. 2367–70

(1941) 'Phylotimos', *ibid.* 20.1: cols. 1030–2

(1950) Review of E. Wenkebach, F. Pfaff, edd., *Galeni In Hippocratis Epidemiarum Librum VI Commentaria I–VIII* (Corpus Medicorum Graecorum v. 10, 2, 2, Leipzig, 1940), in *Gnomon* 22: 226–35; repr. in Diller, 1973: 223–33

(1959a) 'Der innere Zusammenhang der hippokratischen Schrift De victu', *Hermes* 87: 39–56; repr. in Diller, 1973: 71–88

(1959b) 'Stand und Aufgaben der Hippokratesforschung', *Jahrbuch, Akademie der Wissenschaften und der Literatur, Mainz*, 271–87; repr. in Diller, 1973: 89–105

(1967) Review of H. Flashar, *Melancholie und Melancholiker*, in *Gnomon* 39: 651–7; repr. in Diller, 1973: 256–61

(1973) *Kleine Schriften zur antiken Medizin*, edd. G. Baader and H. Grensemann (Ars Medica II.3, Berlin/New York)

Dilthey, W. (1922) *Gesammelte Schriften* I (Leipzig/Berlin)

Dittenberger, W., ed. (1903–5) *Orientis Graeci Inscriptiones Selectae*, 2 vols. (Leipzig/Berlin)

Dobson, J.F. (1925) 'Herophilus of Alexandria', *Proceedings of the Royal Society of Medicine* 18: 19–32

(1926–7) 'Erasistratus', *Proceedings of the Royal Society of Medicine* 20: 825–32

Dodds, E.R. (1951) *The Greeks and the Irrational* (Berkeley/Los Angeles)

Döring, K. (1972) *Die Megariker* (Amsterdam)

Douglas, M. (1966) *Purity and Danger* (London)

Drabkin, I.E. (1944) 'On medical education in Greece and Rome', *Bulletin of the History of Medicine* 15: 333–51

(1957) 'Medical Education in ancient Greece and Rome', *Journal of Medical Education* 32: 286–95

Drabkin, M.F. and I.E. (1951) *Caelius Aurelianus: Gynaecia* (Supplements to *Bulletin of the History of Medicine* 13)

Drachmann, A.B. (1948) *Ktesibios, Philon and Heron* (Copenhagen)

(1963) *The Mechanical Technology of Greek and Roman Antiquity* (Copenhagen/Madison/London)

Droysen, J.G. (1952–3) *Geschichte des Hellenismus*, rev. edn E. Bayer, 3 vols. (Basel; 1st edn 1836–43)

Duckworth, W.L.H. (1962) *Galen on Anatomical Procedures: The Later Books*, edd. M.C. Lyons and B. Towers (Cambridge)

Düring, I. (1961) 'Aristotle's method in biology', in *Aristote et les problèmes de méthode: Symposium Aristotelicum, 1960*, ed. S. Mansion (Louvain/Paris), 213–21

Dulière, W.-L. (1965) 'Les "Dictyaques" de Denys d'Égée ou les dilemmes du "sic et non" de la médecine antique. Histoire d'un procédé dialectique', *L' Antiquité Classique* 34: 506–18

Duminil, M.-P. (1983) *Le sang, les vaisseaux, le coeur dans la Collection hippocratique* (Paris)

Dupuis, J. (1892) *Théon de Smyrne* (Paris)

Durrbach, F., Roussel, P., and Launey, M. (1926–37) *Inscriptions de Délos*, 5 vols. (Paris)

Dustmann, M. (1938) *Die Geschichte der Ernährungstherapie im Altertum* (Diss. Düsseldorf)

Ebbell, B. (1937) *The Papyrus Ebers* (Copenhagen/London)

Ebstein, E. (1911) 'Geschichtliche Entwicklung der Therapie', in P. Krause und C. Garré (eds.), *Lehrbuch der Therapie innerer Krankheiten* 1 (Jena), 776–815

Edel, E. (1976) *Ägyptische Ärzte und ägyptische Medizin am hethitischen Königshof: neue Funde von Keilschriftbriefen Ramses' II. aus Bogazköy* (Opladen)

Edelstein, E.J. and L. (1945) *Asclepius*, 2 vols. (Baltimore)

Edelstein, L. (1931a) 'Antike Diätetik', *Die Antike* 7: 255–70; transl. by L. Temkin in Edelstein, 1967: 303–16

(1931b) ΠΕΡΙ ΑΕΡΩΝ *und die Sammlung der hippokratischen Schriften* (Problemata 4, Berlin)

(1932) 'Die Geschichte der Sektion in der Antike', *Quellen und Studien zur Geschichte der Naturwissenschaften und der Medizin* 3.2: 50–106; transl. by L. Temkin in Edelstein, 1967: 247–301

(1935a) 'Hippokrates (16), Nachträge', *Pauly-Wissowas Realencyclopädie der classischen Altertumswissenschaft*, Suppl. 6: cols. 1290–1345

(1935b) 'Methodiker', *ibid.*, cols. 358–73; transl. in Edelstein, 1967: 173–91

(1935c) 'The development of Greek anatomy', *Bulletin of the Institute of the History of Medicine* 3: 235–48

(1939) 'The genuine works of Hippocrates', *Bulletin of the History of Medicine* 7: 236–48; repr. in Edelstein, 1967: 133–44

(1940) Review of Jaeger, 1938a, in *American Journal of Philology* 61: 483–9; repr. in Edelstein, 1967: 145–52

(1967) *Ancient Medicine: Selected Papers of Ludwig Edelstein*, eds. O. and C.L. Temkin (Baltimore)

Edelstein, L., and Kidd, I.G. (1972) *Posidonius* I (Cambridge)

Edgar, C.C. (1925–40) *Zenon Papyri*, 5 vols. (Catalogue géneral des Antiquités Égyptiennes du Musée du Caire 79)

Ellenberger, W., and Baum, H. (1943) *Handbuch der vergleichenden Anatomie der Haustiere*, 18th edn (Berlin)

Englert, L. (1929) *Untersuchungen zu Galens Schrift Thrasybulos* (Studien zur Geschichte der Medizin, eds. K. Sudhoff and H. Sigerist, 18)

Erbse, H. (1950) *Untersuchungen zu den attizistischen Lexika* (Abhandlungen der deutschen Akademie der Wissenschaften, Berlin, phil.-hist. Kl.) 1949.2)

(1953) 'Homerscholien und hellenistische Glossare bei Apollonios Rhodios', *Hermes* 81: 163–96

(1961) Überlieferungsgeschichte der griechischen klassischen und hellenistischen Literatur', in Hunger et al. (1961–4), 1:207–83

Ermerins, F.Z. (1840) *Anecdota medica Graeca* (Leiden; repr. Amsterdam 1956)

Evans, J.A.S. (1962) 'A Social and Economic History of an Egyptian Temple in the Greco-Roman Period', *Yale Classical Studies* 17: 143–283

Fabricius, C. (1972) *Galens Exzerpte aus älteren Pharmakologen* (Ars Medica II.2, Berlin)

Fabricius, J.A. (1716–54) *Bibliotheca Graeca*, 14 vols. (Hamburg; 4th edn, 12 vols. (1790–1809))

Ferngren, G.B. (1982) 'A Roman declamation on vivisection', *Transactions and Studies of the College of Physicians in Philadelphia* ser.5, 4.4: 272–90

Fick, A., and Bechtel, F. (1894) *Die griechischen Personennamen*, 2nd edn (Göttingen)

Finlayson, J. (1893) 'Herophilus and Erasistratus: A bibliographical demonstration', *The Glasgow Medical Journal* 39.5: 321–52

Flashar, H. (1966) *Melancholie und Melancholiker in den medizinischen Theorien der Antike* (Berlin)

(1971) ed., *Antike Medizin* (Wege der Forschung 221, Darmstadt)

Forbes, C.A. (1955) 'The education and training of slaves in antiquity', *Transactions and Proceedings of the American Philological Association* 86: 321–60

Forster, E.M. (1961) *Alexandria*, 3rd edn (Garden City) (1st edn, Alexandria, 1922)

Forster, E.S., see Peck, A.L., and Forster, E.S. (1937)

Foucault, M. (1966) *Les mots et les choses* (Paris)

(1969) *L'Archéologie du savoir* (Paris)

Fränkel, H.F. (1915) *De Simia Rhodio* (Diss. Göttingen)

Fraser, P.M. (1960) 'Inscriptions from Ptolemaic Egypt', *Berytus* 13.2: 123–61

(1969) 'The career of Erasistratus of Ceos', *Rendiconti del Istituto Lombardo, Classe di lettere e scienze morali e storiche* 103: 518–37

(1972) *Ptolemaic Alexandria*, 3 vols. (Oxford)

Frede, M. (1980) 'The original notion of cause', in Schofield et al., 1980: 217–49

(1981) 'On Galen's epistemology', in Nutton, 1981: 65–86

(1982) 'The method of the so-called Methodical school of medicine', in Barnes et al., 1982: 1–23

Fredrich, C. (1899) *Hippokratische Untersuchungen* (Philologische Untersuchungen 15)

French, R.K. (1978) 'The thorax in history', *Thorax* 33: 10–18, 153–66, 295–306, 439–56, 555–64, 714–27

von Fritz, K. (1971a) *Grundprobleme der Geschichte der antiken Wissenschaft* (Berlin)

(1971b) ed., *Pseudepigrapha* (Fondation Hardt, Entretiens 18)

(1972) 'Zenon (2)', *Pauly-Wissowas Realencyclopädie der classischen Altertumswissenschaft* II.19: cols. 83–121

Fuchs, R. (1892a) *Erasistratea* (Diss. Berlin; Leipzig)

(1892b) 'Die Plethora bei Erasistratos', *Jahrbücher für klassische Philologie* 38 = *Neue Jahrbücher für Philologie und Pädagogik*, Jg. 62, Bd 145: 679–91

(1894a) 'De Erasistrato capita selecta', *Hermes* 29: 171–203

(1894b) 'Der cod. Paris. supplem. Graec. 636: Anecdota medica Graeca', *Rheinisches Museum* N.F. 49: 532–58

(1897) 'Lebte Erasistratos in Alexandreia?', *Rheinisches Museum* N.F. 52: 377–90

Fuhrmann, M. (1960) *Das systematische Lehrbuch* (Göttingen)

(1967) 'Xenokritos (4)', *Pauly-Wissowas Realencylopädie der classischen Altertumswissenschaft* II.18: col. 1533

Furley, D.J. (1957) 'Empedocles and the Clepsydra', *Journal of Hellenic Studies* 77: 31–4

(1971) 'Knowledge of atoms and void in Epicureanism', in J.P. Anton and G.L. Kustas, eds., *Essays in Ancient Greek Philosophy* (Buffalo, N.Y.), 607–19

Furley, D.J., and Wilkie, J.S. (1972) 'An Arabic translation solves some problems in Galen', *Classical Review* N.S. 22: 164–7

(1984) *Galen on Respiration and the Arteries* (Princeton)

Gadamer, H.G. (1965) *Wahrheit und Methode* 2nd edn (Tübingen)

Gärtner, H. (1962) *Rufus von Ephesos: Die Fragen des Arztes an den Kranken* (Corpus Medicorum Graecorum, Suppl. 4, Berlin); Teubner edn (Leipzig, 1970)

García Ballester, L. (1974) 'De la anatomía alejandrina al "Corpus Galenianum" ', *Medicina e Historia* 37: I–XVI

Gardiner, A.H. (1935) *Hieratic Papyri in the British Museum*. Third Series: Chester Beatty Gift, 2 vols. (London)

Gask, G.E. (1940) 'Early medical schools. III: The School of Alexandria', *Annals of Medical History*, 3rd ser., 2: 383–92

Gelzer, M. (1907) 'Zwei Prinzipien der antiken Traumdeutung', in *Juvenes dum sumus: Aufsätze zur klassischen Altertumswissenschaft der 49. Versammlung deutscher Philologen* (Basel), 40–51

Georgiades, T. (1949) *Der griechische Rhythmus* (Hamburg)

Geurts, P. (1941) *De erfelijkheid in de oudere Grieksche wetenschap* (Nijmegen/Utrecht)

Ghalioungui, P. (1960) 'Des papyrus égyptiens à la médecine grecque', *XVIIe Congrès international d'histoire de la médecine, Athènes–Cos*, I: *Communications*, 296–305

(1968) 'The relation of Pharaonic to Greek and later medicine', *Bulletin of the Cleveland Medical Library* 15.3: 96–107

(1973) *The House of Life: Per Ankh. Magic and Medical Science in Ancient Egypt* (Amsterdam)

Giannantoni, G., & Vegetti, M., eds. (1984) *La scienza ellenistica* (Elenchos IX, Naples)

Gil, L. (1973) 'Ärztlicher Beistand und attische Komödie. Zur Frage der *demosieuontes* and Sklaven-Ärzte', *Sudhoffs Archiv* 57: 255–74

Glucker, J. (1978) *Antiochus and the late Academy* (Hypomnemata 56)

Gombrich, E. (1961) *Art and Illusion*, 2nd edn (New York)

Gorteman, C. (1957) 'Médecins de cour dans l'Égypte du IIIe siècle avant J.-C', *Chronique d'Égypte* 32: 313–36

Gossen, H. (1912) 'Herophilos (4)–(5)', *Pauly-Wissowas Realencyclopädie der classischen Altertumswissenschaft* 8.1: cols. 1104–10

  (1919) 'Kallianax', *Pauly-Wissowas Realencyclopädie der classischen Altertumswissenschaft* 10.2: col. 1613

  (1956) 'Nachtrag, Herophilos (4)', *ibid.* Suppl. 8: col. 179

Gotfredsen, E. (1942) *Oldtidens laere om hjerte, kar og puls* (Acta Historica Scientiarum Naturalium et Medicinalium, ed. Bibliotheca Universitatis Hauniensis, 1, Copenhagen)

Gottschalk, H.B. (1980) *Heraclides of Pontus* (Oxford)

Gourevitch, D. (1980) 'Le dossier philologique du nyctalope', in *Hippocratica. Actes du Colloque hippocratique de Paris, 1978*, ed. M. D. Grmek (Paris), 167–88.

Graindor, P. (1938) 'Le nom de l'université d'Athènes sous l'Empire', *Revue Belge de Philologie et d'Histoire* 17: 307–12

  (1939) *Terres cuites de l'Égypte gréco-romaine* (Rijksuniversiteit te Gent: Werken uitg. door de Faculteit van de Wijsbegeerete en Letteren 86, Antwerp)

Grapow, H., von Deines, H., Westendorf, W. (1954–62) *Grundriss der Medizin der alten Ägypter*, 7 vols. in 9 (Berlin)

Greenhill, W.A. (1843) 'Professor Marx's Herophilus', *British and foreign medical review* 15: 106–14

  (1873a) 'Erasistratus', *Dictionary of Greek and Roman Biography* 2 (London), 42–4

  (1873b) 'Herophilus', *Dictionary of Greek and Roman Biography* 2 (London), 438–9

Grenfell, B.P., Hunt, A.S., et al (1898–) *The Oxyrhynchus Papyri* (London)

Grensemann, H. (1964) 'Zu den Hippokratesglossaren des Erotian und Galen', *Hermes* 92: 505–7

  (1968a) *Der Arzt Polybos als Verfasser hippokratischer Schriften* (Abhandlungen der Akademie der Wissenschaften und der Literatur, Mainz, geistes- und sozialwissenschaftliche Kl., 1968.2)

  (1968b) 'Weitere Bemerkungen zu den Hippokratesglossaren des Erotian und Galen', *Hermes* 96: 177–90

  (1968c) *Die hippokratische Schrift 'Über die heilige Krankheit'* (Ars Medica II.1, Berlin)

  (1974) 'Polybos', *Pauly-Wissowas Realencyclopädie der classischen Altertumswissenschaft*, Suppl. 14: cols. 428–36

  (1975) *Knidische Medizin, I. Die Testimonien zur ältesten knidischen Lehre und Analysen knidischer Schriften im Corpus Hippocraticum* (Ars Medica II.4.1, Berlin)

Grmek, M.D. (1962) *Les reflets de la sphygmologie chinoise dans la médecine occidentale* (Biologie medicale 51, 60ᵉ année, no. hors série)

von Grot, R. (1887) *Über die in der hippokratischen Schriftensammlung enthaltenen pharmakologischen Kentnisse* (Dorpat)

Guéraud, O., ed. (1931–2) *Publications de la Societé Royale Égyptienne de Papyrologie, Textes et documents*, 1. 'Εντεύξεις (Cairo) (= P. Enteux.)

Guillemean, Jacques (1597) *Guillemean's French chirurgerye or the manualle operations of chirurgerye*, transl. A.M. (London)

Habicht, C. (1958) 'Die herrschende Gesellschaft in den hellenistischen Monarchien', *Vierteljahrschrift für Sozial- und Wirtschaftsgeschichte* 45: 1–16

Haeser, H. (1875–82) *Lehrbuch der Geschichte der Medicin und der epidemischen Krankheiten*, 3rd edn, 3 vols. (Jena)

Hahm, D. (1977) *The Origins of Stoic Cosmology* (Columbus, Ohio)

Hall, T.S. (1974) 'Idiosyncrasy: Greek Medical Ideas of Uniqueness', *Sudhoffs Archiv* 58: 283–302

Hanson, A.E. (1985) 'Papyri of medical content', *Yale Classical Studies* 28: 25–47

Harig, G. (1968) 'Die Medizin der Sklavenhaltergesellschaft: Griechisch-römische Antike', in Mette & Winter, 1968: 41–126

(1974) *Bestimmung der Intensität im medizinischen System Galens* (Berlin)

(1976) 'Methodische Medizin und gesellschaftliche Entwicklung in der Antike', *Acta Congressus Internationalis XXIV. Historiae Artis Medicinae, 1974* (Budapest), 2: 1139–43

Harless, J.C.F. (1816) *Analecta historico-critica: De Archigene medico et de Apolloniis medicis eorumque scriptis* (Erlangen/Bamberg)

Harris, C.R.S. (1973) *The Heart and the Vascular System in Ancient Greek Medicine* (Oxford)

Havet, J. (1889) *Lettres de Gerbert (983–997)* (Paris)

Heath, T.L. (1912) *Archimedes*, 2nd edn (Cambridge; repr. New York, 1957)

(1926) *The Thirteen Books of Euclid's Elements*, 2nd edn, 3 vols. (Cambridge; repr. New York, 1956)

Heiberg, J.L. (1879) *Quaestiones Archimedeae* (Copenhagen)

(1882) *Litterargeschichtliche Studien über Euklid* (Leipzig)

(1901) 'Anatolius sur les dix premiers nombres', *Annales internationales d'histoire*, Congrès de Paris, 1900, 5e section: Histoire des sciences (Paris), 27–41

(1912) *Pauli Aeginetae libri tertii interpretatio latina antiqua* (Leipzig)

Heidegger, M. (1963) *Sein und Zeit*, 10th edn (Tübingen)

Heidel, W.A. (1911) 'Antecedents of Greek corpuscular theories', *Harvard Studies in Classical Philology* 22: 111–72

Heinen, H. (1966) *Rom und Ägypten von 51 bis 47 v.Chr.* (Diss. Tübingen)

Heinimann, F. (1955) 'Diokles von Karystos und der prophylaktische Brief an König Antigonos', *Museum Helveticum* 12: 158–72

Helmreich, G. (1914) *Handschriftliche Studien zu Galen* III (Gymnasial-Programm Ansbach)

Herbst, W. (1911) *Galeni Pergameni de Atticissantium Studiis Testimonia* (Diss. Leipzig)

Herrmann, J. (1957–8) 'Vertragsinhalt und Rechtsnatur der ΔΙΔΑΣΚΑΛΙΚΑΙ', *Journal of Juristic Papyrology* 11/12: 119–39

Herzog, R. (1928) *Heilige Gesetze von Kos* (Abhandlungen der preussischen Akademie der Wissenschaften, Berlin, phil.-hist. Kl., 1928.6)

 (1931) *Die Wunderheilungen von Epidauros* (Philologus Suppl. 22.3)

 (1935) *Urkunden zur Hochschulpolitik der römischen Kaiser* (Sitzungsberichte der preussischen Akademie der Wissenschaften, Berlin, phil.-hist. Kl., 967–1019)

Hirschberg, J. (1899) 'Geschichte der Augenheilkunde I: Geschichte der Augenheilkunde im Alterthum', in A. Graefe and T. Saemisch (eds.), *Handbuch der gesamten Augenheilkunde* XII.2, 2nd edn (Leipzig), 53–419; repr. Hildesheim/New York, 1977; transl. F.C. Blodi, *The History of Ophthalmology*, I: *Antiquity* (Bonn, 1982)

 (1919a) 'Die Bruchstücke der Augenheilkunde des Demosthenes', *Archiv für die Geschichte der Medizin* 11: 183–8

 (1919b) 'Galen und seine zweite Anatomie des Auges', *Berliner klinische Wochenschrift* 610–12, 620–3

Hobein, H. (1929) 'Sphairos (3)', *Pauly-Wissowas Realencylopädie der classischen Altertumswissenschaft* II.6: cols. 1683–93

Hoff, H.E. (1964) 'Nicolaus von Cusa, van Helmont, and Boyle: The first experiment of the Renaissance in quantitative biology and medicine', *Journal of the History of Medicine and Allied Sciences* 19: 99–117

Hohenstein, H. (1935) *Der Arzt Mnesitheos aus Athen* (Diss. Berlin)

Hondius, J.J.E., et al., eds. (1923–) *Supplementum epigraphicum Graecum* (Leiden)

Horine, E.F. (1941) 'An epitome of ancient pulse lore', *Bulletin of the History of Medicine* 10: 209–49

Howell, J. (1644) *England's teares for the present warres* (London)

Huchzermeyer, H. and H. (1974) 'Die Bedeutung des Rhythmus in der Musiktherapie der Griechen von der Frühzeit bis zum Beginn des Hellenismus', *Sudhoffs Archiv* 58: 113–48

Hultsch, F. (1896) 'Archimedes (3)', *Pauly-Wissowas Realencyclopädie der classischen Altertumswissenschaft* 2: cols. 538–9

Hunger, H., et al. (1961–4) *Geschichte der Textüberlieferung der antiken und mittelalterlichen Literatur*, 2 vols. (Zurich)

Hunt, A.S., Smyly, J.G., Edgar, C.C. (1938) *The Tebtunis Papyri*, III, Part II (London)

Hurlbutt, F.R., Jr (1939) 'Peri Kardiēs: A treatise on the heart from the Hippocratic Corpus. Introduction and translation', *Bulletin of the History of Medicine* 7: 1104–13

Huxley, T.H. (1879) 'On certain errors respecting the structure of the heart attributed to Aristotle', *Nature* 21: 1–5

Ilberg, J. (1890) 'Die Hippokratesausgaben des Artemidoros Kapiton und Dioskurides', *Rheinisches Museum* N.F. 45: 111–37

(1893) *Das Hippokrates-Glossar des Erotianos und seine ursprüngliche Gestalt* (Abhandlungen der Königlich sächsischen Gesellschaft der Wissenschaften, Leipzig, 34, phil.-hist. Kl. 14.2: 101–48)

(1895) 'De Hippocratis Epidemiorum libri tertii characteribus', *Philologus* 54, N.F. 8: 396–402

(1905) 'Aus Galens Praxis', *Neue Jahrbücher für das klassische Altertum* 15: 276–312

(1924) *Die Ärzteschule von Knidos* (Berichte über die Verhandlungen der sächsischen Akademie der Wissenschaften, Leipzig, phil.-hist. Kl. 76.3)

(1930) *Rufus von Ephesos* (Abhandlungen der sächsischen Akademie der Wissenschaften, Leipzig, phil.-hist. Kl., 41.1)

Inscriptiones Graecae, eds. A. Kirchhoff, W. Dittenberger, F. Hiller von Gaertringen, G. Kaibel, J. Kirchner, W. Kolbe, et al. (1873–) (Berlin)

Iversen, E. (1939) 'Papyrus Carlsberg No. VIII. With some remarks on the Egyptian origin of some popular birth prognoses', *Historisk-filologiske Meddelelser udgivet af det Kgl. Danske Videnskabernes Selskab*, XXVI.5 1939.5: 1–31

(1953) 'Wounds in the head in Egyptian and Greek medicine', in *Studia orientalia Ioanni Pedersen Septuagenario* (Copenhagen), 163–71

Jacoby, F. (1923–58) *Fragmente der griechischen Historiker*, 15 vols. (Berlin/Leiden)

Jaeger, W. (1913) 'Das Pneuma im Lykeion', *Hermes* 48: 29–74; repr. in Jaeger, 1960: I, 57–102

(1938a) *Diokles von Karystos. Die griechische Medizin und die Schule des Aristoteles* (Berlin; repr. 1963)

(1938b) *Vergessene Fragmente des Peripatetikers Diokles von Karystos nebst zwei Anhängen zur Chronologie der dogmatischen Ärzteschule* (Abhandlungen der preussischen Akademie der Wissenschaften, Berlin, phil.-hist. Kl. 1938.3; 1–46); repr. in Jaeger, 1960: vol. II, pp. 185–241

(1940) 'Diocles of Carystus: A new pupil of Aristotle', *Philosophical Review* 49: 393–414; repr. in Jaeger, 1960: II, 243–65

(1945) *Paideia*, trans. G. Highet, 3 vols., 2nd edn (New York)

(1947) 'Praise of law: The origin of legal philosophy and the Greeks', in

Interpretations of Modern Legal Philosophies. Essays in Honor of Roscoe Pound
New York), 352–75

(1957) 'Aristotle's use of medicine as model of method in his Ethics',
Journal of Hellenic Studies 77: 54–61; repr. in Jaeger, 1960; vol. II, pp.
491–509

(1960) *Scripta Minora*, 2 vols. (Rome)

Joly, R. (1961) 'La question hippocratique et le témoignage du *Phèdre*', *Revue
des Études Grecques* 74: 69–92; transl. in Flashar, 1971: 52–82

(1966) *Le niveau de la science hippocratique* (Paris)

(1969) 'Esclaves et médecins dans la Grèce antique', *Sudhoffs Archiv* 53:
1–14

(1970) Review of H. Grensemann, *Der Arzt Polybos* (1968) in *Gnomon* 42:
190–2

Jonckheere, F. (1947) *Le papyrus médical Chester Beatty* (Brussels)

(1951a) 'La place du prêtre de Sekhmet dans le corps médical de
l'ancienne Égypte', *Actes du VIᵉ Congrès d'histoire des sciences*, Amsterdam,
1950 (Paris), I, 324–33

(1951b) 'À la recherche du chirurgien égyptien', *Chronique d'Égypte* 26:
28–45

(1951c) 'Le cadre professionel et administratif des médecins égyptiens',
Chronique d'Égypte 26: 237–68

(1952) 'Médecins de cour et médecine palatine sous les Pharaons',
Chronique d'Égypte 27: 51–87

(1958) *Les médecins de l'Égypte pharaonique: Essai de prosopographie* (Brussels)

Jones, W.H.S. (1947) *The Medical Writings of the Anonymus Londinensis*
(Cambridge)

Jouanna, J. (1969a) 'Le médecin Polybe, est-il l'auteur de plusieurs ouvrages
de la Collection hippocratique?', *Revue des Études Grecques* 82: 552–62

(1969b) Review of Grensemann, 1968a, in *Revue des Études Anciennes* 71:
475–8

(1974) *Hippocrate, Pour une archéologie de l'école de Cnide* (Paris)

(1975) *Hippocrate, La Nature de l'homme* (Corpus Medicorum Graecorum
I.1.3, Berlin)

Junker, H. (1928) 'Die Stele des Hofarztes 'Irj', *Zeitschrift für ägyptische
Sprache und Altertumskunde* 63: 53–70

Kalbfleisch, C. (1892), *In Galeni De Placitis Hippocratis et Platonis Libros
Observationes Criticae* (Diss. Berlin)

Karpp, H. (1934) 'Sorans vier Bücher Περὶ ψυχῆς und Tertullians Schrift
De Anima', *Zeitschrift für die Neutestamentliche Wissenschaft* 33: 31–47

Keil, J. (1905) 'Ärzteinschriften aus Ephesos', *Jahreshefte des Österreichischen
Archäologischen Instituts* 8: 128–38

Kessels, A.H.M. (1969) 'Ancient systems of dream-classification', *Mnemosyne*, ser. 4, 22: 389–424.

Kidd, I.G. (1971) 'Stoic intermediates and the end for man', in Long, 1971: 150–72

Kind, F.E. (1920) Review of Wenkebach, 1920, in *Berliner philologische Wochenschrift* Jg. 40, 1920.51: cols. 1201–9

(1927a) 'Lucius (7)', *Pauly-Wissowas Realencyclopädie der classischen Altertumswissenschaft* 13.2: cols. 1652–3

(1927b) 'Lysias (14), *ibid*.: col. 2543

(1927c) 'Soranos', *Pauly-Wissowas Realencyclopädie der classischen Altertumswissenschaft* 11.5: cols. 1113–30

(1928) 'Mantias (4)', *Pauly-Wissowas Realencyclopädie der classischen Altertumswissenschaft* 14.1: col. 1257

Klein, J. (1865) *Erotiani Vocum Hippocraticarum conlectio* (Leipzig)

Kleingünther, A. (1933) ΠΡΩΤΟΣ ΕΥΡΕΤΗΣ (*Philologus* Suppl. 26.1)

Kollesch, J. (1966) 'Zur Geschichte des medizinischen Lehrbuchs in der Antike', in *Aktuelle Probleme aus der Geschichte der Medizin. Verhandlungen des XIX. Internationalen Kongresses für Geschichte der Medizin, 1964*, ed. R. Blaser, H. Buess (Basel), 204–8.

(1968) 'Zur σημείωσις-Lehre der empirischen Ärzteschule', *Verhandlungen des XX. Internationalen Kongresses für Geschichte der Medizin, Berlin, 22.–27. August 1966* (Hildesheim), 273–7

(1973) *Untersuchungen zu den pseudogalenischen Definitiones Medicae* (Akademie der Wissenschaften der DDR, Zentralinstitut für Alte Geschichte und Archäologie, Schriften zur Geschichte und Kultur der Antike 7, Berlin)

(1975a) 'Zenon (12)', *Der kleine Pauly* 5: col. 1506

(1975b) 'Zeuxis (2)', *Der kleine Pauly* 5: col. 1527

(1976) 'Zur Säftelehre in der Medizin des 4. Jahrhunderts v.u.Z.', *Acta Congressus Internationalis XXIV Historiae Artis Medicinae, 1974* (Budapest), 2: 1339–42

(1979) 'Ärztliche Ausbildung in der Antike', *Klio* 61: 507–13

Kotrč, R.F. (1973) 'Critical notes on Galen's *De venae sectione adversus Erasistrateos Romae degentes*', *Classical Quarterly* n.s. 23 (1973), 369–74.

Kremmer, M. (1890) *De catalogis heurematum* (Diss. Leipzig)

Kroll, W. (1930) 'Marullus (5)', *Pauly-Wissowas Realencyclopädie der classischen Altertumswissenschaft* 14.2: col. 2053

(1951) 'C. Plinius (5) Secundus der Ältere', *Pauly-Wissowas Realencyclopädie der classischen Altertumswissenschaft* 21.1: cols. 271–439

Krug, A. (1985) *Heilkunst und Heilkult* (Munich)

Krumbacher, K. (1897) *Geschichte der byzantinischen Literatur von Justinian bis zum Ende des oströmischen Reiches (527–1453)*, 2nd edn (Munich) (Handbuch der klassischen Altertumswissenschaft IX.1)

Kuchenmüller, W.E. (1928) *Philetae Coi Reliquiae* (Diss. Berlin)

Kudlien, F. (1962) 'Poseidonios und die Ärzteschule der Pneumatiker', *Hermes* 90: 419–29

(1963a) 'Die Datierung des Sextus Empiricus and des Diogenes Laertius', *Rheinisches Museum* N.F. 106: 251–4

(1963b) 'Probleme um Diokles von Karystos', *Sudhoffs Archiv für Geschichte der Medizin* 47: 456–64; repr. in Flashar, 1971: 192–201

(1964a) 'Bakcheios', *Der kleine Pauly* 1: col.808

(1964b) 'Demosthenes (3)', *Der kleine Pauly* 1: col. 1487

(1964c) 'Herophilos und der Beginn der medizinischen Skepsis', *Gesnerus* 21: 1–13; repr. in Flashar, 1971: 280–95

(1964d) 'Nomenklaturgeschichtliche Addenda zur "Nachgeburt"', *Sudhoffs Archiv für Geschichte der Medizin* 48: 86–8

(1965) 'Dogmatische Ärzte', *Pauly-Wissowas Realencyclopädie der classischen Altertumswissenschaft*, Suppl. 10: cols. 179–80

(1967a) *Der Beginn des medizinischen Denkens bei den Griechen* (Zurich/ Stuttgart)

(1967b) 'Xenophon (13)', *Pauly-Wissowas Realencyclopädie der classischen Altertumswissenschaft* II.18: cols. 2089–92

(1967c) 'Dioskurides (6) Phakas', *Der kleine Pauly* 2: col. 91

(1968a) 'Anatomie', *Pauly-Wissowas Realencyclopädie der classischen Altertumswissenschaft*, Suppl. 11: cols. 38–48

(1968b) 'Der Arzt des Körpers und der Arzt der Seele', *Clio Medica* 3: 1–20

(1968c) *Die Sklaven in der griechischen Medizin der klassischen und hellenistischen Zeit* (Forschungen zur antiken Sklaverei, eds. J. Vogt and H.U. Instinsky, II, Wiesbaden)

(1968d) 'Pneumatische Ärzte', *Pauly-Wissowas Realencyclopädie der classischen Altertumswissenschaft*, Suppl. 11: cols. 1097–108

(1969a) 'Antike Anatomie und menschlicher Leichnam', *Hermes* 97: 78–94

(1969b) 'Lysimachos (5)', *Der kleine Pauly* 3: col. 842

(1969c) Review of H. Grensemann, *Der Arzt Polybos* (1968), in *Clio Medica* 4: 150–1

(1970) 'Medical education in classical antiquity', in C.D. O'Malley, ed., *The History of Medical Education* (Berkeley/Los Angeles)

(1972a) 'Medicina helenístico-romana (300 a.c.–100 d.c.)', in P. Laín Entralgo, ed., *Historia Universal de la Medicina* II (Barcelona), 153–99

(1972b) 'Praxagoras', *Der kleine Pauly* 4: col. 1122

(1972c) 'Zenon (13)', *Pauly-Wissowas Realencyclopädie der classischen Altertumswissenschaft* II.19: col. 146

(1972d) 'Zeuxis (7)–(8)', *ibid.*: cols. 386–7

(1974a) 'Dialektik und Medizin in der Antike', *Medizinhistorisches Journal* 9: 187–200

(1974b) 'Die stoische Gesundheitsbewertung und ihre Probleme', *Hermes* 102: 446–56

(1979) *Der griechische Arzt im Zeitalter des Hellenismus. Seine Stellung in Staat und Gesellschaft* (Abhandlungen, Akademie der Wissenschaften und der Literatur, Mainz, geistes- und sozialwissenschaftliche Kl., 1979.6)

Kühn, C.G. (1826) *Additamenta ad elenchum medicorum veterum* III (Leipzig)

Kühner, R. (1898–1904) *Ausführliche Grammatik der griechischen Sprache*, Teil 2: *Satzlehre*, 3rd edn rev. B. Gerth, 2 vols. (Hannover/Leipzig; repr. 1966)

Kümmel, W. (1977), *Musik und Medizin. Ihre Wechselbeziehung in Theorie und Praxis von 800 bis 1800* (Freiburger Beiträge zur Wissenschafts- und Universitätsgeschichte 2)

Kuhn, T.S. (1970) *The Structure of Scientific Revolutions*, 2nd edn (Chicago)

Laín Entralgo, P. (1962) 'Die ärztliche Hilfe im Werk Platons', *Sudhoffs Archiv für Geschichte der Medizin* 46: 193–210

Lammert, F. (1940/41) 'Hellenistische Medizin bei Ptolemaios und Nemesios', *Philologus* 94: 125–41

Latte, K. (1931) Review of F. Hiller von Gaertringen, ed., *Inscriptiones Graecae*, vol. IV, ed. minor, fasc. 1: *Inscriptiones Epidauri* (1929), in *Gnomon* 7: 113–35

Lattin, H.P. (1961) *The Letters of Gerbert with his Papal Privileges as Sylvester II* (New York)

LeBas, P., and Waddington, W.H. (1870) *Voyage archéologique en Grèce et Asie Mineure*, II. Partie: *Inscriptions grecques et latines* III (Paris)

Leboucq, G. (1944), see Bidez and Leboucq (1944)

Leca, A.-P. (1971) *La médecine égyptienne au temps des Pharaohs* (Paris)

Lefebvre, G. (1952) 'Prêtres de Sekhmet', *Archiv Orientální* 20: 57–64

(1956) *Essai sur la médecine égyptienne de l'époque pharaonique* (Paris)

Leflon, J. (1946) *Gerbert: Humanisme et Chrétienté au Xe siècle* (Abbaye S. Wandrille)

Leo, F. (1901) *Die griechisch-römische Biographie* (Leipzig)

Le Page Renouf, P. (1873) 'Note on the medical papyrus of Berlin', *Zeitschrift für ägyptische Sprache und Alterthumskunde* 11: 123–5

Lesky, E. (1950) *Die Zeugungs- und Vererbungslehren der Antike und ihr Nachwirken* (Akademie der Wissenschaften und der Literatur, Mainz, Abhandlungen der geistes- und sozialwissenschaftlichen Kl. 1950.19)

Letronne, [A.J.,] (1842–8) *Recueil des inscriptions grecques et latines de l'Égypte*, 2 vols. (Paris)

Lewis, N. (1986) *Greeks in Ptolemaic Egypt* (Oxford)

Lloyd, A.C. (1962) 'Genus, species, and ordered series in Aristotle's biology', *Phronesis* 7: 67–90

Lloyd, G.E.R. (1961) 'The development of Aristotle's theory of the classification of animals', *Phronesis* 6: 59–81

(1964) 'Experiment in early Greek philosophy and medicine', *Proceedings of the Cambridge Philological Society* 190, N.S. 10: 50–72

(1966) *Polarity and Analogy* (Cambridge)

(1968) 'Ancient Medicine and Modern Controversies', review of Edelstein, *Ancient Medicine* (1967), *History of Science* 7: 125–9

(1973) *Greek Science After Aristotle* (London)

(1975a) 'Alcmaeon and the early history of dissection', *Sudhoffs Archiv* 59: 113–47

(1975b) 'A note on Erasistratus of Ceos', *Journal of Hellenic Studies* 95: 172–5

(1975c) 'The Hippocratic Question', *Classical Quarterly* N.S. 25: 171–92

(1979) *Magic, Reason and Experience* (Cambridge)

(1982) 'Observational error in later Greek science', in Barnes et al., 1982: 128–64

(1983) *Science, Folklore and Ideology. Studies in the Life Sciences in Ancient Greece* (Cambridge)

(1984) 'Hellenistic Science', in *The Cambridge Ancient History* VII.1, ed. A. E. Astin, M. Frederiksen, R. M. Ogilvie, 321–52 (Cambridge)

Long, A.A., ed. (1971) *Problems in Stoicism* (London)

Longrigg, J. (1963) 'Philosophy and medicine: some early interactions', *Harvard Studies in Classical Philology* 67: 147–75

(1965) 'ΚΡΥΣΤΑΛΛΟΕΙΔΩΣ' *Classical Quarterly* 59, N.S. 15: 249–51

(1971) 'Erasistratus', *Dictionary of Scientific Biography* 4: 382–6

(1972) 'Herophilus', *ibid.* 6: 316–19

(1975a) 'Praxagoras', *ibid.* 11: 127–8

(1975b) 'Elementary Physics in the Lyceum and Stoa', *Isis* 66, no. 232: 211–29

(1981) 'Superlative achievement and comparative neglect: Alexandrian medical science and modern historical research', *History of Science* 19: 155–200

(1985a) 'A seminal "debate" in the fifth century B.C.?', in *Aristotle on Nature and Living Beings. Studies presented to D.M. Balme*, ed. A. Gotthelf (Pittsburgh/Bristol): 277–87

(1985b) 'Herophilus and the arterial vein', *Liverpool Classical Monthly*, 10.10: 149–50

Lonie, I.M. (1964) 'Erasistratus, the Erasistrateans, and Aristotle', *Bulletin of the History of Medicine* 38: 426–43

(1965a) 'Medical theory in Heraclides of Pontus', *Mnemosyne*, ser. 4, 18: 126–43

(1965b) 'The Cnidian Treatises of the Corpus Hippocraticum', *Classical Quarterly* N.S. 15: 1–30

(1973) 'The paradoxical text "On the Heart" ', *Medical History* 17: 1–15, 136–53

(1978) 'Cos versus Cnidus and the historians, I, II', *History of Science* 16: 42–75, 77–92

(1981) *The Hippocratic Treatises 'On Generation', 'On the Nature of the Child', 'Diseases IV'* (Ars Medica II.7, Berlin)

Loria, G. (1914) *Le Scienze esatte nell' antica Grecia*, 2nd edn (Milan)

Lucas, A., and Harris, J.R. (1962) *Ancient Egyptian Materials and Industries*, 4th edn (London)

Luck, G. (1953) *Der Akademiker Antiochus* (Noctes Romanae 7)

Maas, P. (1927) 'Simias (6)', *Pauly-Wissowas Realencyclopädie der classischen Altertumswissenschaft* II.5: cols. 155–8.

MacKinney, L. (1964) 'The concept of Isonomia in Greek medicine', in Mau and Schmidt, 1964: 79–88

McMinn, J.B. (1956) 'Fusion of the gods', *Journal of Near Eastern Studies* 15: 201–13

Magnus, H. (1876) *Geschichte des grauen Staares* (Leipzig)

(1878) *Die anatomie des Auges bei den Griechen und Römern* (Leipzig)

(1901) *Die Augenheilkunde der Alten* (Breslau)

Majno, G. (1975) *The Healing Hand. Man and Wound in the Ancient World* (Cambridge, Mass.)

Mani, N. (1959–67) *Die historischen Grundlagen der Leberforschung*, 2 vols. (Basler Veröffentlichungen zur Geschichte der Medizin und der Biologie, 9 and 21, Basel)

Mansfeld, J. (1975) 'Alcmaeon: "Physikos" or Physician?', in *Kephalaion: Festschrift C.J. de Vogel*, eds. J. Mansfeld and L.M. de Rijk (Assen), 26–38

Manuli, P. (1980) 'Fisiologia e patologia del femminile negli scritti ippocratici dell' antica ginecologia greca', in M.D. Grmek, ed., *Hippocratica. Actes du Colloque hippocratique de Paris, 1978* (Paris)

Marganne, M.-H. (1981) *Inventaire analytique des papyrus grecs de médecine* (Centre de recherches d'histoire et de philologie de la IVᵉ section de l'École Pratique des Hautes Études. Hautes études du monde greco-romain (Geneva), vol. 12)

Mariotti, I. (1966) *Aristone d'Allessandria* (Bologna)

Marx, K.F.H. (1838) *Herophilos: Ein Beitrag zur Geschichte der Medizin* (Karlsruhe/Baden)

(1840) *De Herophili celeberrimi medici vita scriptis atque in medicina meritis* (Göttingen)

Mau, J., and Schmidt, E.G., eds. (1964) *Isonomia* (Deutsche Akademie der Wissenschaften, Berlin, Institut für griechisch-römische Altertumskunde, Arbeitsgruppe für hellenistisch-römische Philosophie, Veröffentlichungen Nr. 9)

May, M.T. (1968) *Galen on the Usefulness of the Parts of the Body*, 2 vols. (Ithaca, N.Y.)

Mayer, A. (1912) 'Die Chronologie des Zenon und Kleanthes', *Philologus* 71, N.F.25: 211–37

Meier, C.A. (1967) *Ancient Incubation and Modern Psychotherapy*, transl. M. Curtis (Evanston, Illinois)

Merle, H. (1916) *Die Geschichte der Städte Byzantion und Kalchedon* (Diss. Kiel)

Mette, A., and Winter, I., eds. (1968) *Geschichte der Medizin* (Berlin)

Mewaldt, J. (1909) 'Galenos über echte und unechte Hippocratica', *Hermes* 44: 111–34

Meyer, J.B. (1855) *Aristoteles' Thierkunde* (Berlin)

Meyerhof, M. (1928) 'Eine Augenbehandlung durch Galen, nach arabischen Quellen', *Klinische Monatsblätter für Augenheilkunde* 80 (1928.1): 819–21

Meyer-Steineg, T. (1910) 'Thessalos von Tralles', *Archiv für Geschichte der Medizin* 4: 89–108

(1916) *Das medizinische System der Methodiker* (Jena)

Meyer-Steineg, T., and Sudhoff, K. (1921) *Geschichte der Medizin im Überblick* (Jena; 4th edn 1950)

Michler, M. (1968) *Hellenistische Chirurgie, Teil I: Die alexandrinischen Chirurgen. Eine Sammlung und Auswertung ihrer Fragmente* (Wiesbaden)

Mokhtar, G., Riad, H., and Iskander, Z. (1973) *Mummification in Ancient Egypt* (Cairo)

Mola, T. (1962) *La scuola di Erofilo: Apollonio Erofileo e gli altri medici che ebbere nome Apollonio* (Istituto di storia della medicina, Università di Roma)

(1963) 'La scuola di Erofilo: Andrea', *Atti e memorie dell' Accademia di Storia dell' Arte Sanitaria*, ser. II.a, 29: 71–83

Most, G.W. (1981) 'Callimachus and Herophilus', *Hermes* 109: 188–96

Mudry, P. (1982) *La préface du 'De medicina' de Celse* (Bibliotheca Helvetica Romana 19, Rome)

Müller-Graupa (1933) 'Mouseion' 4. Das alexandrinische Mouseion', *Pauly-Wissowas Realencylopädie der classischen Altertumswissenschaft* 16.1: cols. 801–21

Münzer, F. (1897) *Beiträge zur Quellenkritik der Naturgeschichte des Plinius* (Berlin)

(1903) 'Dioskurides (4)', *Pauly-Wissowas Realencylopädie der classischen Altertumswissenschaft* 5.1: col. 1125

(1930) 'C. Marius (16)', *ibid.* 14.2: cols. 1815–17

Mugler, C. (1970–2) *Archimède*, 4 vols. (Paris)

Nachmanson, E. (1917), *Erotianstudien* (Uppsala/Leipzig)

Nanetti, O. (1944) 'τὸ Ιατρικόν', *Aegyptus* 24: 119–25

Neuburger, M. (1906) *Geschichte der Medizin* I (Stuttgart); trans. E. Playfair (London, 1910)

(1926) *Die Lehre von der Heilkraft der Natur* (Stuttgart)

Neuburger, M., and Pagel, J., eds. (1902–5) *Handbuch der Geschichte der Medizin*, begründet von T. Puschmann, 3 vols. (Jena)

Neugebauer, O., and Parker, R.A. (1969) *Egyptian Astronomical Texts* III (Providence, Rhode Island/London)

Nussbaum, M.C. (1978) *Aristotle's De Motu Animalium* (Princeton)

Nutton, V. (1975) 'Museums and medical schools in antiquity', *History of Education* 4.1: 3–15

(1977) 'Archiatri and the medical profession in antiquity', *Papers of the British School at Rome* 45: 191–226

(1981) ed., *Galen: Problems and Prospects* (Wellcome Institute for the History of Medicine)

O'Brien, D. (1970) 'The effect of a simile: Empedocles' theories of seeing and breathing', *Journal of Hellenic Studies* 90: 140–79

Oertel, F. (1975) Review of W. Peremans, *Vreemdelingen en Egyptenaren*, in *Kleine Schriften zur Wirtschafts- und Sozialgeschichte des Altertums* (Bonn), 264–70

Oliver, J.D. (1934) 'The Mouseion in late Attic inscriptions', *Hesperia* 3: 191–6

Oliver, J.R. (1935) 'Greek medicine and its relation to Greek civilization', *Bulletin of the History of Medicine* 2: 623–38

Olleris, A. (1867) *Oeuvres de Gerbert, pape sous le nom de Sylvestre* II (Clermont-Ferrand/Paris)

Onians, R.B. (1951) *The Origins of European Thought* (Cambridge)

Oppermann, H. (1925) 'Herophilos bei Kallimachos', *Hermes* 60: 14–32

Otto, W. (1905–8) *Priester und Tempel im hellenistischen Ägypten*, 2 vols. (Leipzig/Berlin)

(1934) *Zur Geschichte der Zeit des 6. Ptolemäers* (Abhandlungen der bayerischen Akademie der Wissenschaften, Munich, phil-hist. Abt., N.F. 11)

Otto, W., and Bengtson, H. (1938) *Zur Geschichte des Niederganges des Ptolemäerreiches* (Abhandlungen der bayerischen Akademie der Wissenschaften, Munich, phil.-hist. Abt., N.F. 17)

Ottoson, P.-G. (1984) *Scholastic Medicine and Philosophy. A Study of Commentaries on Galen's 'Tegni' (ca. 1300–1450)* (Naples)

Owen, G.E.L. (1961) 'τιθέναι τὰ φαινόμενα', in *Aristote et les problèmes de méthode: Symposium Aristotelicum, 1960*, ed. S. Mansion (Louvain/Paris, 1961), 83–103

Pagel, J. (1898) *Einführung in die Geschichte der Medizin* (Berlin)

Pais, E. (1922) 'Intorno al tempo ed al luogo in cui Strabone compose la Geografia Storica', *Italia Antica* I (Bologna), 275–91

Panayotatou, A. (1929) 'Terres cuites d'Égypte de l'époque gréco-romaine et maladies', *VIe Congrès international d'histoire de la médecine, Leyde-Amsterdam, 1927* (Antwerp), 41–57

Papiri greci e latini (Pubblicazioni della Società Italiana per la ricerca dei papiri greci e latini in Egitto), ed. G. Vitelli et al. (1912–   ), 15 vols. (Florence)

Parker, R. (1983) *Miasma. Pollution and purification in early Greek religion* (Oxford)

Paton, W.R., and Hicks, E.L. (1891) *The Inscriptions of Cos* (Oxford)

Peacock, T.L. (1831) *Crotchet Castle* (London)

Peck, A.L. (1943) *Aristotle, Generation of Animals*, Loeb edn. (London/ Cambridge, Mass.)

(1965–) *Aristotle, Historia Animalium*, 2 vols., Loeb edn (London/Cambridge, Mass.)

Peck, A.L., and Forster, E.S. (1937) *Aristotle, Parts of Animals, Movement of Animals, Progression of Animals*, Loeb edn (London/Cambridge, Mass.)

Perdrizet, P. (1921) *Les terres cuites grecques d'Égypte de la Collection Fouquet*, 2 vols. (Nancy/Paris Strasbourg)

(1934) 'Le mort qui sentait bon', in *Mélanges Bidez* (Annuaire de l'Institut de philologie et d'histoire orientales 2, Brussels), 719–27

Peremans, W. (1937) *Vreemdelingen en Egyptenaren in Vroeg-Ptolemaeisch Egypte* (Université de Louvain, Conférences d'Histoire et de Philologie, 2ᵐᵉ sér., 43)

Peremans, W., and van't Dack, E., eds. (1950–81) *Prosopographia Ptolemaica* I–IX (=*Studia Hellenistica* 6, 8, 11–13, 17, 20–1, 25 Louvain)

Petersen, J. (1877) *Hauptmomente in der geschichtlichen Entwicklung der medizinischen Therapie* (Copenhagen)

(1903) 'Zur Geschichte der Ernährungstherapie', in E. von Leyden, *Handbuch der Ernährungstherapie* (Leipzig)

Pfaff, F. (1932) 'Die Überlieferung des Corpus Hippocraticum in der nachalexandrinischen Zeit', *Wiener Studien* 50: 67–82

Pfeiffer, R. (1949) *Callimachus*, 2 vols. (Oxford)

(1968) *A History of Classical Scholarship from the Beginning to the end of the Hellenistic Age* (Oxford)

Pfister, F. (1951) *Die Reisebilder des Herakleides* (Sitzungsberichte der österreichischen Akademie der Wissenschaften, Wien, phil.-hist. Kl. 227.2)

Philippson, L. (1831) ΥΛΗ ΑΝΘΡΩΠΙΝΗ (Berlin)

Phillips, E.D. (1970) 'Hippocratica', review of Grensemann, 1968a, et al., *Classical Review* N.S. 20: 23–6

(1973) *Greek Medicine* (London)

Picard, C. (1952) 'Sur quelques représentations nouvelles du Phare d'Alexandrie et sur l'origine alexandrine des paysages portuaires', *Bulletin de correspondance héllenique* 76: 61–95

Picavet, F. (1897) *Gerbert, un pape philosophe* (Paris)

Pigeaud, J.-M. (1978) 'Du rhythme dans le corps. Quelques notes sur l'interprétation du pouls par le médecin Hérophile', *Bulletin de l'Association Guillaume Budé* 1978.3: 258–67

Pinoff, J. (1847) 'Herophilos. Ein Beitrag zur Geschichte der Geburtshilfe', *Janus* 2: 739–43

Platt, A. (1921) 'Aristotle on the heart', in C. Singer, ed., *Studies in the History and Method of Science* II (Oxford), 521–32

Pöhlmann, E. (1960) *Griechische Musikfragmente* (Erlanger Beiträge zur Sprach- und Kunstwissenschaft 8)

Pohl, R. (1905) *De Graecorum medicis publicis*, Diss. phil. Berlin (Leipzig)

Pohlenz, M. (1940) *Grundfragen der stoischen Philosophie* (Abhandlungen der Gesellschaft der Wissenschaften, Göttingen, phil.-hist. Kl., 3.26)

Potter, P. (1976) 'Herophilus of Chalcedon: An assessment of his place in the history of anatomy', *Bulletin of the History of Medicine* 50: 45–60

Poynter, F.L.N., ed. (1958) *The History and Philosophy of Knowledge of the Brain and its Functions* (Oxford/Springfield, Illinois)

Préaux, C. (1939) *L'Économie royale des Lagides* (Brussels)

(1953) 'Les raisons de l'originalité de l'Égypte', *Museum Helveticum* 10: 203–21

Preisigke, F., Bibabel, F., Kiessling, E., Rupprecht, H.-A., eds. (1915–) *Sammelbuch griechischer Urkunden aus Ägypten* (Strassburg/Berlin/Leipzig/Heidelberg/Wiesbaden)

Pusch, H. (1890) *Questiones Zenodoteae* (Dissertationes philologicae Halenses 11: 191–216)

Puschmann, T. (1878–9) *Alexander von Tralles*, 2 vols. (Vienna)

(1886) *Nachträge zu Alexander Trallianus. Fragmente aus Philumenus und Philagrius nebst einer bisher noch ungedruckten Abhandlung über Augenkrankheiten* (Berliner Studien für classische Philologie und Archäologie 5.2)

Raeder, J., Deichgräber K., Kroll, W. (1932) 'Mnemon (3)', *Pauly-Wissowas Realencyclopädie der classischen Altertumswissenschaft* 15.2: col. 2261

Ramsay, W.M. (1895–7) *The Cities and Bishoprics of Phrygia*, 2 vols. (Oxford)

Rawson, E. (1982) 'The life and death of Asclepiades of Bithynia', *Classical Quarterly* N.S. 32:358–70

Reesor, M.E. (1951) 'The "indifferents" in the Old and Middle Stoa', *Transactions and Proceedings of the American Philological Association* 82: 102–10

Regenbogen, O. (1921) 'Hippokrates und die hippokratische Sammlung', *Neue Jahrbücher für das klassische Altertum* 47: 185–97; repr. in Regenbogen, 1961: 125–40

  (1931) 'Eine Forschungsmethode antiker Naturwissenschaft', *Quellen und Studien zur Geschichte der Mathematik, Astronomie, und Physik*, Abteilung B.I.2: 131–82; repr. in Regenbogen, 1961: 141–94

  (1940) 'Theophrastos (3)', *Pauly-Wissowas Realencyclopädie der classischen Altertumswissenschaft*, Suppl. 7: cols. 1354–1562

  (1961) *Kleine Schriften* (Munich)

Reincke, G. (1938) 'Pharos (3)', *Pauly-Wissowas Realencyclopädie der classischen Altertumswissenschaft* 19.2: cols. 1867–9

Reinhardt, K. (1921) *Poseidonios* (Munich)

Rémondon, R. (1964) 'Problèmes du bilinguisme dans l'Égypte Lagide (U.P.Z. I, 148)', *Chronique d'Égypte* 39: 126–46

Rieth, O. (1933) *Grundbegriffe der stoischen Ethik* (Problemata 9, Berlin)

Robert, J. and L. (1965) 'Bulletin épigraphique', *Revue des Études Grecques* 78: 70–204

Robert, L. (1937) *Études anatoliennes* (Paris)

Rose, V. (1863) *Aristoteles Pseudepigraphus* (Leipzig)

  (1864–70) *Anecdota Graeca et Graecolatina*, 2 vols. (Berlin; repr. 1963)

  (1882) *Sorani Gynaeciorum vetus translatio Latina* (Leipzig)

  (1894) *Theodori Prisciani Euporiston libri* III (Leipzig)

Rostovtzeff, M. (1953) *The Social and Economic History of the Hellenistic World*, 2nd imp., 3 vols. (Oxford)

Rousselle, A. (1980) 'Images médicales du corps en Grèce: observation féminine et idéologie masculine', *Annales. Sociétes, Économies, Civilisations* 35: 1089–1115

Rüsche, F. (1930) *Blut, Leben und Seele: Ihr Verhältnis nach Auffassung der griechischen und hellenistischen Antike, der Bibel und der alten Alexandrinischen Theologen* (Studien zur Geschichte und Kultur des Altertums, Ergänzungsbd 5, Paderborn)

Ruge, W. (1919) 'Kalchedon (1)', *Pauly-Wissowas Realencylopädie der classischen Altertumswissenschaft* 10.2: cols. 1555–9

Rydbeck, L. (1967) *Fachprosa, vermeintliche Volkssprache und Neues Testament* (Acta Universitatis Upsaliensis: Studia Graeca Upsaliensia 5)

Saake, H. (1974) 'Pneuma', *Pauly-Wissowas Realencyclopädie der classischen Altertumswissenschaft*, Suppl. 14: cols. 387–412

Samuel, A.E. (1962) *Ptolemaic Chronology* (Münchener Beiträge zur Papyrusforschung und antiken Rechtsgeschichte 43)

Sarton, G. (1927–48) *Introduction to the History of Science*, 3 vols. in 5 (Baltimore)
  (1952–9) *A History of Science*, 2 vols. (Cambridge, Mass./London)

Sattler, P. (1963) *Griechische Papyrusurkunden und Ostraka der Heidelberger Papyrus-Sammlung* (Veröffentlichungen aus der Heidelberger Papyrussammlung, N.F. 3)

Saunders, J.B. de C.M. (1963) *The Transition from Ancient Egyptian to Greek Medicine* (Logan Clendening Lectures, 10th series, Lawrence, Kansas)

Scarborough, J. (1969) *Roman Medicine* (London, 1969)
  (1970) 'Diphilus of Siphnos and Hellenistic Medical Dietetics', *Journal of the History of Medicine and Allied Sciences* 25: 194–201
  (1975) 'The drug lore of Asclepiades of Bithynia', *Pharmacy in History* 17: 43–57
  (1976) 'Celsus on human vivisection at Ptolemaic Alexandria', *Clio Medica* 11: 25–38

Schadewald, O. (1866) *Sphygmologiae historia inde ab antiquissimis temporibus usque ad aetatem Paracelsi* (Diss. med. Berlin)

Schelenz, H. (1904) *Geschichte der Pharmazie* (Berlin)

Scherer, V. (1976) *Die Epistula de ratione ventris vel viscerum* (Diss. Berlin)

Schmidt, A. (1927) *Drogen und Drogenhandel im Altertum*, 2nd edn (Leipzig)

Schmidt, M.C.P. (1912) *Kulturhistorische Beiträge zur Kenntnis des griechischen und römischen Altertums*, 2 vols. (Leipzig)

Schneider, C. (1967–9) *Kulturgeschichte des Hellenismus*, 2 vols. (Munich)

Schöne, H. (1893) *De Aristoxeni ΠΕΡΙ ΤΗΣ ΗΡΟΦΙΛΟΥ ΑΙΡΕΣΕΩΣ libro tertio decimo a Galeno adhibito* (Diss. Bonn)
  (1903) 'Bruchstücke einer neuen Hippokratesvita', *Rheinisches Museum* N.F. 58: 56–66
  (1907) 'Markellinos' Pulslehre. Ein griechisches Anekdoton', *Festschrift zur 49. Versammlung deutscher Philologen und Schulmänner* (Basel), 448–72
  (1910) 'Echte Hippokratesschriften', *Deutsche medizinische Wochenschrift* 36: 418–66
  (1911) *Galeni De partibus artis medicativae* (Universitätsprogram Greifswald); Latin text repr. in *CMG, Supplementum Orientale* II (Berlin, 1969), pp. 117–29

Schöner, E. (1964) *Das Viererschema in der antiken Humoralpathologie* (Sudhoffs Archiv, Beiheft 4)

Schofield, M., Burnyeat, M., Barnes, J., eds. (1980) *Doubt and Dogmatism. Studies in Hellenistic Epistemology* (Oxford)

Schott, H.A. (1891) *De septem orbis spectaculis* (Diss. Munich)

Schrijvers, P.H. (1977) 'La classification des rêves selon Hérophile', *Mnemosyne* ser. 4, 30: 13–27

Schubring, K. (1962) 'Epistula Paraxagorae', *Sudhoffs Archiv für Geschichte der Medizin* 46: 295–310

Schwartz, E. (1903) 'Diodoros (38)', *Pauly-Wissowas Realencylopädie der classischen Altertumswissenschaft* 5.1: cols. 663–703

   (1957) *Die griechischen Geschichtschreiber* (Leipzig)

Sedley, D. (1977) 'Diodorus Cronus and Hellenistic Philosophy', *Proceedings of the Cambridge Philological Society* 203, n.s. 23: 74–120

Shackleton Bailey, D.R. (1965–70) *Cicero's Letters to Atticus*, 7 vols. (Cambridge)

Shaw, J.R. (1972) 'Models for cardiac structure and function in Aristotle', *Journal of the History of Biology* 5: 355–88

Sherwin-White, S.M. (1978) *Ancient Cos* (Hypomnemata 51)

Sigerist, H. (1924) 'Geburt der abendländischen Medizin', in *Essays on the History of Medicine presented to Karl Sudhoff* (Oxford)

   (1927) *Antike Heilkunde* (Munich)

   (1951–61) *A History of Medicine*, 2 vols. (Oxford/New York)

Silvaticus, Matthaeus (1474) *Liber pandectarum medicinae* (Bologna; repr. Venice, 1480)

Simon Ianuensis (1474) *Synonyma medicinae sive Clavis Sanationis* (Padua)

Simon, M. (1906) *Sieben Bücher Anatomie des Galen*, 2 vols. (Leipzig)

Sinclair, T.A. (1951) 'Class distinction in medical practice: a piece of ancient evidence', *Bulletin of the History of Medicine* 25: 386–7

Singer, C. (1928) *A Short History of Medicine* (Oxford); 2nd revised edn E.A. Underwood (1962)

   (1956) *Galen on Anatomical Procedures* (Oxford)

   (1957) *A Short History of Anatomy and Physiology from the Greeks to Harvey* (New York) = 2nd edn of *The Evolution of Anatomy* (London, 1925)

Sisson, S., and Grossman, J.D. (1948) *The Anatomy of Domestic Animals* (Philadelphia)

Sittig, E. (1911) *De Graeorum nominibus theophoris* (Diss. Halle/Wittenberg)

Skeat, T.C. (1954) *The Reigns of the Ptolemies* (Münchener Beiträge zur Papyrusforschung und antiken Rechtsgeschichte 39)

Smith, G.E. (1914) 'Egyptian mummies', *Journal of Egyptian Archaeology* 1: 189–96

Smith, W.D. (1973) 'Galen on Coans versus Cnidians', *Bulletin of the History of Medicine* 47: 569–85

   (1979) *The Hippocratic Tradition* (Ithaca, N.Y./London)

Solmsen, F. (1961) 'Greek philosophy and the discovery of the nerves', *Museum Helveticum* 18: 150–97; repr. in Flashar, 1971: 202–79, and in Solmsen, 1968–82: vol. 1, pp. 536–82

    (1968–82) *Kleine Schriften*, 3 vols. (Hildesheim)

Sorabji, R. (1980) 'Causation, laws, and necessity', in Schofield et al., 1980: 250–82

Souques, A. (1934) 'Que doivent à Hérophile et à Erasistrate l'anatomie et la physiologie du système nerveux?', *Bulletin de la Societé française d'Histoire de la Médecine* 28: 357–65

    (1935) 'Connaissances neurologiques d'Hérophile et d'Erasistrate', *Revue Neurologique* 63: 145–76

    (1936a) 'Connaissances neurologiques d'Hérophile à Galien', *Revue Neurologique* 65: 489–525

    (1936b) *Étapes de la neurologie dans l'antiquité grecque (d'Homère à Galien)* (Paris)

Spoerri, W. (1966) 'Prosopographica', *Museum Helveticum* 23: 44–57

Sprengel, K. (1821–40) *Versuch einer pragmatischen Geschichte der Arzneykunde*, 2nd edn, 5 parts in 8 (Halle)

    (1846) *Geschichte der Arzneikunde* (Halle)

von Staden, H. (1975) 'Experiment and experience in Hellenistic Medicine', *Bulletin of the Institute of Classical Studies* 22: 178–99

    (1976a) 'Die Hippokrateskommentare im Codex Ambrosianus Graecus 473 und Herophilos', *Philologus* 120: 132–6

    (1976b) 'A new testimonium about Polybus', *Hermes* 104: 494–6

    (1978) 'The Stoic theory of perception and its "Platonic" critics', in *Studies in Perception: Interrelations in the History of Philosophy and Science*, ed. P.K. Machamer and R. Turnbull (Columbus, Ohio), 96–136

    (1982) 'Hairesis and heresy: The case of the haireseis iatrikai', in *Jewish and Christian Self-Definition*, III: *Self-Definition in the Graeco-Roman World*, edd. B.F. Meyer and E.P. Sanders (London), 76–100, 199–206

Stadler, H. (1891) *Die Quellen des Plinius im XIX. Buch der Naturalis Historia* (Neuburg a.D.)

Stannard, J. (1961) 'Hippocratic pharmacology', *Bulletin of the History of Medicine* 35: 497–518

Starobinski, J. (1960) *Histoire du traitement de la melancholie des origines à 1900* (Basle)

Steckerl, F. (1958) *The fragments of Praxagoras of Cos and his School* (Philosophia Antiqua 8)

Stengel, P. (1920) *Die griechischen Kulturaltertümer*, 3rd edn (Handbuch der Altertumswissenschaft 5.3, Munich)

Steudel, J. (1943) 'Der vorvesalische Beitrag zur anatomischen Nomenklatur', *Sudhoffs Archiv für Geschichte der Medizin und der Naturwissenschaften* 36: 1–42

Steuer, R.O., and Saunders, J.B. de C.M. (1959) *Ancient Egyptian and Cnidian Medicine* (Berkeley/Los Angeles)

Sudhoff, K. (1909) *Ärztliches aus griechischen Papyrusurkunden. Bausteine zu einer medizinischen Kulturgeschichte des Hellenismus* (Studien zur Geschichte der Medizin, Puschmann-Stiftung, Heft 5/6)

(1913) 'Die Lehre von den Hirnventrikeln in textlicher und graphischer Tradition des Altertums und Mittelalters', *Archiv für Geschichte der Medizin* 7: 149–205

Susemihl, F. (1891–2) *Geschichte der griechischen Litteratur in der Alexandrinerzeit*, 2 vols. (Leipzig; repr. Hildesheim, 1965)

Switalski, W. (1902) *Des Chalcidius Kommentar zu Platons Timäus* (Münster/Westfalen)

Talamonti, R. (1968) 'Lo "Stato neutro" di Erofilo e la "Opportunitas ad Morbum" di Giovanni Brown', *Collana di Pagine di Storia della Medicina*, Miscellanea 17, 133–9

Tallmadge, G.K. (1939) 'Pierre Gassendi and the *Elegans de septo cordis pervio observatio*', *Bulletin of the History of Medicine* 7: 429–57

Tannery, P. (1898) 'Ecphante de Syracuse', *Archiv für Geschichte der Philosophie* 11, N.F. 4: 263–9

Taton, R. (1966) *Histoire générale des sciences I: La science antique et médiévale (des origines à 1450)*, 2nd edn (Paris)

Temkin, O. (1928) 'Der systematische Zusammenhang im Corpus Hippocraticum', *Kyklos* 1: 9–43

(1932) 'Geschichte des Hippokratismus im ausgehenden Altertum', *Kyklos* 4: 1–80; pt 2 transl. in Temkin, 1977: 167–77

(1935a) 'Celsus' "On Medicine" and the ancient medical sects', *Bulletin of the Institute of the History of Medicine* 3: 249–64

(1935b) 'Studies on late Alexandrian medicine: 1. Alexandrian commentaries on Galen's *De Sectis ad Introducendos*', *Bulletin of the Institute of the History of Medicine* 3: 405–30; repr. in Temkin, 1977: 178–97

(1951) 'On Galen's pneumatology', *Gesnerus* 8: 180–9; repr. in Temkin, 1977: 154–61

(1953) 'Greek medicine as science and craft', *Isis* 44: 213–25; repr. in Temkin, 1977: 137–53

(1956) *Soranus' Gynecology* (Baltimore)

(1962a) 'Nutrition from Classical Antiquity to the Baroque', *Human Nutrition Monographs* III (New York), 78–96

(1962b) 'Byzantine Medicine: Tradition and Empiricism', *Dumbarton Oaks Papers* 16: 95–115; repr. in Temkin, 1977: 202–22

(1973) *Galenism* (Ithaca, N.Y.)

(1977) *The Double Face of Janus* (London/Baltimore)

Theiler, W. (1930) *Die Vorbereitung des Neuplatonismus* (Problemata 1, Berlin)

(1982) *Poseidonios*, 2 vols. (Berlin/New York)

Theophanes Confessor (1883) *Chronographia*, ed. C. de Boor, vol. 1 (Leipzig)

Thesleff, H. (1965) *The Pythagorean Texts of the Hellenistic Period* (Acta Academiae Aboensis, Ser. A, 30.1, Åbo)

Thiersch, H. (1909) *Pharos: Antike, Islam und Occident* (Leipzig/Berlin)

Thivel, A. (1981) *Cnide et Cos?* (Paris)

Thompson, D.B. (1966) 'Tanagra', *Enciclopedia dell' arte antica classica e orientale* 7 (Rome), 590–5

Thompson, H.A. (1954) 'Excavations in the Athenian Agora: 1953', *Hesperia* 23: 31–67

Thrämer, E. (1896) 'Asklepios (2)', *Pauly-Wissowas Realencyclopädie der classischen Altertumswissenschaft* 2: cols. 1642–97

(1914) 'Health and gods of healing (Greek)', *Encyclopaedia of Religion and Ethics* 6: 540–53

Till, W.C. (1951) *Die Arzneikunde der Kopten* (Berlin)

von Töply, R. (1898) *Studien zur Geschichte der Anatomie im Mittelalter* (Leipzig/Vienna)

Torraca, L. (1965) 'Diocle di Caristo, il "Corpus Hippocraticum" ed Aristotele', *Sophia* 33: 105–15

Ueberweg, F., Praechter, K. (1926) *Grundriss der Geschichte der Philosophie*, I: *Die Philosophie des Altertums* (Berlin; repr. Darmstadt, 1967)

Uhlirz, M. (1957) *Untersuchungen über Inhalt und Datierung der Briefe Gerberts von Aurillac* (Göttingen)

Unger, F.C. (1923) 'Liber Hippocraticus ΠΕΡΙ ΚΑΡΔΙΗΣ', *Mnemosyne* N.S. 51: 1–101

Usener, H. (1912–14) *Kleine Schriften*, 4 vols. (Leipzig/Berlin)

Usher, A.P. (1954) *A History of Mechanical Inventions*, 2nd edn (Cambridge, Mass.)

Vegetti, M. (1979) *Il coltello e lo stilo* (Milan)

(1984) 'La scienza ellenistica: Problemi di epistemologia storica', in Giannantoni/Vegetti, 1984: 427–70

Verbeke, G. (1945) *L'évolution de la doctrine du pneuma du stoïcisme à S. Augustin* (Paris, Louvain)

Viano, C.A. (1984) 'Perché non c'era sangue nelle arterie: la cecità epistemologica degli anatomisti antichi', in Giannantoni/Vegetti, 1984: 297–352

von Vilas, H. (1903) *Der Arzt und Philosoph Asklepiades von Bithynien* (Vienna)

Vitelli, C. (1900) 'Studiorum Celsianorum particula prima', *Studi Italiani di filologia classica* 8: 449–88

Vogel, K. (1967) 'Byzantine Science', in *The Cambridge Medieval History* IV.2, ed. J.M. Hussey (Cambridge), 264–305

Volker, W. (1938) *Fortschritt und Vollendung bei Philo von Alexandrien* (Texte und Untersuchungen 49.1, Leipzig)

Von der Mühll, F. (1912) 'Herophilos (1)', *Pauly-Wissowas Realencyclopädie der classischen Altertumswissenschaft* 8.1: col. 1104

Waddington, W.H., Babelon, E., Reinach, T. (1904–25) *Recueil général des monnaies grecques d'Asie Mineure*, 4 vols. (Paris)

Walbank, F.W. (1957–79) *A Historical Commentary on Polybius*, 3 vols. (Oxford)

Walsh, J. (1927) 'Galen's studies at the Alexandrian School', *Annals of Medical History* 9: 132–43

Waszink, J.H. (1941) 'Die sogenannte Fünfteilung der Träume bei Chalcidius und ihre Quellen', *Mnemosyne*, 3rd ser. 9: 65–85

(1947) *Q. Septimi Florentis Tertulliani De anima* (Amsterdam)

Watermann, R. (1958) 'Die altägyptischen Augenärzte', *Sudhoffs Archiv für Geschichte der Medizin* 42: 117–41

Wehrli, F. (1967–9) *Die Schule des Aristoteles, Texte und Kommentare*, 10 vols., 2nd edn (Basel/Stuttgart)

Weinreich, O. (1909) *Antike Heilungswunder* (Religionsgeschichtliche Versuche und Vorarbeiten 8.1, Giessen; repr. Berlin, 1969)

Wellmann, M. (1888) 'Zur Geschichte der Medicin im Alterthume', *Hermes* 23: 556–66

(1891) 'Die Medicin bis in die zweite Hälfte des zweiten Jahrhunderts', in Susemihl, 1891–2: vol. I, pp. 777–828

(1892a) 'Die späteren Ärzte', in Susemihl, 1891–2: vol. II, pp. 414–47

(1892b) 'Zur Geschichte der Medicin im Altertum', *Neue Jahrbücher für Philologie und Pädagogik*, eds. Fleckeisen und Masius, Jg. 62, Bd 145: 677–8

(1894) 'Andromachos (18) der Jüngere', *Pauly-Wissowas Realencyclopädie der classischen Altertumswissenschaft* 1.2: col. 2154

(1895a) *Die pneumatische Schule bis auf Archigenes* (Philologische Untersuchungen 14)

(1895b) 'Apollonios (99)–(111)', *Pauly-Wissowas Realencyclopädie der classischen Altertumswissenschaft* 2.1: cols. 148–51

(1895c) 'Aristoxenos (8)', *ibid.*: col. 1065

(1896a) 'Asklepiades (39)', *ibid.* 2.2: col. 1632

(1896b) 'Asklepiades (43) ὁ νεώτερος', *ibid.*: cols. 1633–4

(1897) *Krateuas* (Abhandlungen der Königlichen Gesellschaft der Wissenschaften, Göttingen, phil.-hist. Kl., N.F. 2.1, Berlin)

(1898) 'Das älteste Kräuterbuch der Griechen', in *Festgabe für Franz*

Susemihl. *Zur Geschichte griechischer Wissenschaft und Dichtung* (Leipzig), 1–31

(1899) 'Chrysippos (15)–(19)', *Pauly-Wissowas Realencyclopädie der classischen Altertumswissenschaft* 3: cols. 2509–11

(1900a) 'Zur Geschichte der Medicin im Alterthum', *Hermes* 35: 349–84

(1900b) Review of J. Hirschberg, *Geschichte der Augenheilkunde* 1: *Geschichte der Augenheilkunde im Alterthum* (1899), in *Deutsche Literaturzeitung* 21. Jg.: Nr. 24, 1587–90

(1901) *Fragmentsammlung der griechischen Ärzte*, 1: *Die Fragmente der sikelischen Ärzte Akron, Philiston und des Diokles von Karystos* (Berlin)

(1903) 'Demosthenes' ΠΕΡΙ ΟΦΘΑΛΜΩΝ', *Hermes* 38: 546–66

(1905a) 'Dionysios (132)', *Pauly-Wissowas Realencyclopädie der classischen Altertumswissenschaft* 5: col. 976

(1905b) 'Dioskurides (10)', *ibid.*: cols. 1129–30

(1907a) 'Erasistratos (2)', *ibid.* 6.1: cols. 353–50

(1907b) 'Eudemos (17)', *ibid.*: col. 904

(1908) 'Asklepiades aus Bithynien von einem herrschenden Vorurteil befreit', *Neue Jahrbücher für das klassische Altertum* 21: 684–703

(1910) 'Zu Apollonios Mys' Schrift περὶ εὐπορίστων φαρμάκων', *Hermes* 45: 469

(1913) *A. Cornelius Celsus, Eine Quellenuntersuchung* (Philologische Untersuchungen 23, Berlin)

(1919) 'Eine pythagoreische Urkunde des IV. Jahrhunderts v. Chr.', *Hermes* 54: 225–48

(1922) 'Der Verfasser des Anonymus Londinensis', *Hermes* 57: 396–429

(1924–5) 'Über Träume', *Archiv für Geschichte der Medizin* 16: 70–2

(1929) 'Hippokrates des Herakleides Sohn', *Hermes* 64: 16–21

(1930) 'Beiträge zur Geschichte der Medizin im Altertum', *Hermes* 65: 322–31

(1931) *Hippokratesglossare* (Quellen und Studien zur Geschichte der Naturwissenschaften und der Medizin 2)

Wenkebach, E. (1917) *Pseudogalenische Kommentare zu den Epidemien des Hippokrates* (Abhandlungen der Königlichen preussischen Akademie der Wissenschaften, Berlin, phil.-hist. Kl., 1917.1)

(1920) *Eine alexandrinische Buchfehde um einen Buchstaben in den hippokratischen Krankengeschichten* (Sitzungsberichte der preussischen Akademie der Wissenschaften, Berlin, 241–53)

(1925) *Untersuchungen über Galens Kommentare zu den Epidemien des Hippokrates* (Abhandlungen der preussischen Akademie der Wissenschaften, Berlin, phil.-hist. Kl., 1925.1)

West, S. (1973) 'Cultural Interchange over a Water-Clock', *Classical Quarterly* 67, N.S. 23: 61–4

Westphal, R. (1883–93) *Aristoxenus von Tarent. Melik und Rhythmik des classischen Hellenentums*, 2 vols. (Leipzig)

Wickersheimer, E. (1966) *Les manuscrits latins de médecine du Haute Moyen Age dans les Bibliothèques de France* (Paris)

Wiedemann, W. (1976) *Untersuchungen zu dem frühmittelalterlichen medizinischen Briefbuch des Codex Bruxellensis 3701–15* (Diss. Berlin)

Wiersma, W. (1942) 'Das Referat des Alexandros Polyhistor über die pythagoreische Philosophie', *Mnemosyne*, ser. 3, 10: 97–112

Wilcken, U. (1899) *Griechische Ostraka aus Ägypten und Nubien*, 2 vols. (Leipzig/Berlin)

(1927–37) *Urkunden der Ptolemäerzeit*, 2 vols. in 3 (Berlin/Leipzig)

Wilson, J.A. (1962) 'Medicine in Ancient Egypt', *Bulletin of the History of Medicine* 36: 114–23

Wilson, L.G. (1959) 'Erasistratus, Galen, and the Pneuma', *Bulletin of the History of Medicine* 33: 293–314

Wolters, P. (1906) ' 'Αρχιατρὸς τὸ δ'', *Jahreshefte des österreichischen archäologischen Instituts* 9: 295–7

Woodhead, A.G. (1952) 'The state health service in ancient Greece', *Cambridge Historical Journal* 10.3: 235–53

Woollam, D.H.M. (1958) 'Concepts of the brain and its functions in classical antiquity', in F.L.N. Poynter, ed., *The History and Philosophy of Knowledge of the Brain and its Functions* (Springfield, Illinois/Oxford), 5–18

Wunderer, C. (1898–1909) *Polybiosforschungen*, 3 vols. (Leipzig)

Yahuda, A.S. (1947) 'Medical and anatomical terms in the Pentateuch in the light of Egyptian medical papyri', *Journal of the History of Medicine and Allied Sciences* 2: 549–74

Yoyotte, J. (1968) 'Une théorie étiologique des médecins égyptiens', *Kêmi* 18: 79–84

Zervos, S. (1909) 'Über die Einführung des ersten Thermometers und der ersten Uhr in die medizinische Praxis', *Mitteilungen zur Geschichte der Medizin und der Naturwissenschaften* 8: 468–70

Zuntz, G. (1959) 'Aristeas Studies I: "The Seven Banquets" ', *Journal of Semitic Studies* 4: 21–36

(8.188; 8.219–20) 385; (9.210;
9.227–36) 137; (9.363) 304 n. 230;
(10.48; 10.85–101; 10.112–17;
10.142–3) 63; (10.318) 533 n. 11,
534 n. 12; (10.347) 63; (11.46) 93
n. 12; (11.47ff.) 94 n. 15; (11.50)
81, 407; (11.57–9) 94 n. 15;
(11.61) 94; (11.186) 103; (11.187)
93 n. 11
P. (1.84) 528; (2.94) 93 n. 11;
(2.245) 56; (2.247) 93 n. 11;
(3.32) 533 n. 11, 534 n. 12; (3.71–
5) 63; (3.245) 59; (3.280) 112

SILVATICUS, MATTHAEUS
Pandect. 577
SIMIAS RHODIUS
(frr. 29–32 Fr.) 492 n. 34
SIMON IANUENSIS
Clavis 576–7
SIMONIDES
PMG (604) 94
SIMPLICIUS
In Arist. Ph. (*CAG* IX, pp. 151.28–9;
153.15–6) 170 n. 91
SOPHOCLES
Tr. (1054) 173 n. 109
SORANUS
Fract. (9) 510
Gyn. (1.10.3) 217; (1.12.2–3) 214;
(1.12.3) 500; (1.14.2) 239;
(1.27.2–3) 81, 373; (1.29.1, 4) 373;
(1.44) 395; (1.57) 63, 229;
(1.57.3–4) 218; (2.55[124].1) 510;
(3.pr.2) 366, 510, 537 nn. 32 &
34, 538, 552; (3.pr.3.4) 80, 365;
(3.pr.4.2–3) 366; (3.19) 510;
(3.26–9) 517 n. 20, 518 n. 21;
(3.29) 518; (3.38.2–3) 114; (3.43)
510, 538; (4.1) 510; (4.1.4) 81;
(4.1.4–5) 367; (4.1.6) 476;
(4.1.6ff.) 509 n. 24; (4.2) 510;
(4.2) 394, 511; (4.5.4) 469; (4.9–
13) 404 n. 36; (4.14ff.) 518 n. 22;
(4.14.5) 518; (4.35–40) 395;
(4.36.1–2) 371; (4.39.3) 114
Quaest. (ps.-Sor.) (23) 102 n. 52;
(103) 374; (172) 346
Vit. Hp. (4) 477; (15) 64
SOTADES
(fr. 1 Powell) 29 n. 98

STEPHANUS (PHILOSOPHUS)
In Hp. Prog. (1.4; p. 40 Duffy) 435
STOBAEUS, IOANNES
Ecl. (1.19.1) 319; (2.7.7c) 94;
(2.7.11s) 309 n. 240; (4.36.24)
135; (4.38.9) 125–6
STRABO
Geo. (12.4.3; 563–4c) 508 n. 18;
(12.8.20; 580 c) 531, 538;
(14.1.34; 645c) 525 n. 17, 526 n.
19, 552, 557; (17.1.6; 791–2c) 161
n. 66; (17.1.8; 793–4c) 460 n. 74,
524 n. 7; (17.1.10; 795c) 150 n.
30; (17.1.12; 797c) 524 n. 5
STRATO (PHILOSOPHUS)
(frr. 54–67 Wehrli) 304 n. 229; (frr.
119–21) 389
SUDA
(α.691) 391; (α.4107) 282 n. 150;
(δ.1206) 522; (κ.1113) 391
SUETONIUS
Tib. (8) 462 n. 81
SUPPLEMENTUM EPIGRAPHICUM
GRAECUM
(VIII.621) 150 n. 32; (XI.414.23;
XVII.540; XVII.827) 35 n. 1;
(XIX.467) 42 n. 17; (XX.509) 566
n. 1; (XXIV.1166) 96 n. 24;
(XXVI.1241) 38 n. 7; (XXXIII.1211)
59
SUPPLEMENTUM HELLENISTICUM
(18; pp. 7–8) 576, 582–4
SVF
(1.45–6) 92 n. 10; (1.190) 93 n. 13;
(1.190–5) 96 n. 27; (1.192–4) 95 n.
20; (1.359) 93 n. 13; (1.409–21)
584; (1.622) 96 n. 25; (II.35–44) 92
n. 10; (II.48; II.122; II.123) 93 n.
11; (II.227; II.229) 562 n. 16;
(II.439–40) 465; (II.509ff.) 393;
(II.716) 253 n. 52, 254 n. 53;
(II.838–9) 390; (II.876; II.877) 527
n. 23; (II.879; II.889; II.945) 275 n.
125; (II.1198) 309 n. 240; (III.70)
93 n. 13; (III.96) 93 n. 12; (III.104–
5) 114; (III.106–8) 101 n. 48;
(III.117ff.) 93 nn. 13–14; (III.121)
94; (III.122) 94 nn. 18–19, 95 n.
20; (III.127–39) 95 n. 20; (III.138–
9) 93 n. 13; (III.605) 309 n. 240;

SELECT INDEX OF GREEK WORDS

GENERAL INDEX

(IL = see also Index Locorum)

liver, 153, 162–4, 169, 180–3, 219–20, 226, 227–30, 234, 241, 389, 423–4, 426
lizard, 18
lobes (of liver), 182–3, 227–8
lozenge, 527
Lucius, Asclepiadean (?), 537
Lucius, pharmacologist, 537 n. 34
Lucullus, 567 n. 4
lung, 178, 192–3, 221–3, 240–1, 260–2, 303, 320–2, 378–80
Lycus, 60 n. 40, 189, 370, 452, 470
lymphatic vessels, 180–1, 226, 241
Lysimachus of Cos, 493 n. 41, 564

Magendie, François, 402
magic, 4, 6–9
Magnus of Ephesus, Pneumatist, 587
male, see reproductive organs: male; reproductive theory; seed
malnutrition, 544
Manetho of Sebennytus, 25
Manilius, 572
Mantias, 300 n. 209, 401, 450–1, 453, 459, 509 n. 26, 515–18, 546–7, 561 n. 15
Marcellinus, physician, 282–4, 392, 512, 557 n. 18, 582, (IL)
mare, 184–5, 233
Marinus, 159–60, 191–2, 201–3, 236–7
Marius, C.—Victorinus, 572
Marius (pseudo-), 38 n. 7, 583
marrow, 201, 474 n. 8
Marseille (Massalia), 574, 575 n. 18
marsh mallow, root of, 17
Martianus Capella, 276, (IL)
Marullus, 147 n. 20, 424
masturbation, 394, 508
materia medica, see pharmacology
matter, 365
measurement, 9, 19, 208–11, 282–3, 347–61, 421–4; see quantification; size; time
meat, 13–14, 467–8
mechanics, 404, 453
Medius, 191–2
melancholy, see bile: black
melilot, 423
membrane, 184–5, 222, 367–8, 371, 378–9; see also meninges; meninx

memory, 502, 502 n. 8
Men Karou, 459–61, 529–30, 559, 575, 582
Menander, 569 n. 16
Menecles of Barca, 68
Menemachus of Aphrodisias, 461
Menemachus Philalethes, 460–1
meninges, 195–6, 223–5, 251, 313–15, 326, 449, 567–8
meninx, chor(i)oid, 251
Menon, Peripatetic, 72, 300–1
menses, 291
menstruation, 297, 299–300, 369–71, 373–4, 436, 450, 507, 537
mental illness, 245, 303, 344–5, 360, 377, 382–3, 399, 413, 473, 506, 563, 567–8
mesentery, 180, 226, 241
method, theory of, 54, 61, 115–37, 148, 348–9, 394, 409, 446, 512–13, 534
Methodists, 58, 62, 235, 301, 375, 457, 461, 465, 542 n. 22; see also Soranus; Themison; Thessalus
metre (and physiology), 276–82, 350–2, 359–60, 393
midwifery, 40–1, 53, 72, 80–1, 90, 155, 296–9, 404, 449; see also obstetrics
milk, see lactation
mind, 449; see also reason
minerals, 417, 438–9
Mithridates VI, 147 n. 18
Mnaseas, 373–4
Mnemon of Side, 502, 556
Mnesitheus, 50, 54, 59, 62, 98–9, 191–2, 311–13, 388, 401, 412–13, (IL)
moisture, 244–7, 312, 367–8, 374, 379–80, 408–9, 449, 537 n. 35
Mondino dei Lucci, 140 n. 4
monkey, 139–40
monster, 368–9
Moschion (Muscio, Mustio), 316–17, 579, (IL)
motion, 200–1, 237, 250–9, 271–2, 296, 318–22, 328, 346–7, 355–6, 358, 372, 389, 567; see also (in)voluntary motion; pulse; respiration
mummification, 29–30, 149–50
muscle, 201, 215, 240–1, 247, 255–7, 262, 319–22, 326–9, 371
Museum (mouseion), 26–7, 29, 39, 458–